WQ
212
PLA

Imperial College London
2407566976

AF805121

Imperial College
London

the Library
www.imperial.ac.uk/library

Please return or renew by the due date.
Fines may be charged on items returned late.

This item belongs to:

- ☐ Central Library
- ☐ Charing Cross
- ☐ Chelsea & Westminster
- ☑ Hammersmith
- ☐ Royal Brompton
- ☐ St Mary's
- ☐ Silwood Park

14 JUL 2014

www.imperial.ac.uk/library

The Placenta

From Development to Disease

To Brian, Emily and Allison for their unwavering support

To Peggy, my childhood sweetheart and wife

To the memory of my grandmother, Fengtong Zhao

The Placenta

From Development to Disease

EDITED BY

Helen H. Kay, MD

Professor
Division of Maternal-Fetal Medicine and Ultrasound-Genetics
Department of Obstetrics and Gynecology
Washington University School of Medicine
St. Louis, MO, USA

D. Michael Nelson, MD, PhD

Virginia S. Lang Professor and Vice-Chairman
Division of Maternal-Fetal Medicine and Ultrasound-Genetics
Department of Obstetrics and Gynecology
Washington, University School of Medicine
St. Louis, MO, USA

Yuping Wang, MD, PhD

Professor
Departments of Obstetrics and Gynecology, and Molecular and Cellular Physiology
Louisiana State University Health Sciences Center – Shreveport
Shreveport, LA, USA

WILEY-BLACKWELL
A John Wiley & Sons, Ltd., Publication

This edition first published 2011, © 2011 by Blackwell Publishing Ltd

Blackwell Publishing was acquired by John Wiley & Sons in February 2007. Blackwell's publishing program has been merged with Wiley's global Scientific, Technical and Medical business to form Wiley-Blackwell.

Registered office: John Wiley & Sons Ltd, The Atrium, Southern Gate, Chichester, West Sussex, PO19 8SQ, UK

Editorial offices: 9600 Garsington Road, Oxford, OX4 2DQ, UK
The Atrium, Southern Gate, Chichester, West Sussex, PO19 8SQ, UK
111 River Street, Hoboken, NJ 07030-5774, USA

For details of our global editorial offices, for customer services and for information about how to apply for permission to reuse the copyright material in this book please see our website at www.wiley.com/wiley-blackwell

The right of the author to be identified as the author of this work has been asserted in accordance with the Copyright, Designs and Patents Act 1988.

All rights reserved. No part of this publication may be reproduced, stored in a retrieval system, or transmitted, in any form or by any means, electronic, mechanical, photocopying, recording or otherwise, except as permitted by the UK Copyright, Designs and Patents Act 1988, without the prior permission of the publisher.

Designations used by companies to distinguish their products are often claimed as trademarks. All brand names and product names used in this book are trade names, service marks, trademarks or registered trademarks of their respective owners. The publisher is not associated with any product or vendor mentioned in this book. This publication is designed to provide accurate and authoritative information in regard to the subject matter covered. It is sold on the understanding that the publisher is not engaged in rendering professional services. If professional advice or other expert assistance is required, the services of a competent professional should be sought.

The contents of this work are intended to further general scientific research, understanding, and discussion only and are not intended and should not be relied upon as recommending or promoting a specific method, diagnosis, or treatment by physicians for any particular patient. The publisher and the author make no representations or warranties with respect to the accuracy or completeness of the contents of this work and specifically disclaim all warranties, including without limitation any implied warranties of fitness for a particular purpose. In view of ongoing research, equipment modifications, changes in governmental regulations, and the constant flow of information relating to the use of medicines, equipment, and devices, the reader is urged to review and evaluate the information provided in the package insert or instructions for each medicine, equipment, or device for, among other things, any changes in the instructions or indication of usage and for added warnings and precautions. Readers should consult with a specialist where appropriate. The fact that an organization or Website is referred to in this work as a citation and/or a potential source of further information does not mean that the author or the publisher endorses the information the organization or Website may provide or recommendations it may make. Further, readers should be aware that Internet Websites listed in this work may have changed or disappeared between when this work was written and when it is read. No warranty may be created or extended by any promotional statements for this work. Neither the publisher nor the author shall be liable for any damages arising herefrom.

Library of Congress Cataloging-in-Publication Data

The placenta : from development to disease / edited by Helen H. Kay, D. Michael Nelson, Yuping Wang.
p. ; cm.
Includes bibliographical references and index.
ISBN 978-1-4443-3366-4 (hardcover : alk. paper)
1. Placenta–Diseases. 2. Placenta. I. Kay, Helen H. II. Nelson, D. Michael. III. Wang, Yuping
[DNLM: 1. Placenta. 2. Placenta Diseases. WQ 212]
RG591.P56 2011
618.3′4–dc22 2010036448

A catalogue record for this book is available from the British Library.

This book is published in the following electronic formats: ePDF 9781444393903; Wiley Online Library 9781444393927; ePub 9781444393910

Set in 9/12 pt Minion by Aptara®, Inc., New Delhi, India
Printed and bound in Singapore by Markono Print Media Pte Ltd

1 2011

Contents

List of Contributors

Jacques S. Abramowicz, MD
The Francis T. and Lester B. Knight Professor
Director, Obstetrics and Gynecology Ultrasound
Department of Obstetrics and Gynecology
Co-Director, Rush Fetal and Neonatal Medicine Center
Rush University
Chicago, IL, USA

William E. Ackerman IV, MD
Assistant Professor
Department of Obstetrics and Gynecology
Ohio State University
Columbus, OH, USA

Mahmoud S. Ahmed, MD
Professor
Director of Maternal-Fetal Pharmacology & Biodevelopment Laboratories
Departments of Obstetrics & Gynecology, Biochemistry & Molecular Biology, and Pharmacology & Toxicology
University of Texas Medical Branch
Galveston, TX, USA

Ray Bahado-Singh, MD
Professor of Obstetrics and Gynecology
Director, Division of Fetal Imaging and Therapeutics,
Department of Obstetrics and Gynecology,
Wayne State University,
Detroit, MI, USA

Marie H. Beall, MD
Professor and Vice Chair
Department of Obstetrics and Gynecology
Harbor-UCLA Medical Center
Torrance CA, USA

and

David Geffen School of Medicine at UCLA
Los Angeles, CA, USA

Louiza Belkacemi, PhD
Assistant Professor
Department of Obstetrics and Gynecology
Los Angeles Biomedical Research Institute at Harbor-UCLA Medical Center
Torrance, CA, USA

and

David Geffen School of Medicine at UCLA
Los Angeles, CA, USA

Mila Cervar-Zivkovic, MD, PhD
Professor
Department of Obstetrics and Gynecology
Medical University of Graz
Graz, Austria

Irene Cetin, MD
Professor of Obstetrics and Gynecology
Department of Clinical Sciences, Hospital Luigi Sacco and Centre for Fetal Research Giorgio Pardi
University of Milan
Grassi, Milan, Italy

Christine H. Comstock, MD
Clinical Professor
Department of Obstetrics and Gynecology
Oakland University William Beaumont School of Medicine
MI, USA

and

Director
Division of Fetal Imaging
William Beaumont Hospital
Royal Oak, MI, USA

Ian P. Crocker, PhD
Senior Scientist
Maternal and Fetal Health Research Centre
School of Biomedicine
University of Manchester
St. Mary's Hospital
Manchester, UK

Mina Desai, PhD
Associate Professor
Department of Obstetrics and Gynecology
Los Angeles Biomedical Research Institute at
Harbor-UCLA Medical Center
Torrance, CA, USA

and

David Geffen School of Medicine at UCLA
Los Angeles, CA, USA

Gernot Desoye, PhD
Professor
Department of Obstetrics and Gynecology
Medical University of Graz
Graz, Austria

Dan Diego-Alvarez, PhD
Research Associate
Department of Medical Genetics
University of British Columbia

and

Child and Family Research Institute
Vancouver, BC, Canada

and

Professor
School of Biology
IE University
Segovia, Spain

Julia Froehlich, MSc
PhD Student
Department of Obstetrics and Gynecology

and

Institute of Histology, Embryology and Cell Biology
Medical University of Graz
Graz, Austria

Hilary S. Gammill, MD
Assistant Professor
Maternal-Fetal Medicine
Department of Obstetrics and Gynecology
University of Washington School of Medicine
Seattle, WA, USA

and

Research Associate
Fred Hutchinson Cancer Research Center
University of Washington School of Medicine
Seattle, WA, USA

Thaddeus G. Golos, PhD
Professor
Departments of Comparative Biosciences, Obstetrics, and Gynecology
The Wisconsin National Primate Research Center
University of Wisconsin-Madison
Madison, WI, USA

Ian A. Greer, MD, FRCP, FRCOG, FMedSci
Professor
Department of Health and Life Sciences
University of Liverpool
Liverpool, UK

Gilad A. Gross, MD
Professor
Department of Obstetrics, Gynecology and Women's Health,
Division of Maternal-Fetal Medicine and Ultrasound-Genetics
St. Louis University School of Medicine
Assistant Director, MFM Fellowship Program
Medical Director, Labor and Delivery and Antepartum Service,
St. Mary's Health Center
St. Louis, MO, USA

Katja Gwin, MD, PhD
Assistant Professor
Department of Pathology
University of Chicago
Chicago, IL, USA

Christina S. Han, MD
Clinical instructor
Department of Obstetrics, Gynecology and Reproductive Sciences
Yale University School of Medicine
New Haven, CT, USA

Gary D. V. Hankins, MD
Professor
Department of Obstetrics and Gynecology
University of Texas Medical Branch
Galveston, TX, USA

Sonia S. Hassan, MD
Associate Professor
Director, Center for Advanced Obstetrical Care and Research
Perinatology Research Branch, NICHD, NIH, DHHS, Bethesda, MD, USA/Detroit, MI, USA
Director, PRB/WSU Maternal-Fetal Medicine Fellowship Program
Division of Maternal-Fetal Medicine and Ultrasound-Genetics
Department of Obstetrics and Gynecology
Wayne State University, School of Medicine, Hutzel Women's Hospital
Detroit, MI, USA

Ursula Hiden, MSc, PhD
Junior Scientist
Department of Obstetrics and Gynecology
Medical University of Graz
Graz, Austria

Wolfgang Holzgreve, MD, MBA
Professor
Department of Obstetrics/Department of Biomedicine
University of Basel
Basel, Switzerland

and

Institute for Advance Study
Wallotstrasse, Berlin, Germany

Shahzya S. Huda, MBChB, MD, MRCOG, MRCP
Clinical Lecturer in Obstetrics and Gynaecology
Department of Reproductive and Maternal Medicine
University of Glasgow
Glasgow, UK

Joan S. Hunt, PhD, DSc(HON)
University Distinguished Professor
Department of Anatomy and Cell Biology
University of Kansas Medical Center
Kansas City, KS, USA

Berthold Huppertz, PhD
Professor of Cell Biology
Institute of Cell Biology, Histology and Embryology
Medical University of Graz
Graz, Austria

Aliya N. Husain, MD
Professor
Department of Pathology
University of Chicago
Chicago, IL, USA

Nicholas P. Illsley, DPhil
Professor
Department of Obstetrics, Gynecology, and Women's Health
UMDNJ-New Jersey Medical School
Newark, NJ, USA

Daniel L. Jackson, MD
Resident
Department of Obstetrics and Gynecology and Women's Health
Missouri Center for Reproductive Medicine and Fertility
University of Missouri-Columbia
Columbia, MO, USA

Cristiano Jodicke, MD
Fellow
Maternal-Fetal Medicine
Department of Obstetrics and Gynecology
Wayne State University

and

Perinatology Research Branch, NICHD/NIH/DHHS
Detroit, MI, USA

Helen H. Kay, MD
Professor
Division of Maternal-Fetal Medicine and Ultrasound-Genetics
Department of Obstetrics and Gynecology
Washington University School of Medicine
St. Louis, MO, USA

Chong Jai Kim, MD, PhD
Professor
Department of Pathology
Wayne State University School of Medicine
Detroit, MI, USA

and

Perinatology Research Branch, NICHD/NIH/DHHS
Bethesda, MD, USA

Douglas A. Kniss, PhD
Professor
Departments of Obstetrics and Gynecology
Division of Maternal-Fetal Medicine and Biomedical Engineering

and

Director
Laboratory of Perinatal Research
The Ohio State University
Columbus, OH, USA

Frederick T. Kraus, MD
Adjunct Professor
Department of Obstetrics and Gynecology
Washington University School of Medicine
St. Louis, MO, USA

Olav Lapaire, MD
Associate Professor
Department of Obstetrics/Department of Biomedicine
University of Basel
Basel, Switzerland

Fiona Lyall, BSc, PhD, FRCPath, MBA
Professor of Maternal and Fetal Health
Institute of Medical Genetics
University of Glasgow, Yorkhill Hospital
Glasgow, UK

Teng Ma, PhD
Associate Professor
Department of Chemical and Biomedical Engineering
Florida State University
Tallahassee, FL, USA

Chiara Mandò, PhD
Postdoctoral Fellow
Unit of Obstetrics and Gynecology
Department of Clinical Sciences, Hospital Luigi Sacco and Centre for Fetal Research Giorgio Pardi
University of Milan
Grassi, Milan, Italy

Clifford W. Mason, PhD
Research Instructor
Department of Obstetrics and Gynecology
School of Medicine
University of Kansas Medical Center
Kansas City, KS, USA

Jennifer M. McNamara, MD
Fellow
Division of Maternal-Fetal Medicine and Ultrasound-Genetics
Department of Obstetrics and Gynecology
Washington University School of Medicine
St. Louis, MO, USA

Laura Meints, MD
Resident
Department of Obstetrics and Gynecology
Barnes-Jewish Hospital
Washington University School of Medicine
St. Louis, MO, USA

Kenneth J. Moise, Jr, MD
Professor of Obstetrics and Gynecology
Professor of Surgery
Division of Maternal-Fetal Medicine and Ultrasound-Genetics
Department of Obstetrics and Gynecology
Baylor College of Medicine
Texas Children's Fetal Center
Houston, TX, USA

Leslie Myatt, PhD
Professor of Obstetrics and Gynecology
Co-Director, Center for Pregnancy and Newborn Research
Department of Obstetrics and Gynecology
University of Texas Health Science Center San Antonio
San Antonio, TX, USA

Tatiana N. Nanovskaya, DDS, PhD
Assistant Professor
Department of Obstetrics and Gynecology
University of Texas Medical Branch
Galveston, TX, USA

D. Michael Nelson, MD, PhD
Virginia S. Lang Professor and Vice-Chairman
Division of Maternal-Fetal Medicine and Ultrasound-Genetics
Department of Obstetrics and Gynecology
Washington University School of Medicine
St. Louis, MO, USA

J. Lee Nelson, MD
Professor
Department of Rheumatology
University of Washington School of Medicine
Seattle, WA, USA

and

Member
Fred Hutchinson Cancer Research Center
University of Washington School of Medicine
Seattle, WA, USA

Thinh Nguyen, MD
Fellow
Division of Maternal-Fetal Medicine and Ultrasound-Genetics
Department of Obstetrics, Gynecology, and Women's Health
St. Louis University School of Medicine
St. Mary's Health Center
St. Louis, MO, USA

Anthony O. Odibo, MD, MSCE
Associate Professor
Division of Maternal-Fetal Medicine and Ultrasound-Genetics
Department of Obstetrics and Gynecology
Washington University in St. Louis
St. Louis, MO, USA

Michael J. Paidas, MD
Associate Professor
Co-Director, Yale Women and Children's Center for Blood Disorders
Co-Director, National Hemophilia Foundation-Baxter Clinical Fellowship Program at Yale
Division of Maternal-Fetal Medicine and Ultrasound-Genetics
Department of Obstetrics, Gynecology and Reproductive Sciences
Yale University School of Medicine
New Haven, CT, USA

Ramesha Papanna, MD, MPH
Fellow
Division of Maternal-Fetal Medicine and Ultrasound-Genetics
Department of Obstetrics, Gynecology and Reproductive Sciences, Yale University
School of Medicine
New Haven, CT, USA

Samuel Parry, MD
Professor
Director
Department of Maternal-Fetal Medicine
University of Pennsylvania
Philadelphia, PA, USA

Suzanne E. Peterson, MD
Fellow
Maternal-Fetal Medicine
Department of Obstetrics and Gynecology
University of Washington School of Medicine
Seattle, WA, USA

Margaret G. Petroff, PhD
Associate Professor
Department of Anatomy and Cell Biology
University of Kansas Medical Center
Kansas City, KS, USA

Roxane Rampersad, MD
Assistant Professor
Division of Maternal-Fetal Medicine and Ultrasound-Genetics
Department of Obstetrics and Gynecology
Washington University School of Medicine
St. Louis, MO, USA

Raymond W. Redline, MD
Professor of Pathology and Reproductive Biology
Case Western Reserve University School of Medicine
Cleveland, OH, USA

and

Co-Director
Pediatric and Perinatal Pathology
University Hospitals Case Medical Center
Cleveland, OH, USA

Gregory E. Rice, PhD, MHA, MAICD
Professor
Deputy Director (Translation)
Center for Clinical Research
University of Queensland, Royal Brisbane and Women's Hospital Campus
Brisbane, QLD, Australia

John M. Robinson, PhD
Professor
Department of Physiology and Cell Biology
Ohio State University
Columbus, OH, USA

Wendy P. Robinson, PhD
Professor
Department of Medical Genetics
University of British Columbia

and

Child and Family Research Institute
Vancouver, BC, Canada

Roberto Romero, MD
Chief, Perinatology Research Branch
Program Director for Obstetrics and Perinatology
Intramural Division, NICHD, NIH, DHHS
Bethesda, MD, USA/Detroit, MI, USA
Professor of Molecular Obstetrics and Genetics
Center for Molecular Medicine and Genetics
Wayne State University, School of Medicine, Hutzel Women's Hospital
Detroit, MI, USA

and

Professor of Epidemiology
Michigan State University
East Lansing, MI, USA

Michael G. Ross, MD, MPH
Professor and Chair
Department of Obstetrics and Gynecology
Los Angeles Biomedical Research Institute at Harbor-UCLA Medical Center
Los Angeles Biomedical Research Institute at Harbor-UCLA Medical Center
Torrance, CA, USA

and

David Geffen School of Medicine at UCLA
Los Angeles, CA, USA

Yoel Sadovsky, MD
Scientific Director, Magee-Womens Research Institute
Elsie Hilliard Hillman Chair of Women's Health Research
Professor of Obstetrics, Gynecology, Microbiology and Molecular Genetics
Department of Obstetrics, Gynecology, and Reproductive Sciences
University of Pittsburgh
Pittsburgh, PA, USA

Danny J. Schust, MD
Associate Professor
Department of Obstetrics, Gynecology and Women's Health
Missouri Center for Reproductive Medicine and Fertility
University of Missouri-Columbia
Columbia, MO, USA

Christina Scifres, MD
Assistant Professor of Obstetrics, Gynecology, and Reproductive Sciences
Magee-Womens Research Institute
Department of Obstetrics, Gynecology, and Reproductive Sciences
University of Pittsburgh
Pittsburgh, PA, USA

Colin P. Sibley, PhD
Professor of Child Health and Physiology
Maternal and Fetal Health Research Centre
School of Biomedicine and Manchester Academic Health Sciences Centre
University of Manchester
St. Mary's Hospital
Manchester, UK

Christina Stern, MD
Resident
Department of Obstetrics and Gynecology
Medical University of Graz
Graz, Austria

Toshihiro Takizawa, MD, PhD
Professor
Department of Molecular Medicine and Anatomy
Nippon Medical School
Tokyo, Japan

Methodius G. Tuuli, MD, MPH
Fellow
Division of Maternal-Fetal Medicine and Ultrasound-Genetics
Department of Obstetrics and Gynecology
Washington University in St. Louis
St. Louis, MO, USA

Ignatia B. Van den Veyver, MD
Professor
Department of Obstetrics and Gynecology

and

Department of Molecular and Human Genetics
Baylor College of Medicine
Houston, TX, USA

Marion S. Verp, MD
Associate Professor
Departments of Obstetrics and Gynecology, and Human Genetics
The University of Chicago
Chicago, IL, USA

Yuping Wang, MD, PhD
Professor
Departments of Obstetrics and Gynecology, and Molecular and Cellular Physiology
Louisiana State University Health Sciences Center – Shreveport
Shreveport, LA, USA

Carl P. Weiner, MD, MBA
KE Krantz Professor and Chair
Professor, Molecular and Integrative Physiology
Department of Obstetrics and Gynecology
School of Medicine
University of Kansas Medical Center
Kansas City, KS, USA

Shu Wen, MD, PhD
Postdoctoral Associate
Department of Obstetrics and Gynecology
Baylor College of Medicine
Houston, TX, USA

Caroline Wright, MBBS
Obstetric Clinical Research Fellow
Maternal and Fetal Health Research Centre
School of Biomedicine and Manchester Academic Health Sciences Centre
University of Manchester, St. Mary's Hospital
Manchester, UK

Stacy Zamudio, PhD
Senior Scientist, Director of Research
Division of Maternal-Fetal Medicine and Surgery
Department of Obstetrics and Gynecology
Hackensack University Medical Center
Hackensack, NJ, USA

Preface

The human placenta is central to the important events that influence not only development and growth of the fetus but also the risks for multiple adult diseases in both the mother and offspring. Diabetes mellitus, obesity, and cardiovascular disease, among others, have origins in utero where the placenta plays a pivotal role. Our goal as editors of The Placenta: From Development to Disease was to create a comprehensive, yet succinct, resource for new investigators and clinicians, while also providing a manual for senior investigators and experienced clinicians who mentor trainees at all educational levels.

With this ambitious goal in mind, we selected topics of interest to both clinicians and researchers. We first introduced the contemporary concepts about the placenta's central position in the developmental origins of human adult disease (DOHAD) and in the cardiovascular health and maternal placental syndromes (CHAMPS). We then described the developmental biology of the placenta and the further dissection by molecular analyses for the structure and function of this organ, including assessments of metabolic, secretory and transport functions. We have highlighted key techniques used to study the placenta, both in the laboratory and in the clinical setting. Indeed, our authors provide some chapters with step-by-step instructions for study of the placenta by newcomers. From there we move to specific clinical disorders that influence pregnancy outcomes, underscoring the pivotal role the placenta plays in each. We conclude with topics that are at the forefront of clinical and research applications, including proteomics, stem cell development, and prenatal diagnosis by analysis of cell-free RNA and DNA from trophoblast.

The chapters are designed to be reader friendly, and the clinical pearls, research spotlights, and teaching points are targeted at the novice. For seasoned investigators, we hope the overviews of topics outside their area of research and the technique chapters will be especially useful for training. For experienced clinicians, we aimed to heighten awareness of the diverse functions performed by the placenta and to provide insights into how the placenta can be a window to current and future disease(s).

Most importantly, The Placenta: From Development to Disease would not be possible without the committed efforts of the authors of the chapters. Clinicians and investigators; students, trainees, and postdoctoral fellows; and junior and senior investigators from around the world – all have contributed to this endeavor. We owe tremendous gratitude to each of them for their insightful contributions, their attention to deadlines, and their willingness to allow us to edit their chapters, sometimes brutally, for uniformity of style. Without these talented authors, we as editors would not have been able to produce a book with the breadth and depth, yet succinct writing style, that we feel has blossomed. Last but clearly not least, we thank the publishers at Wiley-Blackwell for their recognition of the importance of the placenta as a subject for a book and for their editorial support throughout this endeavor.

Sincerely,
Helen Kay
D. Michael Nelson
Yuping Wang

PART I

Fetal Origins of Adult Disease/Programming

1

CHAPTER 1

Maternal Undernutrition and Fetal Programming: Role of the Placenta

Louiza Belkacemi[1,2], *D. Michael Nelson*[3], *Mina Desai*[1,2], *and Michael G. Ross*[1,2]

[1]Department of Obstetrics and Gynecology, Los Angeles Biomedical Research Institute at Harbor-UCLA Medical Center, Torrance, CA, USA
[2]David Geffen School of Medicine at UCLA, Los Angeles, CA, USA
[3]Division of Maternal-Fetal Medicine and Ultrasound-Genetics, Department of Obstetrics and Gynecology, Washington University School of Medicine, St. Louis, MO, USA

Introduction

What is developmental origins of health and disease (DOHaD)?

DOHaD is an area of research that emerged following retrospective cohort studies of David Barker and colleagues during the late 1980s. These investigators studied the association of geographical distribution of heart disease in the United Kingdom to a person's birthplace, irrespective of the place where individuals develop disease [1]. Their data suggested that environment in early life causes permanent changes in fetal physiology that predisposes the adult to disease later in life. Association of early undernutrition with low birth weight is a major component of fetal programming of the Barker hypothesis. The key contention of the Barker hypothesis is that the undernourished fetus is programmed to exhibit a "thrifty phenotype," and this predisposes to a lifetime of increased food intake and fat deposition. Such individuals develop obesity, diabetes, and hypertension as adults, due to alterations in homeostatic regulatory mechanisms as a fetus.

The placenta is a multifunctional organ that synthesizes, metabolizes, and transports nutrients required by the fetus. The placenta is also a source of hormones that influence fetal, placental, and maternal metabolism and the course of fetal development. By virtue of these roles, the placenta plays a pivotal role in fetal programming.

Scope of problem

Four hundred thousand children in the United States alone are born annually with low birth weight resulting from intrauterine growth restriction (IUGR). IUGR is variably defined, but a common definition is a fetal weight below the 10th percentile for gestational age as determined by antenatal ultrasound (hence the phrase IUGR) or by newborn birth weight percentiles (hence the phrase small for gestational age). IUGR babies exhibit aberrant development and require higher neonatal intensive care. In addition to the short-term risks, the long-term risk of developmental programming includes metabolic disorders later in life. Up to 63% of adult diabetes, hypertension, and heart disease may be attributed to low-birth-weight conditions in conjunction with an accelerated newborn-to-adolescent weight gain and obesity. Therefore, the DOHaD field is increasingly recognized as an important contributor to the epidemic of obesity and metabolic syndrome in Western populations.

The Placenta: From Development to Disease, First Edition. Edited by Helen H. Kay, D. Michael Nelson and Yuping Wang.
© 2011 Blackwell Publishing Ltd. Published 2011 by Blackwell Publishing Ltd.

Why should we care?

We as scientists

The DOHaD field is now unequivocally established, yet still in its infancy. There is still a lack of specific mechanisms to explain the effects for most of the epidemiological observations described for adult human disease. Fetal growth is directly related to placental growth and placental phenotype, which are regulated by the genetic background. We as scientists have great potential to study the signals for fetal nutrient demand that control placental transfer capacity. Importantly, there are great opportunities to dissect molecular mechanisms that regulate placental nutrient transfer in early pregnancy and that program nutrient transfer closer to term.

We as clinicians

Clinicians should aim to identify IUGR placentas and fetuses early enough to institute appropriate monitoring, and ideally, interventions that can limit adverse outcomes for the offspring. Examination of the maternal diet prior to and during pregnancy together with early detection of "placental disease" may help improve outcomes in IUGR.

We as patients with a "placental disease"

Patients should improve life style, including a healthy diet, physical exercise, and prenatal care to optimize fetal and neonatal outcomes.

Importance of maternal nutrients for fetal development

During normal pregnancy, the primary determinant of fetal growth is the concentration of nutrients in the maternal circulation and the blood supply to the placenta. Glucose, amino acids (AA), and fatty acids (FA) are among the nutrients vital for fetal growth and development. Collectively, the data show that deficiency of nutrients in the mother causes alterations in placental nutrient transport and reduced body weight in the offspring.

Glucose

The majority of fetal glucose derives from maternal metabolism of carbohydrate in the diet. Glucose supply to the fetus is a facilitated process mediated by members of the glucose transporter (GLUTs) family. Four isoforms GLUT1, GLUT3, GLUT4, and GLUT8 have been identified in human and rodent placentas. Glucose deprivation leads to hypoglycemia. This suggests that less glucose availability affects fetal growth. In rats, severe maternal glucose deprivation reduces placental transfer and fetal uptake of glucose, which results in fetal growth restriction.

AA

Fetal AA come from maternal AA pools derived from the diet. Fetal concentrations of nearly all AA are greater than maternal concentrations, suggesting that the placenta actively transfers AA from the maternal compartment to the developing fetus. Essential AA must be supplied in food, while nonessential AA are synthesized by the fetus from essential AA. Several AA transporter systems have been identified in human and rat placentas. Abnormalities in AA transport may be the reason that total AA concentrations are lower than controls in IUGR babies. AA transport by the placenta is downregulated following maternal protein deprivation and may contribute to fetal growth restriction.

Fatty acids

FA content and character in fetal plasma directly correlates with the FA composition of maternal plasma and with the maternal diet. Essential FA cannot be synthesized and are dietary essentials (e.g., linoleic and linolenic acid). Essential FA in human pregnancy are transported from maternal to fetal circulations as triglyceride-rich lipoproteins, which are hydrolyzed by placental lipases. This results in free FA (FF) release, which are transported by saturable plasma membrane FA-binding proteins, FA translocase, and a family of FA transport proteins. Low birth weight in both human and rat pregnancy correlates with low intake of essential FA.

Clinical Pearl

Balanced diets containing complex carbohydrates, essential AA, and essential FA optimize the substrates needed for normal fetal growth and development.

Factors affecting placental capacity for nutrient transfer

Multiple factors interact to influence the placental delivery of nutrients to the fetus. Size, histopathology, blood flow, transporter abundance, and organ consumption are factors responsive to environmental changes. Key studies address placental size, morphology, and transport abundance.

Size

Placental size affects the capacity for nutrient transport through changes in surface area, and placental weight correlates with fetal weight at term in many species. Timing, duration, and etiology of nutritional restriction yield variable phenotypes for placental mass. The Dutch Famine of 1944–45 reflects a highly cited example of this premise. Exposure to famine only during the first trimester of pregnancy enhanced placental weight at delivery without any impact on newborn weights when compared to control women, resulting in an increased placental-to-birth-weight ratio. In contrast, women subjected to starvation in their third trimester of pregnancy had reduced weight placentas and low-birth-weight newborns but an unaltered ratio of placental-to-birth-weight as compared with nonstarved women [1]. These results suggest that human placental adaptations in early pregnancy can overcome some environmental stressors such that fetal nutrition is maintained in late gestation. Collectively, these data suggest the placenta may compensate for insults to minimize fetal growth restriction. The histomorphology of the placenta ultimately determines placental function.

Histomorphology

Small placentas exhibit altered histopathology and ultrastructure compared to normal size placentas. Notably, the maternal undernutrition that yields IUGR in human pregnancy generates placentas with a reduced surface area for nutrient exchange, a lower volume density of trophoblasts, and increased placental apoptosis at term. In IUGR placentas, absent or reversed end-diastolic flow in the umbilical artery, as assessed by Doppler velocity waveform analysis, is indicative of poorly branched and capillarized villi, and thickened exchange barrier. In these placentas, vascular resistance occurs as a result of inadequate trophoblast invasion of the spiral arteries. In contrast, in less severe IUGR, positive end-diastolic umbilical artery flow is associated with a normal stem artery development, increased capillary angiogenesis, and adequate terminal villous development. Thus, the thicker placental exchange barrier and the increased placental vascular resistance in severe IUGR may correspond to alterations in placental structure directly involved in fetal programming of cardiovascular disease.

These structural alterations in the human placenta are mirrored in the guinea pig exposed to global maternal undernutrition compared to control diets. The nutrient deprived gestations exhibit a labyrinthine placenta with a 70% lower surface area and a barrier thickness 40% higher in late gestation. A reduction in the length of the labyrinthine vessels and decreased expression of vascular endothelial adhesion molecules in the murine placenta in response to maternal protein malnutrition are compatible with the possibility that alterations in maternal nutrition changes placental vascular function [2]. These histopathological changes predispose to lower nutrient transfer to the fetus. Our work in the rat exposed to maternal undernutrition showed enhanced apoptosis in junctional and labyrinthine zones of the placenta [3], suggesting that both hormone production and maternal–fetal exchange are impacted. Taken together, these data indicate that restriction of nutrients impairs the functional capacity of the placenta disproportionately compared to the reduction in placental weight alone.

> **Clinical Pearl**
>
> Doppler velocimetry techniques may be used to detect increased placental vascular resistance and predict adverse pregnancy outcome.

Transport abundance

Reductions in maternal–fetal nutrient transfer may derive from an inadequate maternal supply, inadequate placental blood flow, impaired placental transport, or a combination of these processes. Maternal nutritional status affects transporters in the placenta, which is time dependent. For example, rats fed 50% less food during the last week of gestation have lower than control glucose levels in maternal plasma, a lower maternal-to-fetal glucose concentration gradient, and downregulation of GLUT3 expression, suggesting a mechanism for placental glucose transport dysfunction. These changes suggest that transport-mediated mechanisms may effectively reduce fetal levels of glucose.

Placental transport of AA is affected by the activity and location of AA transporter systems. In humans, circulating essential AA concentrations are decreased in growth-restricted human fetuses, likely from reduced AA transport activity. In rats, maternal protein restriction downregulates placental nutrient transport prior to the onset of fetal growth restriction, suggesting that a reduced placental supply of AA is a causal factor for IUGR, not simply a consequence of this malady.

Undernourished women exhibit placental and offspring deficiency in essential FA, leading to altered placental FA metabolism and IUGR. These placentas not only have decreased levels of arachidonic acid and docosahexaenoic acid, but also show an altered ratio of both these FA relatives to their essential FA precursors, linoleic and α-linolenic, consistent with abnormal metabolism [4].

Taken together, these studies show the pivotal role played by the placenta in assuring that multiple nutrients are available to sustain normal fetal growth.

Placental nutrient synthesis and metabolism

Uteroplacental tissues in humans, ruminants, and equids metabolize glucose derived from the maternal circulation. Placental glucose consumption is reduced during short periods of maternal undernutrition, but this reduction has no effect on the partitioning of glucose between the uteroplacental and fetal tissues in humans [5]. Conversely, prolonged maternal hypoglycemia induces uteroplacental tissues to use less of the more limited supply of glucose available, thereby sparing glucose for the fetus. These adaptations correlate with reduced GLUT1 expression, offering a mechanism for the effect. The placenta metabolizes glucose to lactate during normal pregnancy [5], and this event increases the maternal-to-fetal concentration gradient for glucose. Placental lactate production decreases in response to maternal undernutrition in sheep, making glucose less readily available for fetal consumption [5].

The placenta synthesizes some of the AA required for fetal growth. For example, fetal glycine in sheep and human placentas are from endogenous synthesis. Serine derived from the fetus is converted in the placenta to glycine, and this AA is released back to the fetus. Interestingly, explant cultures from IUGR human placentas accumulate less serine in vitro than normal term villous explants. Besides placental synthesis of AA, uteroplacental tissues metabolize AA, supplying the fetus with essential AA [5].

The placenta synthesizes significant concentrations of FA in humans, sheep, and pigs. FA synthesis in term human placenta is lower than its oxidation. IUGR placentas commonly show a deficiency in oxidative enzymes, resulting in excess lipid peroxidation and free radical formation, both of which are harmful to maternal endothelial cells when released.

Collectively, these data show that placental nutrient synthesis and metabolism influence fetal growth and development.

Placental hormone synthesis and metabolism

The placenta releases hormones into both the maternal and fetal circulations, and synthesis and secretion of these hormones are responsive to environmental changes. Human placental lactogen, progesterone, insulin-like growth factors (IGF), and glucocorticoids play critical regulatory roles in fetal homeostasis.

Human placental lactogen and progesterone influence maternal metabolism to favor glucose delivery to the fetus [6]. Concentrations of both hormones are lower in undernourished mothers, and this may contribute to limited delivery of glucose to the fetus. This suggests that changes in placental endocrine dysfunction may be a cause and not a consequence of altered fetal growth.

Clinical Pearl

Maternal plasma concentration levels of lactogen and progesterone may be used to predict adverse outcomes for the offspring.

The IGF family of hormones modulates growth, cell division, and differentiation. The action of the IGFs is regulated by IGF-binding proteins (IGFBPs), and together may modulate fetal growth. IGF-I is mitogenic for placental stromal fibroblasts and has insulin-like effects to increase AA transport in human placental cells. The ovine placenta clears IGF-I from the umbilical circulation when fetal IGF-I concentrations are high but secretes IGF-I when fetal concentrations are low. Fetal IGF-I concentrations positively correlate with fetal body weight to suggest that hormone production, metabolism, or both adjust to conditions prevailing in utero to yield optimal fetal growth. IGF-II modulates trophoblast development at the feto–maternal interface. Disturbances in IGF-II expression and activity associate with IUGR in human pregnancy [7].

Research Spotlight

There are fetal sex differences in the IGF axis. IGF-II concentrations in umbilical cord serum from male neonates are significantly higher than those in female neonates, and cord plasma IGF-I and IGFBP-3 are higher in female neonates than in males.

Glucocorticoids are key regulators of organ development and maturation. The placenta is not a site for synthesis of glucocorticoids, but the placental 11β-hydroxysteroid dehydrogenase type 2 (11β-HSD2) converts active glucocorticoids to inactive metabolites. This enzyme is affected by exogenous exposure to glucocorticoids and by fetal and maternal glucocorticoid concentrations. The human 11β-HSD2 enzyme is localized to the syncytiotrophoblast and is thus positioned to limit glucocorticoids transfer to the fetus. Extended periods of maternal undernutrition downregulates placental 11β-HSD2 activity, increasing placental exposure to glucocorticoids. This leads to feto–placental growth restriction and abnormalities in cardiovascular and metabolic function in the adult offspring. Therefore, changes induced by elevated glucocorticoids may have beneficial effects on the offspring viability, but they also impact negatively on fetal growth and development [8]. Thus, 11β-HSD2 enzyme plays a vital role to protect the fetus from exposure to excess maternal glucocorticoids.

Research Spotlight

Synthetic glucocorticoids such as dexamethasone and betamethasone are not extensively metabolized by placental 11β-HSD2, possibly due to protection from their 9-halogen group.

Collectively, these studies show that hormone synthesis and metabolism by the placenta are affected by maternal nutritional status and that the biological effects of the hormones influence fetal growth and development.

Mechanisms of placental programming

The placenta regulates fetal development by regulating nutrient transfer to the fetus and by controlling the bioavailability of specific hormones important to fetal growth and development. The placenta therefore plays a pivotal role in mediating the programming effects of suboptimal conditions during development. Mechanisms likely involved in programming the effects of maternal undernutrition include modulation of placental vascular resistance, regulation of the nutrient supply, epigenetic, gene imprinting, and metabolism of glucocorticoids.

Maternal undernutrition increases placental vascular resistance, and this subjects the fetal heart to an excess workload. This observation provides a direct link between altered placental structure and programming the risk for cardiovascular diseases in IUGR fetuses. The placenta functions as a nutrient sensor and directly regulates the nutrient supply available for fetal growth. Genomic imprinting is an epigenetic phenomenon whereby the expression of a gene depends on the parent of origin. For example, IGF-I is an imprinted gene and is crucial to fetal development as described above. IGF-I is downregulated in placentas exposed to nutrient restriction [7]. Moreover, a placenta-specific transcript (P0) for the IGF-II gene is expressed exclusively in the labyrinthine trophoblast of the mouse, and deletion of this transcript yields diminished placental growth, reduced placental nutrient transfer, and fetal growth restriction. Methylation of DNA restricts the genes available for transcription in cells. Maternal undernutrition affects the methylation status of the placental IGF-II gene and, in so doing, may control placental supply of maternal nutrients to the fetus. Imprinted genes in the placenta may be modified by perturbations of the maternal environment and altered fetal programming results. Moreover, the placenta strongly influences fetal endocrinology and metabolism. A well-documented example is rise in fetal glucocorticoid levels that follows decreased activity in placental 11β-HSD2. The adverse effects of excess fetal glucocorticoids on fetal development of the hypothalamic pituitary axis may program the fetus to be at higher risk for metabolic diseases as an adult.

Intervention strategies targeting the placenta to prevent altered fetal growth, fetal programming, or both should dissect in more detail how placental growth, nutrient transport function, and placental oxidative stress are modulated by maternal administration of IGFs or pharmacological levels of methyl donors. Targeted upregulation of the activity of placental 11β-HSD2 may also beneficially modulate feto–placental health.

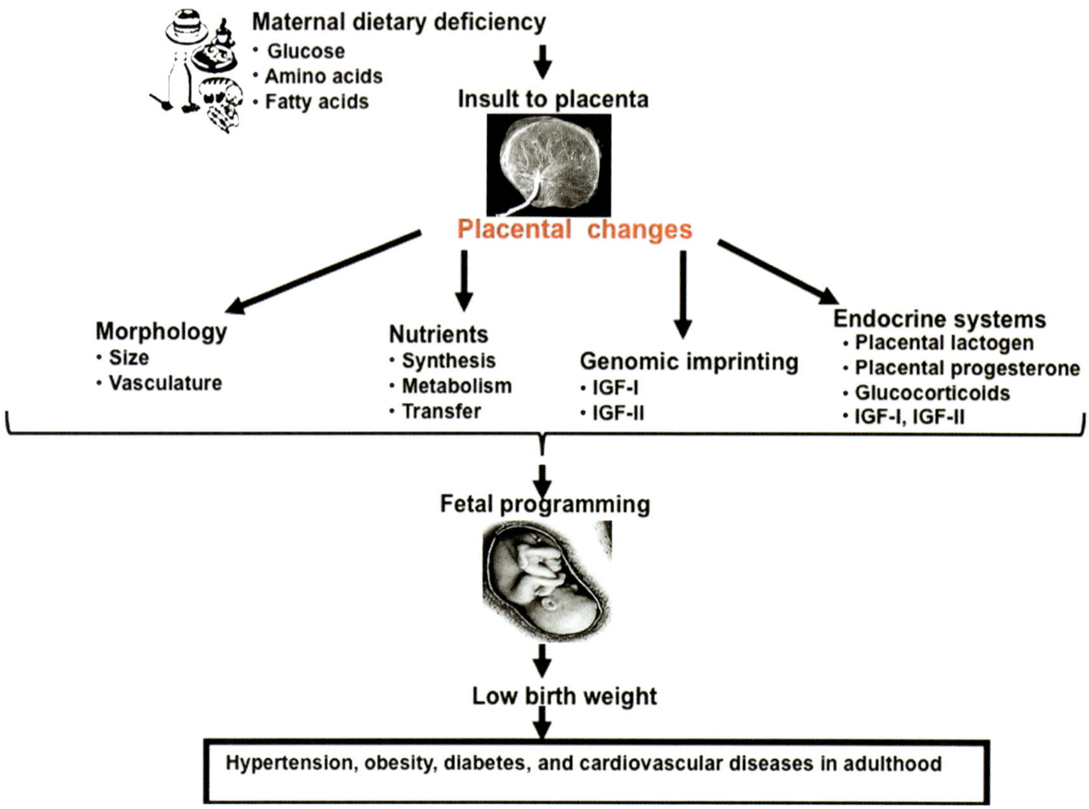

Figure 1.1 The role of the placenta in fetal programming resulting in diseases of adulthood.

Summary

Maternal nutrition during pregnancy is an important determinant of optimal fetal development, pregnancy outcome, and ultimately, life-long health. Barker's epidemiological studies have stimulated new ideas about both in utero development and risks for adult diseases. Animal models of programming have shown that most fetal organs are vulnerable to the effects of maternal undernutrition during critical periods of development. Importantly, these studies show that programming the placenta, as illustrated in Figure 1.1, may mediate effects on the fetus.

Maternal undernutrition reduces fetal growth in part by impairing placental development and function. Placental alterations include decreases in placental weight, altered vascular development, reductions in glucose, AA, and FA transport, and hormone synthesis and metabolism. The plasticity of the placenta allows this pivotal tissue to respond to exogenous insults and to compensate for many environmental influences. Moreover, maternal diet may alter the placental genome through gene imprinting, an effect that may affect future generations. When the placental response is not sufficient to maintain fetal growth, IUGR results and suboptimal outcomes result (Table 1.1). The elucidation of further roles for the placenta in fetal programming will increase our understanding of DOHaD and hopefully will provide new strategies to prevent and treat suboptimal fetal development in the future.

☞ Teaching Points

1. Fetal programming may occur following natural or experimental environmental changes in both humans and animals.
2. Maternal undernutrition-mediated fetal programming results in different outcomes depending on species, sex, and type of diet. It is dependent on time and length of insult.

Table 1.1 Consequences of maternal nutrient restriction on adult offspring.

Natural or Controlled Diet	Species	Adult Offspring Outcome
Poor living conditions: Low-birth-weight baby	Human	Coronary heart disease, hypertension, obesity
Twin pregnancies: The growth restricted baby	Human	Noninsulin-dependent type (II) diabetes mellitus
Food restriction due to increased litter size	Pig	Hypertension, glucose intolerance
	Guinea-pig	Glucose intolerance, insulin deficiency
Global nutrient restriction	Ovine	Hypertension
	Sheep	Hypertension, smaller livers, females have reduced progesterone secretion during the luteal phase of their estrous cycles and markedly reduced fertility
	Guinea-pig	Modification of pituitary–adrenal axis function
	Rat	Glucose intolerance, hypertension, hypercholesterolemia, obesity
	Rat-like hamster	Delay in physical and neurodevelopment
Protein deprivation	Rat	Glucose intolerance, relative insulin resistance, hyperinsulinemia, hypertension
	Mice	Longevity affected
Global mineral (calcium, copper, iron, magnesium, zinc) or vitamin restriction	Rat	Glucose intolerance, insulin resistance, obesity
Chromium restriction	Rat	Obesity
Low-sodium diet	Rat	Hypertension and reduced creatine
Iron deficiency	Rat	Hypertension

3 Placental development during pregnancy has a major impact on pregnancy outcome. Thus, small-for-gestational-age placentas are more likely to result in offspring with metabolic diseases later in life.

4 Genetic imprinting has a major role in placental development. Maternal undernutrition during pregnancy significantly decreases placental Igf2, which negatively affects placental growth.

5 Glucocorticoid treatment changes placental handling and fetal delivery of lactate and selected AA. Glucocorticoids also impact placental expression of GLUTs (GLUT1 and GLUT3) in a dose- and time-dependent manner in both human and rat placentas.

References

1. Barker DJP and Osmond C (1986) Infant mortality, childhood nutrition, and ischemic heart disease in England and Wales. *Lancet* 1: 1077–81.
2. Rutland CS, Latunde-Dada AO, Thorpe A et al. (2007) Effect of gestational nutrition on vascular integrity in the murine placenta. *Placenta* 28: 734–2.
3. Belkacemi L, Chen CH, Ross MG et al. (2009) Increased placental apoptosis in maternal food restricted gestations: Role of the Fas pathway. *Placenta* 30: 739–51.
4. Cetin I, Giovannini N, Alvino G et al. (2002) Intrauterine growth restriction is associated with changes in polyunsaturated fatty acid fetal–maternal relationships. *Pediatric Research* 52: 750–5.
5. Hay WW Jr (1995) Regulation of placental metabolism by glucose supply. *Reproduction, Fertility and Development* 7: 365–75.
6. Fowden AL and Forhead AJ (2004) Endocrine mechanisms of intrauterine programming. *Reproduction* 127: 515–26.
7. Fowden AL (2003) The insulin-like growth factors and feto-placental growth. *Placenta* 24: 803–12.
8. Fowden AL and Forhead AJ (1998) Glucocorticoids and the preparation for life after birth: Are there long-term consequences of the life insurance? *Proceedings of the Nutrition Society* 57: 113–22.

2

CHAPTER 2
Cardiovascular Health and Maternal Placental Syndromes

Shahzya S. Huda[1] *and Ian A. Greer*[2]

[1]Department of Reproductive and Maternal Medicine, University of Glasgow, Glasgow, UK
[2]Department of Health and Life Sciences, University of Liverpool, Liverpool, UK

Introduction

Pregnancy is a time of great maternal metabolic, anatomical, and physiological challenges in order to adapt the mother to the needs of the developing fetus. Adverse maternal outcomes and, in particular, placental complications can occur if the mother or fetus fails to rise sufficiently to these challenges. The maternal placental syndromes (MPS) encompass a spectrum of diseases associated with placental dysfunction, including the hypertensive disorders of pregnancy, placental infarction, and fetal growth restriction (FGR) secondary to placental insufficiency. Although their etiology is both multifactorial and incompletely understood, these conditions share some common pathological mechanisms and predisposing risk factors. Increasing evidence suggests that these women are more likely to develop cardiovascular disease (CVD) in later life. This chapter explores the relationships between the predisposition of women who develop these MPS and their future cardiovascular health.

Maternal placental syndromes

Hypertensive disorders of pregnancy

Hypertension is the most common medical problem encountered in pregnancy and remains an important cause of maternal and fetal morbidity and mortality worldwide. Although both chronic and gestational hypertension have significant adverse effects on pregnancy outcomes, the development of preeclampsia (PE) is associated with the highest risk. PE is a multisystem disorder complicating 2–3% of pregnancies and is characterized by hypertension and proteinuria. The risks to the fetus from PE include growth restriction, iatrogenic preterm delivery, hypoxic-neurologic injury, perinatal death, and long-term risks associated with low birth weight and prematurity.

Although the pathogenesis of PE is not fully understood, endothelial dysfunction, as part of a generalized inflammatory reaction, is a hallmark of PE and involves the maternal circulation to the placenta and the maternal systemic vasculature. Healthy pregnancy is associated with a state of relative systemic inflammation, and therefore, PE may represent the culmination of the maternal systemic inflammatory responses engendered by the pregnancy itself. Notably, all the inflammatory changes of normal pregnancy are exaggerated in PE, and features of the disease include not only endothelial dysfunction but a wider stress response, including the acute phase response and metabolic effects of dyslipidemia and increased insulin resistance (IR). Physiologically, this may be an attempt by the mother to compensate for the deficient placental function.

The Placenta: From Development to Disease, First Edition. Edited by Helen H. Kay, D. Michael Nelson and Yuping Wang.
© 2011 Blackwell Publishing Ltd. Published 2011 by Blackwell Publishing Ltd.

There is increasing support for the theory that PE is, fundamentally, two separate pathological processes that occur based on the gestational age at onset of disease. This concept remains an area of ongoing research. More than 80% of all cases comprise the late-onset type, which is generally associated with a normally grown baby with normal placentation manifested by normal or only slightly altered behavior of the uterine spiral arteries. In contrast, early onset disease represents a smaller, but more severe, subset of cases. Early onset PE is associated with abnormal placentation, inadequate and incomplete trophoblast invasion of maternal spiral arteries, increased vascular resistance in the uterine arteries and within the placental bed, as well as FGR. As a consequence of poor placentation, oxidative and endoplasmic reticulum (ER) stress of the placenta occur to yield endothelial dysfunction and inflammation. The early onset disease is a subgroup associated with severe complications, and this fact has made this phenotype the focus of much basic and clinical research.

Clinical Pearl

Early onset PE is associated with a much higher incidence and severity of fetal and maternal complications and requires increased antenatal surveillance in order to optimize administration of steroids and timing of delivery.

Fetal growth restriction

FGR is the failure of the fetus to reach its genetically predetermined growth potential due to adverse genetic or environmental factors. The clinical impact of increased perinatal mortality and morbidity is further exaggerated in the presence of prematurity. Although the etiology is multifactorial, placental insufficiency is the most common cause. Diagnosis of placental insufficiency can be based on ultrasound parameters, but FGR is often a diagnosis of exclusion. Currently, no in utero treatment can improve or reverse established growth restriction, and management is based on antenatal surveillance to determine judicious timing of steroid administration and the gestational age at delivery. In normal pregnancy, there is effective first trimester invasion of maternal trophoblasts, resulting in the formation of a low-impedance and high-capacitance circulatory interface between the maternal and fetal circulations. The fetus, however, is vulnerable to nutrient deprivation even in the presence of minor placental insufficiency or abnormal placental development.

Epidemiology

There is increasing epidemiological evidence to suggest that adverse pregnancy outcomes such as PE, preterm delivery, and low birth weight are associated with increased risk for the affected women for CVD in later life. In a retrospective cohort study in Scotland using discharge data of almost 130,000 women, PE was associated with a twofold increased risk of subsequent ischemic heart disease (IHD) (RR 2.0;1.5–2.5) [1]. More alarmingly, if a woman had a combination of PE, preterm delivery, and a baby of low birth weight, she has a risk of IHD or death seven times that of controls (95% CI 3.3–14.5). A recent meta-analysis combining eight studies (2,346,997 women), with a mean follow-up of 11.7 years, demonstrated a relative risk of 2.16 (1.86–2.52) of IHD in women with PE, substantiating previous evidence [2]. This doubling of risk remains robust even after adjusting for pre-pregnancy hypertension, diabetes mellitus, obesity, dyslipidemia, metabolic syndromes, and smoking. Furthermore, there is an inverse relationship between birth weight and the incidence of adult CVD, with offspring birth weight also inversely related to maternal CVD, suggestive of an intergenerational influence. Although low birth weight may result from preterm delivery or FGR, both are independently associated with an increased risk of maternal cerebrovascular disease and CVD, with double the risk of developing CVD if the mother delivered a baby in the lowest birth weight quintile for gestational age [1]. These epidemiological links are biologically plausible as women who develop either MPS or CVD share many features such as endothelial dysfunction, inflammation, and oxidative stress. Common risk factors, either genotypic or phenotypic, appear to underlie both conditions. We have previously proposed a model whereby pregnancy with its concomitant digression into a metabolic syndrome is a "stress test" of maternal metabolic response (Figure 2.1) [3]. Women who develop adverse pregnancy outcomes such as PE or FGR make greater excursions into metabolic disturbances during pregnancy and are predisposed to metabolic and vascular disease in later life.

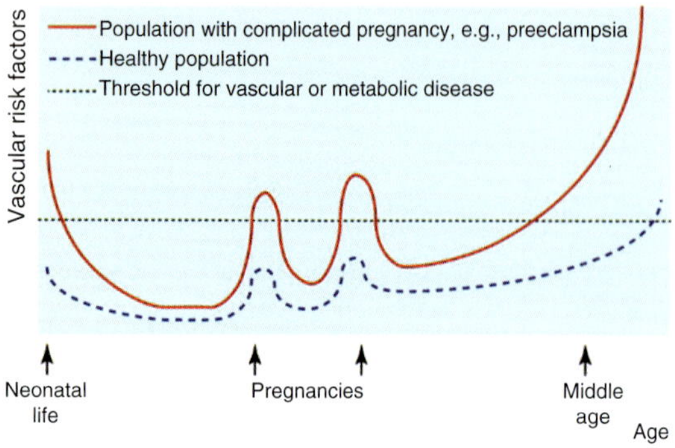

Figure 2.1 Risk factors for vascular disease are identifiable during excursions into the metabolic syndrome of pregnancy. (Reproduced by permission of Sattar N and Greer IA (2002) Pregnancy complications and maternal cardiovascular risk: Opportunities for intervention and screening? *British Medical Journal* 325(7356): 157–60.)

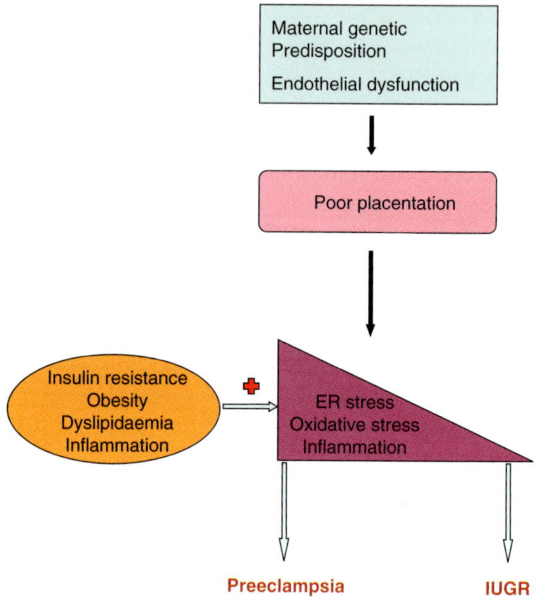

Figure 2.2 Diagram of proposed pathogenesis of FGR and PE. Contributions of both maternal and placental factors determine the clinical syndrome. There is a greater systemic maternal inflammatory response as well as greater ER and oxidative stress in women who develop PE.

Research Spotlight

Women with a combination of PE, preterm delivery, and SGA are up to seven times more likely to develop CVD. The use of adverse pregnancy outcome history as part of risk assessment for future CVD requires evaluation.

Maternal placental syndromes—common pathology?

FGR and early onset PE are associated with infarction of the placenta and are different clinical manifestations of placental insufficiency that have common features in the placental pathology. Both conditions exhibit abnormal histopathology of spiral arterioles in the basal plate. Notably, both conditions also share multiple predisposing maternal risk factors, including race, pre-existing hypertension, inflammation, and nongestational diabetes. Interestingly, the latter characteristics are also important risk factors for CVD in later life. The manifestation of different clinical phenotypes despite similar placental pathology may be due to a variable maternal response products released from a stressed placenta. Alternatively, the similarities in placental pathology may be more apparent than real, and the placental dysfunction in the two phenotypes may indeed be different. Contributions from both maternal and placental factors likely determine the ultimate clinical manifestations (Figure 2.2).

Patterns of placental disease

Failure of trophoblastic invasion and differentiation necessary for remodeling of the spiral arteries has long been implicated in both FGR and PE. The myometrial portion of the artery is most significantly affected with a graduated increase in severity from FGR cases that are normotensive to those that are hypertensive. This results in reduced placental perfusion, increased placental ischemia, and subsequent oxidative stress. Accumulation of lipid-laden macrophages surrounded by areas of fibrinoid necrosis in the spiral arteries is called acute atherosis, and this histopathology is comparable to atherogenesis in nonpregnant women (Figure 2.3). These plaques project into the vessel lumen to further restrict uteroplacental blood flow. Acute atherosis is more pronounced in the cases of PE associated with FGR compared to FGR alone. Indeed, placental morphological changes are more prominent in pregnancies complicated by PE with FGR than in PE alone. This is consistent with data that show that the mean birth weight is lower in pregnancies complicated by FGR secondary to PE than in the cases of unexplained

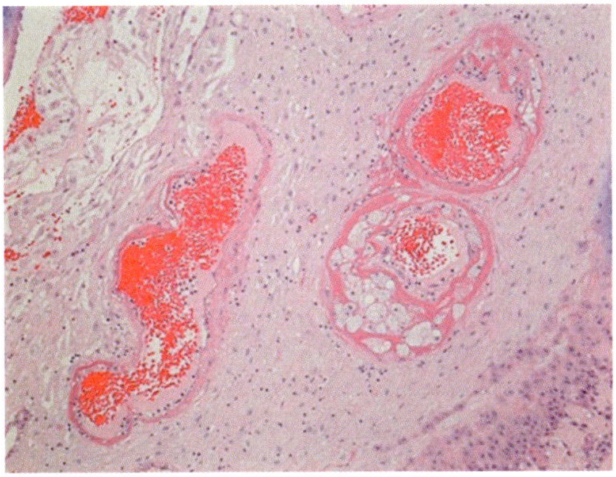

Figure 2.3 Histology of acute atherosis in the spiral arteries within the decidua. The arterial lesion is histologically characterized by fibrinoid necrosis of the vessel walls (eosinophilic staining) with infiltration of foam cells into the damaged vessel wall. On light microscopy, it appears similar to that seen in atherosclerosis. (Reproduced by permission of PathologyOutlines.com, Inc., and Dr. Yan Lemeshev.)

FGR without PE. The placental pathology in both FGR and PE is explored in further detail in Chapters 31 and 32.

Metabolic syndrome of pregnancy

The common and disparate metabolic, pathological, and constitutional risk factors for the development of MPS and future CVD are examined in the following.

Obesity and insulin resistance

The prevalence of obesity has risen exponentially in the last 20 years. Obesity is a significant risk factor in the development of gestational hypertension and PE, with the risk of PE doubling for every 5–7 kg/m^2 increase in BMI. Although the contribution of increased adiposity to the pathogenesis of PE is not fully understood, the increased inflammation, IR, and endothelial dysfunction attributed to obesity are likely contributing factors.

In contrast, FGR is less common in obese women with normal glucose tolerance, as they have a tendency to have neonates with an increased percentage of body fat as well as a metabolic profile consistent with IR. However, in common with obese offspring, babies of low birth weight are more likely to suffer from metabolic diseases, such as type 2 diabetes and CVD in later life. The factors for this are unknown but are thought to be either secondary to genetic predisposition to IR or to in utero programming as a result of the adverse maternal metabolic environment.

Dyslipidemia

In PE, the hyperlipidemia of normal pregnancy is compounded by marked increases in free fatty acids (FFA) and triglycerides (TG). Increased TG drives production of small, dense LDL to enhance oxidative stress and to create an atherogenic environment where small, dense LDLs are preferentially ingested by the macrophages in the vessel wall of the spiral arteries. A reduction in HDL cholesterol limits endothelial protection. Elevated FFA leads to systemic hyperinsulinemia, impaired peripheral insulin sensitivity, and endothelial dysfunction. Interestingly, there is no predisposition to dyslipidemia in women who develop unexplained FGR without PE.

Inflammation and endothelial dysfunction

Normal pregnancy evokes a systemic inflammatory response that is exaggerated in PE. The inflammation involves both the acute phase response of leukocytosis and the activation of complement and the clotting cascades. There are increases of proinflammatory cytokines, including TNF-alpha and IL-6, and PAI-1. Upregulation of the inflammatory response is also apparent in FGR, although not as exaggerated as that seen in PE. There is an increase in activation of circulating neutrophils together with an increase in placental and circulating levels of proinflammatory cytokines relative to uncomplicated pregnancies. Indeed, evidence of chronic inflammation in the placenta in pregnancies complicated by FGR is similar to that seen in preterm deliveries and PE.

Endothelial cells are key mediators of both local and systemic inflammatory responses. Features of endothelial dysfunction are accentuated in pregnancies complicated by both PE and FGR. There is upregulation of adhesion molecule expression on the endothelium, and these anchor marginated leukocytes to facilitate perivascular accumulation. There are also abnormalities of uterine and brachial artery blood flow prior to the clinical manifestation of the phenotypes. These findings suggest that the endothelial dysfunction may precede both FGR and PE, albeit more pronounced in women who develop PE.

Oxidative and endoplasmic reticulum stress

The ER is central to many cellular functions and is the major subcellular site for protein folding and trafficking. Failure of the ER's adaptive capacity results in activation of the unfolded protein response (UPR), which intersects with inflammatory and stress signaling pathways. ER stress may thus be the link between inflammation and metabolic disease, including obesity, IR, and type 2 diabetes mellitus. ER stress is a major component of the pathophysiology in FGR and PE, resulting in reduced cell proliferation and increased apoptosis in placentae of both conditions [4]. ER stress and oxidative stress are closely linked as both are stimulated by vascular malperfusion and ischemia reperfusion. UPR generates reactive oxygen species (ROS), and together, they activate similar intracellular inflammatory signaling pathways such as the NF-κB pathways.

Research Spotlight

ER stress links inflammation and metabolic disease and is a major determinant of the pathophysiology of IUGR and PE [4].

Angiogenic factors

The altered release of placental factors into the maternal circulation as a result of placental oxidative stress and inflammation is pivotal in the pathogenesis of MPS. Soluble fms-like tyrosine kinase-1 (sFlt-1), an antagonist of vascular endothelium-derived growth factor (VEGF) and placental growth factor (PlGF), is upregulated in PE to increase systemic concentrations of sFlt-1 and lower circulating concentrations of the anti-inflammatory and vasodilatory VEGF and PlGF-1. They, in turn, lead to an imbalance in circulating angiogenic factors [5]. One of the key elements involved in VEGF and sFlt-1 gene transcription is the transcription factor, hypoxia-inducible factor 1 alpha (HIF1alpha), which is stimulated by hypoxia and inflammation. Soluble endoglin (sEng) is upregulated in PE, induces endothelial dysfunction and hypertension in vivo, and correlates with the severity of the clinical syndrome. In combination with sFlt-1, sEng augments vascular damage. Parallels again exist between PE and CVD, with higher sFlt-1 levels following acute MI, and higher levels correlate with increased morbidity [6]. Statins have anti-inflammatory effects and reduce the release of antiangiogenic factors including sFlt-1 in normal healthy term placentae. Further research into the use of statins as a potential modifying therapeutic agent in the prevention of PE is ongoing.

Research Spotlight

An imbalance of the angiogenic factors sFlt-1, VEGF, and PlGF-1 is implicated in the pathogenesis of both FGR and PE. Imbalances of these growth factors correlate with the myocardial damage post myocardial infarction.

Long-term vascular and metabolic changes

Epidemiological evidence for the increased risk of CVD in women with pregnancies complicated by PE and FGR is consistent, but there remains uncertainty as to the degree of adjustment for potential confounders; there is little direct evidence for this increased risk. Furthermore, there are minimal data on the underlying mechanisms for this apparent increase in risk of CVD. Women with a history of PE have persistent dyslipidemia, increased inflammation, higher concentrations of C-reactive protein, abnormal microvascular function, and vascular dilatation up to 30 years after the sentinel pregnancy. Features of metabolic dysregulation are not as apparent in women with a history of a delivery complicated by FGR. However, there remains an inverse relationship between delivery of a low-birth-weight infant and later life higher maternal systolic blood pressure, IR, dyslipidemia, and inflammatory markers, including CRP and IL-6. All are important predictors of vascular events outside of pregnancy. Moreover, mothers with small-for-gestation offspring at term exhibit disruption of both endothelial-dependent and endothelial-independent vascular function remote from the index pregnancy [7], even when controlled for maternal obesity and smoking. The variations in maternal metabolic and vascular phenotype, apparent in women with a history of MPS, may be directly responsible for the relationship with future CVD risk.

Long-term health strategies

Coronary heart disease (CHD) is the most common single cause of death among women in the Western world with growing evidence of some unique sex-specific features of CHD. Women with CHD present atypically, with a greater frequency of nonexertional chest pain. Primary and secondary prevention initiatives for CHD in women are often limited because they do not acknowledge this atypical presentation. Importantly, women with established CVD are twice as likely as men to have associated metabolic syndrome, and women with CVD and metabolic syndrome have a tenfold increased risk for death while men with both conditions have up to a threefold higher risk of death. Proactive risk assessment approaches in women are needed to identify those at high risk at early stages in life so that intervention can be effective. Primary preventative strategies may include lifestyle modifications in diet and exercise, which have been shown to significantly reduce long-term cardiovascular risk. Pharmacological therapy to reduce dyslipidemia and vascular inflammation may also play a preventative role in the future.

In summary, women with a history of MPS are at higher risk of future vascular-related events, compared to women with normal pregnancies. The pathological mechanisms for this higher risk are not elucidated. Whether primary interventions can influence future cardiovascular health is a pressing question that is yet to be answered.

☞ Teaching Points

1. The MPS share similar pathological mechanisms and predisposing maternal risk factors
2. The systemic inflammatory response and metabolic dysregulation are more pronounced in PE compared to FGR alone.
3. Women with a history of MPS are at increased future risk of cardiovascular disease.
4. Mechanisms for this increased risk may be due to a maternal predisposition to endothelial dysfunction, inflammation, dyslipidemia, and IR.
5. Future studies should clarify whether knowledge of obstetric outcomes adds to CVD risk factor prediction models, and whether primary intervention strategies will modify this risk.

References

1. Smith GC, Pell JP, and Walsh D (2001) Pregnancy complications and maternal risk of ischaemic heart disease: A retrospective cohort study of 129,290 births. *Lancet* 357(9273): 2002–6.
2. Bellamy L, Casas JP, Hingorani AD et al. (2007) Pre-eclampsia and risk of cardiovascular disease and cancer in later life: Systematic review and meta-analysis. *British Medical Journal* 335(7627): 974.
3. Sattar N and Greer IA (2002) Pregnancy complications and maternal cardiovascular risk: Opportunities for intervention and screening? *British Medical Journal* 325(7356): 157–60.
4. Burton GJ, Yung HW, Cindrova-Davies T et al. (2009) Placental endoplasmic reticulum stress and oxidative stress in the pathophysiology of unexplained intrauterine growth restriction and early onset pre-eclampsia. *Placenta* 30(Suppl. A): S43–8.
5. Maynard S, Epstein FH, and Karumanchi SA (2008) Pre-eclampsia and angiogenic imbalance. *Annual Review of Medicine* 59: 61–78.
6. Onoue K, Uemura S, Takeda Y et al. (2009) Usefulness of soluble fms-like tyrosine kinase-1 as a biomarker of acute severe heart failure in patients with acute myocardial infarction. *American Journal of Cardiology* 104(11): 1478–83.
7. Kanagalingam MG, Nelson SM, Freeman DJ et al. (2009) Vascular dysfunction and alteration of novel and classic cardiovascular risk factors in mothers of growth-restricted offspring. *Atherosclerosis* 205(1): 244–50.

II

PART II

Placental Development, Physiology, and Immunology

3

CHAPTER 3
Development and Anatomy of the Human Placenta

Roxane Rampersad[1], *Mila Cervar-Zivkovic*[2] *and D. Michael Nelson*[1]

[1]Division of Maternal-Fetal medicine and Ultrasound-Genetics, Department of Obstetrics and Gynecology, Washington University School of Medicine, St. Louis, MO, USA
[2]Department of Obstetrics and Gynecology, Medical University of Graz, Graz, Austria

Overview

The human placenta interfaces the mother and fetus to prevent immune rejection, to transfer nutrients, to dispose fetal wastes, and to secrete hormones that sustain pregnancy. We describe key aspects of the development and anatomy of this vital organ.

The placenta at delivery: Starting at the end to understand the beginning

The placenta is formed from the merger of the chorion and the allantois in early pregnancy, and thus, the "afterbirth" delivered in the third stage of labor is called the *chorioallantoic placenta*. This is a discoid organ that weighs an average of 470 g [1]. Placental weight is directly proportional to fetal weight, and at term, a typical fetal to *placental ratio* is seven when determined by weight. Alteration of this ratio associates with pregnancy pathologies and placental dysfunction. The endometrium of pregnancy is called the *decidua* and the attachment site of the chorioallantoic placenta onto the uterus is at the *decidua basalis*, or basal plate, sometimes called the maternal surface. The basal plate viewed on the delivered chorioallantoic placenta exhibits about 10–40 irregularly shaped indentations that define *cotyledons* (Figure 3.1). Major branches of the umbilical circulation supply each cotyledon, and the demarcations that define cotyledons are formed by *placental septae*, which are invaginations of the maternal decidua into the chorioallantoic placental disc. The cotyledons consist of villous trees that are bathed in maternal blood, hence the designation *villous hemochorial placenta*, that are outgrowths from immature intermediate villi on the chorionic plate, and that branch to form progressively smaller diameter intermediate and terminal villi.

Research Spotlight

The only nonhuman primate with a villous hemochorial placenta is the armadillo.

The fetal facing surface where the umbilical cord inserts is the *chorionic plate* (Figure 3.1). The edges of the placenta converge where the chorionic and basal plates meet to form the *chorioamnion* membrane that houses the amniotic fluid. The amnion faces the fetus as a single layer of epithelium with a subjacent basement membrane and an avascular connective tissue base. The *chorion leave*, or smooth chorion, consists of mesenchyme, mononuclear cytotrophoblasts, and vessels that are an extension of the spiral arterioles of the decidua basalis.

The Placenta: From Development to Disease, First Edition. Edited by Helen H. Kay, D. Michael Nelson and Yuping Wang.
© 2011 Blackwell Publishing Ltd. Published 2011 by Blackwell Publishing Ltd.

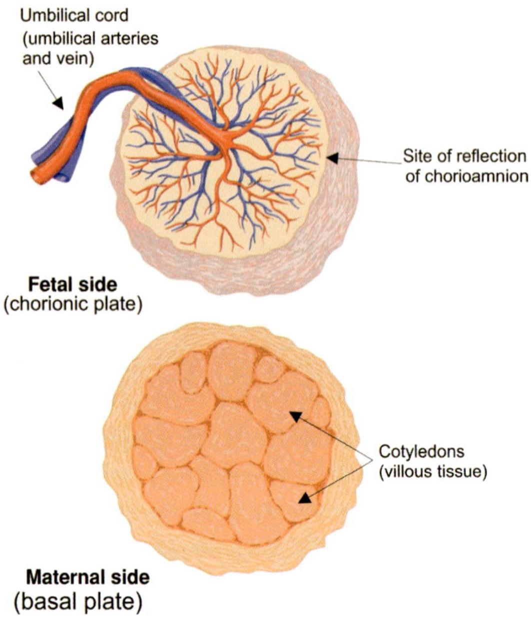

Figure 3.1 Illustration of the term human placenta: The upper illustration depicts the chorionic or fetal side of the placenta. The umbilical cord inserts within the chorionic plate and the chorionic vessels are shown supplying each cotyledon. The veins carry oxygenated blood, shown in red, while arteries carry deoxygenated blood, shown in blue. The basal or maternal side seen in the lower illustration is in contact with the uterine endometrium and divided into cotyledons.

Clinical Pearl

A single umbilical vein and two umbilical arteries ramify over the chorionic surface, with the arteries passing over the veins. As the placenta is rarely circular in shape, the umbilical cord inserts eccentrically into most placentas.

Back to the beginning with decidualization

The decidua, or endometrium of pregnancy, changes in structure in anticipation of implantation, and this change is called *decidualization*. Endometrial stromal cells transform into an epithelioid appearance, and the endometrial glands secrete nutrients called *histiotroph*, which will be used by a successful conceptus for growth and development in the first few weeks of pregnancy. The decidua is invaded with immune cells comprising 50% of the population, including macrophages, T-lymphocytes, and a unique population of natural killer (NK) cells that have reduced cytotoxicity compared to circulating NK cells.

Placental development from implantation through the first trimester

The fertilized egg, called a *zygote* traverses the Fallopian tube while a series of mitotic divisions yield a ball of cells called a *morula*. This ball of cells partitions into a peripheral layer called the *trophectoderm* that circumscribes the perimeter of the *blastocyst* and forms the placenta and extraembryonic membranes (Figure 3.2(a)). An asymmetric group of cells within the blastocyst form the inner cell mass, or *embryoblast*, that develop into the fetus and are on the side proximal to the site of attachment of the blastocyst to the epithelium of the uterus.

The formation of the amniotic cavity and chorioamnion begins on the fourth post-conception day as the inner cell mass ultimately differentiates into a bilaminar disc composed of cuboidal hypoblast and columnar epiblast (Figure 3.2(b)). The epiblast is delineated by a collection of fluid within the inner cell mass. Amnioblasts derived from the epiblast will line the *amnion*. The hypoblasts that are most distant from the endometrium become displaced by endoderm and migrate to line the blastocyst cavity, transforming this into the primitive yolk sac. The formation of the primitive yolk sac separates this cavity from a second transformation that occurs with migration and proliferation of extraembryonic endoderm, resulting in the definitive secondary *yolk sac*. The yolk sac will ultimately form the primitive blood vessels and red blood cells of the early embryo, among other entities.

The *amniotic membrane* consists of a single layer of cuboidal epithelial cells loosely connected to the chorion at this stage. The *chorion* is composed of a spongy layer of loose collagen, fetal blood vessels, and chorionic mesoderm [1]. A blastocoel results when fluid appears internally to form a cavity, and the blastocyst that evolves bursts out of the zona pellucida because a gang of cells on the blastocyst surface, dubbed the *zona breaking cells*, release the blastocyst to seek an implantation site on the uterine epithelium of the decidua. Defining the contour of the blastocyst and containing the fluid is a single layer of flattened cells called the trophectoderm, as mentioned

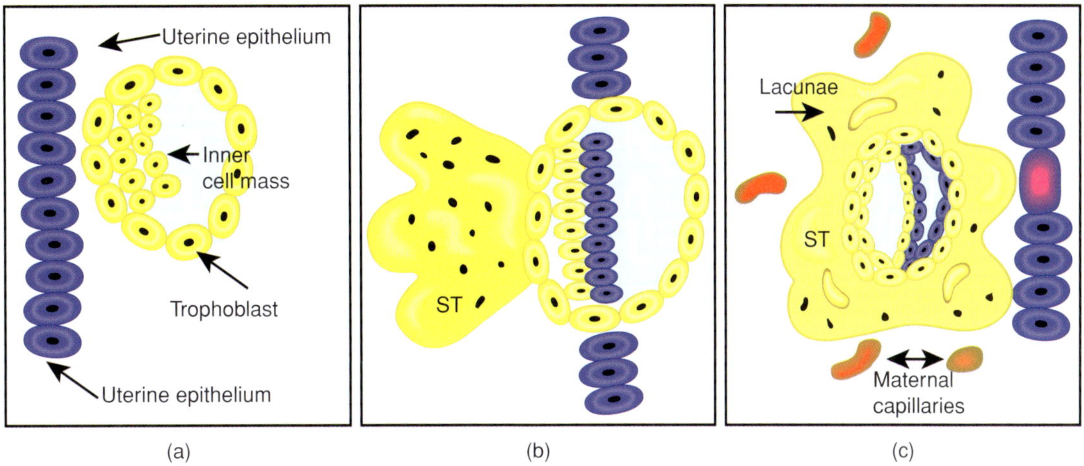

Figure 3.2 Implantation of the blastocyst: (a) Apposition of the blastocyst is the first step in implantation. The trophectoderm is the outer layer of cells comprised of trophoblast cells seen in yellow. Adhesion of the blastocyst occurs with the inner cell (green) mass closest to the decidua (purple). (b) During invasion of the blastocyst, the cytotrophoblast proliferate (c) to form an invasive multinucleated syncytiotrophoblast (ST). The inner cell mass also differentiates into a bilaminar disk of embryoblast (green) and amnioblast (pink). (c) Following invasion, vacuoles are formed within the syncytiotrophoblast. The vacuoles coalesce to form lacunae. The lacunae are the primitive intervillous space that will be filled with maternal blood with erosion of maternal capillaries (red).

earlier. The trophectoderm cells ultimately form the multiple cytotrophoblast lineages that are described below. *Interstitial implantation* in the human is one of the most aggressive implantation processes described among animal species and evolves through prelacunar and lacunar stages.

The prelacunar stage begins on the seventh day post conception as microvilli emanating from trophectoderm make initial contact with the luminal epithelium of the uterus, a process known as *apposition* (Figure 3.2(a)). Attachment of the blastocyst soon follows through a complex interplay between the trophoblast cells and the decidua, both secreting multiple mediators that include prostaglandins, proteolytic enzymes, chemokines, cytokines, selectins, and integrins to name but a few [2]. Trophectoderm invades the endometrium after attachment and these cells penetrate the uterine epithelium to reside within the decidua. The human blastocyst thereby yields interstitial implantation within the connective tissue and adjacent to the maternal vessels that will ultimately provide blood flow to the placenta (Figure 3.2(b)). As the blastocyst invasion proceeds, the mononucleated trophoblast cells, or *cytotrophoblasts*, proliferate and fuse to form a double layer, with the outer cells forming a true syncytium as a terminally differentiated *syncytiotrophoblast* that comes in direct contact with the maternal tissue.

At the lacunar stage, ongoing proliferation and fusion of cytotrophoblasts yield abundant syncytiotrophoblasts that surround the majority of the implanted blastocyst and that develop spaces within the syncytium (Figure 3.2(c)). These vacuoles coalesce to form lacunae and columns of syncytiotrophoblast form trabeculae. The lacunae are the primitive forms of what will become the intervillous space in the chorioallantoic placenta where maternal blood will circulate.

Clinical Pearl

The human conceptus develops in an extremely low oxygen environment until 10 weeks' gestation, with a $pO_2 <$ 15 mm Hg.

The intervillous spaces are fluid filled without maternal blood until 10–12 weeks of gestation, as the spiral arterioles are plugged with specialized *endovascular cytotrophoblasts* [3]. The low oxygen environment may protect the fetus from reactive oxygen species during the time of organogenesis. The spiral arterioles begin to perfuse the intervillous space at the end of the first trimester to

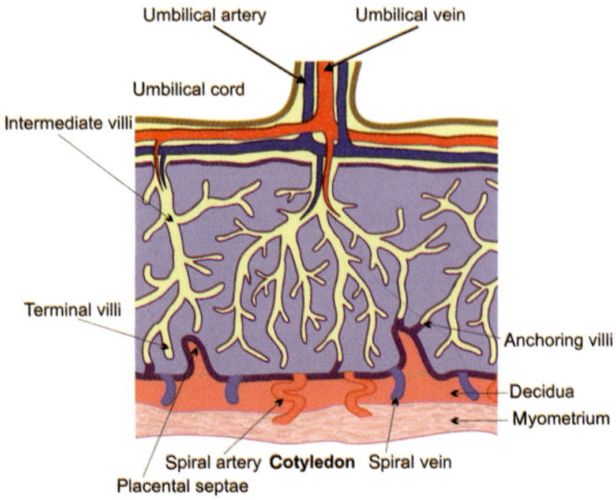

Figure 3.3 Villous tree: Representation of the branching villous tree where intermediate villi give rise to terminal villi.

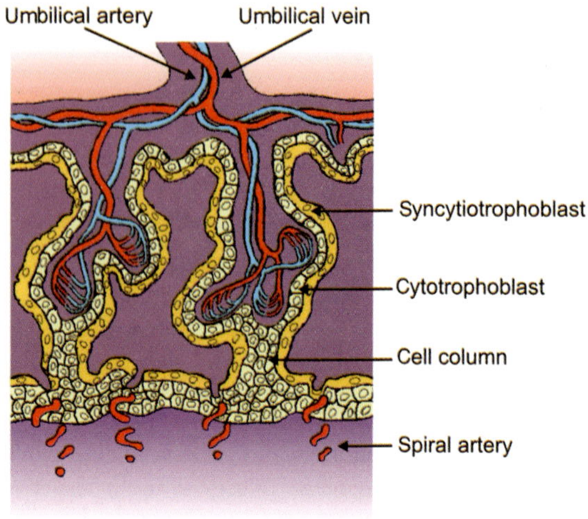

Figure 3.4 Placenta circulation: Representation of villi within a cotyledon. The outer layers of villi are lined with multinucleated syncytiotrophoblast and mononucleated cytotrophoblast. Fetal vessels are shown within the villous core. Surrounding the villi is the intervillous space.

allow feto–maternal exchange of oxygen and nutrients (Figure 3.3).

A villous tree develops

Villi are finger-like projections that form a treelike structure that generally contain an outer surface layer of multinucleated syncytiotrophoblast and a subjacent layer of mononucleated cytotrophoblasts (Figure 3.4). The two trophoblast phenotypes share a basement membrane that delimits a loose connective tissue core through which fetal vessels ramify and where fetal macrophages called *Hofbauer cells* are a prominent feature of the histology. Despite the fact that nucleated fetal red blood cells are seen in the primitive villous vessels by about 20 days post conception, the maternal and fetal circulations do not initially exchange nutrients and wastes until about 10 weeks' gestation, as this cannot occur until spiral arterioles perfuse the intervillous space. Interestingly, the early conceptus is nourished from the secretions of the endometrial glands called *histiotroph*.

Types of villi

Early villus development is characterized by the invasion of cytotrophoblasts into the columns of syncytiotrophoblast trabeculae. These villi are sequentially invaded by mesenchyme and then fetal vessels. A *primary villus* is thus one formed by trophoblastic trabeculae with a central core of cytotrophoblasts. A *secondary villus* is one with mesenchyme also in the core. A *tertiary villus* is formed from a secondary villus penetrated by fetal vessels. Also called a *mesenchymal villus*, a tertiary villus has both a surface of syncytiotrophoblasts and a complete layer of cytotrophoblasts that rest on a basement membrane.

Mesenchymal villi from 5 weeks' post conception differentiate into four villus types. *Immature intermediate villi* contain abundant mesenchyme, edema, and matrix channels that provide a path for the Hofbauer cells to patrol the villous core. *Stem villi* derive from immature intermediate villi through transformation of the villous core into a dense stroma containing an extensive arcade of fetal vessels. *Terminal villi* bud from the surface of mesenchymal and immature intermediate villi (Figure 3.3). Ongoing proliferation of cytotrophoblasts indented with mesenchyme yields outgrowths of syncytiotrophoblast called *syncytial sprouts* (Figure 3.5(a)). As these protrude into the lacunae, which soon will be occupied by maternal blood, they form the precursors of the tertiary villi that are critical to nutrient exchange in the second half of pregnancy. *Mature intermediate villi* become prominent beyond 20 weeks' gestation and yield *tertiary villi*, which

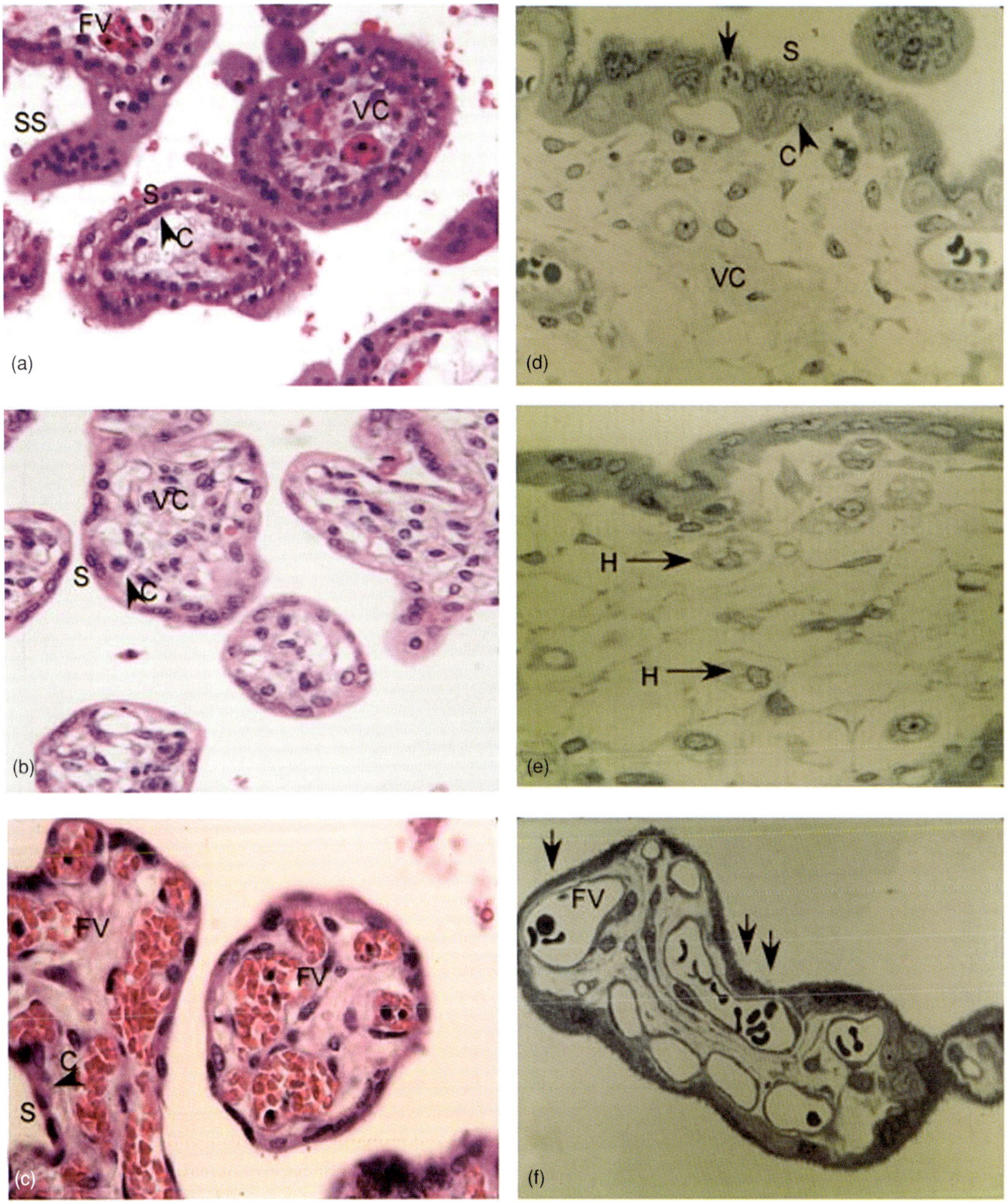

Figure 3.5 Placental Villi: (a) H&E staining of a first trimester villi composed of an outer layer of syncytiotrophoblast (S) and cytotrophoblast (C with arrowhead). The intervillous space surrounding the villi is devoid of maternal blood. A syncytial sprout (SS) is seen extending from a mesenchymal villi. Within the villous stroma are fetal vessels (FV) with nucleated fetal red blood cells. (b) H&E staining of second trimester villi with less dense villous core (VC). (c) H&E staining of terminal villi with several fetal vessels. (d and e) Toluidine blue staining of a first trimester villi with edematous villous core. Hofbauer cells are labeled within the villous core (H). (f) Vasculosyncytial membrane of a terminal villus. (Images courtesy of Dr. Frederick Kraus and Dr. Raymond Redline.)

are formed as villous sprouts that are relatively small in diameter and are also composed of syncytiotrophoblast, cytotrophoblasts, and fetal capillary loops. Mature intermediate villi differ from their precursor (i.e., immature) namesake that dominate the placenta of less than 20 weeks' gestation, as they have a thinner layer of syncytiotrophoblast, a discontinuous layer of cytotrophoblasts, a well-developed fetal vasculature, and no villous core channels.

Components of the villous core

The above description indicates that the core of placental villi evolves over gestation. Early villi are edematous with fluid channels, limited fetal vessels, and minimal connective tissue, which make Hofbauer cells prominent with their large size and vacuolated cytoplasm (Figure 3.5 (d & e)). Undifferentiated stromal cells, fibroblasts, pericytes, and myofibroblasts contribute to the cellular composition of the stroma. The villous core in later gestation is more cellular, contains lesser amounts of collagen, is more vascular, and generally offers a diminished diffusion barrier for gases and nutrients to transfer between the maternal and fetal circulations (Figures 3.5(b & c)).

Fetal vessels are composed of a monolayer of nonfenestrated endothelial cells that line the lumen of capillaries, sinusoids, and larger vessels (Figures 3.5(a, c, & f)). The latter have smooth muscle in their vessel walls and are located in the *stem villi* that originate from the chorionic plate. The vessel endothelium and smooth muscle walls produce multiple vasoactive proteins, among which are endothelial-derived relaxing factor, atrial natriuretic peptide, and endothelin-1.

Anchoring villi that rest on the decidua basalis result from multiple ramifications of stem villi that ultimately connect to the basal plate through the cytotrophoblastic cell columns (Figure 3.3). The cells of the column proliferate at the origin of their basement membrane attachment on the villus, and cytotrophoblastic daughter cells extend into the decidua. These cells differentiate into a spectrum of variably *invasive extravillous cytotrophoblasts*, as described below. Terminal villi are prominent in the last trimester and form the ultimate branches of the villous tree (Figure 3.3). These are bathed in maternal blood in the intervillous space, offer a high ratio of surface to cross-sectional area, and are critical for nutrient and gas exchange. Extremely thin areas that interface the maternal blood space and the fetal vasculature in the last trimester are called *vasculosyncytial membranes*, which are comprised of a thin, non-nucleated segment of syncytiotrophoblast cytoplasm, the trophoblast and endothelial basement membranes, and the endothelium (Figure 3.5(f)). The circulations are separate, but their proximity may be within a few microns of each other.

Multiple phenotypes of trophoblast evolve from the trophectoderm

The trophectoderm of the blastocyst is the origin of all trophoblastic cell lineages. Cytotrophoblasts fuse to form syncytiotrophoblasts while also differentiating into extravascular cytotrophoblasts in the cell columns as well as endovascular cytotrophoblasts within maternal vessels. Cytotrophoblasts form a continuous layer beneath the syncytiotrophoblast in the immature intermediate villi before 20 weeks' gestation. The villous cytotrophoblast layer becomes discontinuous as gestation advances and cross-sections of cytotrophoblast cell bodies ultimately occupies about one-fifth of the shared basement membrane that supports the syncytiotrophoblast. The villous cytotrophoblasts emanate multiple cytoplasmic extensions to yield a stellate structure, and multiple infoldings of the basal plasma membrane substantially enhance surface area above that of the basement membrane on which the cytotrophoblasts rest. Despite the changes in morphology over gestation, the ratio of nuclei in the syncytiotrophoblast compared to the subjacent cytotrophoblasts on villi remains constant at 10:1 from the first trimester through term, a fact commonly overlooked in textbooks. Villous and extravillous cytotrophoblasts are mitotically active, while syncytiotrophoblast are not (Figure 3.5(d)). The cytotrophoblasts provide a stem cell population with daughter cells fusing with overlying syncytiotrophoblasts to replenish this terminally differentiated layer on villi. Both villous cytotrophoblasts and syncytiotrophoblasts produce protein and steroid hormones critical for pregnancy, including the alpha and beta subunits of HCG, HPL, members of the transforming growth factor family of proteins, progesterone, and estriol.

Extravillous cytotrophoblasts are invasive and mediate penetration of the decidua. There are a variety of extravillous trophoblast phenotypes, some of which proliferate, others express selective integrins important to invasion into the interstitium, some mimic an endothelial phenotype to modify the spiral arterioles, and while still others form multinucleated giant cells characteristic of the placental bed at term.

The syncytiotrophoblast of term placenta is a multinucleated, continuous layer surrounding the surface of the villous tree. The syncytium is formed by membrane–membrane fusion of cytotrophoblasts with the overlying syncytiotrophoblast. The outer syncytial layer is exposed to the intervillous space and thus is bathed in maternal blood. Maintenance of this layer depends on the continued proliferation of the villous cytotrophoblast layer, as syncytiotrophoblast is mitotically inactive. Aging nuclei in the syncytium are prominent in the last trimester and collections of effete nuclei form *syncytial knots* that bulge off the apical surface of villi. Turnover of the syncytium is controversial, but one hypothesis poses knots as a source of nuclei for release into the maternal vasculature. What is for sure is that thousands of fragments of syncytiotrophoblasts and villous cytotrophoblasts are released into the maternal circulation daily in normal pregnancy, and these trophoblast components occur with an even higher frequency in complicated pregnancies. Some of these fragments likely derive from areas of discontinuity in the syncytiotrophoblast layer on villous surfaces. Such areas are commonly marked by the presence of a surface matrix of fibrin, fibrin-type fibrinoid described later, which is used as a scaffold for re-epithelialization of the denuded areas [4]. The apical surface of the syncytiotrophoblast is covered with microvilli, and there is up to 12 m^2 of surface area exposed to the maternal vasculature at term in normal pregnancies. The microvilli containing actin are adjacent to microtubules and microfilaments that are intermixed as a network in the apical surface abutting the intervillous space. This cytoskeleton is important for the structural integrity of the trophoblast layer as mechanical insults from perfusion of maternal blood likely cause some of the routine injury noted in the histopathology of placentas from uncomplicated pregnancies. The cytoskeleton of both the syncytiotrophoblasts and the cytotrophoblasts of villi contain multiple intermediate filaments, including cytokeratins 7 and 18, commonly used in studies of isolated villous trophoblasts. In contrast, vimentin intermediate filaments are reliable markers of mesenchymal components such as endothelial cells.

Intermediate trophoblasts are a distinct population of terminally differentiated, mononucleated cytotrophoblasts that are rather large with a clear cytoplasm immunoreactive for HPL but not HCG. When they are found within the margin of anchoring villi, they are known as villous intermediate trophoblasts. Implantation site intermediate trophoblasts can also be seen in the decidua, the myometrium and the maternal spiral arterioles. A third subtype of intermediate trophoblasts is found in the chorionic leave, and these possess a high activity of 15-hydroxyprostaglandin dehydrogenase that inactivates the prostaglandins produced in high amounts by the amnion.

Placental fibrinoid

Fibrinoid is a nonspecific descriptor for an acellular matrix component found in multiple tissues that exhibit a characteristic eosinophilic staining with hematoxylin and eosin. The appearance is not dissimilar from the tinctorial qualities of fibrin deposited in tissues, but fibrinoid connotes the presence of multiple proteins without specificity for one. Multiple locations in the placenta have fibrinoid deposits, including the villous tree and throughout the basal plate. Fibrin-containing fibrinoid deposits on the surface of villi mark discontinuities of the syncytiotrophoblast at sites of presumed trophoblast turnover by apoptosis. *Fibrin-type fibrinoid* is composed predominantly of fibrinogen and fibrin and is derived from maternal blood. *Intravillous fibrinoid* is descriptive of the deposit that appears in the midst of a villus, commonly apparent in placentas of normal pregnancies. *Matrix-type fibrinoid* contains multiple matrix proteins, including fibronectin, laminin, type IV collagen, vitronectin, and fibrillin. These extracellular matrix components substitute for the fibrin and fibrinogen that characterize the above fibrin-type fibrinoid. Fibrinoid in the basal plate at the junction of anchoring villi has an eponym, called *Rohr's striae*. A well-known fibrinoid, called *Nitabuch's layer* historically, was incorrectly assigned immune functions for survival of the fetal allograft, but this matrix instead is merely *matrix-type fibrinoid* distributed discontinuously throughout the basal plate at the interface between the chorioallantoic placenta and the maternal decidua.

Conclusion

The placenta is indeed an interesting structure not only for the functionality exhibited but the importance the placenta has played in the ontogeny and phylogeny of animal species. More knowledge of the human placental structure and function will surely be rewarded by improved understanding of normal and abnormal pregnancies.

Teaching Points

1 A fertilized egg is a zygote that evolves into a ball of cells called the morula and a cavity containing blastocyst.

2 After interstitial implantation of the blastocyst, the trophectoderm as the outer layer of the blastocyst evolves into the human placenta.

3 The endometrium of pregnancy is called the decidua, which undergoes decidualization in preparation for implantation.

4 The human conceptus develops in a low oxygen environment until about 10–12 weeks' gestation when maternal blood perfuses the intervillous space.

5 Maternal spiral arterioles undergo a transformation through influences of invading trophoblasts to loose their smooth muscle coats and dilate to accommodate a tenfold increase in blood flow that enters the chorioallantoic placenta where there is an open circulation.

6 A treelike structure evolves from immature intermediate villi to ramify from the stem villi of the chorionic plate to attach at the decidua basalis via anchoring villi. The smaller diameter terminal villi provide a high surface exchange area within the hemochorial, chorioallantoic disc.

7 The basic villous structure consists of a surface layer of syncytiotrophoblast, a subjacent layer of villous cytotrophoblasts, a basement membrane that delimits a connective tissue villous core, which contains tissue macrophages called Hofbauer cells and an arcade of fetal vessels.

8 The syncytiotrophoblast is unique in human biology as the only true syncytial epithelium that functions as an endothelium when bathed in maternal blood, occupying the intervillous space.

9 Multiple phenotypes of trophoblast perform different functions within the human placenta. The villous trophoblast mediates maternal–fetal exchange, invasive trophoblasts penetrate the decidua basalis, endovascular trophoblasts transform spiral arterioles, and trophoblasts of the chorion leave modulate prostaglandin activity.

10 Fibrinoid is a nonspecific term that relates an eosinophilic staining pattern to hypocellular areas of extracellular materials on villi as fibrin-type fibrinoid and in the decidua basalis as matrix-type fibrinoid.

References

1. Benirschke K, Kaufmann P, and Baergen RN (2006) *Pathology of the Human Placenta*. 5th edn. New York: Springer; p. 1050.
2. Aplin JD and Kimber SJ (2004) Trophoblast-uterine interactions at implantation. *Reproductive Biology and Endocrinology* 2: 48.
3. Hustin J and Schaaps JP (1987) Echographic and anatomic studies of the maternotrophoblastic border during the first trimester of pregnancy. *American Journal of Obstetrics and Gynecology* 157(1): 162–8.
4. Nelson DM, Crouch EC, Curran EM et al. (1990) Trophoblast interaction with fibrin matrix. Epithelialization of perivillous fibrin deposits as a mechanism for villous repair in the human placenta. *American Journal of Pathology* 136(4): 855–65.

4

CHAPTER 4
Immunologic Aspects of Pregnancy

Joan S. Hunt and Margaret G. Petroff
Department of Anatomy and Cell Biology, University of Kansas Medical Center, Kansas City, KS, USA

Introduction

Pregnancies in humans and some other mammals are characterized by intimate juxtapositioning of maternal and fetal cells and their products. In most instances of such close positioning of genetically different cells and molecules, the immune system of the host—in this case, the mother—would be expected to produce an immune rejection response. Oddly, but providentially, in the pregnancies of women and certain experimental animals such as rodents, not only are the "foreign" embryos/fetuses tolerated by the mother, but emerging evidence indicates active encouragement of fetal growth and development via classical immune system components.

Understanding the potential importance of these unexpected and diametrically opposed observations requires a brief explanation of the innate and adaptive immune systems as both are operative in the pregnant uterus. Both participate in the immunological reshuffling that takes place in the modified endometrium of pregnancy (i.e., decidua) following implantation, which culminates in a predominance of innate immunity. Furthermore, rather to be in a fighting mode where immune cells are primed for action, as is the case in the nonpregnant uterus and other mucosal sites, leukocytes in the pregnant uterus are in a becalmed state of immune tolerance when they meet the foreign invaders (fetal cells). This chapter presents some of the well-documented mechanisms underlying utero-placental tolerance together with intriguing evidence for proactive support of pregnancy by components of the immune system. Finally, the phenomenon of maternal/fetal chimerism is discussed as are pathological situations in which the delicate immunological balance between the mother and embryo/fetus is disturbed.

Basic elements of innate and adaptive immune responses

The innate immune system

From the time of Metchnikoff working in the late 19th century to the present day, investigators have been intrigued with the migratory leukocytes of the innate immune system. Originating in the bone marrow, these cells either circulate continuously in the blood, ready to respond to chemokines, indicating tissue destruction, or constitutively infiltrate normal tissues and form a first line of defense, lying in wait for microbial or other invaders.

The major leukocyte subtypes in the innate immune system, where cells are designed for immediate action against invading pathogens, are granulocytes (neutrophils, eosinophils, basophils) and mast cells (basophil relatives), antigen-presenting cells (APC; monocytes, macrophages, dendritic cells, B cells), and a special lymphocyte lineage termed natural killer cells (NK cells; Figure 4.1). The adaptive immune system comprised other types of lymphocytes, which are preprogrammed to respond to specific antigens during maturation in the thymus (T cells) and bone marrow (B cells). Their activation most often requires interaction with APC and takes several days to peak.

The Placenta: From Development to Disease, First Edition. Edited by Helen H. Kay, D. Michael Nelson and Yuping Wang.
© 2011 Blackwell Publishing Ltd. Published 2011 by Blackwell Publishing Ltd.

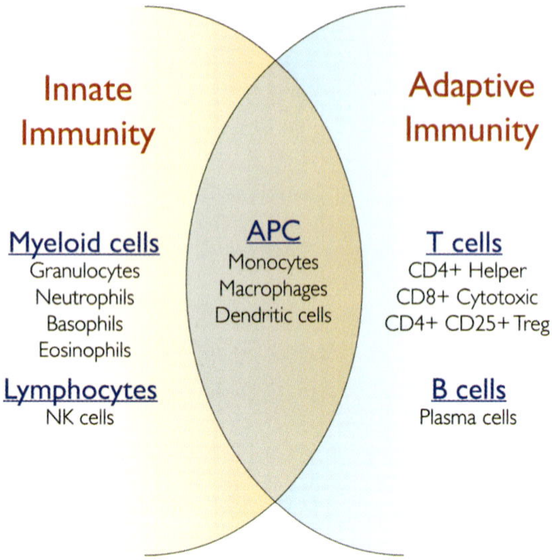

Figure 4.1 Cells of the innate and adaptive immune systems. On the left, cells generating only innate immune responses are shown, and on the right, cells generating only adaptive immune responses are shown. In the center are cells of the innate immune system, antigen presenting cells (APC), which bridge these two types of responses, providing cell surface and secreted molecules that stimulate adaptive immunity.

Although the granulocytes are dedicated to immediate killer action and are comparatively short-lived, both APC and NK cells respond to environmental signals and are capable of long life as inhabitants of organs and tissues. APC and NK cells have receptors that recognize debris, microbes, and their products and respond to stimulatory as well as inhibitory signals. For example, APC recognize products of dying cells and microbes and present these to preprogrammed T lymphocytes to stimulate the adaptive immune response pathway. The NK cells participate in this process by providing interferon-γ (IFNγ), which activates the APC and stimulates production of certain growth and differentiation factors. Both macrophages and NK cells have activating and inhibiting receptors that boost or diminish their ability to produce inflammatory cytokines and other proteins.

The adaptive immune system

APC bridge the gap between the innate and adaptive immune systems (Figure 4.1). These cells include macrophages, dendritic cells, and B cells, all of which continuously sample their local surrounding environment by phagocytosis, endocytosis, and pinocytosis. Proteins internalized by APC are degraded, and products of this degradation combine with major histocompatibility complex (MHC) molecules, after which the complex is transported to and presented at the cell surface. It is only in this context that T lymphocytes, the master regulators of the adaptive immune system, become aware of foreign invaders through the interaction of the MHC/foreign antigen complex with the T cell receptor.

Because the extracellular environment is constantly ingested by APC, many harmless self proteins are placed together with MHC molecules. In the homeostatic condition, the resulting interaction with self-reactive T cells that may have escaped deletion during their development in the thymus leads to tolerance. In contrast, APC are alerted to the presence of pathogens by highly conserved pathogen-associated molecular patterns (PAMPs), such as endotoxin or double-stranded RNA, through constitutively expressed receptors. These PAMPs serve to signal "danger" to APC, alerting them to rapidly upregulate their antigen presenting functions and produce factors such as IFNγ that will ultimately lead to immunity against the foreign invader.

The nature of the ensuing immune response depends on both the features of the antigens and the local tissue milieu. T lymphocytes activated in this way are called "helpers" in that they provide the signals that direct the effector responses. Effector responses can be mediated by cytotoxic T lymphocytes or by B cells, which differentiate into antibody-producing plasma cells. Further, these responses can be pro- or anti-inflammatory. Researchers are beginning to understand the molecular and environmental cues in pregnancy that direct the adaptive arm of the immune system towards its unique, largely anti-inflammatory, and tolerance-inducing features.

Immunological aspects of normal pregnancy

In human pregnancies, the major organs involved in the immunological changes that take place to accommodate the fetus are uterus, particularly the portion lining the lumen called the endometrium of pregnancy or decidua, and the chorioallantoic placenta together with the amniochorion membranes.

The pregnant uterus

Although the nonpregnant uterus contains many cells of the maternal adaptive immune system, the pregnant uterus is flooded with cells of the maternal innate immune system [1]. Generally speaking, all of these cells demonstrate immunosuppressive characteristics. Bulmer et al. have studied the distribution of uterine leukocytes in depth [2]. They show that implantation a phenotypically distinct subset of NK cells ($CD56^+/CD16^-$) predominates. These cells comprise more than 50% of endometrial cells during the first two trimesters. The uterine NK cells are poor killers of foreign cells, whether fetal or tumor.

Macrophages are an abundant (20%) population that is stable throughout pregnancy. Although macrophages in other locations are capable of producing a vast array of inflammatory molecules, macrophages in the pregnant uterus are phenotypically immunosuppressive [3,4]. Also present but in small numbers are two types of powerful cells, dendritic cells, a highly effective APC, and $CD4^+/CD25^+/Foxp3^+$ T lymphocytes with a regulatory function that are known as Treg. The dendritic cells are less than effective participants in uterine development of adaptive immune responses, being negatively affected by one or more placental product [5]. Although few in number, the uterine Treg may function as on–off regulators of many immune responses at the maternal–fetal interface [2].

Research Spotlight

Dendritic cells are normally potent antigen presenters that initiate immune responses. However, in the pregnant uterus, these cells are tuned down by HLA-G proteins emanating from the trophoblast cells of the placenta. This immunoregulatory substance may also be produced by the dendritic cells themselves [5]. This is one of the many ways in which the maternal uterus is programmed for tolerance to the feto–placental allograft.

Clinical Pearl

The innate immune system predominates in the pregnant uterus, likely to secure tolerance to the fetus. Dependence on the innate immune system alone, instead of as a partner with the adaptive immune system, may predispose the pregnant uterus to infections and contribute to mid-trimester fetal loss [6].

The placenta

The placenta and extraplacental membranes are the major guardians of the fetus, shuttling water and nutrients into the fetus, removing wastes, producing hormones such as progesterone that support the condition of pregnancy, and acting as active and passive barriers to maternal anti-fetal immunological activity. The outermost trophoblast cell layers of the villous placenta and the extraplacental chorion membrane, both of which are derived from the trophectoderm of the blastocyst, serve as immunological defenders. They form the maternal face of the fetal tissues and constitute a sac within which fetal embryonic tissues are safely encased. Trophoblast cells are therefore essentially the only fetal cells "seen" by the mother.

Subpopulations of trophoblast cells are readily identifiable by anatomic location as described in the chapter on placental anatomy in this book. Villous cytotrophoblast cells (vCTB) serve as precursors for the syncytiotrophoblast (sTB) and extravillous CTB (xvCTB) (Figure 4.2). The first subset (vCTB) resides subadjacent to the second subset (sTB) and serves as the source of the third subset (xvCTB). Although each subpopulation has specific functions, all, unlike other eukaryotic cells, are negative for the classical HLA class Ia (HLA-A, -B) and HLA class II (HLA-D) antigens that are the main targets of killer cytotoxic lymphocytes.

In terms of active defense, placental trophoblast cells exhibit or secrete molecules such as progesterone, HLA-G and B7H1 that thwart potential maternal anti-fetal immune cell attacks either directly or indirectly [7–9]. HLA-G is believed by some to be a marker for highly viable pre-implantation embryos but this remains controversial. Figure 4.3 shows serial sections of the human placental bed where all subpopulations of trophoblast cells exhibit cytokeratin-7 (Figure 4.3(a)), HLA-G is expressed on invasive xvCTB (Figure 4.3(c)), and B7H1 is prominent on sTB as well as the vCTB and xvCTB cells (Figure 4.3(d)). As for passive defense, the sTB cell layer is syncytialized, forming a seamless, single-cell presence that blocks much of the traffic of migrating maternal leukocytes accustomed to squeezing between cells.

Research Spotlight

Recent studies predict that members of the B7 family of immune costimulatory molecules exhibited by trophoblast cells may divert harmful maternal immune responses [8] and

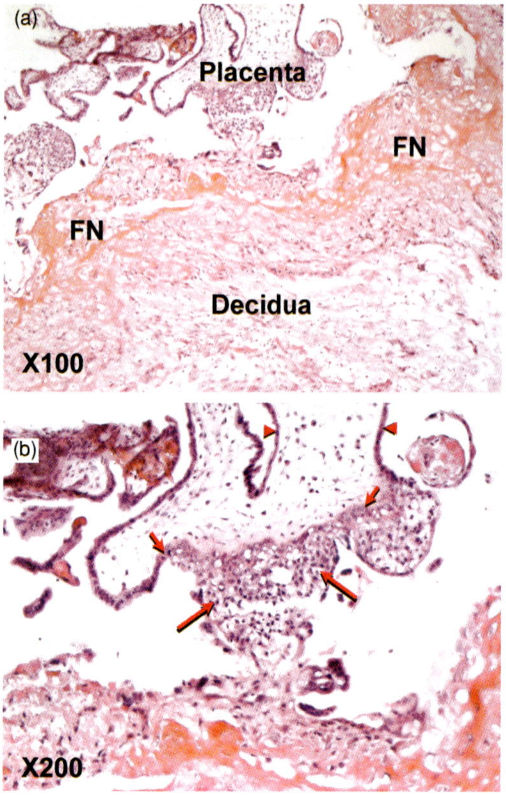

Figure 4.2 The maternal–fetal interface at 13 weeks of normal pregnancy. (a) Hematoxylin and eosin stain, 100× original magnification. (b) Hematoxylin and eosin stain, 200× original magnification. Trophoblast cells (villous cytotrophoblast, short arrows; syncytiotrophoblast, arrowheads; extravillous cytotrophoblast, long arrows) are shown as they are positioned within the villus, emerging from the villus and invading the maternal uterine decidua. Between the placental villi and the decidual is an area of fibrinoid necrosis (FN).

that unusual HLA proteins produced by trophoblast cells inhibit production of cytotoxic molecules by resident and circulating maternal immune cells [7–9].

Clinical Pearl

Human pregnancy is invariably marked by genetic differences between the fetus and mother, but safety of the fetus from immune rejection is provided by multiple, highly diverse systems operating mainly at the maternal–fetal interface. The mechanisms mentioned above and other more subtle processes carry out this mission effectively without compromising systemic immunity or the overall health of the mother.

Beneficial aspects of immunity

Helpful functions of maternal uterine immune cells

Either directly or indirectly, fetal tissues program the maternal uterine cells for tolerance. The predominance of the innate immune system in the pregnant uterus is one example of the successful mammalian accommodations for avoiding destruction of the fetus made by an outraged maternal immune system. The observation that the maternal leukocytes are in suppressive rather than attack mode is consistent with the postulate that resident and incoming leukocytes are environmentally programmed to avoid killing fetal cells.

The products of these same decidual leukocytes may have beneficial effects on pregnancy. Some of these are known; both implantation and parturition are accompanied by reactions in the uterus that include production of inflammatory cytokines such as interleukin-1 (IL-1) and IL-6. Maternal leukocytes are the major contributors of these inflammation-associated cytokines at implantation, as shown in mice, but both maternal and placental macrophages are sources of tumor necrosis factor-α (TNF), a potent inflammatory cytokine, as human pregnancy concludes [10,11]. Possibly, the mild inflammatory process of implantation alerts the mother to the presence of the fetus in early pregnancy, and the major inflammatory process at the end of pregnancy facilitates release of the placenta from the uterus via induction of matrix metalloproteinases.

Other observations made in mice that benefit our understanding of human pregnancy include evidence for production of IFNγ by uterine NK cells, which has many effects that include induction of maternal spiral artery modification [12] and activation of uterine macrophages. Mice with genetic alterations have been useful in these and other experiments by showing that products of the uterine NK cells facilitate placental growth and development.

Helpful functions of fetal cells at the maternal–fetal interface

Considerable hard evidence supports the idea that fetal tissues program the maternal uterine cells for tolerance, either directly or indirectly. Alterations in the uterine leukocyte subpopulations and their products simply do not occur until the blastocyst has entered the uterus and

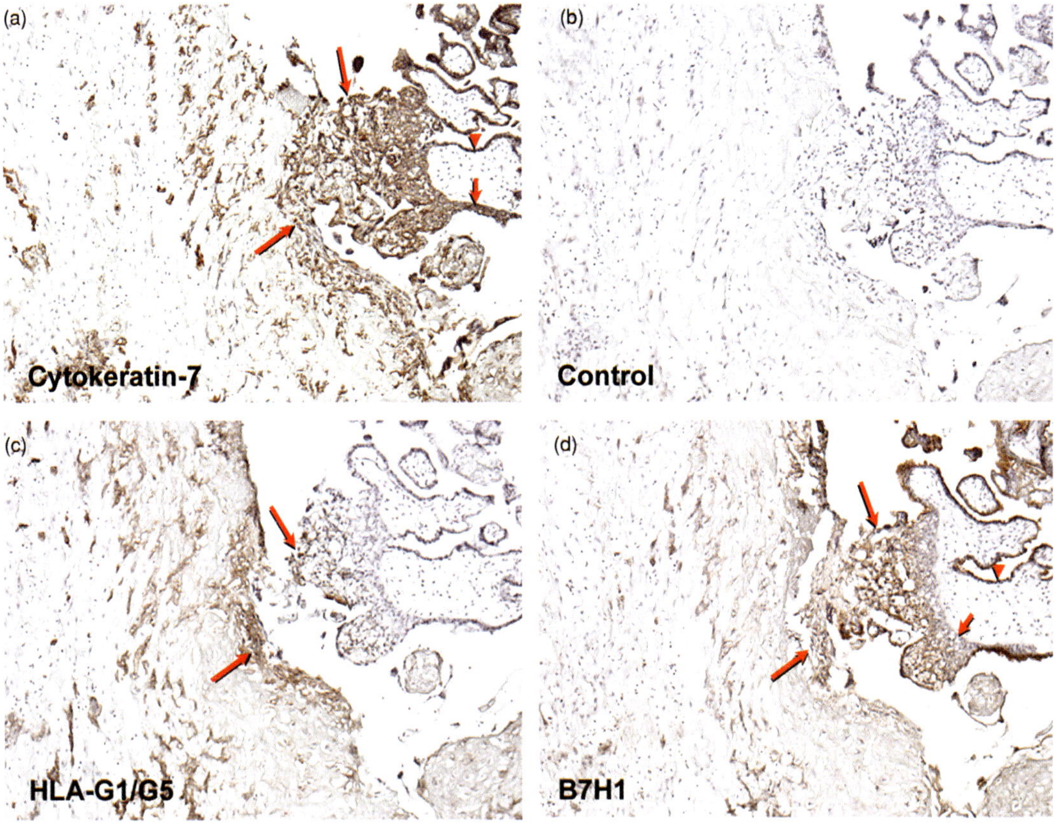

Figure 4.3 Expression of marker proteins by trophoblast subpopulations. Immunohistologic results illustrate (a) expression of a trophoblast-specific marker, cytokeratin-7, by all three subpopulations of trophoblast, (b) lack of staining with an isotype specific control IgG, (c) restricted expression of HLA-G1 and HLA-G5 to extravillous cytotrophoblast cells as identified by MEM-G9 (ExBio), (d) expression of B7H1 on syncytiotrophoblast, villous cytotrophoblast, and migrating extravillous cytotrophoblast cells identified by MIH1, eBiosciences. Original magnification, ×100.

breached the epithelium. Moreover, grafts to the pregnant uterus of experimental animals survive significantly longer than grafts to the nonpregnant uterus [13].

Fetal cells are held responsible for driving the process leading to graft acceptance. Among the products of fetal trophoblast cells that contribute to the highly beneficial new tolerogenic program characterizing pregnancy are progesterone, HLA-G, anti-inflammatory cytokines (transforming growth factor-β, IL-10), and B7 family proteins [7–9]. Within the villous placenta, the stromal cells are home to many members of the TNF superfamily of ligands as well as their receptors [14]. Some of these may contribute to modeling of the placenta as they are responsible for apoptosis. For example, FasL, first identified in the immune system, may be used by migrating xvCTB cells to forcefully invade the maternal spiral arteries.

Other members of these TNF ligand and receptor families that are incapable of stimulating apoptosis may contribute to development and/or differentiation of placental cells [15]. Members of the B7 family have been postulated also to contribute similarly [8]. Finally, HLA-G facilitates uterine and placental vascular development [7–9].

Research Spotlight

Production of an HLA-G-like substance in monkey placentas has a major influence on development of the vasculature of the monkey placenta [16].

Clinical Pearl

Substances such as IL-10, TNF family ligands, and HLA class Ib proteins, all of which were first identified in the immune system, establish tolerance, encourage the development and differentiation of the fetus and membranes, and stimulate modification of the maternal spiral arteries during pregnancy.

Chimerism: Fetal cells in maternal blood and tissue

Active movement of fetal cells into the mother begins in the first trimester in all pregnancies. The pregnant human uterus itself becomes an example of natural chimerism; fetal and maternal cells reside side by side without evidence of immune reaction [3]. As surprising as this intimate juxtapositioning of maternal and fetal cells in the uterus, equally unexpected is the fact that fetal cells traffic into the maternal blood, lodge within maternal organs and, in some women, persist for decades [17]. Several types of cells can inhabit maternal tissues, including fetal hematopoietic cells and trophoblast cells. The astonishing aspect of this is that in some women, these fetal cells persist in spite of multiple genetic disparities that would otherwise be expected to trigger their demise via the maternal immune system. Fetal microchimerism in mothers is most commonly observed in highly vascular organs such as the lung, spleen, liver, and the blood itself. This issue is the subject of another chapter in this book.

Whether these cells participate in the normal function of their resident organ, contribute to local pathogenesis and disease, or assist with tissue repair following pathogenic insult is still a matter of debate. The presence of fetal cells and DNA has been suggested to play a role in the remittance of rheumatoid arthritis during pregnancy, but also may play an adversarial role in the development of autoimmunity. The observation that these cells can take on the properties of surrounding parenchymal cells of a given organ in the absence of tissue pathology also suggests that these cells could mimic the normal properties of the neighboring indigenous cells.

Research Spotlight

Recent research has shown an association between fetal microchimerism and a reduced risk of cancer. These findings raise the exciting possibility that persistence of fetal cells in maternal tissue play a role in immune surveillance for cancer cells.

Clinical Pearl

Highly sensitive mechanisms for detection of fetal cells and DNA in maternal blood are key technical innovations in noninvasive prenatal genetic diagnosis. Fast-moving progress is being made in implementing such technology in the clinic, and uses of this technology include detection of genetic disorders and fetal sex determination.

Interrupted pregnancy

Maternal anti-fetal immunity

At this point in time, the scientific literature does not contain any convincing evidence that mothers ever reject their embryo/fetuses because of differences in maternal and fetal HLA antigens. Activities of the cytotoxic T lymphocytes programmed to kill cells expressing paternal HLA are muted. Yet there is abundant evidence for maternal anti-fetal immunity in the form of antibodies. Stimulation of antibody production may occur at the termination of pregnancy when fetal blood is released into the maternal blood circulation. Fortuitously, the maternal anti-fetal antibodies cause no damage as the placenta has many defense mechanisms that prevent damaging antibodies from reaching the embryo. These include expression of proteins interfering with complement-mediated cell lysis and trapping of antigen–antibody complexes by placental macrophages (Hofbauer cells).

On occasion, the seeding of foreign fetal blood cells into the mother results in anti-fetal erythrocyte, leukocyte, and platelet antibodies. In subsequent pregnancies, high levels of these antibodies may cause damage to the fetus. The best known syndrome, erythroblastosis fetalis, has long been recognized and remedial measures are routinely taken to avoid stimulation by fetal erythrocyte Rh antigens at delivery. Fetal phospholipids may also be targets of maternal antibodies. Anti-phospholipid syndrome remains difficult to diagnose and difficult to treat. Under some, but not all, profiles of this disease, antibodies to specific lipids impede the course of pregnancy. However, despite decades of study, the underlying mechanism(s) for pregnancy failure remain unclear. For a recent review, see Pasquali et al. [18].

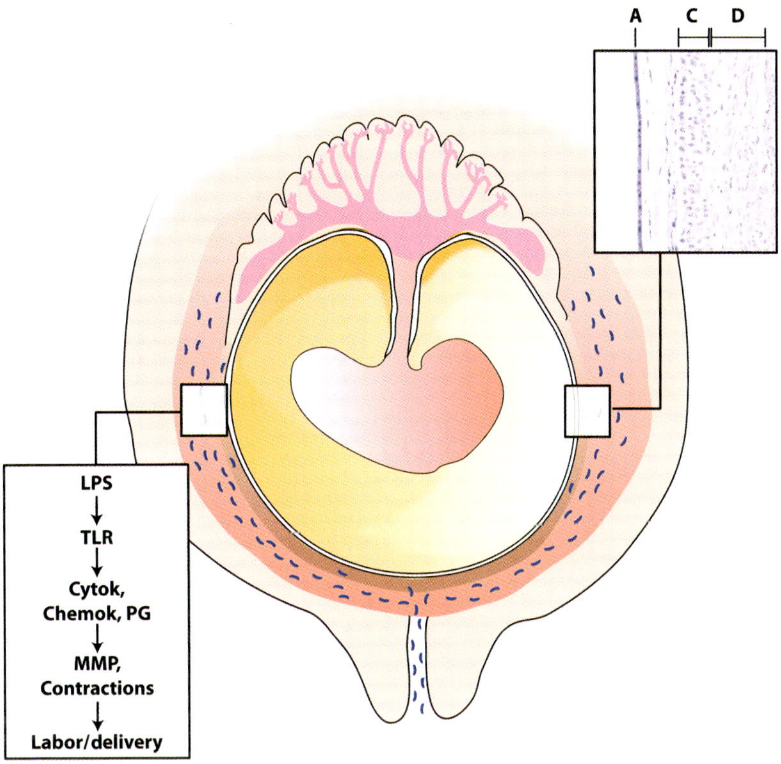

Figure 4.4 Ascending infections of the amniochorion. Pathogenic microorganisms ascending through the female reproductive tract encounter resident maternal APC such as macrophages and dendritic cells in the decidua adjacent to the chorion membrane. These may be stimulated to produce molecules associated with inflammation and pregnancy loss. LPS, lipopolysaccharide from Gram-negative microorganisms; TLR, toll-like receptors for LPS on APC; Cytok, cytokines; Chemok, chemokines; PG, prostaglandins; MMP, matrix metalloproteinases; A, amnion membrane; C, chorion membrane; D, decidua.

Infections

Preterm birth—that which occurs prior to 37 complete weeks of gestation—is the most common cause for perinatal morbidity and mortality. Worldwide, the prevalence of preterm birth ranges from 5% to 25%, being highest in low-income countries. In the United States, recent estimates of preterm birth have approached 13%. Intrauterine infection is thought to account for nearly half of preterm births that occur prior to the 28th week of gestation.

Intrauterine infections precipitating preterm birth may be acquired as a result of ascension of vaginal bacteria (Figure 4.4). Bacterial vaginosis, a marker for pathogenic fastidious bacteria, is associated with a 50% increase in risk of preterm birth; systemic infections are also associated with higher risk for premature birth. Furthermore, the maternal immune response to these infections may vary due to polymorphisms in cytokine genes such as TNF. Gene differences could influence the magnitude of the immune response, and women predisposed to a heightened inflammatory cytokine production may be at elevated risk for premature birth.

The cells responding to infection are likely to derive from maternal immune and decidual cells as well as fetal trophoblast, amnionic epithelial cells, and macrophages. The cytokine response to bacterial product precipitates premature uterine release of prostaglandins and matrix metalloproteases, events that overlap with normal parturition. These effectors lead to cervical remodeling and ripening, as well as weakening of the extraplacental membranes. Furthermore, prostaglandin productions stimulate uterine contractions, and in the absence of effective tocolytic intervention, premature birth ensues.

> **Research Spotlight**
> The molecular events mediating the response to bacterial products are beginning to be understood; the prevention of these responses may prove to be an effective intervention to preterm birth in certain patient cohorts [19].

Other abnormalities of pregnancy

Preeclampsia (PE) is among the common problems that have deleterious effects on the progress of pregnancy. Here, women have dangerous rises in blood pressure and proteinuria. Immune phenomena have been implicated in this condition as certain cytokines such as TNF are elevated. Higher densities of blood-born placental trophoblast cells are observed, which may play a role in the elevations [20], and a lack of $CD4^+Foxp3^+$ Treg cells in PE pregnancy compared to healthy pregnancy have been reported [21]. These results suggest that a delicate balance of regulatory and proinflammatory molecules required for healthy pregnancy is disturbed in PE, with disastrous consequences. The same problems appear when intrauterine growth restriction (IUGR) is associated with PE and are even more dangerous.

> **Research Spotlight**
> Lower levels of $CD4^+Foxp3^+$ Treg cells and higher levels of $CD4^+$IL-17-producing T cells in PE pregnancy compared to healthy pregnancy have been reported, suggesting a role for Treg cells in PE.

> **Clinical Pearl**
> Comparative studies on normal, healthy pregnant women, age-matched nonpregnant women exposed to fetal blood cell antigens or infectious microorganisms, and women with PE demonstrate clearly that excesses of mediators associated with both healthy pregnancy and normal immunity can negatively influence the progress and quality of gestation.

Summary

Attempts to transplant organs and tissues between genetically disparate individuals prompted the discovery of the immunological paradox of pregnancy by Billingham, Brent, and Medawar in 1953. The conundrum of such close apposition of maternal and fetal tissues despite their genetic dissimilarities sparked an intense interest in the immunology of reproduction to elucidate the mechanisms of fetal evasion of the maternal immune system. It is now clear, however, that the maternal immune system is the foe in only rare cases, for example, those eliciting erythroblastosis fetalis or preterm labor and birth. More often the maternal immune system is an ally. The role of the fetus, and more specifically, the trophoblast, as an ambassador to the mother in order to mediate the peaceful transition of her immune system towards acceptance has emerged as a result of intensive research. Furthermore, in several cases, the maternal immune system is commandeered by the state of pregnancy, as in the case of assignment of highly specific functions of maternal immune cells in the remodeling of the maternal–fetal interface towards an acceptable haven in which the fetus can flourish.

Acknowledgements

The authors thank the National Institutes of Health for financial support (PO1 HD049480, Hunt and Petroff; HD24212, Hunt; HD045611, Petroff) and the Kansas Institutional Network for Biomedical Research Excellence (P20 RR016475, J.S. Hunt, P.I.). We thank S. Fernald, U54 HD055763 (J. Tash, P.I.), Center, for Male Contraceptive Research and Drug Development, for assistance with figures.

> **Teaching Points**
> 1 The innate immune system predominates over the adaptive immune system in the pregnant uterus so as to secure tolerance to the fetus. But dependence on the innate immune system alone instead of as a partner to the adaptive immune system may predispose the pregnant uterus to infections, a major cause of fetal loss.
> 2 Human pregnancy is invariably marked by genetic differences between the fetus and mother, but safety of the fetus from immune rejection is provided by multiple, highly diverse systems operating mainly at the maternal–fetal interface. These systems do not markedly compromise systemic immunity or the overall health of the mother.
> 3 Substances first identified in the immune system are useful in the establishment of tolerance, the development and differentiation of the fetus and its accompanying membranes, and the processes by which maternal spiral arteries are modified during pregnancy.

4 Highly sensitive mechanisms for detection of fetal cells and DNA in maternal blood have been established and represent a key technical innovation in noninvasive prenatal genetic diagnosis. Clinical usefulness of these technologies includes detection of genetic disorders and fetal sex determination.

5 Comparative studies on normal, healthy, pregnant women and age-matched women exposed to fetal blood cell antigens or infectious microorganisms as well as women suffering common problems of pregnancy such as PE demonstrate clearly that when in excess, substances associated with normal immunity and healthy pregnancy can impede the progress and quality of gestation.

References

1. Hunt JS and McIntire RH (2006) Inflammatory cells and cytokine production. In: Peebles DM and Myatt L (eds) *Inflammation and Pregnancy*. Abington, United Kingdom: Informa Healthcare;pp. 1–12.
2. Bulmer JH, Williams PJ, and Lash GE (2010) Immune cells in the placental bed. *International Journal of Developmental Biology* 54: 281–94. PMID: 19876837.
3. Hunt JS and Petroff MG (2008) Molecular immunology of the maternal–fetal interface. In: Aplin JD, Fazleabas AT, Glasser SR, and Giudice LC (eds) *The Endometrium*. 2nd edn. New York, NY: Informa Healthcare; pp. 524–45.
4. Nagamatsu T and Schust DJ (2010) The immunomodulatory roles of macrophages at the maternal–fetal interface. *Reproductive Sciences* 17: 209–18.
5. Bahri R, Naji A, Menier C et al. (2009) Dendritic cells secrete the immunosuppressive HLA-G molecule upon CTLA4-Ig treatment: Implication in human renal transplant acceptance. *The Journal of Immunology* 183: 7054–62. PMID: 19915057.
6. Moffett A and Loke YW (2006) Immunology of placentation in eutherian mammals. *Nature Reviews Immunology* 6: 584–94. PMID: 16868549.
7. Hunt JS, McIntire RH, and Petroff MG (2006) Immunobiology of human pregnancy. In: Neill JD (ed.) *Knobil and Neill's Physiology of Reproduction*. Vol. 2, 3rd edn. St. Louis, MO: Elsevier/Academic Press; pp. 2759–85.
8. Petroff MG and Perchellet AL (2010) Review: B7 family molecules as regulators of the maternal immune system in pregnancy. *American Journal of Reproductive Immunology*, 63: 506–19.
9. Hunt JS (2006) Stranger in a strange land. *Immunological Reviews* 213: 36–47. PMID: 16972895.
10. McMaster MT, Dey SK, and Andrews GK (1993) Association of monocytes and neutrophils with early events of blastocyst implantation in mice. *Journal of Reproduction and Fertility* 99: 561–9. PMID: 8107041.
11. Chen HL, Yang YP, Hu XL et al. (1991) Tumor necrosis factor alpha mRNA and protein are present in human placental and uterine cells at early and late stages of gestation. *American Journal of Pathology* 139: 327–35. PMID: 1867321.
12. Ashkar AA, Di Santo JP, and Croy BA (2000) Interferon gamma contributes to initiation of uterine vascular modification, decidual integrity, and uterine natural killer cell maturation during normal murine pregnancy. *The Journal of Experimental Medicine* 192: 259–70. PMID: 10899912.
13. Beer AE and Billingham RE (1971) Immunobiology of mammalian reproduction. *Advanced Immunology* 14: 1084. PMID: 4927660.
14. Phillips TA, Ni J, and Hunt JS (2001) Death-inducing tumour necrosis factor (TNF) superfamily ligands and receptors are transcribed in human placentae, cytotrophoblasts, placental macrophages and placental cell lines. *Placenta* 22: 663–72. PMID: 11597186.
15. Hunt JS, Pace JL, and Gill RM (2010) Immunoregulatory molecules in human placentas: Potential for diverse roles in pregnancy. *International Journal of Developmental Biology* 54: 457–67. PMID: 19757386.
16. Bondarenko GI, Burleigh DW, Durning M et al. (2007) Passive immunization against the MHC class I molecule Mamu-AG disrupts rhesus placental development and endometrial responses. *Journal of Immunology* 179: 8042–50. PMID: 18056344.
17. Khosrotehrani K and Bianchi DW (2005) Multi lineage potential of fetal cells in maternal tissue: A legacy in reverse. *Journal of Cell Science* 118: 1559–63. PMID: 15811948.
18. Pasquali JL, Poindron V, Korganow AS et al. (2008) The antiphospholipid syndrome. *Best Practice and Research Clinical Rheumatology* 22: 831–45. PMID: 19028366.
19. Gravett MG, Rubens CE, Nunes TM, and GAPPS Review Group (2010) Global report on preterm birth and stillbirth: Discovery science. *BMC Pregnancy and Childbirth* 10(Suppl 1): S2. DOI: 10.1186/1471-2393-10-S1-S2.
20. Redman CW and Sargent IL (2008) Circulating microparticles in normal pregnancy and pre-eclampsia. *Placenta* 29(Suppl A): S73–77. PMID: 18192006.
21. Santner-Nanan B, Peek MJ, Khanam R et al. (2009) Systemic increase in the ratio between Foxp3^{+} and IL-17-producing CD4^{+} T cells in healthy pregnancy but not in pre-eclampsia. *Journal of Immunology* 183: 7023–30. PMID: 19915051.

5

CHAPTER 5
Vascular Development in the Placenta

Berthold Huppertz
Institute of Cell Biology, Histology and Embryology, Medical University of Graz, Graz, Austria

Introduction

Development of the placental vasculature is key for normal embryogenesis and growth of the fetus in utero. Maternal oxygen and nutrients that reach the placenta are transported to the fetus through the umbilical cord that connects to a vascular arcade within the villous tree. Thus, effective and appropriately regulated growth and branching of the placental vasculature is required for adequate growth of the fetus. This vascularization throughout pregnancy controls the shape of the placental villous trees and optimizes maternal–fetal transfer.

Vasculogenesis and angiogenesis

Vessel development in an avascular tissue is called vasculogenesis, which is defined as formation of new blood vessels from differentiation of pluripotent mesenchymal progenitor cells. Hence, vasculogenesis takes place in the absence of pre-existing vessels. In the human placenta, there is no sprouting of embryonic vessels through the umbilical cord into the placental villi. Instead, as blood vessels form by vasculogenesis within the connective tissues of the placenta, a new process called angiogenesis connects preformed vessels with each other. Different modes in growth of vessels are known and are described below.

Vasculogenesis early in placental development

The very earliest development of the placenta starts at the time of implantation when the mononucleated trophoblasts of the blastocyst differentiate. The trophoblasts, in direct contact with the inner cell mass and the uterine epithelium, fuse with each other to generate the first syncytiotrophoblast. This multinucleated structure penetrates the uterine epithelium to allow invasion of the early embryo into the decidual stroma of the uterus.

Over the following days, the syncytiotrophoblast, cytotrophoblasts, and extra-embryonic mesenchyme grow and differentiate to establish the first organ of the embryo, the placenta. The first 3 weeks of development are characterized by the absence of blood or endothelial cells within the placenta. The primary villi are mere trophoblastic structures, while secondary villi contain a mesenchymal core surrounded by villous trophoblast.

Placental vasculogenesis starts in the cores of secondary villi at the four somite embryo stage, at day 21 post conception (pc) [1]. Hemangiogenic progenitor cells differentiate within the mesenchymal core of placental villi, prior to the formation of the first vessels. Such progenitor cells are derived from mesenchymal cells rather than embryonic blood cells. Placental macrophages (Hofbauer cells) also derive from progenitor cells within the villous core prior to the establishment of a vascular connection between placenta and embryo.

The Placenta: From Development to Disease, First Edition. Edited by Helen H. Kay, D. Michael Nelson and Yuping Wang.
© 2011 Blackwell Publishing Ltd. Published 2011 by Blackwell Publishing Ltd.

With the onset of vasculogenesis, new cell types differentiate within the mesenchymal stroma of placental villi, now referred to as tertiary villi. Recruitment of pluripotent mesenchymal cells leads to the formation of hemangiogenic stem cells, which in turn differentiate into two different cell populations:

1 Hematopoietic cells are the precursors of blood cells, which are formed within the placenta independent of embryonic blood cells—at least during very early stages of human development.

2 Angioblastic cells further differentiate into endothelial precursor cells and subsequently form the first vessels.

Research Spotlight

In the placenta, both hematopoietic cells and angioblastic cells are derived from hemangiogenic stem cells, which are differentiated from villous core mesenchymal stem cells.

Angiogenesis in the placenta

At this stage of development, vasculogenesis evolves into angiogenesis. From the newly formed vessels, additional vessels emanate to create a vascular network. This network is achieved by multiple aspects of vessel growth (Figure 5.1):

1 Nonbranching angiogenesis is growth by extension in length of an existing vessel.

a *Elongation* (Figure 5.1(a)) is longitudinal growth of a vessel at one end. The vessel otherwise remains unaltered except at the end that accrues new cells to extend and vascularize new tissues. This type of angiogenesis results in extended capillaries.

b *Intercalation* (Figure 5.1(b)) is the longitudinal growth of a vessel within an existing vessel excluding the ends. This type of longitudinal growth will expand an existing network of vessels and will increase the distance between connecting points and branches of vessels. This type of angiogenesis results in capillary loops.

2 Branching angiogenesis. This type of vessel growth leads to the development of vascular branches and a ramified appearance.

a *Sprouting* (Figure 5.1(c)) occurs when endothelial cells from existing vessels degrade their basement membrane and migrate into the surrounding connective tissue. Proliferation yields a new vessel to form a new branch. This type of angiogenesis results in multiple capillaries.

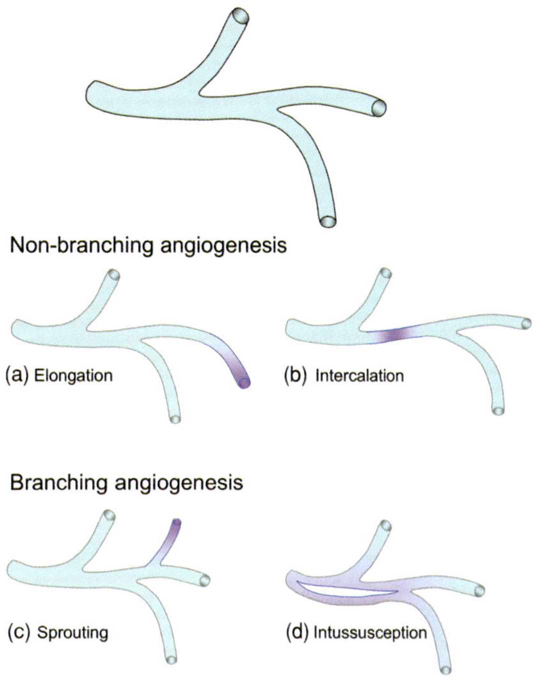

Figure 5.1 Modes of angiogenesis. Angiogenesis is the development of new vessels from already existing vessels. The newly formed endothelial parts of the vessels are highlighted in pink. Nonbranching angiogenesis leads to vessel growth in length without the formation of branches. (a) Elongation is characterized by longitudinal growth of a vessel at one end. (b) Intercalation is characterized by longitudinal growth of a vessel somewhere within the vessel rather than at its end. Branching angiogenesis leads to the formation of new branches from already existing vessels. (c) Sprouting is characterized by outgrowth of endothelial cells from a vessel to form a new branch. (d) Intussusception is characterized by the formation of a dividing new wall in the center of an existing vessel. By this means two new parallel vessels are formed and are separated by a new endothelial wall.

b *Intussusception* (Figure 5.1(d)) occurs when endothelial cells grow into the lumen of an existing vessel to generate a branch from the center. This process allows one vessel to branch into two from an existing vascular wall. This type of angiogenesis results in parallel capillaries.

New vessels that form from outgrowing endothelial cells require stabilization and modulation into arteries or veins. This is achieved by recruitment of perivascular cells such as pericytes and smooth muscle cells. How the new vessel matures depends on where the vessel was formed and the influence of the intravillous microenvironment.

> **Research Spotlight**
>
> Changes in the fetoplacental blood flow impact on the ratio of branching and nonbranching angiogenesis within the placenta.

Growth factors regulate vasculogenesis and angiogenesis

While vasculogenesis occurs during days 21–32 pc, angiogenesis continues from day 32 pc until delivery [1]. The growth factors below are involved with both processes.

1 Vascular endothelial growth factor (VEGF)
2 Placental growth factor (PlGF)
3 Fibroblast growth factor (acidic and basic FGF, aFGF, and bFGF)
4 Epidermal growth factor (EGF)
5 Angiopoietin (Ang-1 and Ang-2).

Vasculogenesis occurs in the cores of secondary villi in an environment where undifferentiated mesenchymal cells are surrounded by villous cytotrophoblasts and syncytiotrophoblast. The villous trophoblast plays a major role in the induction of this process within the villous core by secretion of the growth factors VEGF, PlGF, and bFGF. These proteins not only induce differentiation of hematopoietic and angioblastic cells but also yield the first placentally derived macrophages. These so-called Hofbauer cells are placenta-specific macrophages that can be found in each villus throughout pregnancy. As soon as the fetoplacental circulation is established, fetal bone marrow-derived monocytes enter the placental stroma to become local macrophages and thus add to the population of Hofbauer cells. The population of placental macrophages thereby becomes a heterogeneous mixture of placental-derived and systemic-derived cells. Importantly, Hofbauer cells secrete several angiogenic growth factors, most notably VEGF. Smooth muscle cells that have differentiated to form the walls of large vessels also secrete VEGF, FGF, and angiopoietin. This switch in angiogenic control from trophoblasts to stromal cells is an important transition in pregnancy, which allows the microenvironment to precisely control vascularization in the stromal core of placental villi.

Capillary growth throughout pregnancy

After the vascular network develops in early pregnancy, capillary growth continues until delivery, but formation of vascular beds changes as the placenta grows and develops. Total capillary length in a given placenta changes little during the first half of pregnancy [2]. After midgestation, there is an exponential growth in length of vessels that correlates well with the appearance of terminal villi and that continues until delivery. Similarly, volume growth of placental vessels shows an exponential rise after midgestation [2]. There is a 14-fold increase in total villous volume between 10 and 40 weeks of gestation. Within this expansion, there is also a 14-fold expansion of trophoblast volume, but only a tenfold increase in villous stroma. Remarkably, the volume of placental vessels increases the most, expanding 56-fold. Volumes increase in all compartments of villi over gestation (Figure 5.2 (a)), but the relative growth of the compartments differ. For example, the relative volume of the villous trophoblast does not change between 10 and 40 weeks of gestation, while the relative volume of the stroma decreases during pregnancy from 65% at 10–13 weeks to 47% at 37–40 weeks. In contrast, the relative volume of the placental vessels continuously increases from 6% at 10–13 weeks to 25% at 37–40 weeks (Figure 5.2 (b)). This increase in placental vessel volume clearly illustrates the adaptation of the placenta to the needs of the growing fetus.

Oxygen influences capillary growth

The early development of the human placenta takes place in a low oxygen environment. The placenta is perfused with maternal plasma, not maternal blood, during the first trimester. Consequently, the intraplacental partial oxygen pressure (pO_2) is about 15 mm Hg until 10–12 weeks of gestation [3] when the clusters of extravillous trophoblasts plugging the maternal spiral arteries resolve to allow the onset of placental perfusion with maternal blood [2].

There is no direct comparison between intraplacental oxygen concentrations and vessel evolution between weeks 5 and 15 in literature. Nonetheless, very early vascular development likely depends on the intraplacental oxygen tension. Higher than normal oxygen levels associate with premature perfusion of the placental villi as viewed with ultrasound, and this abnormal perfusion correlates with a marked reduction in capillary growth to the point of avascularity in some villi. In contrast, chronic hypoxemia due to maternal anemia shows increased villous capillary growth even in the first trimester of pregnancy.

There is little information about in vivo oxygen values in the placenta in the second and third trimesters. The

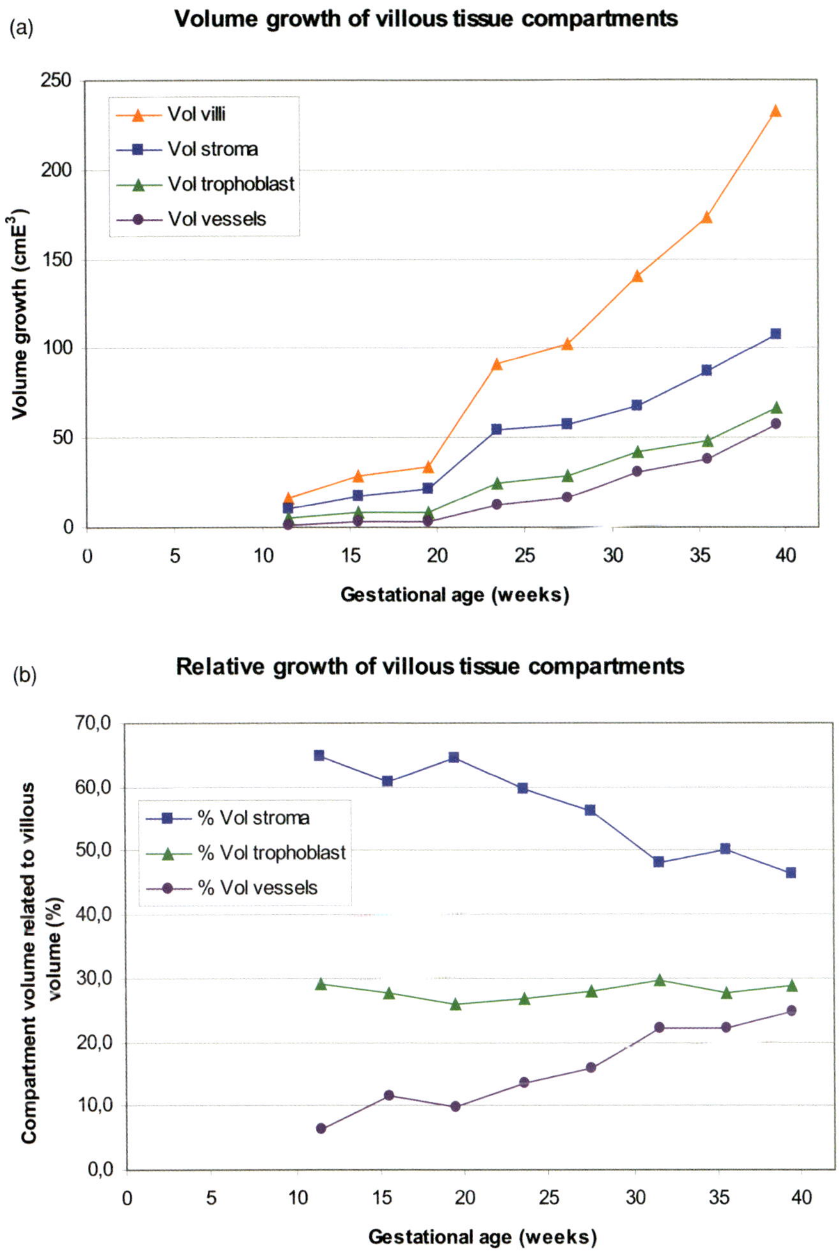

Figure 5.2 Volume growth of placental villous tissue compartments. (a) The growth in volume is shown for the three villous tissue compartments, villous trophoblast, stroma, and vessels. The volumes of all compartments increase from 10 to 40 weeks of gestation and thus the total volume of villi increases as well. (Data are plotted from values given in Mayhew TM (2002) Fetoplacental angiogenesis during gestation is biphasic, longitudinal and occurs by proliferation and remodelling of vascular endothelial cells. *Placenta* 23: 742–50.) (b) Growth of villous tissue compartments is related to total villous volume. The three tissue compartments show complementary relative growth during gestation. (Data are calculated and plotted from values given in Mayhew TM (2002) Fetoplacental angiogenesis during gestation is biphasic, longitudinal and occurs by proliferation and remodelling of vascular endothelial cells. *Placenta* 23: 742–50.)

available data include measurements of pO_2 in retroplacental uterine veins, which is a surrogate measurement for placental oxygen concentrations. The second half of gestation is characterized by the expansion and growth of the whole placenta, laterally with expanding villous trees arranged as placentomes. Maternal spiral arteries are recruited, and their numbers are directly related to the frequency of placentomes. Oxygen content in the intervillous compartment also fluctuates, with the highest oxygen levels in the maternal blood of the intervillous space at outlets of the spiral arteries. The blood disperses through the intervillous space and follows the clefts and channels of the densely packed villous trees. Maternal blood oxygen levels are lowest where this blood is drained from the intervillous space at the uteroplacental veins. Vessel growth within the placental villi continually evolves in response to growth factors that adapt to the local oxygen concentrations, and the villous morphology reflects all of these parameters.

Research Spotlight

The morphology and branching pattern of placental villi is a direct consequence of growth of placental vessels, i.e., of branching and nonbranching angiogenesis.

Heterogeneity of placental endothelial cells

The placental endothelium is derived from the villous stroma, which in turn is derived from the extraembryonic mesoderm. Similar to the systemic vascular endothelium, the placental endothelium is a highly dynamic system involved in angiogenesis, cell trafficking, nutrient transport, and maintenance of vascular tone. Endothelial cells are no longer considered a passive conduit for blood but instead are now accepted to be a cell population with a high level of heterogeneity and plasticity [4]. The plasticity of placental endothelial cells depends on their genotype and whether they are from an arterial or venous bed. Cells differ in their genotypic, phenotypic, morphologic, and functional characteristics. Isolated placental arterial endothelial cells express genes such as *hey-2*, *connexin 40*, and *depp*. Moreover, VEGF stimulates proliferation only in arterial endothelial cells, while PlGF is only effective on venous endothelial cells [5] where cells express development-associated genes such as *gremlin*, *mesenchyme homeobox 2*, and *stem cell protein DSC54*.

Research Spotlight

Recent research highlights differences not only in endothelial cells of arteries and veins but also between endothelial cells from placentas of males versus females due to the influence of sex hormones [6].

Blood flow changes and oxygen delivery to the fetus

The placenta is a unique human organ where the oxygen content is balanced by two independent vascular systems, the maternal and fetal circulations. Maternal blood supplies the organ with oxygen, while fetal blood extracts oxygen from the placenta and supplies the fetus with this essential gas. Variations in one or both vascular systems will result in alterations to the delicate balance of placental oxygen supply and demand [7].

Intraplacental hypoxia

Maternal conditions such as chronic anemia or hypobaric hypoxia (high altitude) result in a reduced oxygen supply to the placenta, so-called preplacental hypoxia [8]. The placental response to chronic hypoxia/hypoxemia is an increase in endothelial proliferation, which in turn leads to an increased number of both capillary loops and terminal villi. The enhanced villous branching increases villous surface area to maximize transfer of oxygen and nutrients from the maternal to the fetal circulation.

In nonplacental tissues, low oxygen levels induce new formation of capillaries, which increases the exchange area. Concomitantly, higher numbers of capillaries also reduce vascular resistance as the new capillaries are positioned in parallel with the already existing capillaries. The ensuing drop in perfusion pressure induces dilation of precapillary arterioles to preserve perfusion pressure. The vasculature in the placenta does not possess proximal regulatory arterioles or precapillary sphincters. Moreover, the placental vasculature does not form new capillaries in parallel but instead forms capillary loops through intercalation. Such an expansion of capillary loops that are not in parallel will increase, rather than decrease, vascular resistance, and this may have a negative impact on the feto–placental blood flow.

Fetal growth restriction, preeclampsia, or both are described with shallow trophoblast invasion predisposing to an impaired blood supply from the mother to the placenta. This hypothesis is commonly cited, but the presence of hypoxia in the placenta is quite controversial and has never been proven. Interestingly, this hypothesis has recently been challenged [9]. Impaired trophoblast invasion into spiral arteries affects the diameter of the vessels, making them a smaller diameter than expected. However, this does not necessarily affect the blood volume transported through these vessels. Instead, the maternal blood will enter the intervillous space at higher velocity, and this may have a deleterious effect on the fragile villous trees. At the same time, the oxygen concentration delivered over a fixed time period should be similar in placentas with or without abnormal spiral artery invasion [10].

Research Spotlight

Recent data suggest that preeclampsia may not be associated with placental hypoxia due to a failure of trophoblast invasion into the spiral arteries [9]. Placental injury in fetal growth restriction and preeclampsia may instead result from effects of high flow through narrow arteriole vessels [10].

Intraplacental hyperoxia

The intraplacental oxygen concentration is maintained by the inflow via maternal circulation and outflow via the fetal circulation from the placenta. There are pregnancies with increased vascular resistance in the umbilical–placental circulation, with or without fetal circulatory insufficiency, where the transfer of oxygen from the placenta to the fetus is impaired. This scenario may yield relative intraplacental hyperoxia, as maternal oxygen input remains normal, yet exit from the fetoplacental circulation is impaired. Concomitantly, there would be impaired transfer of oxygen to the fetus, described as post-placental fetal hypoxia [8], to paradoxically create placental hyperoxia with fetal hypoxia. Pregnancies with fetal growth restriction and absent or reversed end diastolic flow velocities in the umbilical arteries commonly show hypoxia in the fetus. Interestingly, the placental vasculature adapts to the hyperoxia situation within the placenta by reducing proliferation of endothelial cells, resulting in fewer capillary loops and thus fewer terminal villi. This results in a villous histopathology with long, slender mature intermediate villi, with only a few terminal branches, and the reduced number of terminal villi occupy an intervillous space that contributes a higher volume per unit mass of villi.

Clinical Pearl

In fetal growth restriction, a hypoxic fetus may well be associated with a hyperoxic placenta.

Teaching points

1 Vasculogenesis and angiogenesis are two sequentially occurring processes for the development of a vascular system in the placenta.
2 VEGF, FGF, and PlGF play major roles in placental vasculogenesis and angiogenesis.
3 Placental endothelial cells display major differences in their genotypic and phenotypic characteristics depending on whether they are located in arteries or veins.
4 Oxygen is a major modulator of placental endothelial growth, and a low oxygen environment is crucial for the onset of vasculogenesis early in placental development.
5 Since the placenta is perfused by two independent circulatory systems (maternal and fetal), intraplacental oxygen levels may vary from hypoxia to normoxia and even to hyperoxia depending on the degree of pathology.

References

1. Kaufmann P, Mayhew TM, and Charnock-Jones DS (2004) Aspects of human fetoplacental vasculogenesis and angiogenesis. II. Changes during normal pregnancy. *Placenta* 25: 114–26.
2. Mayhew TM (2002) Fetoplacental angiogenesis during gestation is biphasic, longitudinal and occurs by proliferation and remodelling of vascular endothelial cells. *Placenta* 23: 742–50.
3. Jauniaux E, Watson AL, Hempstock J et al. (2000) Onset of maternal arterial blood flow and placental oxidative stress. A possible factor in human early pregnancy failure. *American Journal of Pathology* 157: 2111–22.
4. dela Paz NG and D'Amore PA (2009) Arterial versus venous endothelial cells. *Cell and Tissue Research* 335: 5–16.

5. Lang I, Schweizer A, Hiden U et al. (2008) Human fetal placental endothelial cells have a mature arterial and a juvenile venous phenotype with adipogenic and osteogenic differentiation potential. *Differentiation* 76: 1031–43.
6. Miller VM (1999) Gender and vascular reactivity. *Lupus* 8: 409–15.
7. Huppertz B and Peeters LL (2005) Vascular biology in implantation and placentation. *Angiogenesis* 8: 157–67.
8. Kingdom JC and Kaufmann P (1997) Oxygen and placental villous development: Origins of fetal hypoxia. *Placenta* 18: 613–21.
9. Huppertz B (2008) Placental origins of pre-eclampsia: Challenging the current hypothesis. *Hypertension* 51: 970–5.
10. Burton GJ, Woods AW, Jauniaux E et al. (2009) Rheological and physiological consequences of conversion of the maternal spiral arteries for uteroplacental blood flow during human pregnancy. *Placenta* 30: 473–82.

6

CHAPTER 6

Hypoxia and the Placenta

Stacy Zamudio

Division of Maternal-Fetal Medicine and Surgery, Department of Obstetrics and Gynecology, Hackensack, NJ, USA

Introduction: Definitions and principles

Basic physiological principles must be reviewed and some definitions clarified to discuss hypoxia within the context of the placenta. Transport of oxygen from ambient air to tissue is via diffusion. Oxygen and all other gases flow from a region of higher partial pressure (P) to one of lower pressure. Oxygen diffuses faster when there is a large pressure difference between the high and low oxygen regions and when there is a thinner tissue barrier. The trophoblast layer on placental villi thins with advancing gestation, which yields enhanced oxygen transfer. A core principle is that oxygen diffuses and reacts according to its partial pressure, and not due to concentration. Oxygen pressure does not equal oxygen content, consumption, or extraction.

The partial pressure of a gas is the pressure that it would exert independently if the gas alone occupies a particular volume. Oxygen comprises 21% of our atmosphere, and barometric pressure at sea level is 760 mm Hg. The partial pressure or oxygen tension (PO_2) at sea level is 160 mm Hg (0.21×760 mm Hg). Ascent to 10,000 feet (3040 m) yields a partial pressure of ~109 mm Hg because barometric pressure is ~520 mm Hg. Clearly, the gradient for oxygen delivery from air to cells is reduced at higher altitudes.

Knowledge of PO_2 is not as useful in clinical circumstances as oxygen content. The latter integrates O_2 tension and hemoglobin characteristics to determine whether a patient's blood is adequately oxygenated for tissue delivery. Arterial oxygen content (CaO_2) is calculated as the amount of oxygen carried within a gram of hemoglobin (carrying capacity = 1.36–1.39 mL/g) multiplied by hemoglobin concentration (g/dL) multiplied by measured O_2 saturation (percent). Arterial oxygen saturation (SaO_2) is the percent of red blood cells carrying oxygen (oxyhemoglobin) and is directly correlated with PO_2. Some investigators also add the quantity of oxygen dissolved in the plasma (0.003 mL O_2/dL $\times$ measured PO_2), but in practice, this amount is negligible and can be ignored. A normal adult CaO_2 at sea level is ~18.5 mL per L (1.36 mL/g $\times$ 14.0 g/dL hgb $\times$ 0.97 SaO_2). Ascent to 10,000 ft would yield a CaO_2 of ~16.9 mL/L, since SaO_2 at this altitude is ~89%. The important principle from the above is that increases or decreases in oxygen concentration do not change the pressure gradient. The concentration is by and large independent of the PO_2 and more dependent on hemoglobin concentration and O_2 saturation.

Oxygen consumption by an organ or tissue is calculated using content, not PO_2. For example, fetal O_2 consumption, also called uptake, is calculated as

[(Δ CaO_2 umbilical vein to umbilical artery) $\times$ umbilical vein blood flow]

We were the first to show that term human fetal oxygen consumption is ~6 mL/min/kg fetal weight. The relevant variables for this calculation were

[(103 mL/L umbilical vein CaO_2 − 39 mL/L umbilical artery CaO_2) $\times$ 93 mL/min/kg blood flow]/1000 = 5.95 mL/min/kg [1].

A final principle is that O_2 extraction is the percentage of oxygen delivered that is removed across the circulation

The Placenta: From Development to Disease, First Edition. Edited by Helen H. Kay, D. Michael Nelson and Yuping Wang.
© 2011 Blackwell Publishing Ltd. Published 2011 by Blackwell Publishing Ltd.

of interest. Extraction may not necessarily equate to consumption if there are other sources of oxygen delivery. In the example above, fetal oxygen extraction is 62% (103 − 39/103) and is equivalent to consumption since the fetus receives oxygen only through the umbilical cord blood vessels. The first fetal defense against hypoxia is to increase extraction, which can reach >90% [1].

Placental hypoxia

Hypoxia is defined as *an inadequate oxygen supply to the cells and tissues of the body*, but what constitutes inadequacy and the means by which oxygen delivery fails to meet demand varies. Hypoxia is caused by anemia (low CaO_2) or excess carboxyhemoglobin (carbon monoxide binding of red blood cells to reduce SaO_2), or by inadequate blood flow, due to infarct or other forms of occlusion. Hypoxemia, defined as *lowered partial pressure of oxygen in the blood* can also cause hypoxia. Hypoxemia is caused by hypoventilation, e.g., from an obstructed airway or depressed respiratory drive, impaired diffusion (commonly due to ventilation–perfusion mismatching), shunting of blood to bypass a site of exchange, or low inspired oxygen, e.g., high altitude or breathing gas mixtures with less than 21% oxygen. The definition of hypoxemia excludes anemia or other primary hemoglobin deficiencies because they do not influence the PO_2 in blood.

To determine what constitutes placental hypoxia, we need to know the normal levels of oxygen. PO_2 is obtained by blood–gas analysis. Arterial blood must be collected anaerobically into heparinized syringes and ideally introduced into the port of an oxygen analyzer immediately. The blood is passed over an oxygen electrode, generally a Clark-type polarographic sensor that measures the pressure of the dissolved oxygen electrochemically.

Research Spotlight

A new generation of techniques relying on oxygen-dependent quenching of phosphorescent fluorophores is used to measure not only PO_2 but also the oxygen dependence of respiration in cells and mitochondria.

Adult arterial PO_2 is 80–100 mm Hg, at which SaO_2 is ≥95%. Clinically, hypoxemia is suspected where hemoglobin saturation falls below 90%, equivalent to ~60 mm Hg PaO_2. The blood leaving systemic capillaries has a PO_2 of 40. Hence, the gradient of oxygen from arteries to veins is ~60 mm Hg. Intracellular PO_2 is tenfold less than capillary PO_2 whilst O_2 tension in the mitochondria, the ultimate destination of oxygen, ranges from <1 mmHg to several mm Hg, depending on measurement technique and diffusion distance. Both intracellular and mitochondrial PO_2 fall in direct proportion to reductions in capillary PO_2.

Clinical Pearl

Near infrared spectroscopy (NIRS) noninvasively measures oxygenation. Transmission and absorption of NIR light contains information about hemoglobin and myoglobin concentration changes that are reflective of blood volume and flow. NIRS has gained favor for measurement of cerebral blood flow and oxygenation, especially in neonates. A similar technique is widely used for measurement of SaO_2. A monitor shines light through the fingernail bed or earlobe and measures SaO_2 based on the spectrophotometric characteristics of the hemoglobin.

Placental PO_2 not only depends on maternal oxygen delivery, but is also influenced by fetal arterial blood returning to the placenta for reoxygenation. Umbilical venous PO_2 is ~30 mm Hg (range 14–42 mm Hg) while fetal arterial blood is ~17 mm Hg (range 5–27 mm Hg) [2]. The average PO_2 gradient within the fetus is thus about 13 mm Hg, whilst the placental to fetal gradient will vary according to the changing oxygen pressure within the intervillous space and the fetoplacental circulation (see Figure 6.2).

Uterine arteries supply 83% of blood flow to the placenta, and the ovarian arteries supply the remainder. Both circulations have PO_2s consistent with the remainder of the arterial circulation at 80–100 mm Hg. In the few studies where PO_2 of the uterine veins draining the placental circulation was measured, values did not differ from the 40 mm Hg reported for venous blood elsewhere. The most reliable human data derive from blood–gas analyses after in vivo sampling of fetal cord blood (cordocentesis) and from oxygen probes used in situ for in vivo measurements of intervillous PO_2 [3]. These data are crucial to research on placental hypoxia, as the findings have refined the methods used to design experiments.

Research Spotlight

Experimental cell culture conditions should attempt to mimic the in vivo situation. O_2 tensions for the placenta are considerably less than 21% O_2, the room air condition used in most studies. Average O_2 tensions are 2.6% (20 mm Hg) in the first trimester, 7.9% (60 mm Hg) in the second trimester, and 5.3% (40 mm Hg) in the late third trimester.

Figure 6.1 summarizes the above literature. PO_2 is much lower in the first trimester than was previously thought. The low PO_2 is adequate for fetal organogenesis and is maintained by trophoblast plugs at the opening of the maternal spiral arteries that lead into the intervillous space. A rise in intervillous PO_2 too early in gestation is associated with pregnancy loss [3]. Loss of the trophoblastic plugs leads to a steep rise in oxygenation at the end of the first trimester that remains relatively constant in the early second trimester. The gradual fall in intervillous PO_2 in the late second and third trimesters has been attributed to increased O_2 extraction by the growing fetus, but the degree of change is questionable, as in vivo measurements at these later stages of pregnancy are limited.

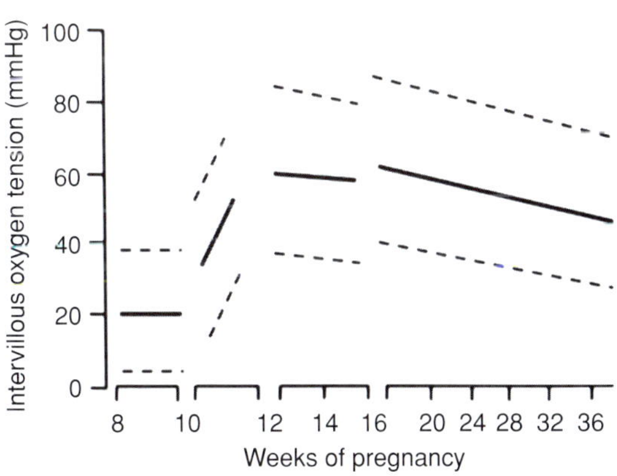

Figure 6.1 The means and 95% confidence intervals of oxygen tension throughout gestation in the intervillous space. (Values are derived from in vivo measurements as reported by Rodesch et al. (1992) *Obstetrics and Gynecology* 80: 283; Soothill et al. (1986) *Fetal Therapy* 1: 168; (1987) *British Medical Journal* 294: 1051; Jauniaux et al. (1999) *Human Reproduction* 14: 2901; (2000) *American Journal of Pathology* 157: 211, (2001) *American Journal of Obstetrics and Gynecology* 184: 998.)

Clinical Pearl

The advent of in vivo fetal or placental blood sampling revealed that near anoxia is present in the first trimester. This has changed the conditions for embryo storage and culture that are used in assisted reproductive technologies with a concomitant enhanced success rate for pregnancy.

The wide confidence intervals in Figure 6.1 are likely due to regional variation in PO_2 within the placenta. PO_2 of blood flowing through the fetoplacental vasculature is constantly equilibrating with the PO_2 in the intervillous space. The range of oxygen tensions present within the blood vessels of the placenta could therefore be as low as 5 mm Hg in the umbilical arterial blood and as high as 80–100 mm Hg in the spiral arterioles. Figure 6.2 illustrates this concept.

Pathophysiology

Placental tissue oxygenation will vary according to the development of the fetal circulation and the degree of fetal extraction of the oxygen provided by the maternal circulation. A useful conceptualization of the causes of placental hypoxia accounts for these dual influences [4].

Preplacental hypoxia is caused by hypoxemia, or by anemia, as discussed above. In this case, there is reduced oxygen tension or content within the maternal blood. *Uteroplacental hypoxia* is caused by limitation of blood flow, most often due to failed trophoblast invasion of the maternal spiral arteries, as described in the chapters on intrauterine growth restriction (IUGR) and preeclampsia (PE). *Postplacental hypoxia* occurs when normally oxygenated blood reaches the intervillous space, but fetoplacental perfusion is compromised. Postplacental hypoxia associates with thrombi and infarcts, velamentous cord insertion, true knots in the umbilical cord, and impaired development of tertiary terminal villi. Figure 6.3 illustrates the third trimester villous tree in normal pregnancies and the altered morphology when placental hypoxia is present.

There are varied explanations for the failed trophoblast invasion and the villous maldevelopment that results in placental dysfunction. These include defects in molecular oxygen sensing, signaling, or both, or the presence of extremes of oxygen content within the intervillous space before antioxidant responses are optimal. Figure 6.3(b)

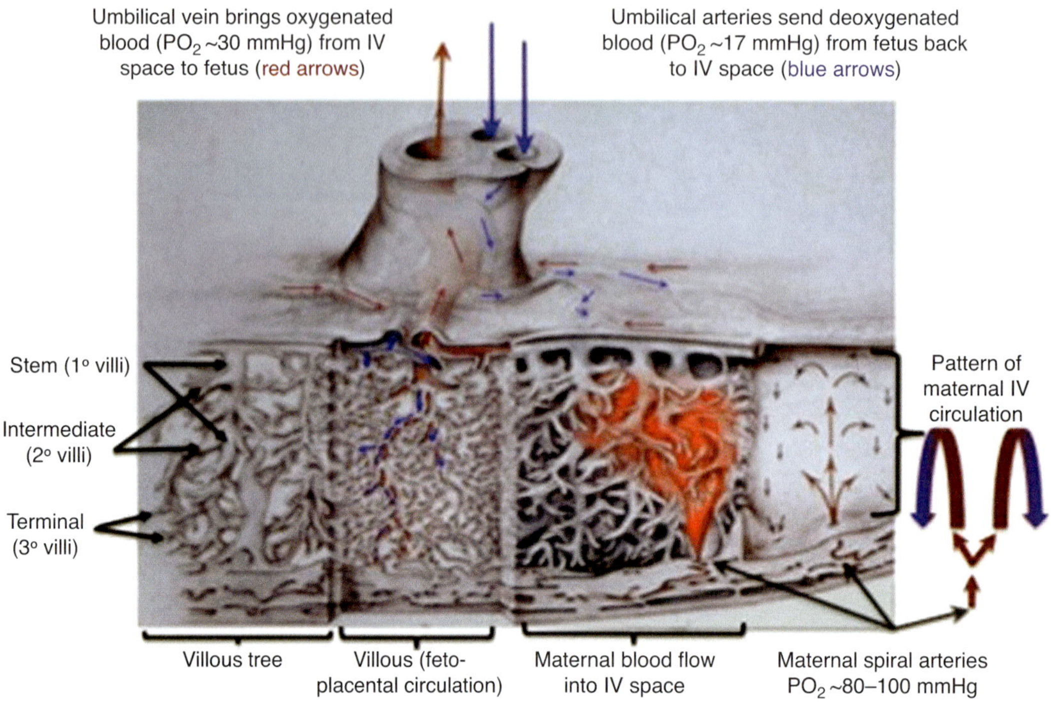

Figure 6.2 Circulation and oxygen tension in the mature human placenta. The left side of the figure shows the villous tree with the stem villi, which form early in placental development, branching into secondary and tertiary (terminal) villi. The latter have thin walls and long arcades of capillary loops to optimize gas exchange. The middle left panel illustrates fetal blood flow within the villous tree. The changing color of the directional arrows shows how PO_2 changes as maternal blood equilibrates with PO_2 in the intervillous space and, ultimately, oxygenates the blood in the vessels coalescing into the umbilical vein. This concept is also illustrated in the right area of the figure where changing oxygen tension of the intervillous blood results from the flow of the maternal blood into and through the intervillous space. (Harris JWS and Ramsey EM (1966) The morphology of human placental vasculature. *Contributions to Embryology* 38: 45–58. Used with permission from Carnegie Institution for Science, Washington, DC, USA.)

shows that fetal vascularization of the placental tree stalls at the developmental phase when the secondary intermediate villi mature and give rise to the terminal tertiary villi. Deranged oxygen sensing contributes to problems in the development of the fetoplacental vasculature and to the failed invasion and remodeling of the maternal spiral arteries. Variation in oxygen content is induced not only by lowered blood flow to the placenta but also by the narrowed lumens of spiral arteries, which results in an increase in blood flow velocity. The increased force of this blood flow can damage the fragile villous tree, to result in excess shedding of aponecrotic trophoblast fragments, inflammation, and oxidative stress, all of which are described in PE [5]. Ischemia results when blood flow ceases for some period of time. This is commonly followed by a resumption of normal flow. Also called hypoxia–reoxygenation or ischemia–reperfusion, this event causes a profound decline in tissue PO_2 followed by rapid reoxygenation. Ischemia, reperfusion, or both associate with apoptosis, inflammation, and oxidative stress. Indeed, some investigators argue that large fluctuations in oxygen are more likely to be causally involved in PE than chronic hypoxemia or a chronic decline in blood flow.

Research Spotlight

Derangement of the molecular pathway for the transcription factor hypoxia-inducible factor (*HIF*) associates with pregnancy pathologies and placental hypoxia. Epigenetic modifications of proteins involved in hypoxia sensing and genetic variations in *HIF* regulatory proteins are under investigation.

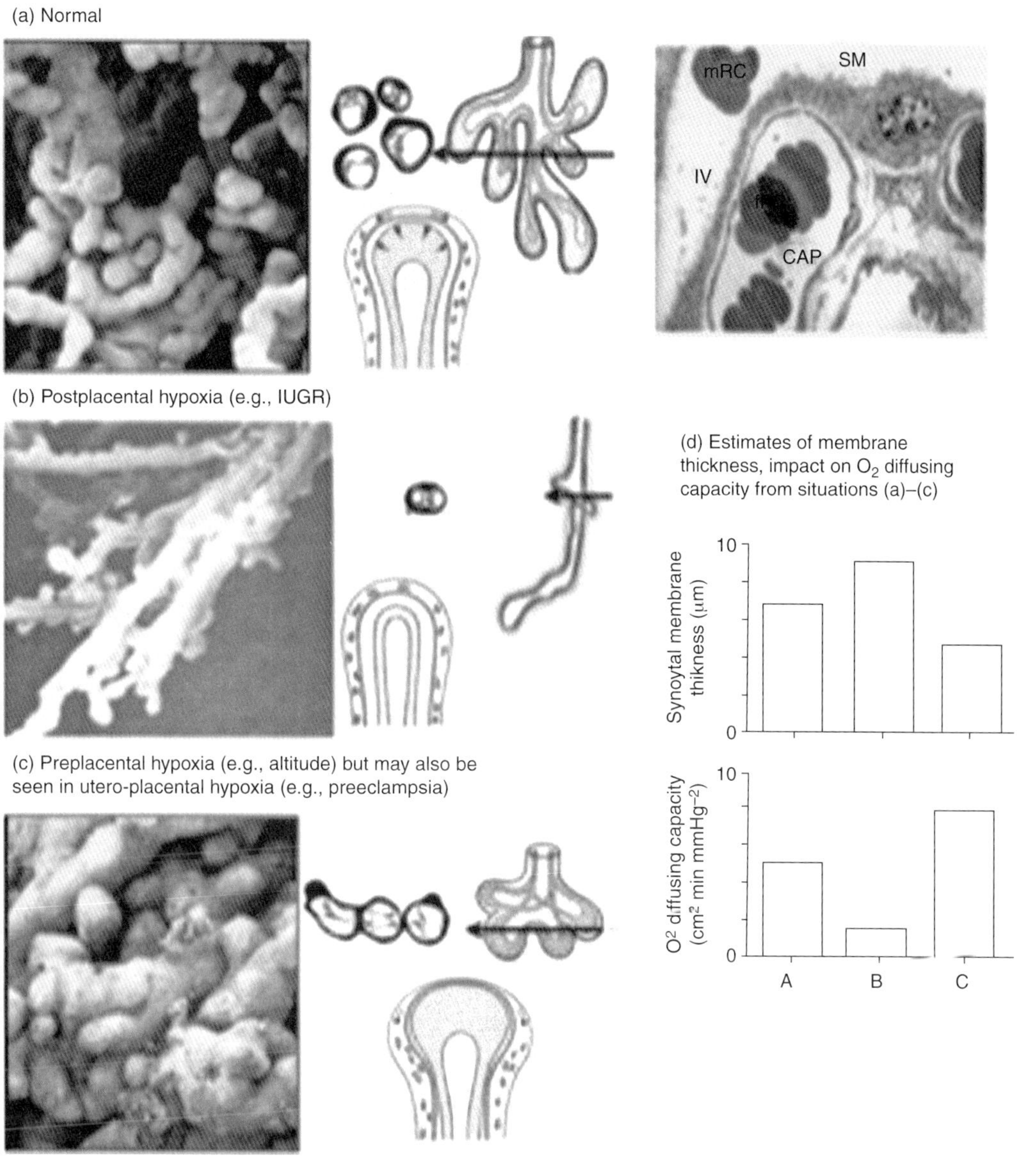

Figure 6.3 Panels (a–c) left side: Scanning electron microscopy of villi from normal and abnormal O_2 conditions. Panel (a), far right, is a photomicrograph of a terminal villus in cross-section, showing the maternal intervillous space (IV), a fetal capillary (CAP), maternal (mRC) and fetal red blood cells (fRC), and the syncytial membrane (SM). Oxygen diffuses from the IV across the SM, the fetal capillary wall (endothelium), and into the fetal red blood cells. Panels (a–c) center top: diagram of the villous tree shown in the photo at left and an associated cross section through the villi, indicated by the arrow through the tree diagram. Panels (a–c) center lower: a longitudinal cross-section of a terminal villus showing the capillary loop, which elongates and pushes the membrane outward during the third trimester. Note the outward growth (arrows), enlarging the diameter of the capillary in (a). This growth is absent in (b) (IUGR) and exaggerated in (c) (preplacental hypoxia). The expansion of the capillary loop reduces the membrane thickness at the point of contact, permitting increased diffusion of oxygen. Panel (d) models the differences in membrane thickness and associated variation in diffusion capacity expected given the terminal capillary loops shown in (a–c). Figures (a and c) from Ali KZM, Burton GJ, Morad N et al. (1996) *Placenta* **17**(8): 678–81. (Longitudinal cross sectional models of capillaries in villi are modified from Karimu and Burton (1994) *Trophoblast Research* 3: 117. Figure (b) is modified from Kaufmann (1987) *Anatomy and Embryology* 173(2): 203–14, Kaufmann et al. Placenta (1987) 8:235.)

Risk factors

Risk factors for placental hypoxia are similar to the risk factors for PE or IUGR. They include medical conditions such as diabetes or multiple gestation where an unusually large mass of placental tissue increases O_2 demand, and conditions where the mother has vasospasm, hypoxemia, or unusually low oxygen carrying capacity, e.g., hypertension, maternal cardiopulmonary disease, altitude residence, or anemia. Inflammatory states predispose to PE and IUGR, but to what extent inflammation can be dissociated from hypoxia-associated placental pathology is as yet unclear. Such conditions include obesity and a variety of autoimmune disorders.

Clinical diagnosis and management

There are few signs within a clinical examination that indicate placental hypoxia is present. Placental hypoxia is commonly assumed to be present in PE or IUGR, often without verification. However, recent data confirm that hypoxia is present in PE and in severe IUGR, based on microarrays and molecular studies of *HIF* and *HIF*-related proteins [6–8]. Placental hypoxia results from perturbations in blood flow, and thus placental hypoxia implicitly or explicitly invokes the concept that blood flow to or within the placenta is inadequate to meet metabolic needs of the feto–placental unit. Doppler blood flow parameters are the most useful tool for clinical diagnosis. Higher than normal bilateral uterine arterial resistance indices are indicative of high placental resistance to blood flow. Abnormal umbilical Doppler parameters, such as elevated umbilical artery resistance indices, or the presence of waveforms in the umbilical vein associate with a greater incidence of PE and IUGR. These Doppler abnormalities indicate that there is increased vascular resistance that impairs flow of both oxygenated umbilical venous blood into the fetus and deoxygenated fetal arterial blood into the villous tree to reach the site of oxygen exchange at the terminal villi. The fetus can increase extraction of oxygen to compensate for lowered maternal blood flow, and thus the PO_2 in the umbilical artery can become very low. As a result, the blood returned to the placenta can lower overall placental PO_2 and contribute to increasing placental hypoxia. Lowered resistance in the fetal middle cerebral artery is indicative of vasodilation in the central nervous system and blood flow redistribution to favor the brain, a response to hypoxia common to all mammalian species. Absent or reversed end-diastolic flow in the umbilical artery is a grave sign, associated with significant fetal mortality and neonatal morbidity. Galan and colleagues 2002 [9] provide an excellent review of the clinical utility of Doppler indices that indicate fetal and by extension placental compromise.

Efforts to treat hypoxia-related placental dysfunction in utero have met with little success. For example, maternal administration of oxygen mixtures higher than 21% to raise maternal PO_2 have shown that fetal oxygen tension either does not change or changes in a clinically insignificant manner and without benefit to the fetus. Moreover, elevating oxygen tension predisposes to oxidative damage to the placenta. Unfortunately, treatment still relies on delivery of the fetus before fetal hypoxemia becomes critical. Therefore, once signs of impaired blood flow are diagnosed, management focuses on monitoring fetal well being and optimizing the timing of delivery. The above overview shows that there are ample opportunities for research into the mechanisms by which placental hypoxia contributes to placental dysfunction and suboptimal pregnancy outcomes.

☞ Teaching Points

1 Hypoxia is defined as an inadequate supply of oxygen supply to the cells and tissues of the body.

2 Oxygen content of the blood is the most clinically relevant indicator of whether oxygen supply is sufficient for metabolic needs, but it does not necessarily reflect oxygen saturation, consumption, extraction, or pressure.

3 Placental intervillous PO2 is ~2–3% in the first trimester, ~7–8% in second trimester, and 5–6% in the third trimester. Second trimester values are closest to what is observed in the capillary/venous circulation elsewhere in the body while first trimester values are lower than in other circulations.

4 Because the placenta is perfused by both the mother and the fetus, perturbations in blood flow in either can contribute to placental hypoxia.

5 Preplacental hypoxia is caused by low maternal arterial PO_2 or by anemia. Uteroplacental hypoxia is caused by limitations in blood flow. Postplacental hypoxia occurs when normally oxygenated blood reaches the intervillous space, but fetoplacental perfusion is compromised.

6 Doppler indices of blood flow and resistance to blood flow are the best clinical indicators of placental compromise that could indicate hypoxia.

References

1. Postigo L, Heredia G, Illsley NP et al. (2009) Where the O_2 goes to: Preservation of human fetal oxygen delivery and consumption at high altitude. *Journal Physiology* 587: 693–708.
2. Lackman F, Capewell V, Gagnon R et al. (2001) Fetal umbilical cord oxygen values and birth to placental weight ratio in relation to size at birth. *American Journal of Obstetrics and Gynecology* 185: 674–82.
3. Jauniaux E, Watson AL, Hempstock J et al. (2000) Onset of maternal arterial blood flow and placental oxidative stress. A possible factor in human early pregnancy failure. *American Journal of Pathology* 157: 2111–22.
4. Kingdom JC and Kaufmann P. (1997) Oxygen and placental villous development: Origins of fetal hypoxia. *Placenta* 18: 613–21; discussion 623–6.
5. Burton GJ, Woods AW, Jauniaux E et al. (2009) Rheological and physiological consequences of conversion of the maternal spiral arteries for uteroplacental blood flow during human pregnancy. *Placenta* 30: 473–82.
6. Soleymanlou N, Jurisica I, Nevo O et al. (2005) Molecular evidence of placental hypoxia in preeclampsia. *Journal of Clinical Endocrinology and Metabolism* 90: 4299–308.
7. Caniggia I, Winter J, Lye SJ et al. (2000) Oxygen and placental development during the first trimester: Implications for the pathophysiology of pre-eclampsia. *Placenta* 21(Suppl A): S25–30.
8. Nevo O, Soleymanlou N, Wu Y et al. (2006) Increased expression of sFlt-1 in in vivo and in vitro models of human placental hypoxia is mediated by HIF-1. *American Journal of Physiology—Regulatory, Integrative and Comparitive Physiology* 291(4): R1085–93.
9. Galan HL, Ferrazzi E, and Hobbins JC (2002) Intrauterine growth restriction (IUGR): Biometric and Doppler assessment. *Prenatal Diagnosis* 22: 331–7.

7

CHAPTER 7
Placental Metabolism

Nicholas P. Illsley
Department of Obstetrics, Gynecology, and Women's Health, UMDNJ-New Jersey Medical School, Newark, NJ, USA

Introduction

Our view of placental metabolism has evolved over time as our understanding of the role of the placenta has increased. Several decades ago, the role of the placenta was seen as a passive barrier, preventing transfer to the fetus of maternal metabolites, proteins and hormones, of bacteria, viruses, xenobiotics, and drugs, while enabling transfer of essential nutrients via specific transporter systems. More recently we have come to understand that the placenta evolves and grows over gestation via a variety of proliferating cell types, requiring high levels of nutrient supply. The rapid expansion of the placenta, especially in the second and third trimesters of human pregnancy, is fueled by uptake and metabolism of nutrients for the purposes of generating cellular energy, synthesizing DNA and RNA, proteins, membranes, and other components crucial for cellular growth. The levels of specific nutrients supplied from the maternal circulation are altered by intraplacental metabolic activity, and thus the nutrient profile presented to the fetus may differ significantly from that taken up from the maternal circulation. The placenta is therefore a metabolically active interface which uses a significant fraction of nutrient uptake for its own purposes.

Most recently we have learned that the placenta plays a dynamic regulatory function by sensing the concentration of available nutrients and adapting placental metabolism to sustain fetal growth. There is evidence to suggest that the placenta can proactively regulate its metabolism to change the profile of nutrients presented to the fetus. The placenta is thus an active and pivotal partner with both the fetus and mother in determining fetal growth.

Placental transfer and metabolism

The placenta plays a unique role with regard to the metabolism of many compounds since a significant number are not only taken up and metabolized by the placenta but are also part of the maternofetal flux, supplying fetal nutrient needs. Alterations in placental metabolism may have an important impact on maternofetal transfer, especially for those nutrients that are both transferred and consumed in large quantities such as glucose, oxygen, and the amino acids. Their intraplacental levels are crucial to the processes of cellular growth and, under conditions of stress or deprivation, to cellular survival. Many of the common pregnancy pathologies are associated with perturbations in the transport and metabolism of these compounds. This review will focus on the placental metabolism of glucose, oxygen, and the amino acids, as not only important metabolic components but also as participatory elements in common pathologies.

Oxygen

Oxygen is frequently omitted from discussions of metabolism because the vast bulk of its utilization takes place through one reaction, as an electron acceptor in the terminal step of the mitochondrial electron transport

The Placenta: From Development to Disease, First Edition. Edited by Helen H. Kay, D. Michael Nelson and Yuping Wang.
© 2011 Blackwell Publishing Ltd. Published 2011 by Blackwell Publishing Ltd.

chain. Nevertheless, availability of oxygen has a profound influence on metabolism within the placenta. Early measures of oxygen consumption by the placenta using indirect calorimetry gave a value of 0.58 mmol/min [1]. Calculations employing our recent direct in vivo measurements [2,3] have given a remarkably similar value of 0.53 $\pm$ 0.09 mmol/min. These values are greater than most of the values obtained from in vitro perfusion studies, which range from 0.1 to 0.5 mmol/min, however in vivo studies also include oxygen consumption by the uterus. The perfusion studies have nevertheless demonstrated a linear relationship between oxygen supply and placental consumption [4], a correlation supported by our in vivo data. Placental oxygen consumption is 37% of the total uterine oxygen consumption of 1.44 $\pm$ 0.07 mmol/min, similar to prior estimates for both human and sheep. On a per kg tissue basis, oxygen consumption by the placenta and uterus (0.36 mmol/min/kg) is clearly above that of the fetus (0.27 mmol/min/kg), demonstrating the high metabolic activity of the placenta.

The most significant regulatory role of oxygen in placental metabolism is the effect of decreased oxygen supply. It is important to remember that oxygen tension in the intervillous space is comparatively low; intervillous PO_2 rises from 3% in the first trimester to 8% in the second, falling to 5% late in pregnancy. Given that hypoxia responses mediated by the HIF-1 (Hypoxia-Inducible Factor-1) transcription factor are initiated at oxygen levels of approximately 5% O_2, it is clear that placental energy metabolism in the placenta is balanced close to the point at which energy generation begins to switch between oxidative metabolism and anaerobic glycolysis. The result is that under conditions of decreased oxygen supply and reduced intervillous PO_2, such as those occurring in preeclampsia or fetal growth restriction, hypoxia responses will be activated in the placenta.

Research Spotlight

Recent research suggests that HIF-1-mediated responses will lead to partial inhibition of placental oxygen consumption, increasing the cellular availability of oxygen in the placenta and providing an increased level of oxygen for transfer to the fetus. Thus initial changes in oxygen metabolism in conditions of placental hypoxia lead to a response that sustains fetal oxygenation.

Glucose

Glucose is the primary substrate for placental energy generation and a source of carbon skeletons for synthetic purposes. The maternal circulation is the only verified source for fetoplacental glucose, as there is no gluconeogenesis in the fetus, and placental gluconeogenesis, if present, contributes minimally. Glucose is transported into the placenta via facilitated diffusion by transporters of the GLUT family, which are embedded in both the microvillous and basal membranes of the syncytiotrophoblast. There is an asymmetric arrangement of transporters between the two opposing faces of the syncytium (microvillous >> basal), resulting in an intrasyncytial concentration of glucose that remains close to that of the intervillous blood. This maximizes the glucose gradient that drives transport across the basal membrane, the rate-limiting step in maternofetal transfer. Intracellular glucose within the trophoblast or placenta does not seem to be compartmentalized between metabolic and transport pools since acute effects that alter cellular glucose consumption produce reductions in both transepithelial and transplacental transport.

The placenta has a very high rate of glucose consumption. Estimates vary depending not only on the methodology utilized, but also on the levels of glucose, degree of oxygenation, and extent of extracellular fluid access to the tissue. In vitro perfusion studies offer the most physiological estimates and assign glucose consumption rates of 0.13–0.33 mmol/min/kg, whereas placental explant rates vary widely, from 0.02 to 0.87 mmol/min/kg. The rate of glucose consumption obtained from our in vivo measurements that include placental and uterine tissue is 0.20 mmol/min/kg, which is consistent with the perfusion measurements. Even assuming a high rate of glucose consumption by uterine tissue, similar to that described for human muscle tissue, placental consumption is still threefold greater than the 0.07 mmol/min/kg rate of fetal glucose consumption measured in our studies [5]. Placental consumption is substantially higher than estimates for skeletal muscle, cardiac muscle, or whole body glucose consumption, highlighting the extremely high rate of glucose metabolism in the placenta. The high glucose consumption is consistent with the low degree of oxygenation and a tendency for placental metabolism to switch to anaerobic metabolism earlier than other tissues. The above estimates also demonstrate that ~55% of the glucose taken up by the pregnant uterus is consumed by placental and uterine tissues.

Research Spotlight

SIRT6, a histone demethylase and co-repressor of the HIF-1 transcription factor, appears to regulate the expression of multiple glycolytic enzymes and may be a master regulator of glucose homeostasis.

Metabolic pathways other than glycolysis are also present in the placenta. Glycogen is synthesized in the placenta although more so in early than late pregnancy. There is increased deposition of glycogen in placentas from diabetic pregnancies at term, mainly around fetoplacental vessels, possibly a response to fetal hyperglycemia. Increased syncytial glycogen is also observed in placentae from preeclamptic pregnancies. Glycogen deposition in preeclampsia takes place in the villous trophoblast instead of fetal vessels. This histopathological finding is likely related to relative cellular immaturity caused by increased villous trophoblast turnover in preeclampsia, rather than a response to metabolite concentrations, consistent with the absence of syncytial glycogen increases in response to glucose or insulin. The pentose phosphate pathway, essential for the production of ribose-5-phosphate for DNA and RNA synthesis and for production of NADPH for reductive biosynthesis, has also been described in the placenta, although higher in first trimester placenta than at term. The utilization of glucose via these different metabolic pathways appears to change over gestation. Earlier in pregnancy, almost 75% of glucose is metabolized through the glycolytic pathway, 15% via non-triose phosphate pathways such as glycogen synthesis and 10% via the pentose phosphate pathway. By term, metabolism has shifted such that consumption via the glycolytic pathway reaches 90%, with non-triose phosphate and pentose phosphate pathways accounting for an additional 5% each (Figure 7.1).

Lactate

One of the consequences of the high rate of placental glucose consumption is that the placenta produces significant quantities of lactate. Some estimates suggest that ≥70% of syncytial glucose consumption ends up as lactate. In vitro explant and perfusion studies show that the placenta produces 0.1–0.3 mmol/min/kg; however, it is likely that lactate is released from the placenta into both fetal and maternal circulations. Under normoxic conditions in vivo, the placenta releases lactate into the fetal circulation at a rate of 0.03 mmol/min/kg, implying a greater release into the maternal circulation. This is consistent with the finding that the lactate transport capacity of the syncytial microvillous membrane is greater than that of the fetal-facing basal membrane. Under hypoxic conditions, however, this arrangement changes; because the fetus becomes a net producer of lactate, the result is placental uptake of lactate from the fetal circulation.

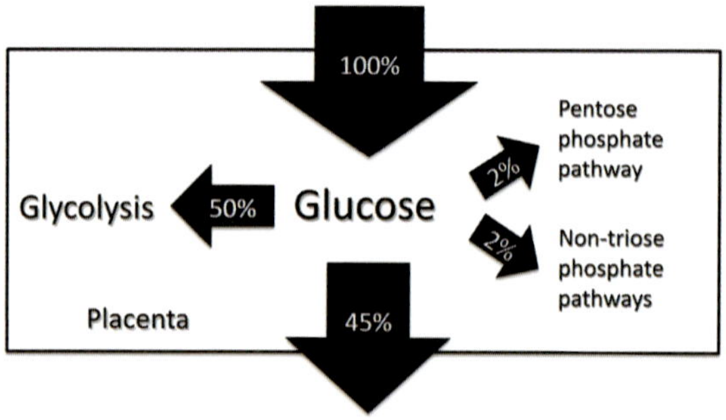

Figure 7.1 *Disposition of placental glucose.* Of the glucose taken up by the human placenta from the maternal circulation, 45% is transported to the fetal circulation, while 50% is metabolized via glycolysis and the remainder is metabolized by the pentose phosphate and non-triose phosphate pathways.

Amino acids

Placental amino acid metabolism is inextricably linked with the maternofetal transfer of amino acids. Transfer of amino acids to the fetus takes place by a concentration gradient from maternal to fetal circulation via transporters in the microvillous and basal membranes of the transporting epithelial layer of the placenta, the syncytiotrophoblast [6]. Amino acid concentrations in the syncytiotrophoblast cells are higher than both maternal and fetal levels; amino acids are transported into the syncytium through transporters operating by secondary active transport. One form of transporter, the sodium-coupled transporter, makes use of the inwardly directed sodium gradient to drive amino acids into the syncytial cells. Another form of transporter, the exchanger, makes use of outwardly directed gradients of certain amino acids to drive the inward movement of other amino acids with related structures. Finally, there appear to be a number of non-exchange efflux transporters that are simple monomolecular transporters, requiring neither exchange nor sodium coupling. Amino acids accumulated in the syncytium are transported into the fetal circulation via exchange and efflux transporters in the basal membrane of the syncytium (Figure 7.2). Many of the amino acid transporters have overlapping specificities and thus the net flux of specific amino acids will depend on the amino acid concentration profile at either side of the membrane across which transport is taking place. Moreover, transporters using a common substrate are coupled; changes in transport through one may then produce intracellular concentration changes that will affect transport through another. The coupled and overlapping nature of these amino acid transporter systems has made analysis of even basic systems extremely complex. Added to this are more recent observations that individual transporters may have several isoforms, differing in kinetic characteristics and cellular distribution.

Much of the research into placental metabolism of amino acids has been carried out in animals, mainly sheep, since it is often difficult to perform in the human the type of measurements necessary to investigate the effect of perturbations. Apart from the simple passage of amino acids across the placenta, the metabolic processes that have been observed thus far can be divided into four types: (1) amino acid metabolism for the purposes of energy generation, (2) amino acid utilization for the synthesis of other components in the placenta, (3) conversion as part of a placental–fetal shuttle system [7], and (4) protein synthesis (Figure 7.3).

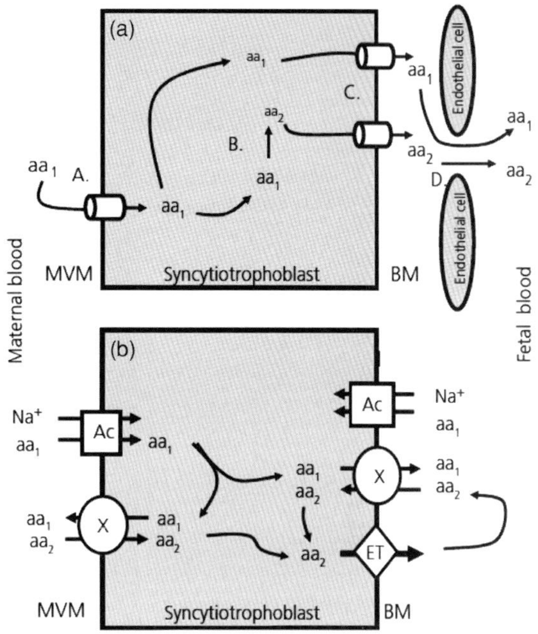

Figure 7.2 *Mechanisms of amino acid transport.* (a) A, amino acids (aa) in maternal blood are taken up by transporters on the apical membrane of the placental syncytiotrophoblast; B, within the syncytiotrophoblast, amino acids are metabolized to produce new amino acids; C, amino acids are transported across the basal membrane by transport proteins; D, amino acids diffuse into fetal blood through fenestrations in the capillary endothelium. (b) Amino acids are taken up by accumulative transporters (Ac) or exchangers (X). Accumulative transporters mediate influx not efflux. Exchangers mediate efflux of specific amino acids but cannot drive net transfer of amino acids. A non-exchange efflux transporter (ET) must exist to allow net transport of amino acids across the basal plasma membrane. (Reproduced, with permission, from the *Journal of Neuroendocrinology* 20: 419–26, 2008.) MVM, microvillous membrane; BM, basal membrane

Energy generation

The utilization of amino acid carbon for oxidative metabolism is a universal phenomenon. However, the amino acid sources and the extent of oxidation differ substantially among cells, tissue, and species. In the placenta, tracer studies have shown that placental uptake of amino acids is in excess of their release into the fetal circulation. These data suggest that there is significant amino acid oxidation within the fetus. For example, branched chain amino acids (BCAA) such as leucine, valine, and isoleucine can be transaminated in the placenta to branched chain keto acids (e.g., leucine to α-keto isocaproic acid, or KIC) and are thence decarboxylated to produce acyl-CoA derivatives, which feed into the tricarboxylic acid cycle. The decarboxylation step, however, is thought to account for a relatively small quantity of the transaminated BCAA (perhaps 10%), and in the human, there is some evidence to suggest that there is actually net uptake of fetal KIC by the placenta. The BCAA deamination reactions also involve transfer of an amino group to a-ketoglutarate, forming glutamate. In turn, the transformation of glutamate back to a-ketoglutarate via the action of glutamate dehydrogenase reduces NAD^+ to NADH, providing reducing equivalents that power ATP generation through the electron transport chain. Conversion of other amino acids such as alanine, glycine, aspartate, phenylalanine, and proline for the purpose of oxidative metabolism has been described in other tissues.

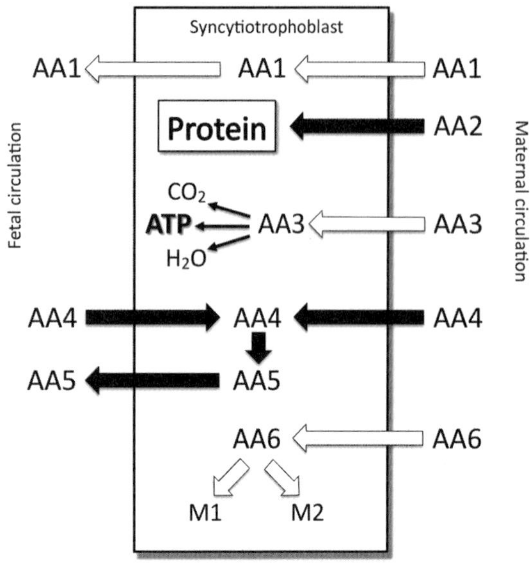

Figure 7.3 *Placental amino acid metabolism.* Apart from amino acids transported to the fetus (AA1), amino acids taken up by the placenta are utilized via a number of other pathways. Amino acids are incorporated into proteins within the placenta (AA2) or used to generate ATP via oxidative metabolism (AA3). Amino acids taken up from the maternal (and fetal) circulation can be transformed to other amino acids for transport to the fetus (AA4/AA5) or metabolized to other compounds (AA6).

While these pathways are likely to be operational in the placenta, their mechanisms have not been elucidated. It is clear however that a significant fraction of placental amino acid uptake is destined for oxidative metabolism, at least under normoxic conditions.

Biosynthesis

Amino acids form an essential part of biosynthetic processes in all cells. In the placenta, leaving aside the primary synthetic route of protein synthesis, a number of such processes have been described. Serine is involved in several transformative processes in the placenta following uptake from maternal and fetal circulations. Serine conversion to glycine forms part of the one-carbon cycle in which tetrahydrofolate is converted to methylene tetrahydrofolate, supplying methyl groups for folate cofactors, which in turn are necessary for nucleotide synthesis as well as homocysteine remethylation to methionine. Serine is also used in the placenta for synthesis of the phospholipid, phosphatidyl serine, a major membrane component. Glycine is not taken up by the placenta from the maternal circulation but is produced in the placenta as the primary source for transfer to the fetus via the action of the enzyme serine hydroxymethyltransferase. Metabolism of proline provides the mechanism for synthesis of a number of polyamines such as spermidine and spermine in the placenta, as does metabolism of arginine to a lesser extent. Arginine is also essential for placental generation of nitric oxide, a key vasodilator, via the action of nitric oxide synthase. Alanine is taken up from the maternal circulation, but tracer studies suggest that a relatively small fraction of alanine uptake is directly transferred to the fetus; production from other substrates such as glutamate and pyruvate may provide a source of alanine for transfer to the fetus. Recent evidence suggests that the transsulfuration pathway responsible for the interconversion of methionine, homocysteine, and cystine/cysteine may be operative in the human placenta, employing serine as a cofactor. It is not known whether the conversion of cystine to taurine also occurs in the placenta however, placental levels of taurine are known to be high. Although these processes have been shown to be functional in the placenta, the extent and significance of these metabolic pathways is still unclear.

Amino acid shuttling

Glutamate is taken up by the placenta from both the maternal and fetal circulations but is not released into the fetal circulation. Instead, placental glutamate is, in part, converted to glutamine, which is released into the fetal circulation. Placentally derived glutamine is then converted by the fetal liver into glutamate, which, when released into the fetal circulation, is shuttled back to the placenta, with net transfer of amino nitrogen into the fetus. Serine is another amino acid that is taken up by the placenta from both circulations but not released into the fetal circulation. Instead, placental conversion of serine to glycine is followed by glycine release into the fetal circulation and hepatic conversion, in part, back into serine, although the purpose of this shuttle is unclear.

Protein synthesis and degradation

Little information is available concerning either placental protein synthesis or degradation. Our laboratory has demonstrated protein synthesis in the syncytiotrophoblast supported by both oxidative and anaerobic metabolism. Under hypoxic conditions, protein synthesis continues to be supported at significant levels by glycolytic generation of energy (unpublished data). Reduced access to energy-generating substrates will decrease placental protein synthesis. However it is unclear whether a reduction in synthesis in conditions such as fetal growth restriction occurs primarily in response to substrate restriction or through decreased endocrine stimulation of growth. Placental protein synthesis in the human is significantly higher in term placenta compared to first trimester and is stimulated substantially in diabetic pregnancy. Even less is known about protein catabolism. Although fetal protein catabolism has been demonstrated under conditions of fetal growth restriction for the purposes of supplying substrates for oxidative metabolism, the absence of gluconeogenic capabilities in the placenta and access to a large maternal pool of amino acid substrates suggests that placental protein catabolism may not be a significant process.

Alterations in maternal and/or fetal circulating amino acid profiles will change the transport characteristics of one or more transporters, leading to changes in the intracellular profile. These alterations will lead not only to direct changes in the efflux of amino acids into the fetal circulation but will also potentially have effects on placental amino acid metabolism, influencing the availability of substrates for metabolic interconversion and further complicating fetal supply.

Supplementation

Given the role of placental metabolism in fetal growth and development, does supplementation of the fetal substrate supply alter the incidence of small-for-gestational age (SGA) pregnancies and other problems associated with fetal growth restriction? A number of animal investigations have shown that the fetal growth restriction produced by placental reduction of substrate supply can be reversed at least in part by supplementation. Successful supplementation studies in animals have for the most part involved provision of nutrients directly to the fetus, via intragastric, intravenous, or intra-amniotic routes. These studies have often shown the generation of a phenotype intermediate to the control and growth-restricted fetuses. Although these studies show the possibilities of supplementation, the impracticality of implementing such procedures in human pregnancy renders them unlikely to be adopted for clinical practice. Other more practical procedures have had poor results. Oxygen administration has shown some improvement in outcomes in human pregnancies. However, this methodology is by its nature restrictive, and significant concerns have been raised regarding the effects of reduced fetal oxygen levels following oxygen administration as well as the effects of hyperoxygenation on parameters such as maternal pulmonary function. Administration of specific nutrients such as glucose or amino acids have not demonstrated significant benefit and have, on the contrary, been associated with problems such as an increased degree of fetal acidosis. Maternal administration of broader nutritional supplements in human pregnancies, including high protein or isocaloric diets, has demonstrated not only an absence of beneficial outcomes in human pregnancies but in some cases increased risks of producing SGA neonates.

Clinical Pearl

Balanced energy/protein supplementation to enhance placental uptake and transport, in which protein provided less than 25% of the total energy content, was associated with small increases in maternal weight (+21 g) and in birth weight (+38 g). Such approaches may have some role in preventing SGA (~30% reduction) although there is no evidence of long-term benefits to the child in terms of growth, neurocognitive development, adiposity, or blood pressure [8].

Teaching Points

1 In the second and third trimesters of normal pregnancy, intervillous PO_2 is 40–60 mm Hg (5–8%), and as a result, placental metabolism is close to the point at which hypoxia responses are initiated. Despite low intervillous PO_2, placental O_2 consumption is high relative to other fetal tissues

2 The placenta exhibits rates of glucose consumption threefold greater than that of the fetus, resulting in >50% consumption of uterine glucose delivery.

3 Placental amino acid utilization can be divided into four broad elements, comprising protein synthesis, metabolism for energy generation, use in the synthesis of other cellular metabolites, and utilization in the placental–fetal shuttling of amino acids.

4 Perturbation of amino acid profiles will cause not only alterations in maternofetal transport, but also changes in intraplacental amino acid metabolism, which can alter the profile of amino acids supplied to the fetus.

5 Although direct fetal administration of nutrients can limit a trajectory of suboptimal fetal growth, balanced energy protein supplementation to the mother is currently the only practical clinical approach to optimize fetal growth.

References

1. Carter A (2000) Placental oxygen consumption. Part I: In vivo studies—A review. *Placenta* 21(Suppl A): S31–7.
2. Postigo L, Heredia G, Illsley NP et al. (2009) Where the O_2 goes to: Preservation of human fetal oxygen delivery and consumption at high altitude. *Journal of Physiology* 587: 693–708.
3. Zamudio S, Postigo L, Illsley NP et al. (2007) Maternal oxygen delivery is not related to altitude- and ancestry-associated differences in human fetal growth. *Journal of Physiology* 582: 883–95.
4. Schneider H (2000) Placental oxygen consumption. Part II: In vitro studies—A review. *Placenta* 21(Suppl A): S38–44.
5. Zamudio S, Torricos T, Fik E et al. (2010) Hypoglycemia and the origin of hypoxia-induced reduction in human fetal growth. *PLoS One* 5: e8551.
6. Cleal JK and Lewis RM (2008) The mechanisms and regulation of placental amino acid transport to the human foetus. *Journal of Neuroendocrinology* 20: 419–26.
7. Cetin I (2001) Amino acid interconversions in the fetal–placental unit: The animal model and human studies in vivo. *Pediatric Research* 49: 148–54.
8. Kramer MS and Kakuma R (2003) Energy and protein intake in pregnancy (Review). *Cochrane Database of Systematic Reviews* (Issue 4). Chichester, UK: John Wiley & Sons.

8

CHAPTER 8

Placental Hormones: Physiology, Disease, and Prenatal Diagnosis

Jennifer M. McNamara and Helen H. Kay

Division of Maternal-Fetal Medicine and Ultrasound-Genetics, Department of Obstetrics and Gynecology, Washington University School of Medicine, St. Louis, MO, USA

Introduction

The placenta is a remarkable organ with diverse functions. One of the most intriguing roles played by the placenta is that as a neuroendocrine organ, producing a wide array of hypothalamic, pituitary, and end organ analogues. Hormones conserve and later mobilize maternal nutrients. Intrauterine growth restriction not only associates with childhood and adult obesity, diabetes, and hypertension, but also with dysregulated placental hormone secretion. This chapter discusses selected placental hormones that have been assigned key roles to ensure a successful pregnancy outcome.

Definition

An endocrine hormone is a secreted substance that acts remote from the site of synthesis to affect a target organ. A paracrine hormone acts locally at the site of production. Many hormones from the placenta have endocrine and paracrine functions. Most placental hormones are protein hormones, but estrogen and progesterone are steroid hormones.

Classification

Placental hormones can be classified into several major groups based on their function in the reproductive axis, the regulation of stress responses, the effects on maternal metabolism, the influence on fetal growth regulation, and vascular development (Table 8.1). Placental proteins have taken a new role in recent years as screening tests for the prenatal diagnosis of fetal aneuploidy (Table 8.2).

Source

Most placental hormones are synthesized and secreted from cytotrophoblasts, syncytiotrophoblasts, or both during pregnancy. Villous stromal cells and macrophages, known as Hofbauer cells, are also a source of hormones and growth factors.

Biology of placental hormones

Reproductive axis hormones

These hormones target maternal reproductive organs, primarily the uterus and the corpus luteum in the ovary.

Human chorionic gonadotropin (hCG)

hCG is a glycoprotein composed of alpha and beta subunits. The alpha subunit is shared with LH, FSH, and TSH, while the beta subunit is unique. Marketed pregnancy tests detect the presence of the beta subunit, both as a dimer form found in serum and a degraded core fragment found in urine. A critical role of hCG is to stimulate the corpus luteum to produce progesterone. Additionally, hCG increases production of testosterone by fetal leydig cells to affect male sexual development before

The Placenta: From Development to Disease, First Edition. Edited by Helen H. Kay, D. Michael Nelson and Yuping Wang.
© 2011 Blackwell Publishing Ltd. Published 2011 by Blackwell Publishing Ltd.

Table 8.1 Placental hormones.[a]

Hormone	Other Common Names	Chemical Category	Location	Primary Function	Production Trend Throughout Gestation	Unique Features
Reproductive axis						
Human chorionic gonadotropin	hCG	Glycoprotein	C,S	Supports corpus luteum, stimulates LH receptor in fetus	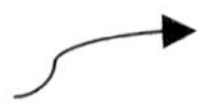	Pregnancy marker for Down syndrome
Estrogen family	Estriol, estrone, estradiol, estetrol, E2, uE3	Steroid	S	Stimulates uterine blood flow and progesterone release, contributes to maternal weight gain	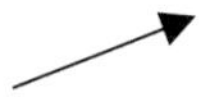	Decreased in fetal steroid production deficiencies
Progesterone	P4	Steroid	S	Endometrial decidualization, myometrial quiescence, decreases insulin sensitivity	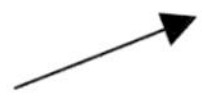	Withdrawal associated with pregnancy loss and labor
Gonadotropin releasing hormone	GnRH, luteinizing-hormone releasing hormone, LHRH, luliberin	Peptide	S	Stimulates hCG release	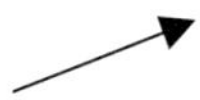	
Oxytocin	Pitocin, syntocinon	Peptide	S	Myometrial contractions	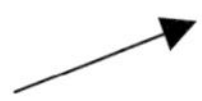	
Inhibin A		Di-peptide, protein complex	C, S, D, A, Ch	Action uncertain but likely counteracts activin	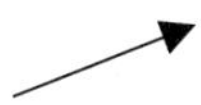	Decreased in early pregnancy loss, increased in preeclampsia and molar pregnancies
Activin A		Di-peptide, protein complex	C, S, D, A, Ch	Local tissue growth	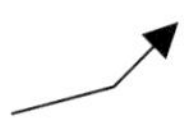	Decreased in early pregnancy loss, increased in preeclampsia and molar pregnancies
Follistatin	Activin A binding protein	Peptide	C, S, D, A, Ch	Inhibits function of TGF-b and activin, promotes release of hCG and progesterone	Uncertain	
Regulate stress response						
Corticotropin releasing hormone	CRH, CRF (former name)	Peptide	C, S, A, Ch, D	Affects uterine blood flow, myometrial contractility, stimulates ACTH release from trophoblasts	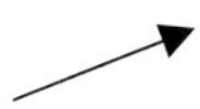	Increased preceding labor and with preeclampsia and IUGR
Chorionic adrenocorticotropic hormone	ACTH	Peptide	S	Stimulates maternal and fetal cortisol synthesis	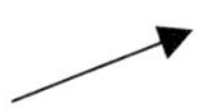	Increased in preeclampsia and IUGR

Table 8.1 *(Continued)*

Hormone	Other Common Names	Chemical Category	Location	Primary Function	Production Trend Throughout Gestation	Unique Features
Urocortin		Peptide	S, A, Ch, D	Similar to CRH	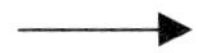	
Maternal metabolism and fetal growth						
Human placental lactogen	hPL, Human chorionic somatomammotropin	Peptide	S	Stimulates insulin production, promotes maternal weight gain	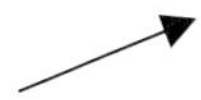	
Prolactin	PRL	Peptide	C, S, D	Promotes maternal weight gain	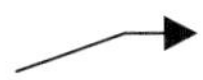	
Human placental growth hormone	hPGH, growth hormone variant, GH-V	Peptide	S	Mobilization of maternal glucose for transfer to fetus, contributes to maternal insulin resistance	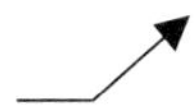	
Growth hormone releasing hormone	GHRH, growth hormone releasing factor, GRF, GHRF, somatocrinin	Peptide	Uncertain	Regulates fetal and placental growth	Uncertain	
Parathyroid hormone-related protein	PTHrP	Peptide	S, A, Ch	Transplacental calcium transfer	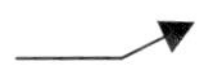	
Leptin		Peptide	C, S, A	Regulates food intake		Decreased with fetal growth restriction
Adiponectin	GBP-28, apM1, AdipoQ, Acrp30	Peptide	C, S	Increases insulin sensitivity		Lower levels in fetal growth restriction
Ghrelin		Peptide	C	Regulates maternal food intake		Increased in fetal growth restriction
Resistin		Peptide	C, S, A	Contributes to insulin resistance		
Visfatin		Peptide	Uncertain	Affects insulin metabolism	Uncertain	May predict metabolic syndrome in adult life, Increased in fetal growth restriction
Insulin-like growth factor-1 and 2	IGF-1, IGF-2	Peptide	C, S, D	Regulates fetal and placental growth	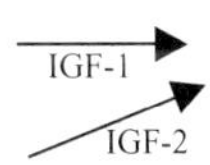	
Vascular development						
Vascular endothelial growth factor	VEGF	Peptide	C, S	Regulates vasculogenesis and angiogenesis	Uncertain	Receptor is VEGFR-1, or "sflt-1"

(Continued)

Table 8.1 (*Continued*)

Hormone	Other Common Names	Chemical Category	Location	Primary Function	Production Trend Throughout Gestation	Unique Features
Placenta growth factor	PlGF	Peptide	C, S	Angiogenic, binds to VEGF receptor, recruits macrophages	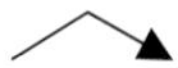	Low levels throughout gestation, decreased in preeclampsia
Fibroblast growth factor	FGF	Peptide	S, Vs	Angiogenesis, regulates placental growth	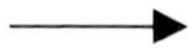	Increased in gestational diabetics
Epidermal growth factor	EGF	Peptide	C, S, Vs	Key role in placental implantation, growth and differentiation	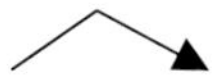	Measured in urine, increased in gestational trophoblastic disease
Transforming growth factor beta	TGF-b	Peptide	S	Anti-cellular proliferation and differentiation, induces apoptosis	Uncertain	Binds receptor "endoglin"
Other hormones						
Thyrotropin releasing hormone	TRH, thyrotropin-releasing factor, TRF, thyroliberin, protirelin	Tripeptide	S, Evt	Releases TSH from fetal pituitary	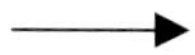	Higher fetal levels than maternal
Neuropeptide Y	NPY	Peptide	S, A, Ch, D	Vasoconstriction	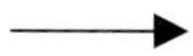	
Relaxin		Peptide	S, A, Ch, D	Promotes uterine blood flow	Uncertain	
Renin	Angiotensinogenase	Peptide	S, A, Ch, D	Regulates maternal blood pressure and uterine blood flow	Uncertain	

C, cytotrophoblast; S, synctiotrophoblast; A, amnion; Ch, chorion; D, decidua; Vs, villous stroma; Evt, extravillous trophoblast.
[a]Table includes collective information from multiple references, not restricted to cited references, and is not inclusive of all published literature.

fetal LH production occurs. LH/hCG receptors have been found throughout the myometrium and uterine vessels, suggesting their involvement in vasodilation and smooth muscle relaxation [1]. Similar to TSH, hCG stimulates thyroxine production within the thyroid [2]. Altered levels of the beta subunit are useful for prenatal screening and diagnosis.

Estrogen

Placental production of estrogen is dependant upon maternal and fetal adrenal production of precursor dehydroepiandrosterone-sulfate (DHEA-S). Estrogens influence uterine blood flow, increase expression of proteins needed for continued progesterone production and steroid metabolism, as well as prepare the breasts for lactation [3].

Progesterone

After the 8th week of gestation, the placenta takes over production of progesterone from the ovary. Production is largely dependant on maternal cholesterol stores. Progesterone is essential for pregnancy to maintain uterine

Table 8.2 Placental hormones in prenatal diagnosis.[a]

Hormone	Tri 21	Tri 18	Tri 13	Preeclampsia	Other
First trimester analytes					
PAPP-A	↓	↓	↓	↓	Decreased in spontaneous abortion, stillbirth, preterm birth, and IUGR
Free or total beta hCG	↑	↓	↓		Decreased in spontaneous abortion
ADAM 12	↓	↓	↓		
PP-13		↓	↓	↓	
Second trimester analytes					
hCG	↑	↓		↑	Increased in placental abnormalities, multiple gestation, or fetal demise
uE3	↓	↓			Decreased in anencephaly and fetal metabolic conditions (SLOS)
Inhibin A	↑	↔		↑	Increased in poor pregnancy outcomes
AFP	↓	↓		↑	Increased in structural fetal or placental anomalies

[a]Table includes collective information from multiple references, not restricted to cited references, and is not inclusive of all published literature. Listed analytes are only used clinically for Down syndrome and trisomy 18 screening; all other uses are still experimental.

quiescence [3]. Withdrawal of progesterone, or an altered response of receptors, allows an otherwise refractory myometrium to become active, which leads to contractions. Additionally, progesterone modulates the maternal immune response to the feto–placental allograft, while also priming the breasts for lactation [3].

Clinical Pearl

Labor initiation in subprimate mammals is related to abrupt progesterone withdrawal. Progesterone's role in humans is not as well known but supplementation with progesterone is used clinically to reduce the risk of recurrent preterm delivery.

Gonadotropin releasing hormone

Gonadotropin releasing hormone functions to stimulate hCG release and is expressed by the placenta throughout pregnancy. Both GnRH and hCG release from the placenta are regulated by activin, inhibin, and follistatin [2].

Oxytocin

Oxytocin levels increase throughout pregnancy. At the onset of labor, there is a marked increase in oxytocin receptors without an increase in maternal circulating hormone levels, suggesting local production of oxytocin, which produces a paracrine effect on the myometrium [2].

Inhibin A, activin A, and follistatin

Inhibin A, activin A, and follistatin belong to a family of inhibin-related proteins that were discovered during investigation of pituitary hormones. Inhibin inhibits while activin stimulates FSH release [2]. These proteins also function as growth factors, embryonic regulators, and immunomodulators during pregnancy. They act in concert with such hormones as EGF, and TGFα, to modulate their own production as well as that of hCG. Their role in early pregnancy loss, placental tumors, preeclampsia, and fetal growth restriction is under investigation [4].

> **Clinical Pearl**
>
> Inhibin A levels are increased in women with a Down syndrome fetus, while both inhibin A and activin A are reduced in early pregnancy loss and increased in molar pregnancy and preeclampsia. Activin A is increased in fetal growth restriction [4].

Hormones that regulate stress response

Corticotropin releasing hormone, urocortin, and adrenocorticotropin

The placenta produces hypothalamic and pituitary analogues of corticotropin releasing hormone (CRH or CRF), urocortin, and adrenocorticotropin (ACTH). CRH and urocortin stimulate ACTH release to yield release of prostaglandins and cortisol. The bioactivity of these three hormones is attenuated by circulating corticotropin releasing factor binding protein (CRF-BP). CRH also stimulates release of fetal DHEA-S, which is aromatized to estrogen. CRH also works locally as a vasodilator, but within the myometrium, it promotes contractility [5].

> **Clinical Pearl**
>
> CRH is elevated in pregnancies complicated by preeclampsia, fetal growth restriction, or abnormal umbilical artery Doppler waveform, likely as a response to stressors [5].

Hormones that regulate maternal metabolism and fetal growth

These hormones induce maternal hyperphagia and nutrient storage while minimizing utilization. Later in pregnancy, they promote fetal and placental growth by mobilizing glucose transfer to the fetus, increasing glucose sensitivity, and increasing calcium absorption.

Human placental lactogen

Along with prolactin and progesterone, human placental lactogen (hPL) early in pregnancy stimulates maternal food intake and maternal weight gain. hPL acts in concert with prolactin to increase circulating insulin levels through increased beta cell proliferation, insulin gene expression, and glucose-independent secretion. hPL also plays a role in calcium absorption and breast development. hPL-deficient women are successful with pregnancy, but women with deficiencies have higher compensatory levels of prolactin [6].

Prolactin

Prolactin likely influences successful implantation, stimulating maternal hyperphagia and regulating fetal growth and development.

> **Research Spotlight**
>
> The mechanisms by which hPL and prolactin stimulate maternal food intake are unclear. These effects may involve induction of the orexigenic agouti-related peptide in the arcuate nucleus, neuropeptide Y in the dorsomedial hypothalamus, or reduction of anorexigenic peptide cocaine and amphetamine-related transcript [6].

Human placental growth hormone

Human placental growth hormone (hPGH) is structurally distinct from pituitary growth hormone, and the *GH-V* gene encoding the protein is expressed solely in the placenta. Secretion is continuous and not regulated by growth hormone releasing hormone, unlike pituitary GH. The production of hPGH increases throughout gestation and substitutes for pituitary growth hormone. hPGH has somatogenic, lactogenic, and lipolytic functions and is a major determinant of maternal insulin resistance in pregnancy. hPGH has also been identified in cord blood, suggesting a direct effect on fetal growth [6].

> **Research Spotlight**
>
> hPL is no longer considered the primary agent of insulin resistance during pregnancy. GH-V is overexpressed in insulin-resistant mouse models, and growth hormone and hPGH are now recognized to play major roles in maternal insulin resistance in human pregnancy [6].

Growth hormone releasing hormone

Placental growth hormone releasing hormone (GHRH) is identical to the hypothalamic product. Rather than stimulate placental release of hPGH, GHRH stimulates the fetal pituitary and likely regulates fetal and placental growth.

Parathyroid hormone-related protein

PTH-rP works with prolactin and hPL to promote maternal gastrointestinal absorption of calcium. Additionally, PTH-rP facilitates transplacental transfer of calcium for fetal bone mineralization. PTH-rP also plays a role in the increased production of insulin in pregnancy and the priming of the breasts for lactation [6].

Adipocytokines

Adipocytokines are a group of metabolically active proteins, produced by adipose tissue that affect maternal metabolism. These hormones are produced by the placenta and thereby may affect fetal growth as well. There are conflicting reports as to how these proteins alter fetal growth and affect maternal metabolism. Leptin regulates maternal food intake and inhibits insulin secretion. Adiponectin levels are lower in insulin-resistant states, whereas resistin potently decreases hepatic insulin sensitivity. Evidence favors that low leptin levels, normal or low adiponectin levels, and high ghrelin and visfatin levels are associated with growth restriction. Elevated levels of visfatin in the fetus are a prognostic marker for development of the metabolic syndrome in adult life [7].

Insulin-like growth factors

The insulin-like growth factors regulate both fetal and placental growth. IGF-2 is the primary growth factor for embryonic development, while IGF-1 levels correlate with birth weight at delivery. IGF-1 and IGF-2 both stimulate placental growth through paracrine functions. Importantly, the IGF-2 gene is imprinted and only expressed from the paternal allele, while the IGF-2 degradation gene is only expressed from the maternal allele. In utero, IGF activity is influenced by other hormones including thyroxine, cortisol, and insulin [8].

Research Spotlight

Beckwith-Wiedemann syndrome associates with macrosomia and is caused by defects of the imprinted 11p15 region of the IGF-2 gene, leading to overexpression of IGF-2. Conversely, Silver-Russell syndrome associates with growth restriction and silencing within the 11p15 region of the IGF-2 gene, which yields diminished expression of IGF-2 [8].

Hormones that regulate vascular development

These hormones promote vasculogenesis (vessel development) in early gestation and angiogenesis (vessel growth and extension) in later gestation.

Angiogenic factors

The placenta is a highly vascular organ and produces many growth factors involved in angiogenesis. Many of these growth factors were discovered as part of efforts to find a cancer cure and now are being investigated as markers for preeclampsia.

Vascular endothelial growth factor (VEGF) initiates vasculogenesis and stimulates angiogenesis while also modulating trophoblast survival and function. The VEGF family consists of several proteins, but the one most commonly studied is VEGF-A, prominent in vascular endothelial cells. Hypoxia promotes placental production of VEGF [9]. Less is known about the regulation of placental growth factor (PlGF), another protein in the same family. PlGF is being investigated as a marker for preeclampsia because PlGF levels tend to be lower than controls before the syndrome is clinically apparent [9]. Both VEGF and PlGF bind to membrane VEGF receptor-1 (VEGFR-1) and soluble VEGFR-1 (sFlt-1), but only VEGF binds to VEGFR-2. Inability of PlGF binding to VEGFR2 differentiates this growth factor from VEGF-mediated angiogenesis.

Clinical Pearl

The VEGF receptor soluble flt-1 is elevated in maternal blood in preeclampsia and the ratio of sflt-1/PlGF may be a marker for detection of preeclampsia [9].

Fibroblast growth factor (FGF) levels correlate with fetal growth and are increased in diabetic patients, which are characterized by a large fetus and placenta [10]. Similarly, epidermal growth factor (EGF) is elevated in serum of patients with gestational trophoblastic disease due to its vasculogenic and angiogenic properties [10]. Conversely,

TGF-β has antiproliferative functions and modulates cell proliferation, differentiation, and apoptosis.

Other hormones

The placenta produces the neuropeptides thyrotropin-releasing hormone (TRH) and neuropeptide-Y (NPY). TRH is released predominantly into the fetal circulation and elicits secretion of TSH from the fetal pituitary. The vasoconstrictor NPY is released into the maternal circulation and acts in a paracrine manner to regulate placental and uterine blood flow and possibly parturition [2].

Relaxin softens the symphysis pubis during pregnancy, reduces collagen synthesis in the cervix, and increases the water, protein, collagen, and glycogen content of the uterus. Relaxin also acts in an autocrine and paracrine manner to increase uterine and placental growth and blood flow, by enhancing angiogenesis.

Renin is a member of the renin–angiotensin system (RAS), which is active within the uteroplacental unit. Renin cleaves angiotensinogen to angiotensin I, which in turn is cleaved by angiotensin converting enzyme to angiotensin II. Renin thereby works in combination with angiotensin to regulate maternal blood pressure and uteroplacental blood flow [2].

Prenatal diagnosis

Altered maternal serum levels of placental hormones are useful for risk assessment in prenatal diagnosis. Table 8.2 displays the most commonly used analytes and the pathology that altered levels may predict. Complex predictive modeling uses the levels of hormones, maternal factors, and gestational age to successfully and sensitively predict the risk for aneuploidy and for adverse pregnancy outcome in an index pregnancy. The function of these hormones in aneuploidy pregnancies remains unknown, but their presence is clinically pertinent because they obviate the need for invasive procedures such as amniocentesis.

First trimester maternal serum analytes include hCG, pregnancy-associated protein peptide A (PAPPA), a disintegrin and metalloprotease 12 (ADAM 12), and placental protein 13 (PP-13). Generally, low levels of any of these proteins are linked with adverse pregnancy outcomes, including aneuploidy, preeclampsia, and fetal demise. An exception is hCG, which is elevated in trisomy 21, molar pregnancy, or abnormal implantation. Low hCG levels associate with nonviable pregnancies. Both hCG and PAPP-A are used clinically, with the fetal nuchal translucency measurement, in first trimester screening for trisomy 21 and 18 [11].

Second trimester maternal serum screening measures hCG, inhibin-A, unconjugated estriol, and alphafetoprotein (AFP). Alterations in these levels allow for a risk assessment of trisomy 21 and 18. Additionally, isolated low estriol levels indicate failure of the fetus to produce adequate substrate for estriol production and facilitate diagnosis of anencephaly, steroid sulfatase deficiency, and Smith-Lemli-Opitz Syndrome [11].

☞ Teaching Points

1. Cytotrophoblasts, syncytiotrophoblasts, decidua, and membranes produce protein and steroid hormones that regulate the reproductive axis, stress responses, maternal metabolism, fetal growth, and angiogenesis throughout gestation.
2. The placenta produces many of the same hormones that are secreted by other organs, but the role of these hormones differs in the pregnant compared to the nonpregnant state.
3. There is little known about the molecular regulation of placental hormones, and this is an area of interest for translational research.
4. Placental hormones are influenced by hypoxia, hyperglycemia, and poor nutrition. The result of these stimuli is alteration of the fetal hypothalamic–pituitary–adrenal axis and the insulin-signaling pathways. In utero stress affects not only fetal outcomes but also adult disease. Imprinting and epigenetic modifications of placental genes affect fetal growth restriction and preeclampsia, and influence the development of diabetes and obesity in later life.
5. Measurement of placental hormone levels in maternal blood contributes to risk assessment in prenatal screening for fetal aneuploidy.

References

1. Kurtzman JT, Wilson H, and Rao CV (2001) A proposed role for hCG in clinical obstetrics. *Seminars in Reproductive Medicine* 19: 63–8.
2. Reis FM, Florio P, Cobellis L et al. (2001) Human placenta as a source of neuroendocrine factors. *Biology of the Neonate* 79: 150–6.
3. Kallen CB (2004) Steroid hormone synthesis in pregnancy. *Obstetrics in Gynecology Clinics of North America* 31: 795–816.

4. Florio P, Luisi S, Ciarmela P et al. (2004) Inhibins and activins in pregnancy. *Molecular and Cellular Endocrinology* 225: 93–100.
5. Florio P, Severi FM, Ciarmela P et al. (2002) Placental stress factors and maternal–fetal adaptive response. *Endocrine* 19: 91–102.
6. Freemark M (2006) Regulation of maternal metabolism by pituitary and placental hormones: Roles in fetal development and metabolic programming. *Hormone Research* 65: 41–9.
7. Briana DD and Malamitsi-Puchner A (2009) Intrauterine growth restriction and adult disease: The role of adipocytokines. *European Journal of Endocrinology* 160: 337–47.
8. Gicquel C and Le Bouc Y (2006) Hormonal regulation of fetal growth. *Hormone Research* 65: 28–33.
9. Grill S, Rusterholz C, Zanetti-Dallenbach R et al. (2009) Potential markers of pre-eclampsia—A review. *Reproductive Biology and Endocrinology* 7: 70.
10. Page NM, Kemp CF, Butlin DJ et al. (2002) Placental peptides as markers of gestational disease. *Reproduction* 123: 487–95.
11. Gagnon A and Wilson RD (2008) Obstetrical complications associated with abnormal maternal serum markers analytes. *Journal of Obstetrics and Gynaecology Canada* 217: 918–32.

9

CHAPTER 9

Placental Transfer in Health and Disease

Caroline Wright and Colin P. Sibley

Maternal and Fetal Health Research Centre, School of Biomedicine and Manchester Academic Health Sciences Centre, University of Manchester, St. Mary's Hospital, Manchester, UK

Introduction

The placenta provides the major route by which all nutrients, ions, gases, water, and other compounds are transferred to the fetus and by which waste products are removed. This organ, therefore, is of fundamental importance for both fetal growth and health. No longer deemed a passive conduit to the fetus, the placenta regulates nutrient transfer, and several aspects of placental structure and function are altered in disease conditions. These are particularly apparent with disorders of fetal growth, both intrauterine growth restriction (IUGR), where a fetus fails to achieve genetic growth potential, and macrosomia, where fetal overgrowth exceeds endogenous genetic growth potential.

Absolute fetal growth rate changes with gestation, very slow in the first trimester and accelerating in the third trimester. The transfer capacity of the placenta accommodates this growth. Changes in transfer capacity are not explained by placental growth alone as macroscopic villous expansion is highest in the first trimester and slows toward term. The increased demands are instead met by one or more of the following: (1) alterations in blood flow into or within the placenta; (2) altered dimensions of the exchange barrier and availability, activity, or both of transporter proteins in the plasma membrane; or (3) alterations in the hydrostatic, osmotic, and electrical gradients and ATP supply of energy for active transport.

In this chapter, we discuss the interaction of these components in the physiology of the healthy placenta and the changes that occur in fetal growth restriction and overgrowth. We underscore the adaptability of the placenta to meet changing fetal demands and to regulate nutrient transfer.

Physiology of placental transfer

A model of placental transfer

Placental transfer can be conceptualized as a three-compartment model consisting of two blood pools separated by the placental exchange barrier. Transfer can occur in two directions: from maternal to fetal blood or fetal to maternal circulations. The net transfer, or flux, of any substance is the arithmetical difference between two unidirectional fluxes. Flux may thus be in either direction depending on concentration, electrical gradients, asymmetric distribution of transporters, and ability to utilize ATP, among other factors that affect the rate of transfer (Figure 9.1).

Extrapolating from Fick's law of diffusion, the placental capacity for diffusional exchange is directly related to the exchange surface area (which increases with gestation involving expansion of villi, formation of terminal villi, and increased number of microvilli on the intervillous space facing membrane (MVM) of the syncytiotrophoblast) and

The Placenta: From Development to Disease, First Edition. Edited by Helen H. Kay, D. Michael Nelson and Yuping Wang.
© 2011 Blackwell Publishing Ltd. Published 2011 by Blackwell Publishing Ltd.

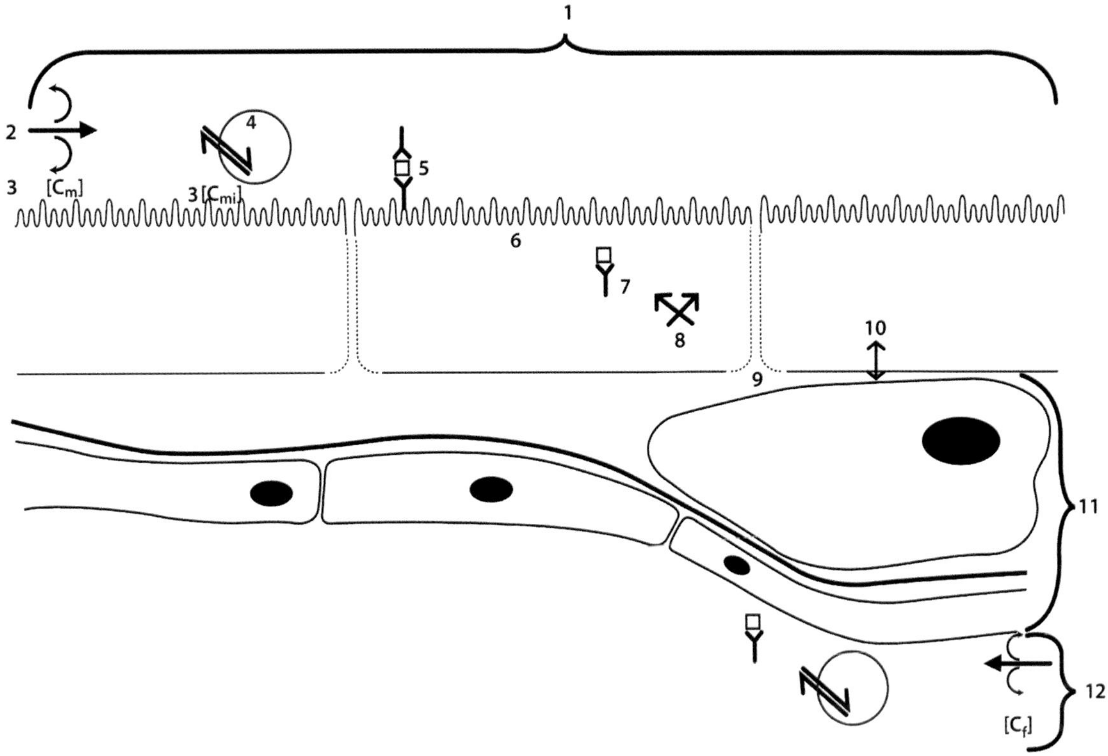

Figure 9.1 Elements contributing to transfer rates in either direction across the placenta. 1. Exchange barrier surface area. 2. Blood flow rate and geometry of flow. 3. Concentration gradients both in whole blood and in unstirred water layer adjacent to microvillous membrane. 4. Transfer rate between erythrocyte and plasma (e. g., respiratory gases). 5. Transfer rate for bound solutes between plasma carrier and membrane receptor and release from membrane receptor. 6. Transfer mechanisms and rate across MVM into syncytiosol. 7. Binding proteins involved in transfer across syncytiosol. 8. Intraplacental metabolic interconversion or catabolism. 9. Aqueous paracyncytial channel pathway. 10. Transporter mechanisms in the BM. 11. Transfer across villous core, cytotrophoblast layer when present, basal lamina, and fetal capillary epithelium. 12. Transfer between placenta and fetal blood combining elements similar to 1–5 above.

is inversely proportional to the thickness of the exchange barrier, which decreases through gestation. Studies in mice demonstrate increased diffusional permeability of inert tracers with increasing gestation and with corresponding alterations in placental dimensions [1]. Similar studies have not been done in humans.

The flow of blood on either side of the exchange barrier enables the delivery, or removal, of a substance. Small lipophilic permeants pass rapidly across the placenta, and transfer rate is therefore dependent upon blood flow, or *flow limited*. Larger hydrophilic permeants transfer slower, are limited by barrier permeability, and are thus described as *diffusion limited*. Therefore, reductions in uterine and umbilical blood flow, as described in IUGR, reduce maternofetal exchange of lipophillic solutes, such as O_2 and CO_2, but will have little effect on the transfer of hydrophilic solutes. By contrast, changes in placental exchange barrier dimensions will have a much greater effect on transfer of hydrophilic solutes such as glucose and amino acids. Such changes occur in IUGR. Transplacental transfer of ions and hydrophilic nutrients occurs by paracellular diffusion (see below) or by a transcellular route, utilizing transporter proteins or endocytosis–exocytosis.

The placenta is permeable to hydrophilic molecules for which no specific transport system has been identified, e. g., creatinine, inulin, and horseradish peroxidise. Permeability to such solutes is not saturable nor is competitively inhibited, suggesting that specific transporters are not involved. The simplest explanation is the existence of extracellular, water-filled, *paracellular* channels that might be formed by syncytiotrophoblastic denudations [2]. Quantitatively, the paracellular route is important for some substances (e. g., calcium and chloride ions) but qualitatively, the *transcellular* route allows fine tuning of maternofetal exchange. Transporter-mediated transfer is likely key, considering the alterations in transporter availability and behavior across gestation. For example, an increase in both the System A amino acid transporter activity for small neutral amino acids and GLUT 1 glucose transporter protein expression is seen towards term.

Electrochemical gradients and polarization of the syncytiotrophoblast

For many nutrients required by the fetus, the fetal plasma concentration is greater than the maternal concentration, suggesting an active transport process. For ions, there is a balancing of both electrical and chemical gradients. The magnitude and polarity of the electrical potential difference (PD) across the placental exchange barrier is controversial, and its measurement poses a number of technical challenges. Further investigation is needed, as the PD is crucial for the transfer of both ions and ion-dependent transport (e. g., sodium coupled amino acid transporters).

Research Spotlight

The only direct microelectrode measurement of human term transplacental PD in vitro yielded −6 mV with the fetus negative. This is small compared to equivalent PDs in other epithelia [3].

Vectorial transfer across an epithelium is usually enabled by the electrochemical gradients, by the localization of transporter proteins on either MVM or basal fetal facing plasma membranes (BM), or both. The syncytiotrophoblast is a true syncytium, and there is a lack of research into how alterations in the location of these transporters and the gradient shifts caused by the mislocations can affect the pathophysiology of diseases. It is noteworthy in this regard that the syncytiotrophoblast Na^+/K^+ATPase is located to the MVM of the syncytiotrophoblast and expression is reduced in IUGR, which may affect ion gradients and activity of other transporters.

Transport of individual substances

Protein and amino acids

Transfer of protein is highly restricted in the placentas of all species. The exception is IgG, which is transferred as immune complexes mediated by the neonatal Fc immunoglobulin receptor, FcRn. Therefore, the placenta is able to maintain fetal plasma concentrations of albumin at 0.1% of maternal plasma concentrations and maternal plasma concentrations of alpha-fetoprotein (AFP) at 0.2% of those in the fetal circulation. A quantitatively small paracellular route is still available for some proteins such as AFP.

Research Spotlight

In the perfused human cotyledon, AFP can be localized to fibrin-containing fibroid deposits, which are known to fill the syncytiotrophblast denudations, suggesting these form a paracellular route of transfer for this large protein [2].

The supply of essential amino acids is key to normal fetal development, and several nonessential amino acids become essential during pregnancy as demand is greater than the ability of the fetus to synthesize them. Transport of amino acids across the human placenta is generally an active process associated with amino acid concentrations in the fetal circulation significantly higher than those in maternal plasma. A multitude of amino acid transporters have now been identified in the placenta. On the MVM, the System A amino acid transporter family transports small neutral amino acids such as glycine and serine and is sodium dependent, utilizing the sodium gradient into the cell maintained by Na^+/K^+ATPase. System A accumulates amino acids in the syncytiotrophoblast that may then be used in energizing transfer of other amino acids via exchange transporters. Transport across the BM is less well understood; both accumulative transporters and amino acid exchangers are present, but neither can drive a net transfer of amino acids to the fetus. This suggests that other transport systems must be present. This is an area of current research.

Glucose

Glucose is essential for the development of the human fetus, and the demand for this substrate is high; in early gestation, there is a lack of fetal gluconeogenesis and towards term the rapid fetal growth significantly increases requirements. Glucose concentrations are lower in the fetal plasma than maternal plasma, and there is strong evidence for transporter-mediated facilitated diffusion down this concentration gradient.

The transfer of glucose is saturable at supraphysiological levels. It is stereo specific and independent of energy sources and sodium, i.e., supporting facilitated diffusion as the mechanism for transfer. A family of 12 facilitated diffusion transport proteins has been identified in mammalian tissues (the GLUT family). GLUT 1 is the predominant isoform expressed in the term human placenta although the importance of the various transporters may alter with gestation, as GLUT 3 protein has been found in first trimester tissue.

Lipids

Marked changes in lipid metabolism occur during pregnancy. Whilst maternal body fat accumulation occurs early in gestation, later in gestation, a more catabolic state develops, providing fatty acids for placental transfer. Maternal plasma lipoproteins can be taken up by the placenta via lipoprotein or other scavenger receptors. Lipoprotein triglycerides may also be hydrolyzed by placental lipases, mainly lipoprotein lipase, localized in the MVM [4]. Free fatty acids are released by this process and diffuse across the plasma membrane. Transfer of nonesterified fatty acids is facilitated by a transporter-mediated mechanism involving plasma membrane fatty acid binding proteins, fatty acid translocase, and a family of fatty acid transport proteins. The precise mechanism of transmembrane passage of fatty acids is still a matter of speculation [5].

Clinical Pearl

Transfer of ketone bodies may become important when there is maternal hyperketonemia, such as during fasting, a high-fat diet, or diabetes. Placental transfer is efficient and may contribute towards fetal lipogenesis, but very high levels may also be toxic to the fetus.

Ions

Sodium

The plasma sodium concentration of the fetus is probably greater than the mother. This cation crosses the placenta both by diffusion through a paracellular route down an electrical gradient and by a transcellular route. The latter is suggested by data that show placental permeability to sodium is greater than would be expected from its diffusion coefficient in water and by the identification of a number of sodium transporters in the human placenta, including the Na^+/H^+ exchanger and Na^+/K^+ ATPase.

Research Spotlight

In human placentas, Na^+/K^+ATPase is predominantly in the MVM [6] rather than the BM. We would predict this ATPase to be in the BM if functioning to pump Na^+ out of the syncytiotrophoblast towards the fetus.

Potassium

Studies into the potassium gradient across the placenta give conflicting results, possibly due to difficulties in measurements as post sampling leakage of the cation occurs from erythrocytes. Transport of potassium in the guinea pig and rat has been demonstrated to be ouabain inhibitable, supporting a transport-mediated process, although this has not been demonstrated in the human placenta. A variety of potassium channels have been identified in human syncytiotrophoblast and cytotrophoblast cells. Although their involvement in placental transfer is not clear, other important functions have been identified, such as the regulation of trophoblast hCG secretion.

Calcium

Total and ionized concentrations of calcium are higher in fetal plasma than maternal plasma in humans. Perfusion experiments with the human placenta show calcium is transported up a concentration gradient and is reduced by inhibitors of metabolism such as cyanide addition or lowering of perfusate temperature. Transporter-mediated active transfer of calcium is therefore a dominant mechanism with the following components. A family of epithelial calcium channels (TRPV5 and TRPV6) is expressed in the placenta and may assist diffusion of calcium down its electrical and concentration gradient from maternal plasma across the MVM into the syncytiotrophoblast. Translocation of calcium across the cytoplasm of the syncytiotrophoblast is achieved by binding to specific proteins, including calbindin-D9 k. On the BM, calcium is transported into fetal extracellular fluid, against its concentration gradient, via Ca^{2+} ATPase–the calcium pump. In studies on isolated BM in vitro, the activity of this transporter increases with gestation in the third trimester, consistent with the increasing demands of the fetus for bone mineralization.

Placental transfer in IUGR

Placental insufficiency is a major cause of human IUGR and accumulating evidence shows that several aspects of placental structure and function are altered, yielding different placental phenotypes. Along with the well-documented alterations in maternal and fetal blood flows in IUGR described by uterine and umbilical Doppler ultrasound measurements, there are changes in the structural variables of the exchange barrier. There is also an ever growing wealth of literature describing a variety of changes in transporter expression and activity. Moreover, these findings relate to preeclampsia, as crossover between these two conditions is well known. Despite this, the placental changes occurring in preeclampsia are often quite different from those in IUGR, even in the presence of a small fetus, supporting differential pathophysiologies.

Research Spotlight

In IUGR, the surface area of the villi and fetal capillaries are significantly reduced [7]. Despite the degree of crossover between IUGR and preeclampsia, these changes are attributable to IUGR when seen in isolation, further supporting differential disease processes [8].

Whether the alterations in placental structure and function seen in IUGR are cause or effect is a difficult issue to answer, but studies from a knockout mouse model, in which the placental-specific transcript of the insulin-like growth factor 2 gene (*Igf2*) was deleted, suggest the former. The altered placental phenotype in mutant mice pregnancies, similar to that seen in human IUGR, was found to precede a decline in fetal growth. Undernutrition in the rat also leads to an altered placental phenotype prior to fetal growth decline.

Research Spotlight

Knockout of the placental-specific transcript of *Igf2* in the mouse leads to a decrease in placental weight with a reduced exchange surface area, an increase in the estimated harmonic mean thicknesses of the barrier, and a strongly correlated decrease in permeability to diffusional markers, as well as fetuses that are 30% smaller than wild type [12]. Furthermore, placental growth restriction occurs at day 14 onwards (term is day 20), but fetal growth restriction does not occur until around day 18 or 19 [9].

The reasons for this delay between placental growth restriction and that of the fetus may be due to a delayed reduction in the diffusional permeability of the mutant placentas to hydrophilic molecules. This effect arises from the altered placental morphology *and* from changes in placental transporter activity or expression in the mutants (see Research spotlight below).

Alterations in specific transporter mechanisms occur in association with human IUGR, as summarized in Table 9.1. General impairment of amino acid transport associates with suboptimal fetal growth and reduced fetal plasma levels of amino acids are seen in IUGR.

Research Spotlight

In IUGR, the activity of the System A amino acid transporter in the placenta is markedly reduced and in the most severe cases of IUGR, as determined by abnormal umbilical artery Doppler and fetal heart tracings, the most profound reductions are seen in System A activity [11].

Interestingly, some placental transporter activities (e.g., System A) go down in IUGR, whereas the Ca^{2+}ATPase increases. The decrease in System A may

Table 9.1 Change in the activity of transporter proteins in syncytiotrophoblast microvillous (MVM) and basal (BM) plasma membranes in IUGR. (Adapted from [10].)

Transporter	MVM Change	BM Change
System A (alanine/glycine)	Decrease	No change
Leucine	Decrease	Decrease
Lysine	No change	Decrease
Na^+-dependent taurine	Decrease	No change
Na^+-independent taurine	No change	Decrease
GLUT1 (glucose)	No change	No change
Na^+/K^+-ATPase	Decrease	No change
$Ca2^+$ (ATP dependent)	(not present)	Increase
Na^+/H^+ exchanger	Decrease	Activity not present
Lipoprotein lipase (cf. FFA transport)	Decrease	Not known
H^+/lactate transporter	No change	Decrease

be causative to IUGR. The increase in Ca^{2+}ATPase may be adaptive to the IUGR: placental supply adapting to specific signals from the fetus.

Research Spotlight

In the *Igf2* knockout mouse model, maternofetal transfer of [14 C]methylaminoisobutyric acid (MeAIB,a specific nonmetabolizable substrate of System A), measured in vivo, was increased by 50% per unit weight of placenta, in the knockout mice at day 16. By day 19, [14 C]MeAIB transfer was similar in knockout and wild-type pups. These data suggest that System A activity in the placenta can be upregulated to increase placental efficiency. However, this upregulation may not be sustainable, so that fetal growth restriction finally ensues [1]. Furthermore, in the same model, fetal calcium accumulation in the fetus of the knockout is reduced but transfer is then upregulated with increased expression of calbindin-9 kd so that fetal calcium content is normal by term [13]. These data indicate that the placenta adapts to fetal growth requirements in this model.

Further evidence for compensatory mechanisms comes from a study of System A transport in the MVM of human placentas from babies across the range of normal birth weights where activity was found to be highest in the smallest babies [14]. This contrasts with IUGR, where downregulation of System A is seen.

Low birth weight infants are often found to be hypoglycemic at birth and may have ongoing problems normalizing glucose levels in the neonatal period. The reasons for this are not entirely clear. Fetal hypoglycemia in IUGR is unlikely to be due to altered placental GLUT 1 function, as protein expression and transport activity are unaltered. The impact of other members of the GLUT family has not been fully established (see Table 9.1).

Lipoprotein lipase is crucial for the process of fatty acid release from lipoproteins to the fetus. Interestingly, the activity of this lipase is reduced in IUGR, in keeping with the altered maternal/fetal lipid ratios also found in the condition (Table 9.1).

Na^+/K^+ATPase activity and expression is decreased in the MVM in IUGR, which may result in a reduced driving force for a range of Na^+-dependent transport mechanisms. The activity and expression of the Na^+/H^+ exchanger (NHE), the primary pH regulating transporter in the syncytiotrophoblast, is reduced in association with IUGR, which could contribute towards acidosis in these fetuses. Note that the activity of a lactate transporter on the BM is also reduced, perhaps contributing further to the fetal acidosis (Table 9.1).

Placental transfer in fetal overgrowth and diabetes

Fetal overgrowth in pregnancies complicated by diabetes is generally thought to be the result of an increased substrate availability, which stimulates fetal insulin secretion and fetal growth. The emphasis in clinical management is therefore rigorous glycemic control. However, despite effective management, macrosomia still occurs and is often unpredictable. Recent studies in vivo provide evidence for increased delivery of some nutrients to the fetus in diabetic states even when metabolic control is strict. For example, umbilical delivery of amino acids is significantly increased even in well-controlled gestational diabetic pregnancies (GDM). These findings suggest that increased maternal substrate levels found in diabetes are insufficient to explain fetal overgrowth, and other mechanisms, such as the upregulation of placental transporters and alterations in placental morphology, contribute to the increased substrate supply.

Research Spotlight

Diabetic pregnancies have placentas with varying degrees of immaturity, with oedema of the stromal villi and focal fibrinoid necrosis. In type-I diabetes, placental weight and volume is increased compared to normals. There is significant reduction in the diffusing capacity of the placenta in diabetic groups, with both an increase in exchange barrier surface area and an increase in barrier thickness seen in association with macrosomia [15].

Mechanisms other than changes in placental morphology are important to the increased nutrient transfer seen in fetal overgrowth. In type-I diabetes, increased expression of the glucose transporter GLUT 1 is seen at the BM, which is the rate limiting step in transfer. GDM with fetal overgrowth, however, is not associated with these changes. Data on the activity of the System A transporter in placentas from diabetic pregnancies are conflicting, with reports of both down- and upregulation. This most likely arises from different phenotypes of the study population. Other nutrient transport systems such as those associated with transplacental calcium (Ca^{2+} ATPase on the BM) and lipid transfer (lipoprotein lipase on the MVM) also show alterations in type-I diabetes but not GDM.

Other mechanisms important in health and disease

There are many other examples of how placental transfer relates importantly to fetal health and disease. Obesity in pregnancy, in the absence of diabetes, is a rapidly increasing problem and is associated with complications such as preeclampsia and fetal overgrowth. There is now preliminary evidence that the latter is associated with alterations in placental transporter expression.

Transplacental transport of maternal IgG to the developing fetus is extremely important in the protection of the newborn from infection. Although the exact mechanisms of the selective and active transfer of IgG across the placental barrier are not fully understood, receptors for the Fc part of IgG (FcgammaRs) in the placenta are believed to play a key role.

Clinical Pearl

In autoimmune thyroid diseases immunoglobulins and goitrogenic drugs can cross the placenta and affect the fetal thyroid. Therefore, careful monitoring of thyroid function, before and during pregnancy, and avoidance of unnecessary drugs are mandatory for optimal fetal growth and development.

Placental transfer can be useful diagnostically. Measurement of AFP in the maternal serum (MS-AFP), is important in antenatal screening for a variety of pregnancy conditions. In the absence of neural tube defects, MS-AFP likely enters the maternal circulation through denudations of the syncytiotrophoblast layer on placental villi. MS-AFP is raised in IUGR and in association with placental infarcts and sonolucencies detected by ultrasound. Interestingly, Toal et al. recently demonstrated placentas with abnormal ultrasound morphology, defined as depth >50% length in the second trimester, had an increased association with IUGR [16] and raised MS-AFP.

Control mechanisms for placental transfer

Our understanding of placental transfer mechanisms remains incomplete but the placenta is able to adapt to changes in the environment. For example, altered substrate levels in the maternal or fetal microcirculations are accompanied by changes in transport functions to coordinate with maternal nutrient or ion availability and fetal demand. Therefore, factors such as malnutrition, reduced blood flow, or hypoxemia may impact upon these regulatory mechanisms and as a consequence be up- or downregulated. Examples of this include the reduction in the expression of System A amino acid transporter, increase in glucose transporters in cultured term trophoblasts during hypoxia, and the effect of metabolic hormones such as insulin, IGF-1, and leptin on nutrient transporters. Disease states such as IUGR and fetal overgrowth may in fact be due to a loss of normal placental sensing of substrates and compensatory up- or downregulation. The patterns seen in the placental specific *Igf2* knockout mice discussed above support this premise.

Excitingly, another candidate "regulator" of transport mechanisms has recently been postulated. mTOR (mammalian target of rampamycin) is a serine threonine kinase and represents an important nutrient sensing pathway in mammalian cells. mTOR is highly expressed in the cytosol of the syncytiotrophoblast and activity is downregulated in IUGR. Although much further research is required, such findings could eventually provide therapeutic targets for use in fetal conditions.

Conclusions

These accumulated observations enable us to describe a series of structural and functional alterations in the placenta that are specific to fetal conditions, even when accepting that groups included in studies may be heterogeneous. Further exploration of these abnormalities together could provide better information on the placental phenotype, allowing more rigorous definitions of conditions such as IUGR and fetal overgrowth and providing better biomarkers for use in clinical practice to identify and diagnose these conditions.

Teaching Points

1 Placental transfer capacity is dependent upon a combination of elements including blood flow in the uterine and umbilical circulations, dimensions of the placental exchange barrier, transport protein activity and expression, and the driving forces across the placenta.

2 The transfer of small lipophilic permeants is "flow limited" and will be affected by alterations in blood flow, whereas transfer of large hydrophilic permeants is "diffusion limited" and will be more affected by changes such as altered exchange barrier dimensions.

3 Differences in exchange barrier dimensions and a range of alterations in transporter activity and expression have been observed in IUGR and fetal overgrowth, both of which are likely to affect nutrient transfer to the fetus in these conditions.

4 Research using mouse knockouts of the placental-specific transcript of *Igf2* gene demonstrated a link between altered exchange barrier dimensions, reduced placental transfer, and IUGR, which seemed causal–restriction of placental size preceded fetal growth restriction.

5 Evidence for placental adaptation to nutrient demand signals was also seen in this model, with improved placental efficiency when placental size is reduced. This adaptability is also supported by studies in the human placenta, where increased amino acid transport occurs in small-for-gestational age babies, but not in frank IUGR, suggesting the initial compensatory mechanism keeps birth weights within a normal range.

6 Alterations in placental transfer differ among the phenotypes for fetal disease. For example, there are differences between macrosomia with type-1 diabetes as compared to macrosomia with gestational diabetes, or small-for-gestational age compared with pregnancies with truly growth-restricted fetuses. These are likely to represent specific *placental phenotypes* that reflect the different etiologies of the fetal conditions.

Acknowledgements

Caroline Wright is funded by a Wellcome Trust Research Training Fellowship. Work in our laboratory is supported by the NIHR Manchester Biomedical Research Centre.

References

1. Sibley CP, Coan PM, Ferguson-Smith AC et al. (2004) Placental-specific insulin-like growth factor 2 (IGF2) regulates the diffusional exchange characteristics of the mouse placenta. *Proceedings of the National Academy of Sciences of the United States of America* 101 (21): 8204–8.
2. Brownbill P, Edwards D, Jones C et al. (1995) Mechanisms of alphafetoprotein transfer in the perfused human placental cotyledon from uncomplicated pregnancy. *The Journal of Clinical Investigation* 96 (5): 2220–6.
3. Greenwood SL, Boyd RD, and Sibley CP (1993) Transtrophoblast and microvillus membrane potential difference in mature intermediate human placental villi. *The American Journal of Physiology* 265 (2 Pt 1): C460–6.
4. Lindegaard ML, Olivecrona G, Christoffersen C et al. (2005) Endothelial and lipoprotein lipases in human and mouse placenta. *Journal of Lipid Research* 46 (11): 2339–46.
5. Haggarty P, Abramovich DR, and Page K (2002) The effect of maternal smoking and ethanol on fatty acid transport by the human placenta. *The British Journal of Nutrition* 87 (3): 247–52.
6. Johansson M, Jansson T, and Powell TL (2000) Na(+)-K(+)-ATPase is distributed to microvillous and basal membrane of the syncytiotrophoblast in human placenta. *American Journal of Physiology* 279 (1): R287–94.
7. Mayhew TM, Manwani R, Ohadike C et al. (2007) The placenta in pre-eclampsia and intrauterine growth restriction: Studies on exchange surface areas, diffusion distances and villous membrane diffusive conductances. *Placenta* 28 (2–3): 233–8.
8. Daayana S, Baker P, and Crocker I. (2004) An image analysis technique for the investigation of variations in placental morphology in pregnancies complicated by preeclampsia with and without intrauterine growth restriction. *Journal of the Society for Gynecologic Investigation* 11 (8): 545–52.
9. Constancia M, Angiolini E, Sandovici I et al. (2005) Adaptation of nutrient supply to fetal demand in the mouse involves interaction between the IGF2 gene and placental transporter systems. *Proceedings of the National Academy of Sciences of the United States of America* 102 (52): 19219–24.
10. Sibley CP (2009) Understanding placental nutrient transfer–Why bother? New biomarkers of fetal growth. *Journal of Physiology* 587 (14): 3431–40.
11. Glazier JD, Cetin I, Perugino G, et al. (1997) Association between the activity of the system A amino acid transporter in the microvillous plasma membrane of the human placenta and severity of fetal compromise in intrauterine growth restriction. *Pediatric Research* 42 (4): 514–9.

12. Constancia M, Hemberger M, Hughes J et al. (2002) Placental-specific IGF-II is a major modulator of placental and fetal growth. *Nature* 417 (6892): 945–8.
13. Dilworth MR, Kusinski LC, Cowley E et al. (2010) Placental-specific IGF2 knockout mice exhibit hypocalcemia and adaptive changes in placental calcium transport. *Proceedings of the National Academy of Sciences of the United States of America* 107 (8): 3894–9.
14. Godfrey KM (1998) Maternal regulation of fetal development and health in adult life. *European Journal of Obstetrics, Gynecology, and Reproductive Biology* 78 (2): 141–50.
15. Jauniaux E and Burton GJ (2006) Villous histomorphometry and placental bed biopsy investigation in Type I diabetic pregnancies. *Placenta* 27 (4–5): 468–74.
16. Toal M, Keating S, Machin G et al. (2008) Determinants of adverse perinatal outcome in high-risk women with abnormal uterine artery Doppler images. *American Journal of Obstetrics Gynecology* 198 (3): 330 e1–7.

10

CHAPTER 10
Placental Fat Trafficking

Christina Scifres and Yoel Sadovsky
Magee-Womens Research Institute, Department of Obstetrics, Gynecology, and Reproductive Sciences, University of Pittsburgh, Pittsburgh, PA, USA

Introduction

Fatty acids are necessary for fetal development [1]. Humans cannot synthesize fatty acids with double bonds three (n-3 or ω-3) or six (n-6 or ω-6) carbons from the methyl terminus, and therefore, these fatty acids must be obtained from the diet. Examples include the n-6 linoleic acid (LA) and n-3 α-linoleic acid (ALA), also known as the essential fatty acids, and their long-chain polyunsaturated fatty acid (LCPUFA) derivatives such as arachidonic acid (AA), eicosapentaenoic acid (EPA), and docosahexaenoic acid (DHA).

In addition to their role as membrane building blocks, regulators of gene expression, and a source of energy, fatty acids are also the precursors of eicosanoids, such as prostaglandins, prostacyclins, thromboxanes, and leukotrienes. These signaling molecules regulate diverse physiological and pathological processes, including gene expression, cell differentiation, immunity, and inflammation. The fatty acids AA and DHA are also important structural components of the nervous system, and inadequate supply of these fatty acids from the mother may be associated with cognitive dysfunction. Transport of fatty acids is highest during the second half of pregnancy, which corresponds to the period of rapid in utero fetal growth and adipose tissue accumulation.

Sterols (e. g., cholesterol) play an essential role in eukaryotic cells [2]. Sterols are precursors for steroid hormones and bile salts. Cholesterol is particularly important during organogenesis, where it governs organ pattern formation via activation of signaling pathways involving the hedgehog protein. Cholesterol is also required for cell mass expansion of the growing fetus and is an integral part of plasma and organelle membranes. Defects of cholesterol metabolism can have profound developmental consequences, such as congenital malformations and learning defects associated with Smith-Lemli-Opitz syndrome, which results from an inability to convert 7-dehydrocholesterol to cholesterol. Although the fetus is capable of synthesizing cholesterol, an exogenous supply is the major source of cholesterol for the developing fetus. In this review, we highlight key pathways in transplacental fat trafficking.

Sources of lipids for placental uptake

LCPUFA derivatives such as AA, DHA, and EPA are consumed by the mother in animal-derived foods. During early pregnancy, these lipids are stored in maternal adipose tissue. Triglycerides, low-density lipoprotein (LDL), cholesterol, and apolipoprotein B are significantly increased in maternal serum during pregnancy. In addition, enhanced lipid catabolism and accelerated breakdown of maternal fat depots occur during the second half of pregnancy in association with relative insulin resistance. These processes, along with hepatic overproduction of triglycerides and elevated postprandial levels of free fatty acid, contribute to increased levels of maternal serum lipids, which are available for transplacental transport to the fetus.

The Placenta: From Development to Disease, First Edition. Edited by Helen H. Kay, D. Michael Nelson and Yuping Wang.
© 2011 Blackwell Publishing Ltd. Published 2011 by Blackwell Publishing Ltd.

Lipid uptake and trafficking in trophoblasts

Substances that are transferred from the maternal to the fetal circulation must cross the villous trophoblast layer that consists of a microvillous membrane facing the maternal circulation and a basal membrane facing the fetal capillary endothelial cells (Figure 10.1). Maternal plasma lipoproteins do not directly cross the placental barrier in significant quantity. Instead, the syncytiotrophoblasts' microvillous membranes express a placenta-specific hydrolase and a lipoprotein lipase, which hydrolyze triglycerides and release them from LDLs and very low density lipoproteins [3]. The activity of trophoblastic lipoprotein lipase increases threefold during pregnancy to meet fetal needs.

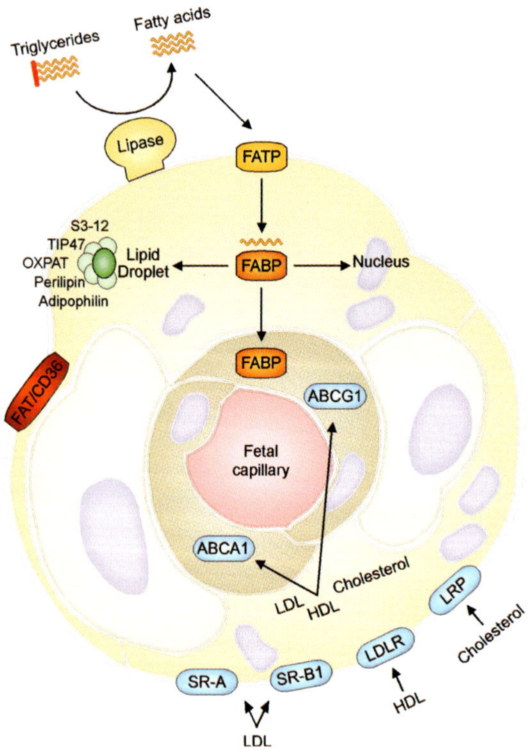

Figure 10.1 Lipid trafficking within placental villi. Triglycerides are cleaved by lipases at the maternal surface of the placenta. Fatty acids are taken up into cells by fatty acid transport proteins (FATPs). These fatty acids are then carried and directed by fatty acid binding proteins (FABPs) to intracellular targets, such as lipid droplets or the nucleus, or shuttled to the fetal circulation. Cholesterol uptake into the syncytiotrophoblast is mediated by LDL receptors (LDLR), LDL-receptor related proteins (LRP), scavenger receptor A (SR-A), and HDL-binding scavenger receptors B1 (SR-B1). ATP-binding cassette (ABC) transporters ABCG1 and ABCA1 mediate cholesterol efflux from fetal capillaries to the fetal circulation.

Clinical Pearl

Regulation of trophoblast lipoprotein lipase is linked to conditions associated with abnormal fetal growth. Indeed, the activity of placental lipoprotein lipase activity is reduced by 47% in preterm intrauterine growth restriction, whereas in diabetic pregnancies, which are commonly associated with fetal overgrowth, the activity of placental lipoprotein lipase is increased by 39% when compared with controls [4].

Fatty acids are unevenly distributed between the maternal and fetal compartments, suggesting that fatty acid transfer across the placenta is highly regulated. For example, LA represents about 10% of the total fatty acids in umbilical cord plasma compared with 30% in maternal plasma, and concentrations of ALA in cord plasma are half of those in maternal plasma. In contrast, AA represents 10% of the total fatty acids in umbilical cord plasma but only 5% in maternal plasma, and concentrations of DHA in umbilical cord plasma are twice those in maternal plasma. Although the precise mechanisms that govern fatty acid transport are unknown, these data suggest that fatty acids are selectively transferred via protein-mediated mechanisms, with passive diffusion playing a minor role. Relevant protein families are described below.

The fatty acid transport proteins (FATPs) are important regulators of cellular fatty acid uptake. The FATPs are a family of integral transmembrane proteins consisting of six identified members that exhibit tissue-specific expression patterns. The FATPs regulate fatty acid transport, and overexpression of these proteins increases the rate of fatty acid internalization, most notably at low concentrations when diffusion is insignificant. FATP1–4 and FATP6 are expressed in the placenta, with subtype-specific expression in the microvillous and basal membranes.

Research Spotlight

The function of placental FATPs remains to be established. FATP4 is expressed in murine trophoblasts and yolk sac. FATP4-null mice exhibit increased midgestation lethality. These data suggest a role for FATP4 in fat absorption during early embryogenesis.

FAT/CD36 is a heavily glycosylated integral membrane protein that is expressed on the cell surface and binds diverse lipids, including oxidized LDLs, lipoproteins, and long-chain fatty acids. FAT/CD36 facilitates the transport of fatty acids, and its activity has been implicated in angiogenesis, atherosclerosis, inflammation, and lipid metabolism. FAT/CD36 expression has been demonstrated in both the microvillous and basolateral membranes of the placenta using both pure trophoblasts and placental membrane preparations [3].

Fatty acid binding proteins (FABPs) play an important role in intracellular transport of fatty acids within the hydrophilic cytoplasm. FABPs are relatively small (14–15 kD) and abundantly expressed proteins that reversibly bind hydrophobic molecules such as saturated and unsaturated fatty acids, eicosanoids, and other lipids. The expression level of FABPs is particularly high in cells that have a large lipid-metabolizing capacity such as hepatocytes, adipocytes, and cardiac myocytes. The main function of these proteins is to import, store, and export fatty acids in cells. FABPs may also transport fatty acids to the nucleus to regulate gene expression [5]. Although little is known about the specific function of FABPs in the placenta, FABP1, -3, -4, -5, and -7 are expressed in the human placenta and in cultured trophoblasts (Figure 10.2). Expression of FABP1, -3, and -4 is upregulated in hypoxic trophoblasts, suggesting that FABPs may support fat accumulation in the hypoxic placenta. FABP pm is expressed at the microvillous plasma membrane and thereby can preferentially bind and facilitate the uptake of selected fatty acids. Blocking of FABPpm causes a reduction in DHA and AA uptake.

In humans, cholesterol crosses from the maternal to the fetal blood through the villous trophoblasts and endothelial cells. Cultured trophoblasts express LDL receptors (LDLR), LDL receptor-related proteins (LRP), scavenger receptors A (SR-A), and HDL (high-density lipoprotein)-binding scavenger receptors BP (SR-B1) on their microvillous membrane. Cholesterol is taken up by trophoblasts via internalization of receptor-bound apoB- or apoE-carrying lipoproteins and oxidized LDL, and from SR-B1-bound HDL. It is subsequently released on the basolateral side. The precise mechanisms regulating cholesterol transport within trophoblasts are largely unknown; whether placental endothelial cells are able to transport cholesterol to the fetal microcirculation is also unknown [2].

The ATP-binding cassette transporters, ABCA1 and ABCG1, are regulators of cholesterol efflux that are predominantly localized to the microvillous surface of human placental endothelial cells. Activation of the liver X receptor (LXR) increases the expression of ABCA1 and ABCG1 and enhances cholesterol efflux from human placental endothelial cells. Inhibition of either ABCA1 or

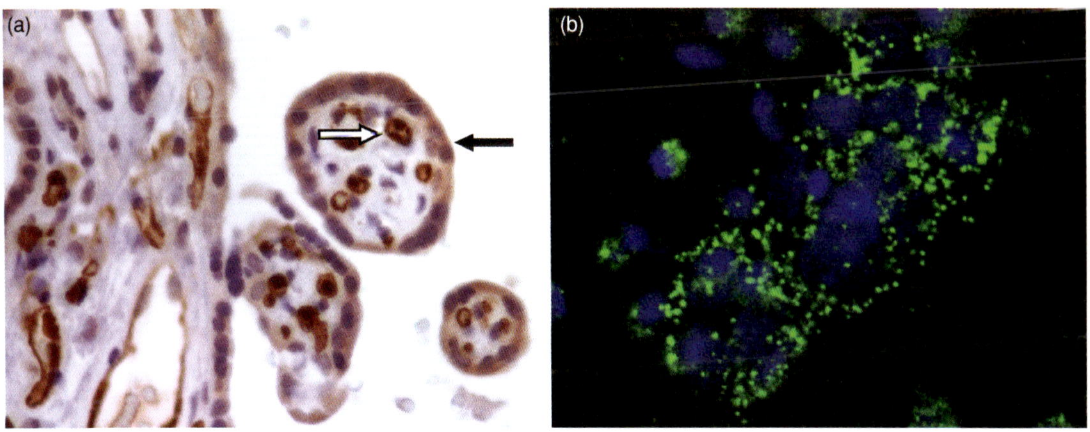

Figure 10.2 FABP4 expression and lipid droplets in human placental trophoblasts. (a) Immunohistochemistry of human placental villi demonstrates FABP4 expression in the syncytiotrophoblast layer (black arrow) and the fetal capillary endothelium (white arrow) within villi (40× magnification). (b) Lipid droplets (green) in cultured primary human trophoblasts are detected using fluorescence from BODIPY fluorophore 493/503, and nuclei (blue) are detected using DAPI.

ABCG1 diminishes cholesterol efflux and fetal lipoprotein levels. These results suggest that human placental endothelial cells contribute to mature lipoproteins in the fetal blood [6].

Placental lipid droplets

Eukaryotic cells store variable amounts of lipid intracellularly in structures commonly referred to as lipid droplets (Figure 10.2). These 1–100 μm droplets are formed in the endoplasmic reticulum and include a core of neutral lipids such as triglycerides, cholesterol esters, and retinol esters. This core is encased in a phospholipid monolayer and a coat of specific proteins, thus resembling the structure of plasma lipoproteins. While serving as a dynamic repository for energy, membrane phospholipids, and signaling molecules, the content of lipid droplets can be rapidly accessed via the activity of lipases and other associated proteins. By serving as a reservoir of bioactive lipids, these droplets protect cells from lipotoxicity [7].

Lipid droplets are associated with a group of conserved proteins termed PAT proteins, which are named after the three original members of the family: perilipin, adipophilin (adipose differentiation-related protein, ADRP), and tail-interacting protein 47 (TIP47). The group now includes additional members such as S3–12 and OXPAT. Perilipin is expressed primarily in adipocytes and steroid-producing cells and functions to control lipolysis. In its hypophosphorylated state, perilipin prevents lipases access to neutral lipid in the droplet core. Once phosphorylated, perilipin facilitates lipase action, in part by recruiting hormone-sensitive lipase to the droplet surface. Adipophilin is a ubiquitous lipid droplet–associated protein, which correlates with intracellular neutral lipid in nonadipocytes.

Research Spotlight

ADRP-null mice have normal lipid droplet formation in adipose cells with unaltered adipose differentiation or lipolysis, possibly a reflection of functional redundancy with the other PAT proteins. The null animals are protected from ectopic lipid deposition in the liver of wild-type animals exposed to a high-fat diet. This suggests that ADRP facilitate the formation of new LD and lipid accumulation.

TIP47 plays an important role in the size and morphology of lipid droplets, where TIP47 knockdown in mice results in smaller, more abundant lipid droplets. S3-12 and OXPAT may facilitate lipid storage. Both S3-12 and OXPAT are stable in the cytosol of cultured cells under lipid-poor conditions but move to the surface of lipid droplets during lipid loading with long-chain fatty acids [8].

Human trophoblasts store lipids in the form of lipid droplets when cultured in hypoxia or when exposed to fatty acids. This accumulation may reflect reduced lipid transport to the fetus, altered placental energy storage and utilization, or protection against lipotoxicity. Lipid droplet–associated proteins (adipophilin, perilipin, S3-12, TIP47, and OXPAT) are expressed in the human placenta as well as in cultured human trophoblasts. Among these proteins, the expression level of adipophilin most closely corresponds to lipid droplet formation.

Regulation of placental fatty acid uptake and metabolism

The processes of lipid transport and metabolism are under the control of complex endocrine signals. One of the most important signals is leptin, which is produced in the maternal, placental, and fetal compartments. Maternal blood levels of leptin are elevated during pregnancy, likely reflecting the production of leptin by the placenta. In addition, the fetus produces leptin and fetal blood leptin levels correlate with birth size. Leptin synthesis is regulated by insulin, glucocorticoids, thyroid hormones, and oxygen availability in utero, suggesting that leptin is a part of the hormonal homeostatic response. The ability of leptin to enhance mobilization of maternal fat stores increases availability of lipids for transplacental transfer.

Adiponectin is primarily produced by adipocytes, and the levels of this hormone are inversely related to accumulation of serum triglycerides in body fat. In skeletal muscle, adiponectin plays an important role in regulating triglyceride accumulation by increasing the expression of proteins that transport lipids (CD36), lipid oxidation (acyl-CoA oxidase), and energy dissipation (uncoupling protein 2). Adiponectin is produced by the placenta, and administration of adiponectin to trophoblast cultures decreases the expression of lipoprotein lipase by trophoblasts. A definitive role for adiponectin in placental lipid trafficking has not been established. Likewise, maternal blood levels of resistin increase as pregnancy progresses, and resistin is also expressed in trophoblasts and amniotic membranes. Although resistin elevates serum triglycerides, attenuates insulin sensitivity, and worsens glucose homeostasis in nonpregnant individuals, the role of this hormone in pregnancy, and specifically in placental lipid trafficking, is uncertain. The peptide hormone ghrelin is produced by the placenta in both first trimester and near term villi. In nonpregnant individuals, ghrelin is secreted mainly from the stomach and circulates as acyl ghrelin (AG) and desacyl ghrelin (DG), which promote adipogenesis. Considered as the counterpart of leptin, ghrelin concentrations increase with fasting and decrease after caloric intake. Hyperglycemia and insulin resistance are independently associated with a decrease in ghrelin concentrations. Serum concentrations of AG are decreased during pregnancy, whereas concentrations of DG remain unchanged.

Several transcriptional regulators modulate the expression of genes involved in lipid trafficking. The peroxisome proliferator–activated receptors (PPARs) and retinoid X receptor alpha (RXRα), the heterodimer partner of the nuclear receptor PPARγ, play a key role in cellular and systemic lipid metabolism. Interestingly, the PPARs and RXR also have an essential role in placental development and function.

Research Spotlight

PPARγ-null murine embryos die at embryonic day 10.5 as a result of maldevelopment of the placental labyrinth. In addition, ablation of RXRα in mice also results in embryonic death with a phenotype similar to that of PPARγ ablation.

PPARγ and RXRα play a role in placental lipid metabolism, and labyrinthine trophoblasts of PPARγ-null or RXRα-null murine embryos lack lipid droplets that are normally present in wild-type placentas. In addition, PPARγ and RXR agonists, alone or in combination, increase fatty acid uptake and accumulation in primary human trophoblasts in culture. This process can be blocked by inhibitors of p38 MAP kinase, which is known to decrease PPARγ activity. PPARγ and RXR activation increase the expression of FATP1 and FATP4 and RXR activation decreases the expression of FABP2 in the murine placenta.

PPARα is expressed in metabolically active tissues including the liver, heart, and skeletal muscle, where protein activity promotes lipid catabolism. In addition, PPARα is highly expressed in the labyrinth and junctional zones of the rat placenta and in human villous trophoblasts.

Research Spotlight

PPARα-null mice do not demonstrate abnormalities of placental development. However, there is an increased rate of abortion and neonatal mortality in these mice, suggesting that PPARα may be involved in mother-to-fetus nutrient exchange.

Research Spotlight

Treatment of rats with a pharmacological dose of PPARα activators throughout pregnancy reduces maternal triglycerides, suggesting that PPARα is involved in the regulation of maternal lipid metabolism.

Teaching Points

1. Pregnancy is characterized by increased levels of maternal serum lipids, including triglycerides, LDL cholesterol, and apolipoprotein B. These lipids are essential for fetal development and growth.
2. Successful transplacental lipid trafficking requires that lipids transverse the placental syncytiotrophoblast layer as well as the fetal endothelial layer. Uptake of these lipids is a highly regulated process. FATP proteins and FAT/CD36 facilitate trophoblast fatty acid uptake, whereas FABPs largely regulate intracellular lipid transport.
3. Trophoblast lipid storage occurs in the form of lipid droplets, which consist of a triglyceride core surrounded by a phospholipid monolayer and associated PAT proteins. This family of proteins regulates the accumulation of lipid droplets. While serving as a reservoir of cellular building blocks and energy, lipid droplets also protect cells against lipotoxicity.
4. Endocrine signals such as leptin and adiponectin are secreted from the maternal, placental, and fetal compartments. These adipokines are important for regulating maternal serum lipids and adipose tissue homeostasis, which serves to ensure the supply of lipids to the developing fetus.
5. Members of the PPAR and RXR family of transcription factors regulate the expression of genes that govern placental lipid uptake and transport.

Acknowledgements

We thank Lori Rideout for assistance with preparation of the manuscript. Work from our laboratory was supported by the ACOG/Ross Products Division Abbott Research Award on Nutrition in Pregnancy (to C. S.) and NIH R01-ES11597 (to Y. S.).

References

1. Haggarty P (2002) Placental regulation of fatty acid delivery and its effect on fetal growth—A review. *Placenta* 23(Suppl A): S28–38.
2. Woollett LA (2008) Where does fetal and embryonic cholesterol originate and what does it do? *Annual Review of Nutrition* 28: 97–114.
3. Duttaroy AK (2009) Transport of fatty acids across the human placenta: A review. *Progress in Lipid Research* 48: 52–61.
4. Magnusson AL, Waterman IJ, Wennergren M et al. (2004) Triglyceride hydrolase activities and expression of fatty acid binding proteins in the human placenta in pregnancies complicated by intrauterine growth restriction and diabetes. *Journal of Clinical Endocrinology and Metabolism* 89: 4607–14.
5. Furuhashi M and Hotamisligil GS (2008) Fatty acid-binding proteins: Role in metabolic diseases and potential as drug targets. *Nature Reviews Drug Discovery* 7: 489–503.
6. Stefulj J, Panzenboeck U, Becker T et al. (2009) Human endothelial cells of the placental barrier efficiently deliver cholesterol to the fetal circulation via ABCA1 and ABCG1. *Circulation Research* 104: 600–8.
7. Farese RV, Jr. and Walther TC (2009) Lipid droplets finally get a little R-E-S-P-E-C-T. *Cell* 139: 855–60.
8. Bickel PE, Tansey JT, and Welte MA (2009) PAT proteins, an ancient family of lipid droplet proteins that regulate cellular lipid stores. *Biochimica et Biophysica Acta* 1791: 419–40.

11

CHAPTER 11

Maternal–Fetal Cell Trafficking and Microchimerism

Hilary S. Gammill[1,2], *Suzanne E. Peterson*[1], *and J. Lee Nelson*[2,3]

[1]Department of Obstetrics and Gynecology, University of Washington School of Medicine, Seattle, WA, USA
[2]Fred Hutchinson Cancer Research Center, University of Washington School of Medicine, Seattle, WA, USA
[3]Department of Rheumatology, University of Washington School of Medicine, Seattle, WA, USA

Introduction

The human placenta was once thought to be an impermeable barrier between mother and fetus. Over time, evidence revealed the physiology of bidirectional exchange of cells between mother and fetus, and the shedding of placental debris and microparticles into the maternal circulation. Cells exchanged between a mother and fetus during pregnancy may durably persist. This phenomenon is called microchimerism (Mc). Broadly defined, Mc is the presence of a small amount of genetically foreign material in an individual, either as cells, cellular debris, DNA, or RNA. Interestingly, Mc associates with both risk for, and protection from, subsequent disease [1].

Historical perspective–Redefining the placental barrier

Our understanding of fetal–maternal cell trafficking during pregnancy is founded upon the 19th century observation of fetal cells in the lungs of pregnant women who had died of eclampsia [2]. In the past several decades, attempts to acquire fetal genetic material for noninvasive prenatal diagnosis have contributed to further understanding of the nature and kinetics of fetal Mc in the mother during pregnancy [3].

Maternal–fetal exchange may also have specific immunologic consequences for the developing fetus. Classic studies by Medawar decades ago showed that in utero exposure to alloantigens results in the development of durable allospecific tolerance in the fetus. Exposure to maternal antigens occurs throughout fetal life and may be responsible for the development of long-lasting tolerance to noninherited maternal antigens in the fetus as well [4].

Detection of Mc

Two primary methodologies have defined the pathophysiology of transplacental trafficking: quantitative polymerase chain reaction (QPCR) and fluorescence in situ hybridization (FISH) (please see Figure 11.1). For identification of Mc from a male fetus, QPCR-based approaches utilize amplification of Y-chromosome-specific sequences. Maternal Mc derived from female fetuses is identified by amplification of either nonshared polymorphisms in the highly polymorphic HLA complex of genes or by amplification of other genetic polymorphisms unique to each family member. QPCR allows for quantification of Mc in DNA extracted from whole blood, peripheral blood mononuclear cells, a particular cell population, plasma, serum, or tissues of interest. Moreover, FISH methodology allows for identification of male cells within a woman (presumed fetal Mc) and female cells within

The Placenta: From Development to Disease, First Edition. Edited by Helen H. Kay, D. Michael Nelson and Yuping Wang.
© 2011 Blackwell Publishing Ltd. Published 2011 by Blackwell Publishing Ltd.

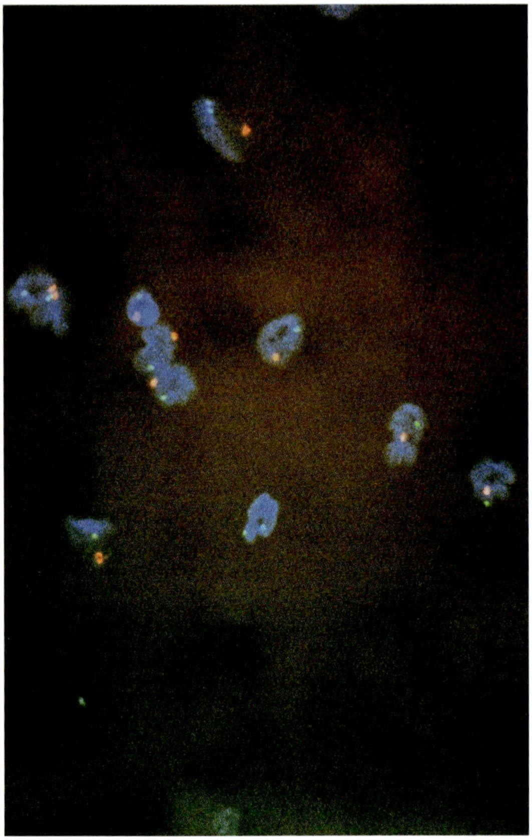

Figure 11.1 Peripheral blood mononuclear cells from a male subject with systemic lupus erythematosus. Fluorescence in situ hybridization used to label the X chromosome in green and the Y chromosome. Cell of female origin (presumably maternal) in center of image with two green probes.

a man (presumed maternal Mc). Combined with techniques such as immunohistochemistry, these approaches allow for both the identification and phenotyping of Mc cells within the host [1].

Research Spotlight

Mc can be detected with QPCR and FISH techniques.

Cellular exchange during pregnancy

Fetal Mc has been detected in the maternal circulation as early as 4 weeks' gestation. Cell-free fetal DNA is likely released from placental microparticles shed by apoptosis. Cell-free DNA is present in the maternal circulation at higher concentrations than fetal cells, but both fetal DNA and cells are commonly detected throughout normal pregnancy. Free fetal DNA is rapidly cleared from the maternal circulation after delivery, with a mean half-life of approximately 16 minutes and complete clearance in the first postpartum day. The kinetics of clearance of fetal cells postpartum is poorly understood, and fetal cells may persist in the mother's circulation for decades in both healthy women and women with disease [1].

Maternal cells and maternal DNA are commonly detected in umbilical cord blood at the time of delivery or at cordocentesis. In humans, circulating maternal Mc within the fetal circulation has been detected by cordocentesis at 19 weeks' gestation. Human studies are limited in the ability to ascertain precise timing of the initial maternal–fetal transfer, although human fetal tissues have contained maternal Mc as early as 14 weeks' gestation. Animal studies suggest that maternal cells reach the fetal system as soon as the placental circulation is established. As is the case with fetal Mc, maternal cells may persist long term [1].

Phenotype and function of fetal Mc acquired by the mother

Fetal Mc has been detected both in circulating cell populations and in tissues of pregnant and parous women. Fetal Mc includes cell subsets such as CD34+38+ progenitors, T cells, B cells, monocyte/macrophages, and NK cells. In tissues, fetal Mc has been identified within the liver, thyroid, cervix, intestine, spleen, lymph nodes, heart, and kidneys of parous women. Tissue-based studies have assessed the phenotype of fetal Mc within maternal liver and heart, demonstrating the expression of tissue-specific surface markers (for example, hepatocyte markers and cardiomyocyte markers) by fetal cells [1]. The role of fetal Mc remains largely unexplored.

Phenotype and function of maternal Mc acquired by the fetus

Similar to fetal Mc, maternal Mc has been detected within T cell and B cell subsets, monocyte/macrophages, NK cells, and CD34+38+ progenitor cells. Within tissues, maternal Mc can reside within fetal liver, lung, heart, thymus, spleen, adrenal, kidney, pancreas, brain, gonads, and lymph nodes [1]. Maternal cells induce the development of fetal regulatory T cells within fetal lymph nodes. These

T_{reg} cells suppress the fetal antimaternal response, and this effect can persist long term [5].

Research Spotlight

The fetus acquires maternal Mc as the immune system develops, and this process influences immune tolerance.

Anatomy of transplacental trafficking

Human placental anatomy suggests two primary pathways by which the mother and fetus exchange material. As detailed in Chapter 3, the human placenta is hemochorial. The layers of cells separating the villous fetal blood from maternal circulation include the fetal endothelium, the villous cytotrophoblast, and the syncytiotrophoblast. Extravillous cytotrophoblasts invade the decidua and remodel the uterine spiral arteries. These two interfaces—the villous tree and the decidua—bring trophoblast directly in contact with maternal cells and, ultimately, the maternal circulation (Figure 11.2). Shedding of apoptotic microparticles from the syncytiotrophoblast directly into the intervillous space yields cell-free fetal DNA in the maternal circulation. Fetal cells may access the maternal circulation through small fetomaternal hemorrhages within injured villi or through invasion of pluripotent extravillous trophoblasts in the arterioles of the basal plate.

Mc and reproductive outcomes

Decades of research have sought to take advantage of the presence of fetal cells and DNA in maternal circulation with the goal of noninvasive prenatal diagnosis. Cell-free fetal DNA has gained attention for diagnostic purposes as the relatively high concentration of cell-free fetal nucleic acids and their rapid clearance allow for sensitivity and specificity of testing during a given pregnancy. However, the fragmented nature of the DNA and the high background of maternal nucleic acids require technological advances to overcome these obstacles before diagnostic use is accepted clinically [3]. See Chapter 43 for a detailed discussion of this area.

Clinical Pearl

Studies of fetal Mc in the maternal circulation may inform techniques for noninvasive prenatal diagnosis.

The process of bidirectional transplacental exchange that occurs physiologically in all pregnancies is exaggerated in certain pathological states of pregnancy, such as fetal aneuploidy and preeclampsia. Higher concentrations of fetal DNA circulate in maternal blood in pregnancies with trisomy 21 compared with euploid pregnancies. Women pregnant with Trisomy 21 fetuses had concentrations of fetal material that were sixfold greater than women with euploid gestations [1]. This difference may result from the influence of fetal aneuploidy on placentation, as placental abnormalities such as hydrops and immature villous histology occur in aneuploidy.

Placental dysfunction underlies preeclampsia, and there is increased oxidative stress in preeclampsia compared with normotensive pregnancies, as described in Chapter 33. Preeclampsia associates with enhanced apoptosis of the syncytiotrophoblast, increased trophoblast fragments and microparticles, and higher concentrations of free fetal DNA in the maternal circulation. Schmorl in the late 1800s first identified trophoblasts in the lungs of women with eclampsia, and fetal cells are now well known to circulate in the mother's blood stream [1,2]. We do not know whether the higher concentrations of fetal Mc in preeclampsia represents increased fetal–maternal trafficking or results from decreased clearance of fetal material.

Clinical Pearl

Higher maternal concentrations of fetal Mc associate with preeclampsia.

Brief review of consequences of persistent Mc

In contrast to free DNA, both fetal and maternal cellular Mc can persist for decades. The health consequences of Mc in the fetus and mother have been explored in epidemiologic studies. Autoimmunity and malignancy are the focus of most studies to date. The autoimmune disease systemic sclerosis (SSc) associates with higher concentrations of fetal Mc in both circulation and tissues. This observation supports the hypothesis that autoimmunity may in fact represent allo-autoimmunity (i.e., Mc antihost reactivity) or auto-alloimmunity (i.e., host anti-Mc reactivity). Higher concentrations of fe-

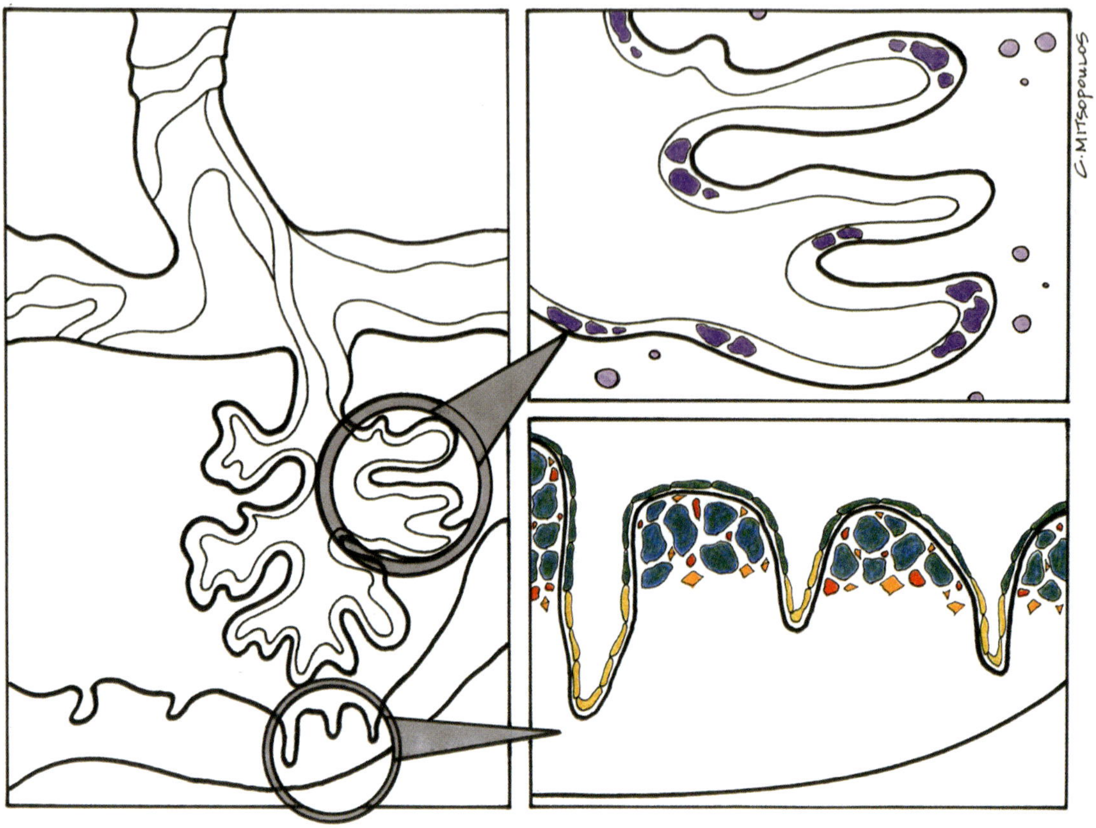

Figure 11.2 Diagram of placenta showing two primary interfaces at which fetal cells may gain access to the maternal circulation. Upper right panel shows syncytiotrophoblast overlying the villous tree. Bottom right panel shows extravillous cytotrophoblast invading the maternal decidua and spiral arteries. (Image created by Christina Mitsopoulos, reproduced with permission.)

tal Mc associate with protection from some malignancies like breast cancer. This supports the hypothesis that Mc may provide allosurveillance, i.e., a graft-versus-tumor effect, to decrease the risk of development of malignancy [1].

Clinical Pearl

Mc has been associated with an increased risk of some autoimmune diseases and with a decreased risk of some malignancies.

Autoimmune disease

The epidemiology of many autoimmune diseases shows a female preponderance, with a notable peak incidence in postreproductive age women. Combined with clinical parallels of some autoimmune diseases with graft versus host disease, these observations prompted investigation of a possible role for fetal Mc in the pathogenesis of autoimmunity, particularly SSc.

Initial studies identified higher concentrations of fetal Mc in the circulation of women with SSc compared with healthy controls. Subsequent investigation showed more fetal Mc in skin biopsies from women with SSc compared with controls. While fetal Mc represents the most common source for Mc in parous women, men and nulliparous women also develop SSc. If low concentrations of allogeneic cells contribute to disease in these situations, alternative means for acquisition of Mc must be explored. Alternative sources for such Mc include early pregnancy losses, including unrecognized pregnancies, twins, maternal Mc, and iatrogenic sources such as blood transfusions. Mc could also originate from an older sibling, passed along with maternal cells, although this has not yet been reported. There is a higher prevalence of maternal Mc with SSc compared with controls [1].

The relationship of Mc with autoimmunity is complex. Similar to transplantation, the HLA relationships of the Mc graft with the host are likely to play a crucial role in determining whether Mc has beneficial, neutral, or adverse consequences. A disease that illustrates this point is rheumatoid arthritis (RA). RA is an autoimmune disease that is ameliorated during pregnancy and that relapses postpartum. HLA disparity of the fetus from the mother is associated with improvement of arthritis during pregnancy. Over the course of pregnancy in women with RA, higher concentrations of fetal Mc in maternal circulation correlate inversely with disease activity [1]. In addition to the clinical improvement in women who have RA and become pregnant, there is also a protective effect of prior pregnancy on the risk of developing subsequent RA. A significant reduction in risk for the development of new RA is observed for parous compared with nulliparous women, and interestingly, this effect wanes with increasing time from the last birth. While the explanation for these observations is not known, a reasonable explanation is that there is an acquisition of HLA disparate fetal Mc carrying HLA alleles that are protective for RA [6]. However, the fetal Mc that a woman acquires could also carry HLA alleles associated with RA-risk. Certain HLA-DRB1 alleles carry a similar sequence referred to as the "shared epitope (SE)" sequence, which is known to be associated with risk of RA. In women who do not themselves genetically carry the SE sequence, acquisition of Mc carrying the SE sequence increases the risk for RA [7]. This illustrates the complexity of potential Mc effects, which depend on multiple factors including the specific HLA alleles carried by the Mc, the HLA alleles of the person who harbors the Mc, and the HLA relationship between the two.

In addition to SSc and RA, Mc has been investigated in Sjogren's syndrome, systemic lupus erythematosus, autoimmune thyroid disease, primary biliary cirrhosis, pruritic urticarial papules and plaques of pregnancy (PUPPP), neonatal lupus syndrome, childhood inflammatory myopathies, and pediatric biliary atresia, with some, but not all studies reporting differences in patient populations compared with controls [1].

Malignancy

A role for fetal Mc has been explored in the association of the reduction in risk for breast cancer among women who have given birth, compared to those who have not. Studies have shown that women with breast cancer are significantly less likely to harbor circulating fetal Mc than healthy controls [1]. Mc cells localize to tissues, but we are unsure if they participate in pathologic processes, contribute to repair or prevention of disease, or simply are bystanders, in colonized organs. Interestingly, there are lower levels of fetal Mc in tissue adjacent to breast cancer cases, compared with healthy controls undergoing benign excisions [8]. Collectively, these data support the hypothesis that fetal Mc functions in an allogeneic surveillance capacity to decrease the risk of developing breast cancer. Similar findings have been reported for a range of other malignancies as well.

Conclusions

The placenta was once thought to be a barrier between two individuals, but this image has changed to one where the placenta is a dynamic gatekeeper for bidirectional exchange of cells and DNA between the mother and fetus. While DNA is rapidly cleared, cells exchanged in this manner may persist long term as Mc and may retain pluripotent capacity. Obstetric factors contribute to the quantity of fetal Mc acquired by the mother. Functional sequelae of Mc are suggested by associations with both risk of and protection from disease later in life, particularly autoimmunity and malignancy. Ongoing investigations aim to clarify the functionality of Mc; such an understanding may ultimately enable us to harness the therapeutic potential of this biologic process.

☞ Teaching Points

1. The human placenta is not an impermeable barrier but instead, allows for exchange of cells and free DNA between mother and fetus.
2. Mc is the presence of a small amount of foreign genetic material in the tissues or circulation of another individual.
3. Cells exchanged between mother and fetus during pregnancy can persist for decades as Mc.
4. Persistent cellular Mc, both maternal and fetal, may influence the risk of certain diseases in later life.

Acknowledgements

NIH: HD-01-264, AI-41721 and AI-45659.

References

1. Gammill H and Nelson J (2010) Naturally acquired microchimerism. *International Journal of Developmental Biology* 54: 531–43.
2. Lapaire O, Holzgreve W, Oosterwijk JC et al. (2007) Georg Schmorl on trophoblasts in the maternal circulation. *Placenta* 28: 1–5.
3. Lo YMD and Chiu RWK (2007) Prenatal diagnosis: Progress through plasma nucleic acids. *Nature Reviews Genetics* 8: 71–7.
4. Dutta P and Burlingham W (2009) Tolerance to noninherited maternal antigens in mice and humans. *Current Opinion in Organ Transplantation* 14: 439–47.
5. Mold JE, Michaelsson J, Burt TD et al. (2008) Maternal alloantigens promote the development of tolerogenic fetal regulatory T cells in utero. *Science* 322: 1562–5.
6. Guthrie K, Dugowson C, Voigt L et al. (2010) Does pregnancy provide vaccine-like protection against rheumatoid arthritis? *Arthritis & Rheumatism*, epub ahead of print.
7. Rak JM, Maestroni L, Balandraud N et al. (2009) Transfer of the shared epitope through microchimerism in women with rheumatoid arthritis. *Arthritis & Rheumatism* 60: 73–80.
8. Gadi V (2010) Fetal microchimerism in breast from women with and without breast cancer. *Breast Cancer Research and Treatment* 121: 241–4.

12

CHAPTER 12
Imprinting in the Human Placenta

Shu Wen[1] *and Ignatia B. Van den Veyver*[1,2]

[1]Department of Obstetrics and Gynecology, Baylor College of Medicine, Houston, TX, USA
[2]Department of Molecular and Human Genetics, Baylor College of Medicine, Houston, TX, USA

What is genetic imprinting?

General concepts

All autosomal chromosomes and genes are present in two copies: one copy is maternally inherited and one is paternally inherited. A small number of genes—about 90 in the mouse and fewer in humans—are imprinted. Genomic imprinting refers to the epigenetic marking of specific genes during germline transmission such that they are mono-allelically expressed in a parent-of-origin-dependent manner. For each imprinted gene, it is always either the maternally inherited or the paternally inherited copy that is expressed. The DNA sequence of the two alleles of an imprinted gene is identical, but they carry other "epigenetic" marks that distinguish from which parent each allele was inherited. Genetic imprinting has been found in eutherian placental mammals and marsupials, identified in plants and insects but not in nonmammalian vertebrates or egg-laying mammals (monotremes), such as the platypus. Most imprinted genes are expressed in placenta, and imprinting may have evolved from specific selective pressures in mammals; consequently, co-evolution of placentation and genetic imprinting has been proposed.

Pronuclear transplantation of mouse germ cells provided early evidence that imprinting is essential for development and of particular importance for trophoblast development. In these experiments, embryos derived from micromanipulated zygotes that contain two male pronuclei survived longer in vitro with better development of extraembryonic tissues, while two female pronuclei generated better embryo differentiation, but earlier developmental arrest and lack of extraembryonic tissues.

Mechanisms and molecules that regulate imprinting

When imprinted genes are transmitted to subsequent generations via male or female haploid gametes, the imprinting marks from the opposite parent must be replaced by those specific for the transmitting parent so that the correct imprinting state is maintained across generations (Figure 12.1). This process requires three phases: *erasure* of the imprinting marks from the previous generation, *establishment* of parent-specific imprints in the germline, and *maintenance*, propagation, and readout of these marks in somatic cells and extraembryonic tissues of the progeny. There has been great progress in uncovering the molecular mechanisms that participate in imprinting, but the regulation of the process is incompletely understood.

No single primary feature of the DNA-sequence distinguishes imprinted genes from nonimprinted, biallelically expressed genes, but many imprinted genes are clustered within larger imprinted domains (Figure 12.2) that contain maternally and paternally imprinted genes interspersed with nonimprinted genes. Within these clusters are one or more imprinting control regions (ICR) (Table 12.1 lists all abbreviations). These are cytosine–guanine (CG)-rich sequences (CpG islands) that are methylated on either the maternally or paternally inherited chromosome, also referred to as differentially methylated regions

The Placenta: From Development to Disease, First Edition. Edited by Helen H. Kay, D. Michael Nelson and Yuping Wang.
© 2011 Blackwell Publishing Ltd. Published 2011 by Blackwell Publishing Ltd.

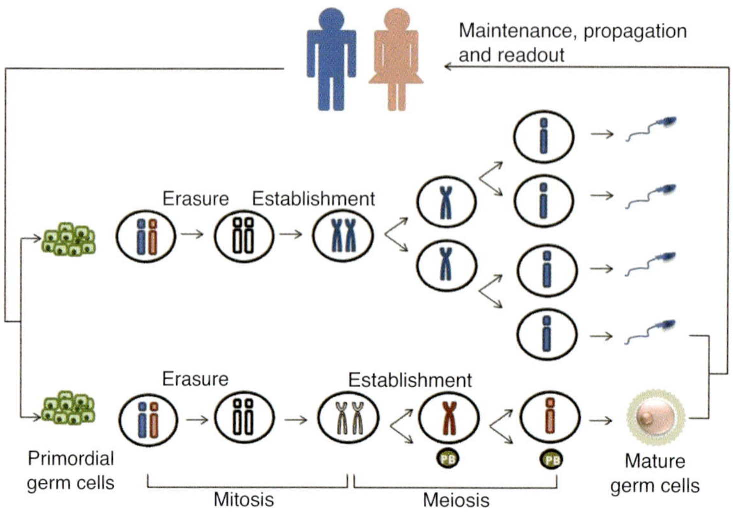

Figure 12.1 Imprinting during the life cycle. In primordial germ cells, imprinting marks from the previous generation are erased and are re-established again in a parent-of-origin specific pattern before germ cell maturation. In male germ cells, this happens during mitosis, while in females, this happens during meiosis. After fertilization, imprinting marks are maintained, propagated, and interpreted (read-out) in somatic cells and extraembryonic tissues of the progeny. Blue, paternal chromosome; pink, maternal chromosome; PB, polar body.

(DMRs). Their methylation status influences the binding of different DNA- or chromatin-binding proteins and transcriptional regulators that determine the expression or silencing of the entire cluster of nearby imprinted genes. DNA methylation works in concert with other mechanisms to regulate imprinting in a combinatorial fashion.

Covalent modification of histones, the components of the nucleosome around which DNA is wound, such as methylation, acetylation, phosphorylation, and ubiquitination of specific residues in the histone-tails can guide the binding of other regulatory proteins, rendering chromatin permissive, or repressive, to transcription of nearby

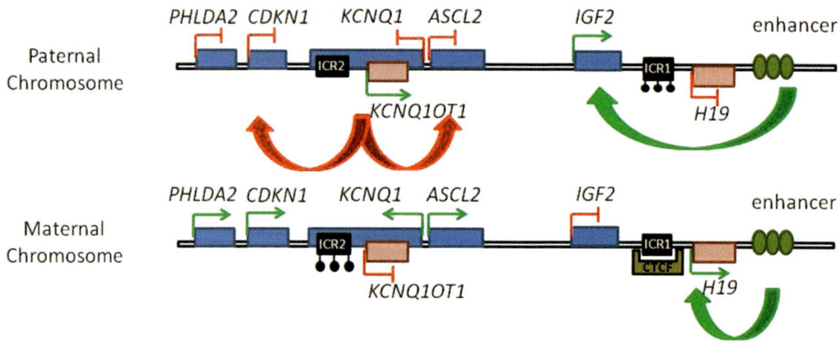

Figure 12.2 Two imprinted gene clusters in human chromosome 11. On the maternal chromosome, the unmethylated ICR1 upstream of *H19* is bound by CTCF, which functions as an insulator and prevents enhancers downstream of *H19* to interact with the *IGF2* gene. The enhancers remain available to interact with the unmethylated ICR1 on maternal chromosome to drive the transcription of *H19*. On the paternal chromosome, methylation of ICR1 is associated with absent CTCF binding and, consequently, insulator function, leaving the enhancers available for interaction with *IGF2* to drive its expression. H19 is silenced because its CpG island (ICR1) is methylated. The *KCNQ1* imprinted locus contains the ICR2 in an intron of *KCNQ1*. On the paternal chromosome, where this ICR2 is unmethylated, it promotes transcription of *KCNQ1OT1* noncoding RNA, resulting in silencing of maternally expressed genes, including *CDKN1*, *ASCL2*, and *PHLDA2*. On the maternal chromosome, the ICR2 is methylated and *KCNQ1OT1* is silenced, thus *CDKN1*, *ASCL2*, and *PHLDA2* are transcribed.

Table 12.1 Abbreviations and gene nomenclature.

Full Name	Abbreviations
Androgenetic complete hydatidiform mole	AnCHM
Angelman syndrome	AS
Assisted reproductive technologies	ART
Beckwith-Wiedemann syndrome	BWS
Biparentally inherited hydatidiform mole	BiHM
Complete hydatidiform moles	CHM
Cytosine-guanine (CG)-rich sequence island	CpG island
Differentially methylated region	DMR
Hydatidiform mole	HM
In vitro fertilization	IVF
Imprinting control region	ICR
Intrauterine growth restriction	IUGR
Loss of imprinting	LOI
MicroRNAs	miRNAs
Noncoding RNAs	ncRNA
Partial hydatidiform mole	PHM
Prader-Willi syndrome	PWS
Silver-Russell syndrome	SRS
Small for gestational age	SGA
Transient neonatal diabetes	TND
X chromosome inactivation	XCI
Gene Nomenclature	**Abbreviations**
Antisense of Igf2r RNA	*Airn*
Achaete-scute complex homolog 2 (Drosophila)	*ASCL2*
CD81 antigen	*CD81*
Cyclin-dependent kinase inhibitor 1	*CDKN1*
CCCTC-binding factor (zinc finger protein)	*CTCF*
DNA (cytosine-5-)-methyltransferase 1	*DNMT1*
DNA (cytosine-5-)-methyltransferase 1 (oocyte-specific transcript)	*DNMT1o*
DNA (cytosine-5-)-methyltransferase 3 alpha	*DNMT3A*
DNA (cytosine-5-)-methyltransferase 3 beta	*DNMT3B*
DNA (cytosine-5-)-methyltransferase 3-like	*DNMT3L*
Growth factor receptor bound protein 10	*GRB10*
H19, imprinted maternally expressed transcript (nonprotein coding)	*H19*
Insulin growth factor 2	*IGF2*
Potassium voltage gated channel, KQT-like subfamily, member 1	*KCNQ1*
KCNQ1 overlapping transcript 1	*KCNQ1OT1*
Neuroendocrine secretory protein 55	*NESP55*
NALP-like receptor (NLR) family, pyrin domain containing 2	*NLRP2*
NALP-like receptor (NLR) family, pyrin domain containing 7	*NLRP7*
Paternally expressed gene 10	*PEG10*
Paternally expressed gene 3	*PEG3*
Pleckstrin homology-like domain, family A, member 2	*PHLDA2*
Pleiomorphic adenoma gene-like 1	*PLAGL1*
Small nuclear ribonucleoprotein polypeptide N	*SNRPN*
Storkhead box 1	*STOX1*
XIST antisense RNA (nonprotein coding)	*TSIX*
X (inactive)-specific transcript (nonprotein coding)	*XIST*
Zinc finger protein 57	*ZFP57*

genes. It has been demonstrated in mouse trophoblast that imprinting can be guided by these mechanisms alone, does not always require DNA methylation, and can be maintained in the absence of the DNA methyltransferase (*Dnmt1*) [1,2]. Other molecular mechanisms that contribute to imprinting regulation involve small noncoding RNAs (ncRNA), such as microRNAs (miRNAs) or long ncRNAs, such as those encoded by the *H19* and the small nuclear ribonucleoprotein-associated polypeptide N (*SNRPN*) genes in humans and mice and antisense of *Igf2r* RNA gene, *Airn* in mice. Similar to their role in gene expression, ncRNAs may regulate imprinted gene expression at the transcriptional or posttranscriptional level. How these molecular mechanisms cooperate has not been studied in detail for all imprinted gene clusters.

A comprehensive discussion of the molecular regulation of imprinting is beyond the scope of this text, but excellent recent reviews exist [3,4]. To illustrate the concepts, we highlight the example of imprinting at the Beckwith-Wiedemann syndrome (BWS) region on chromosome 11p15.5, which is of particular interest for fetal and placental growth. The region contains two imprinted clusters with their two separate ICRs, the insulin-like growth factor 2-encoding gene (*IGF2*)-*H19* cluster and the *KCNQ1* overlapping transcript 1 (*KCNQ1OT1*) cluster (Figure 12.2). A CpG-rich ICR upstream of *H19* is bound by the transcriptional regulator protein CTCF and remains unmethylated on the maternally inherited chromosome. CTCF-binding functions as an insulator, preventing enhancers downstream of *H19* to interact with the *IGF2* gene, which consequently is silenced. The enhancers remain available to interact with the unmethylated CpG-island to drive transcription of *H19* from the maternal allele. On the paternally inherited chromosome, CTCF cannot bind the methylated ICR, allowing enhancers to drive expression of the growth-promoting *IGF2* gene while methylation prevents *H19* transcription. The *KCNQ1* imprinted locus is adjacent to the *IGF2/H19* locus but is regulated separately. It contains an ICR in an intron of *KCNQ1*. This ICR is unmethylated on the paternally inherited chromosome, where it functions as the promoter for transcription of the >60 kb-long ncRNA *KCNQ1OT1*. This results in silencing of maternally expressed genes, including *CDKN1*, *ASCL2*, and *PHLDA2* whose expression limits fetal and placental growth.

Why is there genetic imprinting in mammals?

The conflict hypothesis

Why genetic imprinting has evolved cannot be easily explained because it reduces the advantage of having a diploid genome wherein each gene has two copies that can be expressed. According to the most popular "conflict" or "kinship hypothesis", genetic imprinting evolved because of conflicting needs of parents in placental mammals to ensure optimal reproductive outcomes. Fathers benefit from investing in enhanced fetal growth to maximize fitness of their offspring, while mothers benefit from a longer lifespan and equal allocation of resources between different progeny.

> **Clinical Pearl**
>
> Imprinted genes are expressed in the placenta. The paternally expressed imprinted genes are often growth-promoting for the fetus and placenta, while maternally expressed imprinted genes often limit growth.

This hypothesis explains the growth-related phenotypes of many human imprinting disorders and those that result from inactivation of imprinted genes in mouse models. For example, inactivation in the mouse of maternally expressed imprinted genes, such as *Grb10* and *Igf2r*, leads to embryo overgrowth, whereas inactivation of paternally expressed imprinted genes, such as *Igf2*, restricts embryo growth. In humans, the overgrowth syndrome, BWS, can be caused by unbalanced overexpression of the maternally imprinted *IGF2* by decreased expression due to imprinting abnormalities at the ICR, or it can be caused by inactivating mutations of the maternally expressed *CDKN1* gene. Some cases of Silver-Russell syndrome (SRS), a condition associated with prenatal and postnatal growth restriction, are caused by hypomethylation of the ICR upstream of *H19*, resulting in decreased *IGF2* expression.

Other theories

The parental "nutrient-allocation conflict theory" does not explain all loss-of-function phenotypes of imprinted genes in humans and mice. Mice with loss of *Nesp55* expression grow normally but have anxiety and an abnormal response to novel environmental stimuli. *Cd81*-deficient mice only have an impaired antibody response. The human imprinting disorders Angelman syndrome (AS) and Prader-Willi syndrome (PWS) are associated with neurodevelopmental disability. Some argue that this might be an extension of the conflict to its influence on postnatal behavior. This is supported by the observation that female mice deficient in the paternally expressed gene 3 (*Peg3*) display abnormal nurturing behavior towards their offspring and have fewer oxytocin neurons in the hypothalamus. However, alternative theories have been presented as well. Wolf and Hager proposed that imprinting results from selective co-adaptation of complementary maternal and offspring traits to improve reproductive fitness, whereby loci with more intimate maternal–offspring interaction are predominantly maternally expressed. This may explain the predominance of maternally expressed imprinted genes that are essential for early placental development [5]. The human placenta compared to placentas of other mammals shows selective loss of imprinting of maternally expressed, growth-limiting imprinted genes. It has been proposed that the result of this loss can be explained by evolution towards bipedalism with relatively smaller pelvises in humans compared to other mammals, necessitating shorter gestations and smaller fetuses [6]. These theories are not mutually exclusive, and imprinting may have evolved for a number of different reasons.

Imprinted gene function in development

Timing of imprinting in development

During gametogenesis, the imprinting information from the previous generation must be erased and then re-established according to the sex of the transmitting parent. According to the currently accepted model, all imprints are erased in the primordial germ cells and then re-established again during gametogenesis in a process that in the mouse requires the *de novo* synthesis of methyltransferases Dnmt3a and Dnmt3L. In the male germline, this occurs premeiotically in prospermatogonia, but in the female germline, this process occurs postmeiotically in the growing oocytes during diplotene arrest [7]. In mammals, the entire nonimprinted genome is heavily methylated, but undergoes demethylation shortly after fertilization. This demethylation occurs by a rapid active process in the paternal pronucleus, but by a slower passive process in the maternal genome that continues to the 4-cell stage in mice, after which it is followed by remethylation (Figure 12.1). The methylated ICRs of imprinted loci are protected from the genome-wide wave of demethylation and remethylation, in a process that requires oocyte-specific Dnmt1o and zygotic Dnmt1. Hence, this is a critical and vulnerable developmental stage for the maintenance and propagation of correct imprinting marks. The imprinting marks will be faithfully copied upon mitotic cell division and will be maintained through action of Dnmt1, Dnmt3a, Dnmt3b, and *Zfp57*. Interestingly, in humans, *ZFP57* is the gene mutated in transient neonatal diabetes (TND), which is a disorder associated with variable hypomethylation at imprinted loci. The transcription machinery of somatic cells and extraembryonic tissues interprets this information for proper imprinted gene expression.

Differences in imprinting between human and mice

Most current knowledge of imprinting comes from experiments and observations in mice. The mechanisms of imprinting are largely conserved between mice and humans in the well-studied imprinted regions of the two species. However, some differences exist that are especially relevant for imprinting in the trophoblast, as highlighted below.

Imprinted X inactivation in placenta

X chromosome inactivation (XCI) is a mechanism that assures dosage compensation of X-linked gene expression between XY males and XX females by transcriptional silencing of one X chromosome in female diploid cells. In mice and other animal species, most X inactivation in trophoblast is imprinted, with the paternally inherited X being preferentially inactivated, but this is not the case in humans. In mice, the maternal X chromosome is protected from inactivation in placental tissues because the expression of *Tsix*, a gene involved in regulation of *Xist* is maternally expressed in extraembryonic tissues. Interestingly, *TSIX* expression is not imprinted in humans. Xist is the noncoding RNA that is expressed from and then coats the inactive X chromosome.

Imprinting of Igf2r

Igf2r is an imprinted gene in mice and other mammalian species, but most evidence suggests that *Igf2r* is not imprinted in humans. Disrupted imprinting of *Igf2r* has been implicated in altered fetal and placental growth leading to "large-offspring syndrome," a condition associated with in vitro embryo manipulation in cattle and reproductive cloning in mammals.

Imprinting and bipedialism

Recent studies in the human fetus and placenta on the relationship between imprinted genes and intrauterine growth restriction (IUGR) suggest that the influence of genomic imprinting on fetal growth in mice is incompletely conserved in humans. A reduced selective pressure on imprinting control may have evolved because humans have mostly singleton pregnancies [8] or because they developed bipedalism [6] (see above).

Specific disorders of human placental imprinting

Complete hydatidiform moles

Hydatidiform moles (HM) are abnormal pregnancies with defective embryo development and abnormal hypertrophic trophoblast with malignant potential. The most common forms of sporadic complete hydatidiform moles (CHM) result from fertilization of an oocyte with an inactivated nucleus, sometimes referred to as "empty oocyte." Studies with polymorphic genetic markers have demonstrated that these pregnancies are diploid with a 46,XY or 46,XX karyotype that arises either from duplication of the haploid set of paternal chromosomes from the single fertilizing sperm or, less commonly, from dispermic fertilization [9]. These pregnancies are therefore androgenetic (AnCHM) because their entire genome is paternally derived.

> **Clinical Pearl**
>
> AnCHM can be considered a state of genome-wide uniparental disomy (all chromosome pairs are inherited from one parent) or a genome-wide imprinting disorder (all imprinted loci have paternal epigenetic marks).

Typically complete hypomethylation of maternally methylated DMRs is found, for example in the ICRs regulating the paternally expressed genes *SNRPN* or *PEG3*, while paternally DMRs such as the ICR upstream of the *H19* gene are completely methylated. However, exceptions with relaxation or loss of imprinting can occur. The CHM phenotype is consistent with the maternal and paternal genomes contributing unequally to the development of the extraembryonic derivatives. This observation underscores the importance of imprinted genes in normal trophoblast development.

Interestingly, human dermoid cysts and ovarian teratomas result from parthenogenetic activation and cell division of retained oocytes in an unruptured ovarian follicle. They contain differentiated tissues and structures derived from all three embryonic layers. However, they lack extraembryonic tissues including trophoblast and can thus be regarded as the genetic female equivalent of CHM, with uniparental disomy of the entire maternal genome and a mostly maternal epigenotype at imprinted loci.

Partial HM and diandric versus digynic triploidy

Another form of HM, partial hydatidiform moles (PHM), are usually triploid with a 69,XXX or 69,XXY karyotype wherein two of the haploid sets of chromosomes are paternally derived (diandric) and one is maternally derived. Triploidy is found in 10% of spontaneous abortions and most are diandric, resulting from dispermic fertilization. In diandric triploidy, the fetus typically has relatively normal growth, with either a normal head size or microcephaly, and the placenta is usually a PHM. In the rarer digynic triploidies, the extra haploid set of chromosomes is maternal in origin, the fetus is typically growth-retarded with macrocephaly, and the placenta is small with no HM features.

Biparental HM

A rare class of recurrent HM is pathologically indistinguishable from androgenetic CHM, or in some cases PHM [9]. Surprisingly, these show normal diploid biparental inheritance (BiHM). Analysis of differentially methylated regions (DMRs) at imprinted loci and gene expression studies showed generalized imprinting defects in tissues from BiHM. Absent methylation of imprinted DMRs that normally acquire differential DNA methylation on the maternally inherited allele suggests a defect in the establishment or maintenance of maternal imprints. Autosomal recessive mutations in the NALP-like receptor (NLR) family, pyrin domain containing 7 gene (*NLRP7*) have been found in several familial and sporadic cases of unrelated women with recurrent molar pregnancies. The fact that not all women with these recurrent BiHM have *NLRP7* mutations supports genetic heterogeneity for this disorder. *NLRP7* encodes a protein with a proposed role in apoptosis or immune defense. Whether mutations in *NLRP7* contribute directly or indirectly to defects in the establishment or maintenance of maternal methylation imprints is still unknown.

Clinical Pearl

The phenotypes of uniparental disomy and HM likely result from abnormally imprinted gene expression. Most CHM are diploid androgenetic (46,XX or 46,XY) with all chromosomes paternally derived. PHM are usually triploid pregnancies with 69 chromosomes, of which 46 are paternally inherited. Rare biparentally inherited complete or partial moles also exist and are usually recurrent.

BWS and placentation

BWS is a fetal and neonatal overgrowth syndrome caused by epimutations and paternal deletions of chromosome 11p15.5 (see above). Pregnancies with BWS fetuses are often complicated by polyhydramnios and placentomegaly with placentas of up to twice the normal weight. Interestingly, in a family with recurrent BWS caused by an "epimutation" in 11p15.5, manifested by loss of methylation on the maternally inherited ICR2 in *KCNQ1*, the mother was found to be homozygous for a frameshift mutation in the *NLRP2* gene. Because *NLRP2* is a close homologue of *NLRP7*, this exciting discovery raised the possibility that members of the NLRP family of proteins participate directly in maternal establishment or maintenance of imprinting.

Research Spotlight

The discovery that several NLRP family members are highly or preferentially expressed in germ cells and early embryos, followed by the findings that women with mutations in *NLRP7* have biparental molar pregnancies with global imprinting abnormalities and those with mutations in *NLRP2* have children with BWS caused by an imprinting defect in chromosome 11p15, suggests that several members of the *NLRP* gene family are important for maternal establishment or maintenance of imprinting.

Placental imprinting in other obstetric and reproductive disorders

Imprinting and preeclampsia

Preeclampsia complicates 5% of all pregnancies, and its pathogenesis and progression is tightly linked to the presence of a placenta. Pregnancies with increased placental mass and disturbance in balance of imprinted gene expression such as in CHM, trisomy 13, or BWS are at higher risk for preeclampsia. Furthermore, a mouse model with maternal transmission of an inactivated allele of the maternally expressed imprinted $p57^{KIP2}$ (*Cdkn1*) gene shows several phenotypic and histopathological features of preeclampsia. These observations, as well as familial data that suggest a contribution of matrilineal predisposing genetic factors, have encouraged research into the role of imprinted genes in preeclampsia.

A heterozygous missense variant of *STOX1*, an imprinted gene expressed in the early placenta with a role in trophoblast development, was implicated in a Dutch population as a cause for preeclampsia with matrilineal inheritance, but this association could not be confirmed in other populations.

Yu and colleagues found that there is LOI with biallelic expression of *H19* in normal early pregnancies, but that expression usually becomes mono-allelic with advancing gestation [10]. In contrast, women with preeclampsia, especially those with the most severe hypertension, can have persistent LOI and biallelic expression until later in gestation. This association was again not confirmed in other populations [11].

Imprinting and IUGR

Familial aggregation of IUGR supports a role for genetic factors. Interest in the role of imprinted genes expressed in placenta as contributors to IUGR is sparked by the small placentas seen in digynic triploidy, in SRS, and in some pregnancies conceived via assisted reproductive technologies (ART), all associated with imprinting disorders. Upregulation of *PHLDA2* and *PEG10* and downregulation of *IGF2* and *PLAGL1*, as well as reduced methylation of the BWS ICR1 has been found in human SGA and placentas from IUGR fetuses. Additionally, systematic gene expression screens of placentas from IUGR fetuses show that imprinted genes are altered more often than nonimprinted genes [8,11].

Imprinting and in vitro fertilization (IVF)

Imprinting disorders are rare in the population. Hence, reports of the potential association of IVF with BWS, AS, SRS, and TND, all resulting from methylation defects at ICRs, raised concern that ART may cause abnormal imprinting. IVF in mice can induce alterations of imprinting marks in offspring DNA and aberrant embryonic expression of imprinted genes. Moreover, the superovulation itself can result in abnormal placental expression of imprinted genes in the offspring. What is debated is whether the indications for ART, the manipulation of germ cells and embryos *in vitro*, or the procedure of superovulation are the cause of the abnormally imprinted gene expression. All may contribute to some degree. The contribution of other epigenetic modifications on nonimprinted genes may also contribute to changes in placental function after IVF. Fortunately, imprinting disorders are rare, and the absolute risk to individual patients undergoing ART is low, even though the relative risk in the population is increased.

Clinical Pearl

IVF associates with an increased incidence of imprinting disorders, but a causative role is difficult to prove. The absolute risk for individual patients is low.

Environmental–epigenome interactions and role of imprinted genes in placenta

There is ample epidemiological and animal evidence that intrauterine and early childhood exposures affect disease and health later in life. Adverse intrauterine environments can predispose to hypertension, diabetes, and obesity in adult life. Permanent alterations in gene expression based on epigenetic modifications, such as altered DNA methylation or histone modifications, is a mechanism to impart a permanent memory on cells of the milieu experienced during early development.

Several recent studies explored the interaction between environment and epigenetics. The DMRs of certain imprinted genes are especially sensitive to environmental perturbations. For example, starving of cultured mouse embryonic stem cells alters the expression levels of imprinted genes, such as *Igf2* and *H19*, consequent to changes in methylation. Preimplantation culture of mouse embryos also leads to changes of placental imprinting at multiple genes, and this is affected by the culture media used. This environmental–epigenetic interaction may aid the placenta in adapting to changing physiological conditions, but could also contribute to life-long effects.

Conclusions and future research directions

There are parallels in the evolution of genetic imprinting and placentation and most imprinted genes are expressed in the placenta. Most, but not all, imprinted genes function in the control of fetal and placental growth. Overall, paternally expressed genes are growth promoting while maternally expressed genes are growth reducing, which has led to the most popular "conflict hypothesis" for the evolution of imprinting in placental mammals. Several obstetric disorders may associate with altered imprinting, but the evidence is often conflicting and the underlying mechanisms are poorly understood. We expect that future research will elucidate the role of imprinting in IUGR, in altered growth in IVF-conceived pregnancies, in the predisposition to adult disease from a suboptimal prenatal milieu, and in common obstetric conditions such as preeclampsia. Finally, study of imprinting disorders unique to human placental development, such as CHM and biparental HM, will help identify novel imprinted genes and mechanisms of imprinting in the placenta, some of which likely unique to humans.

Teaching Points

1 Genetic imprinting refers to the expression of a gene from only one allele that is inherited from either the mother or the father.

2 Paternally expressed imprinted genes are often growth-promoting, while maternally expressed imprinted genes are often growth-restricting.

3 The evolutionary role for genetic imprinting is incompletely understood, but may relate to a parental conflict in mammals for survival of the offspring. According to this theory, fathers benefit from larger offspring for reproductive success, while mothers benefit from smaller

offspring and nutritional preservation for reproductive success in successive pregnancies.

4 Mechanisms that modify imprinted gene expression involve differential DNA methylation, histone modifications, and noncoding RNAs that act at the transcriptional and posttranscriptional level.

5 An androgenetic CHM is an example of genome-wide disrupted imprinting because all chromosome pairs are inherited from one parent, in this case, the father, a condition that can be considered as uniparental disomy of all chromosomes.

6 The insulin-like growth factor gene, *IGF2*, is a well recognized and well-studied imprinted gene. Mice with imprinting abnormalities at the *Igf2* locus have altered growth in the fetus and placenta depending on whether the allele is inherited from the father or the mother.

Acknowledgements

Our research on placental imprinting and hydatidiform moles is supported by grants from the National Institutes of Health HD045970, HD058081, and GM081627.

References

1. Wagschal A and Feil R (2006) Genomic imprinting in the placenta. *Cytogenetic and Genome Research* 113: 90–8.
2. Tycko B (2006) Imprinted genes in placental growth and obstetric disorders. *Cytogenetic and Genome Research* 113: 271–8.
3. Bressan FF, De Bem TH, Perecin F et al. (2009) Unearthing the roles of imprinted genes in the placenta. *Placenta* 30: 823–34.
4. Koerner MV and Barlow DP (2010) Genomic imprinting—An epigenetic gene-regulatory model. *Current Opinion in Genetics and Developement* 20: 164–70.
5. Wolf JB and Hager R (2006) A maternal–offspring coadaptation theory for the evolution of genomic imprinting. *PLoS Biology* 4: 2238–43.
6. Isles AR (2009) Evolution of genomic imprinting in humans: Does bipedalism have a role? *Trends in Genetics* 25: 495–500.
7. Trasler JM (2006) Gamete imprinting: Setting epigenetic patterns for the next generation. *Reproduction, Fertility and Developement* 18: 63–9.
8. Diplas AI, Lambertini L, Lee MJ et al. (2009) Differential expression of imprinted genes in normal and IUGR human placentas. *Epigenetics* 4: 235–40.
9. Van Den Veyver IB and Al-Hussaini TK (2006) Biparental hydatidiform moles: A maternal effect mutation affecting imprinting in the offspring. *Human Reproduction Update* 12: 233–42.
10. Yu L, Chen M, Zhao D et al. (2009) The H19 gene imprinting in normal pregnancy and pre-eclampsia. *Placenta* 30: 443–7.
11. Bourque DK, Avila L, Penaherrera M et al. (2010) Decreased placental methylation at the H19/IGF2 imprinting control region is associated with normotensive intrauterine growth restriction but not pre-eclampsia. *Placenta* 31: 197–202.

13

CHAPTER 13

Placental Membranes and Amniotic Fluid Retention

Marie H. Beall[1,2] *and Michael G. Ross*[1,2]

[1]Department of Obstetrics and Gynecology, Los Angeles Biomedical Research Institute at Harbor-UCLA Medical Center, Torrance, CA, USA

[2]David Geffen School of Medicine at UCLA, Los Angeles, CA, USA

Introduction

Successful pregnancy requires the accumulation of significant amounts of water; by term in a normal human pregnancy, the amount of water in the fetal compartments, including fetus, placenta, and amniotic fluid (AF), may approach 5 L. AF fills the gestational sac, surrounding the fetus, allowing for normal musculoskeletal and lung development while protecting the fetus both from trauma and from infection. The water composition of AF is derived primarily across the placenta from the maternal circulation, with a small contribution from fetal metabolic water production. Water then passes into the amniotic sac via the fetal kidneys and lungs and is returned to the fetal circulation by fetal swallowing and by flow across the amnion into the fetal vessels. Abnormalities of any of these processes may influence the amount of AF present; abnormalities of AF volume are associated with a variety of poor perinatal outcomes.

Placental water flux

Water, the primary constituent of AF, flows to the fetus from the mother. Studies in animal models suggest that this flow occurs in the placenta; in late pregnancy, flow directly across the fetal membranes from the decidua is minimal. In biologic systems, the primary mechanism of water flux is passive flow through membrane water channels [1]. The flow of water may be bidirectional (i.e., diffusion) or it may be driven unidirectionally by either hydrostatic or osmotic forces. Within the placenta, hydrostatic forces driving water flow to the fetus would require higher maternal than fetal circulatory pressure. Measurable pressures do not favor maternal-to-fetal flow, so a functional hydrostatic mechanism would require the development of local pressure differences. The direction of maternal blood circulation in the human placental lobule is from central to peripheral, and therefore, at cross-current to the fetal blood flow, directional differences in blood flow could potentially allow local pressure differences to develop that drive water flow.

The relative osmolalities of maternal and fetal plasma also do not favor water flow to the fetus because fetal plasma is hypotonic compared to maternal plasma. Therefore, osmotic water flow in the placenta would also require the development of local osmotic gradients due either to active transport of solutes, such as sodium, or to depletion of solvent from the local perimembrane environment. Either phenomenon may result in a local increase in osmolality due to the "unstirred layer" effect. It has not been possible to directly study pressure or osmotic differences at the level of the syncytium; therefore, only circumstantial evidence is available regarding the forces driving water flow across the placenta.

The Placenta: From Development to Disease, First Edition. Edited by Helen H. Kay, D. Michael Nelson and Yuping Wang.
© 2011 Blackwell Publishing Ltd. Published 2011 by Blackwell Publishing Ltd.

As the fetus defends its intravascular and tissue water volumes, changes in conceptional water are first revealed in the AF volume, and AF volume changes may be an indicator of abnormalities of placental water flow. Although the normal mechanism driving placental water flow is uncertain, pathologic alterations in maternal serum osmolality (20–30 mOsm/kg) have a clear effect on AF volume. Maternal dehydration and increased maternal serum osmolality may be associated with oligohydramnios, while a decrease in maternal serum osmolality is associated with increased AF volume. Therefore, changes in maternal serum osmolality alter maternal-to-fetal water flow across the placenta.

In contrast, there are few reports of alterations in maternal hydrostatic forces affecting AF volume. In particular, there are no reports associating sudden maternal hypertension with fetal polyhydramnios. Studies of perfused human placental lobules suggest that vasoactive substances in the fetal circulation increase fetal venous pressure, inducing loss of fluid to the maternal circulation [2]. These data suggest that *fetal* stress, manifested by an increased production of vasoactive substances, can potentially induce fetal-to-maternal fluid loss (and therefore oligohydramnios) through a hydrostatic mechanism.

Clinical Pearl

Significant maternal dehydration may be associated with oligohydramnios by an osmotic mechanism. Maternal hydration with oral water has been shown to increase AF volume in randomized studies [3].

AF volume and composition

AF volume changes dramatically during human pregnancy (Figure 13.1), increasing from about 20 mL at 10 weeks to 630 mL at 22 weeks and 770 mL at 28 weeks gestation [4]. Between 29 and 37 weeks, there is little change in volume. Beyond 39 weeks, AF volume decreases sharply, averaging 515 mL at 41 weeks and continuing to decrease with post-term pregnancies.

During the first trimester, human AF is isotonic with maternal or fetal plasma [5] but contains minimal protein. These findings suggest that the AF is a transudate of plasma, either from the fetus through nonkeratinized fetal skin or from the mother across the uterine decidua and/or placenta surface. After midgestation, the composition of AF reflects a combination of fetal lung liquid and fetal urine, both fluids with properties different from

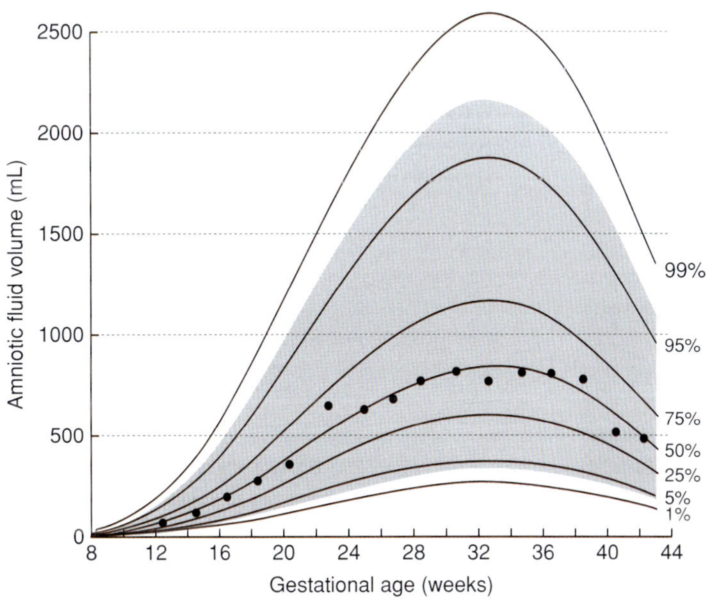

Figure 13.1 Human amniotic fluid volume throughout gestation (From [4]). The range of normal is very large: a 32-week fetus may have more than 2,000 mL of fluid or less than 500 mL.

fetal plasma. Fetal urine is more dilute, with osmolality and sodium and chloride concentrations lower than that of serum, although the near-term fetus can alter its urine volume and osmolality in response to hormonal signals such as vasopressin [6]. By contrast, the osmolality and sodium concentrations of fetal lung liquid are similar to plasma, but lung liquid has a high chloride concentration, 150–169 mEq/L, because the flux of water is driven by the active secretion of chloride into the future airways [7]. In comparison with the first half of pregnancy, human AF osmolality in late pregnancy decreases by 20–30 mOsm/kg to levels approximately 85–90% of maternal serum osmolality. With fetal renal development in the second half of pregnancy, AF urea, creatinine, and uric acid increase until AF concentrations of urinary byproducts are two to three times higher than fetal plasma.

Research Spotlight

Minor components of AF may be useful in the diagnosis of fetal anomalies or pregnancy complications. For example, AF levels of the inflammatory mediators IL-6 and TNF-α may be elevated at midtrimester amniocentesis in patients subsequently delivering preterm [8].

Production of AF

The source of early pregnancy AF has not been well studied; however, first trimester AF is thought to derive from the fetal surface of the placenta, transmembranous flow from the maternal compartment, and transudation from the nonkeratinized fetal skin. The relative contributions from these potential sources are unknown. AF is present in anembryonic pregnancies, indicating that the fetus is likely not the primary AF source in early pregnancy.

By midgestation, the fetus becomes a significant source of AF. Fetal urine begins to enter the amniotic sac, and the fetus begins to swallow AF in conjunction with the transition from embryo to fetus, although the daily volume flows are initially quite small. The fetal lungs also begin to secrete liquid into the AF at this time. By term, the primary sources of AF are the fetal urine and secretions from the fetal lung, and the primary mechanisms for clearance of fluid are fetal swallowing and direct flow of AF across the amnion to the fetal vessels (intramembranous (IM) flow).

IM flow [9] refers to the flow of water and solutes from the amniotic cavity directly across the amnion into the fetal vessels within the placenta. This is thought to occur primarily across microscopic fetal vessels on the surface of the placenta in primates and over the whole membrane surface in species with vascularized membranes. Smaller contributions may come across the umbilical cord and fetal skin, prior to keratinization at 22–24 weeks of gestation. Several lines of investigation, primarily in the sheep, provide indirect evidence of IM flow. For example, injection of distilled water into the AF is followed by a lowering of fetal serum osmolality, which occurs prior to any changes in maternal osmolality, indicating absorption of AF directly into the fetal circulation. In sheep in vivo, the permeability of the amnion to inert solutes such as technetium and inulin is greater from the AF to the fetal circulation than in the other direction. This asymmetry in membrane permeability is not seen in vitro. These findings suggest that there is a continuous flow of water and solutes from AF to the fetal circulation occurring in vivo [10]. Experimental estimates of the net IM flow range from 200 to 400 mL/day in fetal sheep. This, combined with fetal swallowing, approximately equals the flow of urine and lung liquid under homeostatic conditions. In humans, indirect evidence supports the presence of IM flow. For example, intra-amniotic ^{51}Cr appeared in the circulation of fetuses with impaired swallowing [11].

In addition to these major sources of AF, smaller contributions to AF volume are made via secretions from the fetal oral–nasal cavities. A minor source of AF clearance is transmembranous flow, or flow directly from the AF to the maternal blood across the decidua and myometrium.

Daily fetal urine excretion and fetal swallowing are well-described processes for AF production and clearance in both human fetuses and animal models, although there are major differences in current estimates of the volume of human fetal urine production. Other values are derived largely from animal models. We feel the best estimates of daily amniotic volume production and removal in the near term fetus are [12] (Figure 13.2)

- Fetal urine production: 800–1,200 mL/day
- Fetal lung liquid secretion: 170 mL/day
- Fetal swallowing: 500–1000 mL/day
- IM flow: 200–400 mL/day
- Oral–nasal secretions: 25 mL/day
- Transmembranous flow: 10 mL/day.

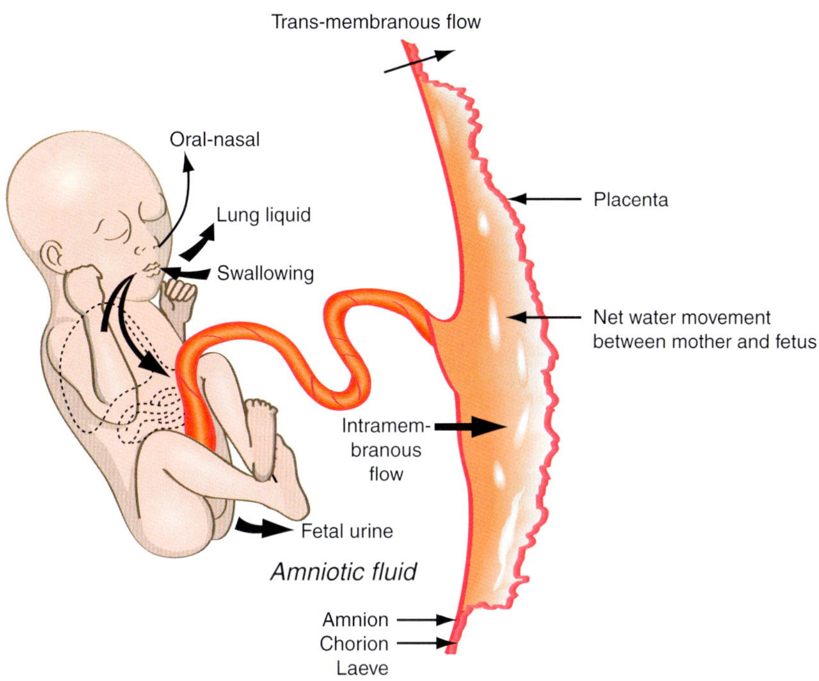

Figure 13.2 Fetus in utero showing major (and minor) sites of amniotic fluid production and removal. Production: fetal urine, lung liquid (oral–nasal secretions). Removal: swallowing, intremembranous flow (transmembranous flow). (Adapted from Seeds AE (1980) Current concepts of amniotic fluid dynamics. *American Journal of Obstetrics and Gynecology* 138(5): 575–86.

Regulation of amniotic fluid volume

In normal pregnancies, the AF volume does not change significantly from day to day, even though the AF itself may be completely exchanged in a 24-hour period. Near term, about 1,000 mL of fluid flows into and out of the amniotic cavity daily; small changes in the balance between inflow and resorption have the potential to rapidly change the AF volume [13]. Thus, a close balance between inflow and resorption must be maintained in order to prevent wide swings in AF volume.

One means of regulating AF volume is by varying the rate of IM flow. In experimental animals, IM absorption of AF may be increased dramatically. For example, ligating the fetal esophagus in sheep did not lead to polyhydramnios despite the absence of fetal swallowing, because of a marked increase in IM flow [14]. The mechanism for upregulation of IM flow has not been identified, although an increase in VEGF and changes in the expression of water channels have been described, suggesting that both angiogenic and permeability factors may be invoked. Although there are a number of studies documenting increased IM flow, no studies have yet found a decrease in IM flow in fetuses with oligohydramnios.

Research Spotlight

Research suggests that aquaporin water channels mediate the passage of water into and out of the AF. The expression of aquaporins is altered in both the amnion and placenta of fetuses with AF abnormalities [15]. There are 13 known mammalian aquaporins (AQPs); placenta and membranes of humans and other species express aquaporins 1, 3, 4, 5, 8, and 9. The relative importance of these aquaporins on maternal-to-fetal water transfer and on AF water circulation is still being worked out. Mouse data suggest a negative correlation of AF volume with amnion AQP1 expression and a positive correlation with placental AQP3 expression.

Mice without AQP1 (knock out mice) have polyhydramnios, while in humans with idiopathic polyhydramnios, AQP1 in the amnion is increased. The human results may be a compensatory response to the increased AF. Similarly, human polyhydramnios is associated with increased AQP3, 8, and 9 expression (RNA and protein) in the amnion and decreased expression of AQP3 and 9 in the placenta. An increase in amnion AQP would have the effect of increasing water flow across the amnion while a decrease in placental AQP expression might slow placental water flow, suggesting that these changes could decrease maternal-to-fetal water flow and increase AF resorption. These actions would prevent polyhydramnios. The increase in AQP8 in the placenta is not consistent with this hypothesis, and remains to be explained. In human oligohydramnios, there is less information available. Amnion AQP1 and 3 expression are decreased, also suggesting a compensatory mechanism. Similar to the findings in polyhydramnios, the placental findings are less clear with AQP3 expression increased, while AQP1 expression may be decreased. These findings may relate to the different locations of the AQPs (AQP1 in the vessels, AQP3 in the trophoblast) or to the specific causes of oligohydramnios in the patients studied. Studies in human amnion explants have shown that the expression of AQP1, 8, and 9 is increased by cyclic AMP, suggesting a mechanism for oligohydramnios with the upregulation of membrane AQPs by stress.

In conclusion, the AQPs appear likely to be involved in the mediation of water passage from mother to fetus across the placenta, as well as in the process of IM flow. It should be acknowledged that AQPs are also involved in other processes involving AF volume, including the production of fluid by both the kidneys and lung, and the effect of altered AQP production is therefore complex. Given the possibility of treatment of AF volume abnormalities with modulation of AQP expression, this remains an area of active research [16].

Abnormalities of AF volume

Abnormalities of AF volume occur when there is an imbalance between AF production and resorption. Either excessive or deficient AF volume is associated with poor perinatal outcome, with greater degrees of abnormality associated with a greater risk of fetal anomalies and perinatal death.

Polyhydramnios affects 1–3% of pregnancies. It may be the result of increased urine production or decreased fetal swallowing. Fetal urine flow can be increased in infants of diabetic mothers as a result of fetal glycosuria. Human fetal urine flow can also be increased in conditions of circulatory overload, as may occur with twin transfusion syndrome or severe fetal anemia. In addition to increased urinary output, absent or reduced fetal swallowing is a common cause of polyhydramnios. Swallowing may be compromised both by neurologic lesions that prevent or impair swallowing activity, i.e., fetal anencephaly, and by anatomic lesions that block passage of the fluid into the fetal upper gastrointestinal tract where AF is normally absorbed, i.e., fetal duodenal atresia. Finally, conditions leading to maternal hypo-osmolality or low serum oncotic pressure can increase water transfer to the fetus across the placenta, with a resultant fetal volume overload, i.e., in cases of maternal syndrome of inappropriate antidiuretic hormone hypersecretion (SIADH) caused by excessive release of vasopressin from the posterior pituitary gland. Although there are no human data, studies on sheep suggest that fetal lung fluid production is normally maintained at the maximum rate. Therefore, increased fetal lung fluid production, at least in the sheep, is not a cause of polyhydramnios. Finally, there is no clinical condition where a defect in IM flow can be shown to cause human polyhydramnios.

Oligohydramnios with intact fetal membranes, affecting 3–5% of pregnancies, is generally a consequence of the reduction of urine flow from the fetal kidney to the amniotic cavity; there are presently no examples of oligohydramnios related to the other sources of AF inflow and resorption. Reduced urine production by the fetal kidney may be caused by reduced renal perfusion, which may in turn be caused by decreased fetal intravascular volume or redirection of fetal blood flow away from the kidney, or by enhanced renal tubular absorption of water. The donor twin in the setting of twin–twin transfusion may demonstrate oligohydramnios due to reduced intravascular volume. Post-term or hypoxic fetuses demonstrate oligohydramnios due to alterations in fetal renal artery flow consistent with the redistribution of fetal blood flow to vital organs. Fetal renal function may also be impaired as a consequence of renal disease, either genetic (i.e., polycystic kidneys) or acquired (i.e., fetal exposure to maternal ingestion of nonsteroidal anti-inflammatory agents). Finally, fetal urine output may be reduced due to an obstruction in the urinary tract downstream from the kidney. The etiology of oligohydramnios varies with gestational age at diagnosis. Oligohydramnios detected in the second trimester is most likely to be due to a fetal anomaly, while fetal growth restriction and idiopathic oligohydramnios are more common in the third trimester.

Distinguishing the etiology of oligohydramnios will separate the fetus with hypoxia from the fetus with a structural anomaly.

Clinical Pearl

Work up for oligohydramnios should include an assessment of the fetal urinary system by careful ultrasound examination. A common scenario in obstetrics is use of Indocin for preterm labor treatment leading to oligohydramnios. The fetal urinary system is normal by scan in this situation.

Teaching Points

1 Water flow across the placenta occurs under osmotic, and possibly hydrostatic, force.

2 AF is largely composed of fetal urine and lung fluid, with the kidneys contributing about 80% of total volume.

3 AF is resorbed via fetal swallowing and directly across the amnion into fetal vessels on the chorionic plate (IM flow). The fetus may be able to modify IM flow to regulate AF volume.

4 Abnormalities of AF volume are associated with abnormalities of AF production or resorption.

References

1. Beall MH, Van Den Wijngaard JP, van Gemert MJ et al. (2007) Amniotic fluid water dynamics. *Placenta* 28(8–9): 816–23.
2. Brownbill P and Sibley CP (2006) Regulation of transplacental water transfer: The role of fetoplacental venous tone. *Placenta* 27(6–7): 560–7.
3. Doi S, Osada H, Seki K et al. (1998) Effect of maternal hydration on oligohydramnios: A comparison of three volume expansion methods. *Obstetrics and Gynecology* 92(4 Pt 1): 525–9.
4. Brace RA and Wolf EJ (1989) Normal amniotic fluid volume changes throughout pregnancy. *American Journal of Obstetrics and Gynecology* 161: 382–8.
5. Campbell J, Wathen N, Macintosh M et al. (1992) Biochemical composition of amniotic fluid and extraembryonic coelomic fluid in the first trimester of pregnancy. *British Journal of Obstetrics and Gynecology* 99: 563–5.
6. Horne RS, MacIsaac RJ, Moritz KM et al. (1993) Effect of arginine vasopressin and parathyroid hormone-related protein on renal function in the ovine foetus. *Clinical and Experimental Pharmacology and Physiology* 20: 569–77.
7. Thurlow RW and Brace RA (2003) Swallowing, urine flow, and amniotic fluid volume responses to prolonged hypoxia in the ovine fetus. *American Journal of Obstetrics and Gynecology* 189: 601–8.
8. Thomakos N, Daskalakis G, Papapanagiotou A et al. (2010) Amniotic fluid interleukin-6 and tumor necrosis factor-alpha at midtrimester genetic amniocentesis: Relationship to intra-amniotic microbial invasion and preterm delivery. *European Journal of Obstetrics and Gynecology and Reproductive Biology* 148(2): 147–51.
9. Gilbert WM and Brace RA (1989) The missing link in amniotic fluid volume regulation: Intramembranous absorption. *Obstetrics and Gynecology* 74: 748.
10. Adams EA, Choi HM, Cheung CY et al. (2005) Comparison of amniotic and intramembranous unidirectional permeabilities in late-gestation sheep. *American Journal of Obstetrics and Gynecology* 193: 247–55.
11. Queenan JT, Allen FH Jr, Fuchs F et al. (1965) Studies on the method of intrauterine transfusion. I. Question of erythrocyte absorption from amniotic fluid. *American Journal of Obstetrics and Gynecology* 92: 1009–13.
12. Brace RA and Ross MG (1998) Amniotic fluid volume regulation. In: Brace RA, Hanson MA, and Rodeck CH (Eds) *Fetus and Neonate—Volume 4: Body Fluids and Kidney Function.* Cambridge University Press; p. 88.
13. Brace RA (1997) Physiology of amniotic fluid volume regulation. *Clinical Obstetrics and Gynecology* 40: 280.
14. Beall MH, van den Wijngaard JP, van Gemert MJ et al. (2007) Regulation of amniotic fluid volume. *Placenta* 28(8–9): 824–32.
15. Zhu XQ, Jiang SS, Zhu XJ et al. (2009) Expression of aquaporin 1 and aquaporin 3 in fetal membranes and placenta in human term pregnancies with oligohydramnios. *Placenta* 30(8): 670–6.
16. Liu H, Zheng Z, and Wintour EM (2008) Aquaporins and fetal fluid balance. *Placenta* 29(10): 840–7.

PART III

Examination of the Placenta, Membranes, and Cord

14

CHAPTER 14
Examination of the Placenta, Membranes, and Cord: Basic Examination

Frederick T. Kraus
Department of Obstetrics and Gynecology, Washington University School of Medicine, St. Louis, MO, USA

Introduction

Chapter 3 on normal placental development and anatomy complements the following description of placental pathology. Briefly, villi early in gestation are called *mesenchymal villi* that have loose stroma, inconspicuous capillaries, and two complete surrounding trophoblast layers consisting of a cytotrophoblast layer surrounding the villous core and an outer syncytiotrophoblast layer on the villous surface. By midtrimester, immature intermediate villi have evolved and exhibit a reticular stroma, more prominent vessels, and a discontinuous cytotrophoblast layer. The outer syncytiotrophoblast layer remains continuous throughout development. Stem villi develop vessels with a smooth muscle investment and central stromal fibrosis. By the end of gestation, terminal villi are smaller, with scant stroma, 4–6 capillary profiles per cross-section, and an inconspicuous, discontinuous cytotrophoblast layer. The fetal capillaries of the villous core abut against thin, attenuated syncytiotrophoblast forming *vasculosyncytial membranes*. The trophoblast layer of stem villi is partly replaced by fibrin-type fibrinoid as gestation proceeds. Mature intermediate villi lose their reticular stroma and become smaller in diameter with a higher surface to cross-section area. Tangential cuts of the villous surface may show clusters of trophoblast nuclei, called syncytial or trophoblastic knots.

Clinical Pearl

A placenta that weighs below the 5th percentile for gestational age is compromised, and any additional lesions add cumulatively toward an adverse prognosis.

Pathological changes of villous tissue

Fetal thrombotic vasculopathy (FTV)

Cessation of fetal blood flow causes degeneration of capillary endothelial cells of terminal villi, which become fragmented ("karyorrhexis") (Figure 14.1(a)). A clot in a fetal vessel produces changes localized to the region supplied by the affected vessel; fetal death results in similar changes throughout the placenta. A later stage of this process leaves villi completely avascular, with fibrotic stroma, still covered by a viable layer of syncytiotrophoblast [1]. The affected areas of the placenta no longer function.

Distal villous hypoplasia (accelerated maturation)

This lesion is a result of reduced uteroplacental blood flow in patients with severe preeclampsia. Terminal villi are extremely small, stem villi are slender with reduced

The Placenta: From Development to Disease, First Edition. Edited by Helen H. Kay, D. Michael Nelson and Yuping Wang.
© 2011 Blackwell Publishing Ltd. Published 2011 by Blackwell Publishing Ltd.

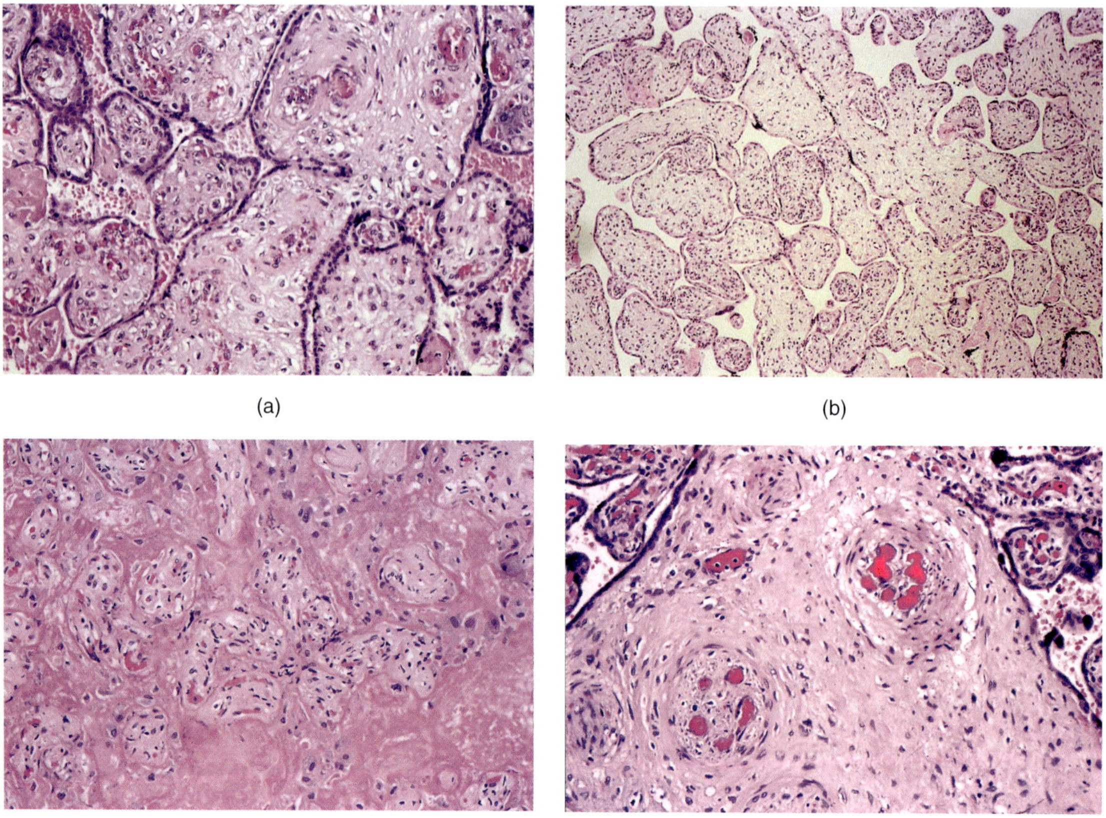

(a) (b) (c) (d)

Figure 14.1 Selected villous pathologic lesions. (a) An early lesion of FTV showing degeneration (karyorrhexis) of the capillary endothelium. (b) Villous edema from the placenta of a fetus with severe edema caused by a severe fetal–maternal hemorrhage. (c) Massive perivillous fibrin from a term placenta. (d) Septation in stem vessels, representing chronic changes of FTV.

branching, and clusters of trophoblast nuclei ("*syncytial knots*") are numerous and more prominent [2].

Chronic villitis; villitis of unknown etiology (VUE)

Noninfectious chronic villitis is characterized by a patchy multifocal infiltrate of lymphocytes and histiocytes in the villous stroma. The lymphocytes are maternal CD8 positive T lymphocytes. The extent is highly variable. Involvement of larger fetal vessels causing thrombosis (obliterative fetal vasculopathy) is a risk factor for neurologic injury to the newborn [3]. Necrosis and fibrin are often present; clusters of villi may become adherent. This is to be distinguished from infectious chronic villitis caused by cytomegalic inclusion virus, vaccinia, toxoplasmosis, syphilis, and other organisms. A component of plasma cells, when present, is strongly suggestive of an infectious process.

Distal villous immaturity, with and without dysmorphic villi

In this disorder, terminal villi and smaller stem villi have enlarged, sometimes very irregular outlines, with mild edema, increased stroma, and irregular vessel distribution. This is found in association with maternal diabetes mellitus and newborns with genetic abnormalities.

Clinical Pearl

Chronic placental FTV or VUE, involving as much as 30–40% of the placenta, is a significant cause of intrauterine growth restriction.

Villous edema

In this disorder, distal villi and immature intermediate villi have swollen outlines resulting from greatly expanded water-filled spaces that compress capillary lumens (Figure 14.1(b)). The most common association of severe villous edema (placental hydrops) is nonimmune fetal hydrops including fetal anemia from severe fetomaternal hemorrhage, congenital heart malformations, and various fetal tumors. This is also a feature in placentas of some extremely low-birth-weight newborns with neurologic disabilities [4]. Effective vascular perfusion is impaired, apparently by compression of the villous capillaries. Villous edema may also occur focally in acute abruption and some cases of acute chorioamnionitis.

Perivillous fibrin

This is seen with scattered clumps of pink amorphous fibrin material normally occurring focally, attached to the denuded surface of some but not all villi, replacing the syncytiotrophoblast cells that may regenerate over the surface of the fibrin. This process may become extensive in preeclampsia. Rarely, massive accumulations of matrix-type perivillous fibrin accumulate in the intervillous space. The resulting lesion, called *massive perivillous fibrin* (Figure 14.1(c)), is associated with loss of the villous syncytiotrophoblast and migration of cytotrophoblast cells into the fibrinoid material, while the villous outlines and stromal cells are preserved [5]. The localized occurrence of such deposits around the villi near the maternal surface of the placenta is called (a misnomer) *maternal floor infarct*. Very extensive lesions (involving 30–50% of the placenta) may result in growth restriction and significant neonatal neurologic impairment [6].

Research Spotlight

Confined placental mosaicism is less important cause of fetal growth restriction; the histopathologie lesions and molecular causes have not been determined.

Mesenchymal dysplasia

This is a rare complex of placental villous enlargement, dilated tortuous chorionic plate vessels, multiple large hydropic villi, myxoid stromal changes, focal chorioangiomatosis, and intravascular thrombi. Growth restriction and IUFD are common outcomes. Variable genetic abnormalities occur with mesenchymal dysplasia, including androgenetic/biparental mosaicism and chimerism, as well as the Beckwith-Wiedemann syndrome in 20% of cases [7].

Clinical Pearl

The ultrasound image of mesenchymal dysplasia of the placenta is similar to that of partial hydatidiform mole; therefore, a common ultrasound interpretation is "suggestive of partial mole."

Histopathology of stem villi and vessels of the chorionic plate

Intimal fibrin cushion

These are seen as a bulging from the inner surface of large fetal vessels, often in or near the chorionic plate. They are large nonocclusive edematous masses of loose connective tissue, usually with a surface coating of fibrin. They may be associated with FTV and older lesions may calcify [1].

Thrombi

Recent thrombi in the cord and larger fetal blood vessels have a layered appearance, with strata of red blood cells alternating with layers of fibrin and platelets. Integrity of the vessel wall around older thrombi breaks down with extravasation of blood into the muscular wall of the vessel and degeneration of the red and white blood cells.

Clinical Pearl

The presence of clots within the fetal circulation of the placenta indicates potential for clots to occur in the fetal circulation such as in the brain or other organs. Cerebral vascular occlusion, with localized infarction, has been demonstrated in this context prenatally as well as neonatally.

Septation

In smaller stem blood vessels, stasis caused by thrombosis or fetal death results in obliteration of the lumen by clumps of fibrin and red blood cells separated by bridging strands of fibroblastic cells forming multiple occluded lumens (Figure 14.1(d)) [8].

Pathological lesions of the interface of decidua and placenta

The implantation site is at the interface between the placenta and the decidualized endometrium, adjacent to the surface of the inner uterine wall. This area includes multiple invasive trophoblasts as described in the chapter on normal placental anatomy. These cells of fetal origin are intermixed with the decidualized endometrium, maternal immune cells, and the spiral arteries that supply maternal blood to the intervillous space of the placenta. The normal anatomy can evolve into pathological lesions, some of which are described below.

Placental site trophoblasts

In patients with preeclampsia, placental site trophoblast cells are increased and have features of immaturity and increased proliferative activity. There may be focal necrosis and increased numbers of lymphocytes and histiocytes in the *decidua*.

Spiral arteries

In patients with preeclampsia, there is a failure in the progression of the physiologic vascular changes in the spiral arteries. The result is called *acute atherosis*, which is characterized by persistence of arterial smooth muscle, reduced expansion of the vascular lumen, and fibrinoid necrosis of the arterial wall (Figure 14.2). Intramural foam cells (macrophages) appear and partial or complete thrombosis may occur [2]. The result is *marked vascular underperfusion* of the placenta, which is often manifested as reduced placental size. Placental infarcts occur in more severe cases, further reducing the amount of functioning placenta. A less frequent abnormality is spiral artery narrowing caused by smooth muscle proliferation with marked thickening of spiral arterial wall. The preeclampsia is often complicated by diabetes mellitus in such cases.

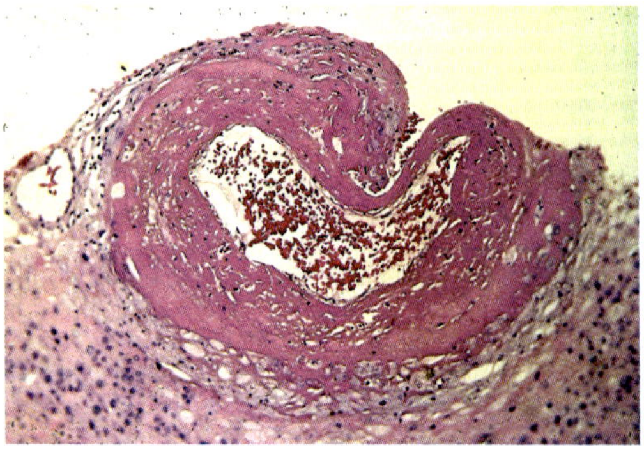

Figure 14.2 A spiral artery from the adherent decidua on the maternal surface of the placenta shows acute atherosis. The mother had severe preeclampsia and the newborn was growth restricted. The vessel is narrow. The lumen is further narrowed by adherent fibrin, and the wall is necrotic.

> **Clinical Pearl**
>
> Acute atherosis and distal villous hypoplasia, the recognized lesions of preeclampsia, are also the most common placental pathologic abnormalities resulting in intrauterine growth restriction.

The chorionic plate

Acute chorioamnionitis

Bacterial infection in the amniotic fluid attracts maternal acute inflammatory cells to infiltrate the chorionic plate, the extraplacental membranes, and the fetal acute inflammatory cells to infiltrate the walls of fetal vessels in the cord and chorionic plate. Thus, there is a *maternal inflammatory response* to amniotic fluid infection in the membranes and chorionic plate and a *fetal inflammatory response* in the blood vessels of the umbilical cord and chorionic plate.

Chorioamnionitis is divided into *stages* of progression and into *grades* of intensity of the inflammatory process [9].

Stage I: The maternal inflammatory response begins with an accumulation of neutrophils in a layer of subchorionic fibrin and may extend into the adjacent lower half of the membranous connective tissue of the chorionic plate.

Stage II: The inflammatory infiltrate extends progressively toward the amnionic basement membrane (Figure 14.3).

Stage III (necrotizing chorioamnionitis): Necrosis of the amnionic epithelium and basement membrane, focal or patchy, occurs.

Grade 1 (mild-moderate): The neutrophilic infiltrate is diffuse but relatively sparse.

Grade 2 (severe): Three or more microabscesses are present (confluent aggregates of neutrophils at least 10 $\times$ 20 cells in extent).

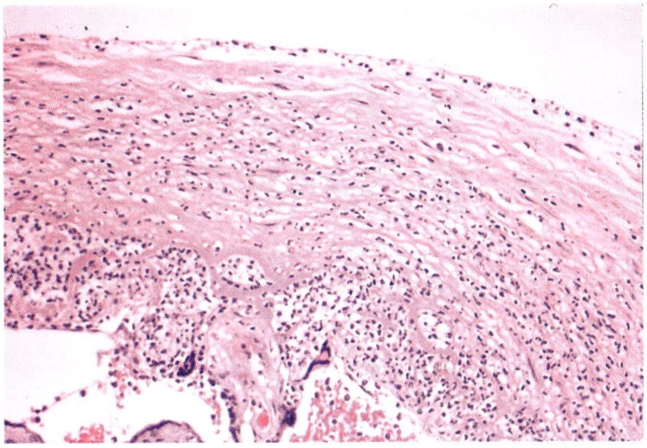

Figure 14.3 Acute chorioamnionitis. The chorionic plate is infiltrated by large numbers of neutrophilic leukocytes. The amnion shows early degenerative changes.

Fetal response in the chorionic plate

Neutrophils from the fetal circulation invade the walls of the fetal blood vessels in the direction of the amnion. Mural or occlusive clots may occur in this context.

> **Clinical Pearl**
>
> The combination of a severe maternal response with a severe fetal response results in a significant increase in the risk of neurologic injury to the newborn.

Amnion nodosum

This is seen as small tan nodules adherent to the fetal surface, replacing the underlying amnion. They are composed of a heterogeneous mixture of vernix squames, eosinophilic debris, and fragments of lanugo hair. The condition occurs in severe oligohydramnios, for instance, with renal agenesis in which fetal urine cannot contribute to the formation of amniotic fluid.

Lesions of the membranes: Amnionic and chorionic layers

Acute chorioamnionitis

The Grades and Stages of the inflammatory response in the membranes resemble the patterns described above in the chorionic plate.

Stage I (early): The neutrophils form a thin layer at the interface between the chorionic membrane trophoblast and the chorionic stroma.

Stage II: Neutrophils infiltrate the stroma of the chorion and amnion.

Stage III: The amnionic epithelium is necrotic.

Grades I and II are identical to the patterns in the chorionic plate.

Umbilical cord

Acute funisitis

The *fetal response* to amniotic fluid infection takes place in the fetal vessels of the umbilical cord and chorionic plate. There are three stages of acute funisitis as below.

Stage I (early): Neutrophils invade the wall of the umbilical vein and/or the walls of the chorionic plate blood vessels.

Stage II: Neutrophils invade the umbilical arteries as well.

Stage III (necrotizing funisitis): Inflammatory cells invade into the Wharton's jelly matrix. There is necrosis, sometimes with calcification, forming a halo around the cord vessels.

Meconium-associated vascular necrosis

This is a rare lesion usually found in association with severe or prolonged meconium staining of the placenta and newborn. Vascular smooth muscle cells of the cord and/or chorionic plate blood vessels develop condensation and fragmentation of nuclei: the cytoplasm becomes swollen and more densely eosinophilic. The nuclear changes may be more accurately characterized as apoptotic [10]. The clinical implications are grave with a high mortality rate and severe neurologic injury to the survivors.

> **Clinical Pearl**
>
> Cord lesions such as velamentous insertion, varices, or torsion may yield repeated partial obstruction to cause stasis and to predispose to thrombosis, hypoxia, and neurologic injury.

Some basics that all should know about processing and evaluation of the human placenta

Clinical data provided to the pathologist with the placenta sent for pathological analysis can greatly enhance the information available in the final pathology report. Useful clinical data include the following:

1 Mother's name, gravidity, parity
2 Clinical diagnoses associated with the pregnancy
3 Gestational age at delivery
4 Antepartum diagnoses and immediate newborn problems
5 Apgar scores
6 Specific indication for submission of the placenta.

Universal safety precautions for transmittal of blood-borne pathogens must be followed routinely.

Post-delivery storage of the placenta should be in a labeled container, which is refrigerated until the examination begins. Routine histologic study is acceptable after 24–48 hours' refrigeration and often is adequate even after 5–7 days of storage.

Fixation in 10% neutral buffered formalin follows the trimming, gross description, and slicing of the placental disc.

Macroscopic examination

Membranes

The closest amnionic rupture to placental margin distance is recorded; the fetal surface and then the maternal surface are described (discoloration, vessel distribution and dilatation, pale, thickened maternal surface, lesions, meconium staining). A strip of the membranes is rolled toward the placental margin, secured with two pins, and placed in formalin. The cord and remaining membranes are trimmed away from the placental margin.

Cord

The cord is measured (length, diameter) detached from the placenta, sliced across at 2–3 cm intervals, recording abnormalities (excessive twisting, tight knot, rupture, clot), and placed in formalin. Identify the proximal and distal segments; a simple method is to cut the proximal end longer and the distal end shorter than the other uniformly cut segments. Characteristics of the cord that should be described include coloration, presence of meconium staining, knots, degree of coiling, and presence of clots.

Placenta

The initial examination of the placenta should focus on its size and thickness; texture includes presence of calcifications and the presence of infarcts or tumors. Any clot on the maternal surface consistent with an abruption should be measured. The membranes and cord are then trimmed away, placenta is weighed, and the placental disc is sliced crosswise at 1–2 cm intervals. The cut surfaces are inspected and abnormalities such as induration, nodularity, and hematomas are described. The slices of placenta are placed in 10% neutral buffered formalin. The volume of fixative must be at least 3× the volume of the placenta itself.

Microscopic examination

The standard examination protocol begins after 12–24 hours' fixation of the strips of placental tissue as described above. Blocks for microscopic sections are prepared as follows:

1 At least two complete cross sections of normal-appearing placenta, central and para-central, from maternal to fetal surfaces should be submitted. These may be divided into two blocks if the placenta is very thick. Ideal thickness of tissue blocks for good histology is 2–3 mm.
2 When additional lesions are identified, at least one section of each type of lesion should be submitted for microscopic study.
3 Two cross sections of cord, one proximal and one distal to placenta plus section of any gross lesion should be submitted in one cassette.
4 Two cross sections of membrane roll should be submitted in one cassette. All sections bear the accession number of the placenta and each is given a unique letter designation listed specifically in the dictated description that accompanies each placenta. For example, these designations could include: A, cord; B, membranes; C, central placenta; D, paracentral placenta; E, a lesion; F, another lesion (see Figure 14.4).

Special analyses of the placenta often use fresh tissue, which requires attention prior to fixation. Some of the common procedures are noted below.

Cytogenetic studies require immediate culture of small tissue fragments. Portions of villous tissue are placed in culture media or a special transport medium, prior to refrigeration or immediate submission to a cytogenetics laboratory. A detailed protocol for tissue handling is available from the cytogenetics laboratory.

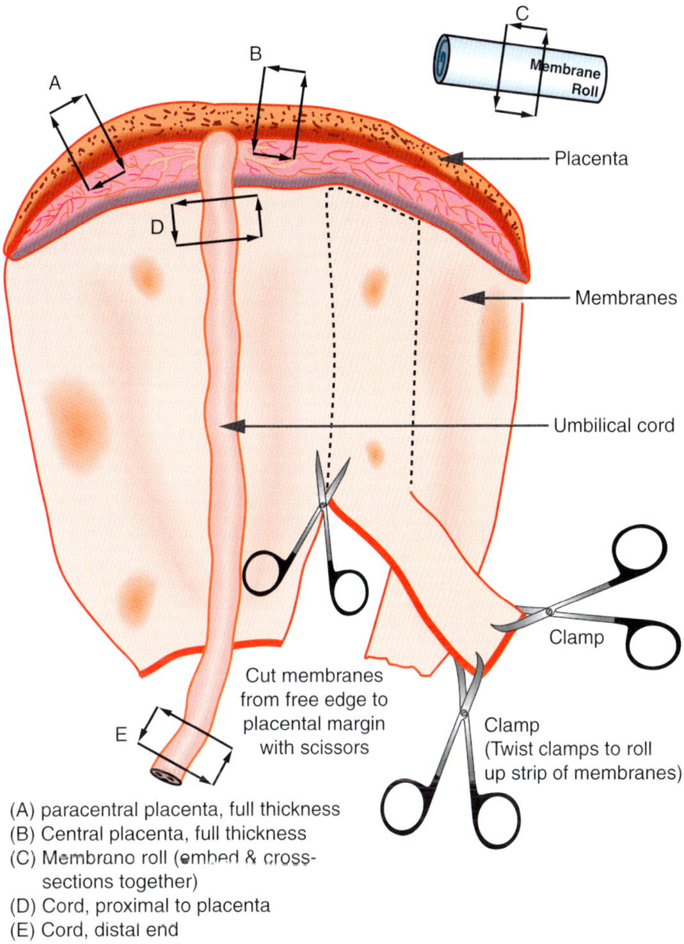

Figure 14.4 Diagram representing locations of standard tissue blocks for microscopic sections. These represent areas of normal-appearing placenta, which should be submitted in every case. Any abnormal areas would require additional sections.

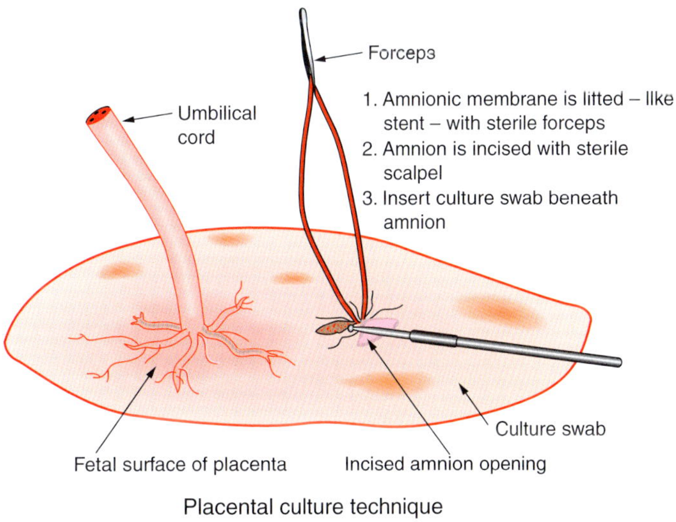

Figure 14.5 Diagram of bacteriologic culture technique. It is important to avoid touching the culture swab to the external surface of the amnion and the margins of the incised opening to avoid contamination of the culture.

Liquid nitrogen storage of placental tissue requires small portions of tissue to be placed in foil or cryo tubes prior to immersion for freezing in liquid nitrogen. Tubes holding such specimens require cryo-resistant labeling, dating of specimen, and storage in a freezer at −70°C. These specimens are useful for studies involving DNA or RNA, including fluorescence in situ hybridization [11], comparative genomic hybridization [11], metabolic disorders, and storage diseases, among others.

Bacterial cultures from the placenta require avoidance of contaminants. A useful technique is to cauterize and then incise the amnionic surface to sample the subchorionic fibrin zone with a sterile swab by sliding it beneath the chorionic plate between it and the amnion. We have found that this approach achieves a significant reduction in the number of contaminants while recovering pathogens successfully [12]. Another technique involves incising the amnion with a sterile scalpel and sliding the swab just beneath the amnion between it and the chorion (Figure 14.5) [13].

Research Spotlight

Several significant bacterial agents can only be identified by polymerase chain reaction (PCR) techniques applied to the 16S rRNA bacterial genes [11].

Electron microscopy can only be done on tiny portions of tissue, dissected with a razor blade or scalpel into a 1–2 mm slice, which are commonly fixed in a glutaraldehyde–formaldehyde fixative.

Immunohistochemistry is best done on tissue blocks no more than 3 mm in minimum diameter and fixed in 10% neutral buffered formalin for 24–48 hours prior to embedding in paraffin. Portions of tissue may be hardened for 12–24 hours initially so that blocks of <3 mm can be more easily cut from the exposed surfaces. The smaller pieces should be further fixed in fresh 10% neutral buffered formalin to complete a 24–48 hour total fixation time. These tissues may also be used for FISH and CGH.

Teaching points

1 If the placental examination cannot be started immediately, store it in the refrigerator. Never fix the entire uncut placental mass directly into formalin because if that is done, most of it will rot.

2 Universal safety precautions must be followed in all cases.

3 Bacterial cultures and portions of frozen tissue for DNA and RNA analysis must be taken as soon as possible before the standard examination procedures are started.

4 The standard sections of the placenta should sample the most normal-appearing and functioning areas. Additional blocks of tissue to determine the nature of grossly evident lesions must be sampled and labeled separately. For instance, record them as "Block D: firm red nodule," or "Block E: irregular tan indurated area."

Bibliography

1. Benirschke K, Kaufmann P, and Baergen R (2006) *Pathology of the Human Placenta*. 5th ed. New York: Springer.
2. Faye-Petersen OM, Heller DS, and Joshi VV (2006) *Handbook of Placental Pathology*. 2nd edn. New York: Taylor and Francis.
3. Fox H and Sebire NJ (2007) *Pathology of the Placenta*. 3rd ed. London: Elsevier.
4. Kraus FT, Redline RW, Gersell DJ et al. (2004) *Placental Pathology. Atlas of Nontumor Pathology, First series, Fascicle 3*. Washington, DC: American Registry of Pathology.

References

1. Redline R, Ariel IB, Baergen RN et al. (2004) Fetal vascular obstructive lesions: Nosology and reproducibility of placental reaction patterns. *Pediatric and Developmental Pathology* 7: 443–52.
2. Redline RW, Boyd T, Campbell V et al. (2004) Maternal vascular underperfusion: Nosology and reproducibility of placental reaction patterns. *Pediatric and Developmental Pathology* 7: 237–49.
3. Redline RW (2007) Villitis of unknown etiology: Noninfectious chronic villitis in the placenta. *Human Pathology* 38: 1439–46.
4. Redline RW, Minich N, Taylor HG et al. (2007) Placental lesions as predictors of cerebral palsy and abnormal neurocognitive function in extremely low birth weight infants (<1kg). *Pediatric and Developmental Pathology* 10: 282–92.
5. Katzman PJ and Genest DR (2002) Maternal floor infarction and massive perivillous fibrin deposition: Histological definitions, association with intrauterine fetal growth restriction, and risk of recurrence. *Pediatric and Developmental Pathology* 5: 159–64.

6. Adams-Chapman I, Vaucher YE, Bejar R et al. (2002) Maternal floor infarction of the placenta: Association with central nervous system injury and adverse neurodevelopmental outcome. *Journal of Perinatology* 22: 236–41.
7. Robinson WP, Lauzon JL, Innes AM et al. (2007) Origin and outcome of pregnancies affected by androgenetic/biparental chimerism. *Human Reproduction* 22: 1114–22.
8. Genest DR (1992) Estimating the time of death in stillborn fetuses: II. Histologic evaluation of the placenta; a study of 71 stillborns. *Obstetrics and Gynecology* 80: 585–92.
9. Redline RW, Faye-Peterson OM, Heller D et al. (2003) Amniotic infection syndrome: Nosology, and reproducibility of placental reaction patterns. *Pediatric and Developmental Pathology* 6: 435–48.
10. King EL, Redline RW, Smith SD et al. (2004) Myocytes of chorionic vessels from placentas with meconium-associated vascular necrosis exhibit apoptotic markers. *Human Pathology* 35: 412–17.
11. Han YW, Shen T, Chung P et al. (2009) Uncultivated bacteria as etiologic agents of intra-amniotic inflammation leading to preterm birth. *Journal of Clinical Microbiology* 47: 38-47.
12. Aquino TI, Zhang J, Kraus FT et al. (1984) Subchorionic fibrin cultures for bacteriologic study of the placenta. *American Journal of Clinical Pathology* 81: 482–6.
13. Kundsin RB, Driscoll SG, Monson RR et al. (1984) Association of Ureaplasma urealyticum in the placenta with perinatal morbidity and mortality. *The New England Journal of Medicine* 310: 941–5.

15

CHAPTER 15
The Umbilical Cord

Raymond W. Redline[1,2]

[1]Case Western Reserve University School of Medicine, Cleveland, OH, USA
[2]Pediatric and Perinatal Pathology, University Hospitals Case Medical Center, Cleveland, OH, USA

Anatomy

The umbilical cord (UC) transmits deoxygenated blood from the fetus to the placenta via paired umbilical arteries that arise from the internal iliac arteries, travel along the lateral margins of the bladder, and flank the urachus to enter the UC at the umbilicus (Figure 15.1). Transitional or glandular epithelial-lined remnants of the urachus are sometimes seen between the arteries in the proximal UC (allantoic duct). The two arteries communicate via Hyrtl's anastomosis in the distal UC within 3 cm of cord insertion into the placenta. Upon reaching the placental insertion site, the umbilical arteries branch into 6–8 major chorionic arteries that send projections into the stem villi to perfuse the cotyledons. Draining veins from the cotyledons in turn gather at the UC to form the umbilical vein, a thin-walled structure that is more easily compressed than the arteries. The connection of umbilical vein to ductus venosus, inferior vena cava, right heart, and foramen ovale allows oxygenated blood to directly enter the fetal arterial circulation. As a consequence of this facilitated pathway, thromboemboli and inflammatory mediators from the placenta have direct access to the microcirculation of fetal organs. Also occasionally seen in the proximal UC are remnants of the enteric epithelial-lined omphalomesenteric duct, which connects the yolk sac to the fetal gastrointestinal tract. The UC is surrounded by a simple squamous epithelium derived from the amnion. Acute stretching is limited by a distinctive "Chinese handcuff toy"- like arrangement of these cells. Vessels and remnants are embedded in Wharton's jelly, a gel-like extracellular matrix that resists compression. Wharton's jelly has a substructure comprised condensed connective tissue sheaths around vessels and surrounding loose collagenous tissue with stromal channels lined by myofibroblasts. Some of these latter cells are pluripotent mesenchymal stem cells that may be useful in therapeutic applications.

Normal development

The UC forms around the body stalk and yolk sac as the embryonic disc folds rostrocaudally and dorsoventrally to herniate into the amnionic cavity (Figure 15.2). The UC initially consists of vasculogenic mesenchyme, believed to be derived from extraembryonic endoderm. Subsequently, a caudal outpouching of embryonic endoderm called the *allantois* projects into the inferior portion of the UC and induces umbilical vessels that will ultimately connect to separately developing vessels of the embryo and placenta. The superior portion of the UC contains the remnants of the secondary yolk sac.

The Placenta: From Development to Disease, First Edition. Edited by Helen H. Kay, D. Michael Nelson and Yuping Wang.
© 2011 Blackwell Publishing Ltd. Published 2011 by Blackwell Publishing Ltd.

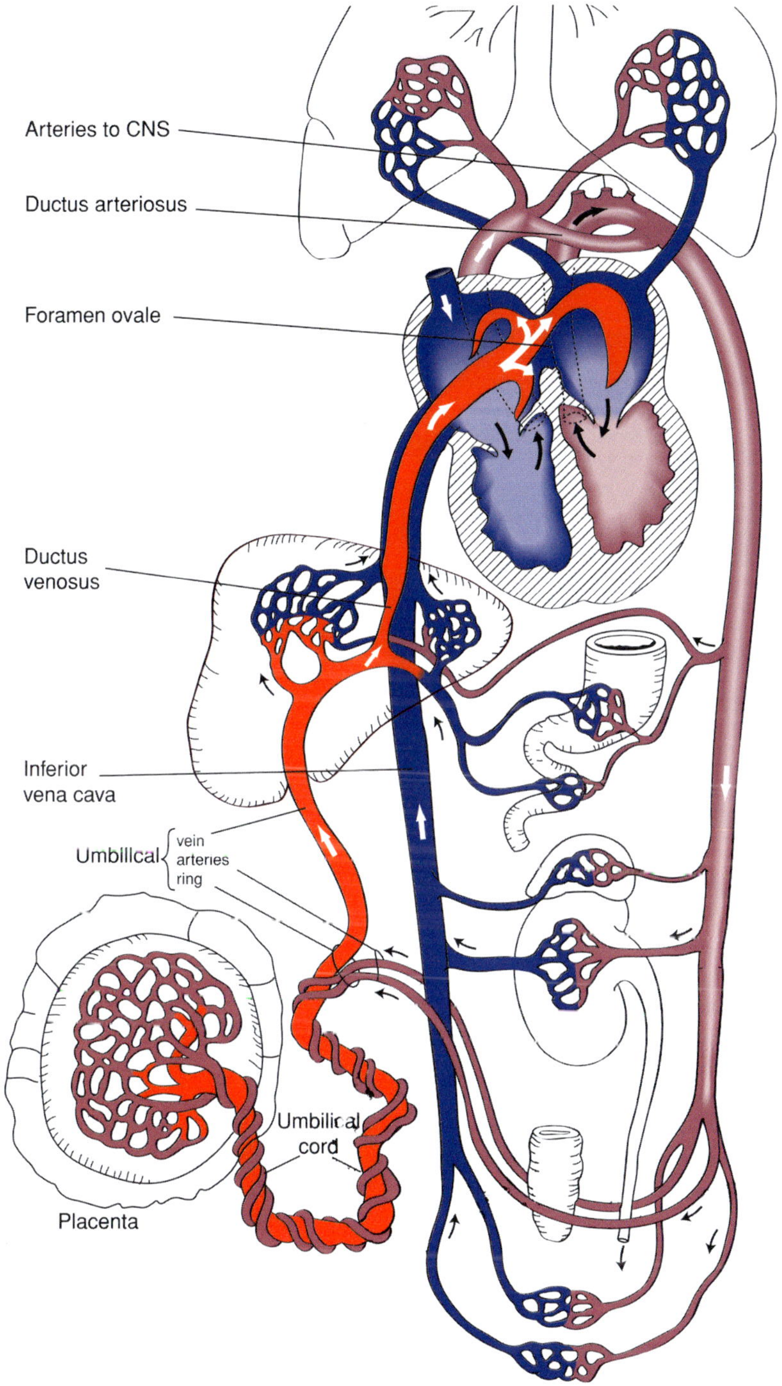

Figure 15.1 Diagram of fetoplacental umbilical circulation (see text for details).

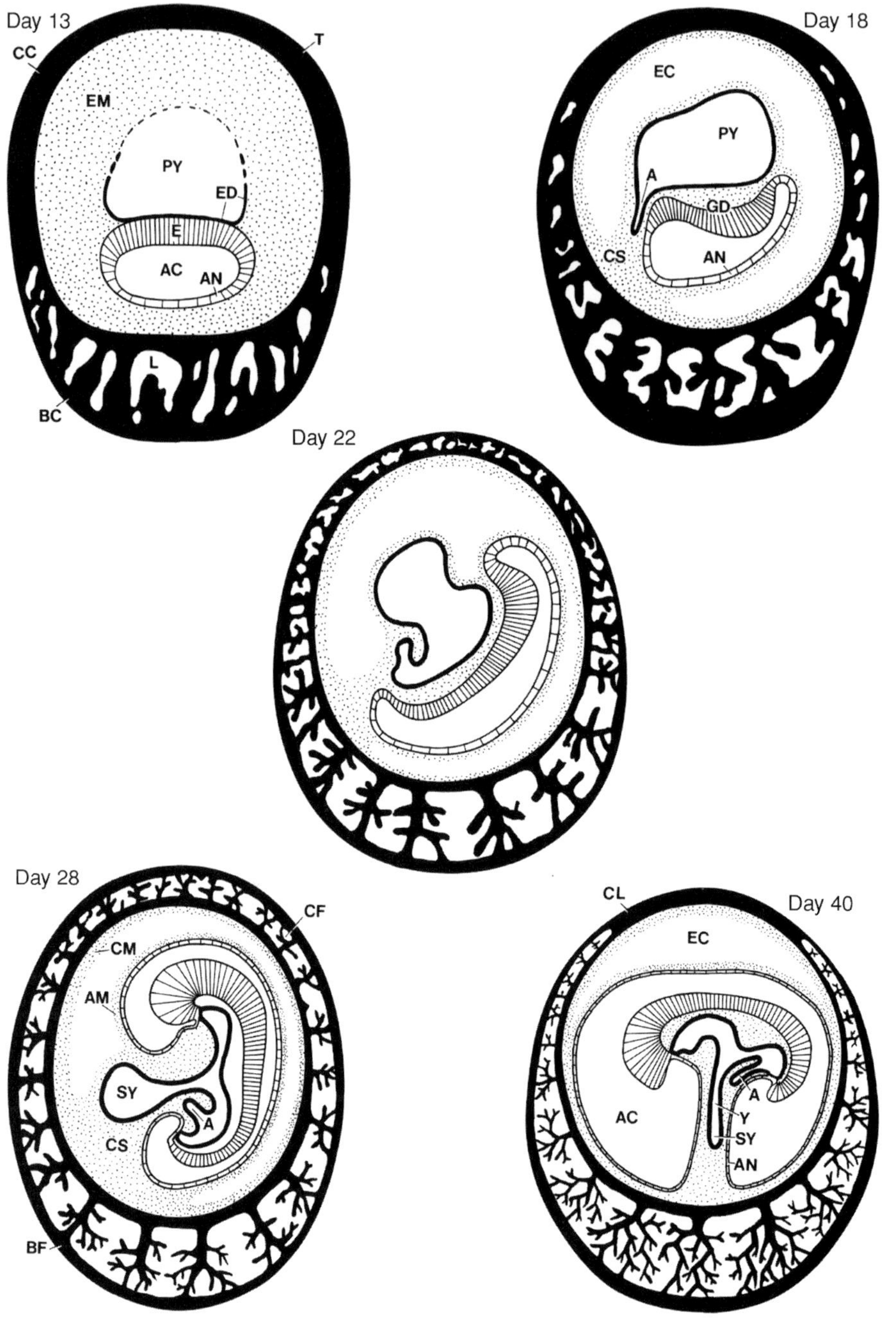

Figure 15.2 Stages of umbilical cord development, embryonic layers with surrounding placenta, day 13 to day 40 postcoitus (see text for details). EM, extra-embryonic mesoderm; PY, primary yolk sac; ED, endoderm; E, embryo; AC, amniotic cavity; AN, amnionic epithelium; CS, connecting stalk; GD, germ disc; CM, chorionic membrane; SY, secondary yolk sac; A, allantois; CF, chorion frondosum; CL, chorion laevae; Y, yolk stalk. (Reproduced with permission, Figure 12.1 from Benirschke K, Kaufmann P, and Baergen R (2006) *Pathology of the Human Placenta* 5th edn. Heidelburg: Springer.)

Research Spotlight

Experiments in the mouse have advanced our understanding of the molecular events involved in UC development [1]. (1) A novel organizer analogous to Henson's node, allantoic core domain, has been identified at the caudal, extraembryonic end of the primitive streak. This organizer expresses T/brachyury, which drives convergent extension of the allantois into UC. (2) Flk1+ angioblasts develop at the distal end of the allantois and migrate proximally. (3) HOX genes *b1* and *b8* are involved in UC patterning. (4) Binding of VCAM-1 at the allantoic tip to $\alpha 4\beta 1$ integrins in the chorion mediates fusion with the placenta while other distinct factors mediate branching and penetration of allantoic vessels into placental parenchyma.

In the human, chorionic vessels are first noted at 4 5/7 weeks. Umbilical veins form shortly thereafter at 5 2/7 weeks from an intraumbilical venous plexus. The right umbilical vein involutes leaving a single left umbilical vein that fuses with the embryonic circulation, completing the fetoplacental circulation at approximately 6 weeks. The UC is short and broad at 6 weeks, becomes elongated and coiled by 8 weeks, and reaches a full coiling pattern by 12–14 weeks.

Malformations

Agenesis

UC agenesis is classified into three types [2] with the first two apparent only in first trimester miscarriages. Type 1 is the classic anembryonic pregnancy detected as an empty sac by ultrasound and usually lacking fetal, amnionic, or yolk sac elements at pathologic examination. Type 2 is similar but also has a stunted or nodular embryo floating free in the extraembryonic coelom. Both types arise when embryonic lethality is inevitable and precludes normal formation of the body stalk and allantoic organizer, e.g., with chromosomal abnormalities. Type 3 UC agenesis, also known as Limb Body Wall Sequence, type 2, is characterized by body stalk vessels that travel outside the UC in a short membranous fold before direct insertion into the placenta. The fetus typically has eventration of the abdominal wall, cloacal abnormalities, and marked deformation of the limbs and spinal column that result secondary to forced apposition of the conceptus to the placenta and membranes (Figure 15.3). The fetus is enclosed in the amnion, but the abdominal contents are free in the extraembryonic coelom.

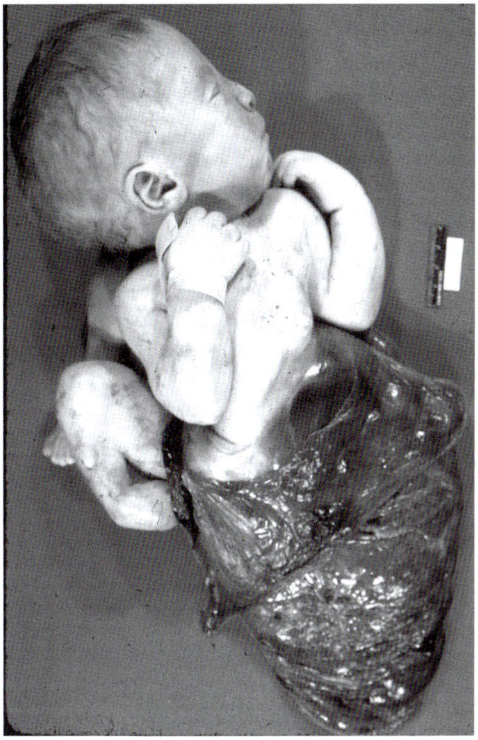

Figure 15.3 Type 3 UC agenesis/Limb Body Wall Sequence, type 2 (see text for details).

Abnormalities of the fetal insertion site

Omphaloceles represent incomplete closure of the lateral embryonic folds resulting in an open defect at the umbilical ring where eventration of abdominal organs into a membranous sac yields a protrusion into the amniotic cavity. Smaller defects measuring <4 cm are termed *umbilical hernias*. The UC arises from the center of the sac. Omphaloceles are found in 1–2/10,000 pregnancies and associate with aneuploidy (particularly trisomy 13), genetic syndromes, or other congenital malformations. *Gastroschisis* deserves mention here because of the frequent confusion of this fetal entity with omphalocele. Gastroschisis is neither a malformation nor an UC anomaly but instead is a disruption of the fetal abdominal wall. This defect is likely secondary to premature obliteration of the right vitelline artery that leads to peri-umbilical infarction with secondary prolapse of the intestines into the amniotic cavity. Gastroschisis is differentiated from omphalocele by the location to the right of the umbilical ring and by the absence of a membranous sac. Gastroschisis occurs in 1/6,000–10,000 births, is not usually associated with other fetal anomalies, and has been increasing in incidence over the past 20 years.

Abnormalities of the placental insertion site

Over 90% of UC insert towards the center of the chorionic plate of the placenta within 3 cm of the margin, another 7–10% insert at or near the junction of the chorionic plate and the chorioamnion, and the remaining 0.2–1.2% insert in the membranes of the chorioamnion. Peripheral UC insertion was once believed to result from abnormal rotation of the blastocyst at nidation. Observations by serial ultrasound now favor a mechanism for UC insertion that results from *trophotropism*, where development of placental tissue preferentially occurs at sites of optimal uterine perfusion and more or less distant from original central UC insertion site. Peripheral UC insertion is associated with a decreased density of vessels on the chorionic plate and a high fetoplacental weight ratio, which may be indicative of a direct effect on placental function and fetal growth [3]. Less common abnormalities include *furcate* UC where the vessels prematurely branch before insertion, *velamentous* interposition of the UC where the umbilical vessels remain intact, but they are without the covering of Wharton's jelly prior to insertion, and *tethered* UC where a fold of amnion fixes the insertion site at an oblique angle to the chorionic plate to restrict cord range of motion.

Umbilical vascular abnormalities

A *single umbilical artery* (SUA) is noted in 0.5–1% of deliveries. Most SUA are classified as type 1 and represent the absence of one of the two umbilical branches from the internal iliac arteries. Most commonly, the absent artery is on the left. Other patterns have been described, e.g., type 2 with a single vitelline artery and umbilical vein, type 3 with a single umbilical artery and two umbilical veins, and type 4 with a persistent right umbilical vein with either a vitelline or umbilical artery. Controversy exists regarding the percentage resulting from primary maldevelopment versus secondary atrophy. Fetal anomalies most frequently associated with type 1 SUA are renal agenesis, imperforate anus, vertebral defects, and cardiac anomalies. Type 2 SUA is usually seen with sirenomelia and caudal regression sequence. *Fused umbilical arteries* result from fusion of the two arteries near the placental insertion site, with an incidence of three percent by ultrasound. *Discordant umbilical arteries* exhibit vessels with different calibers and pulsatility indices by Doppler assessment.

Cysts

True cysts may develop within the umbilical cord from omphalomesenteric or allantoic remnants or on the cord surface (amnion epithelial inclusion cysts). Pseudocysts, those lacking an epithelial lining, may be either single or multifocal. Those measuring <1.0 cm in diameter represent local variations in the composition of Wharton's jelly, while those measuring >2.0 cm associate with aneuploidy, particularly trisomy 18.

Tumors

The majority of tumors in the UC are vascular. Hemangiomas and angiomyxomas (hemangioma with a large associated pseudocyst) can arise from either umbilical or vitelline vessels. Arteriovenous malformations at the fetal UC insertion site can lead to arteriovenous shunting and hydrops fetalis. Teratomas derived from displaced germ cells associated with the yolk sac are most common at the placental insertion site. Interestingly, malignant tumors of the UC do not occur.

Deformation

Length

Animal models suggest that the length of the UC in late pregnancy is primarily determined by fetal movement. This mechanism is supported by the clinical conditions associated with long and short UC in human pregnancy. Conditions associated with a *short cord* of <30 cm may be separated into intrinsic and extrinsic groups. The intrinsic group includes CNS and muscular anomalies, severe limb deficiencies, and urinary tract malformations that lead to decreased production of urine and thereby amniotic fluid. Extrinsic processes include oligohydramnios due to prolonged preterm rupture of membranes or severe uteroplacental insufficiency, a restrictive endometrial cavity due to uterine malformations or large leiomyomas, and amnionic bands that tether the fetus to the placenta. The most extreme example of the latter is early amnion rupture sequence, also called Limb Body Wall Sequence, type 1, which is characterized by a short UC, ventral wall anomalies and disruptions of the face, CNS, or both. Short

UC may predispose to a cord compression pattern on fetal monitoring, but is no longer assigned a causal role in arrest of descent. Long UC of >70 cm associate with conditions that stretch the cord. Pouiselle's law predicts there is an inherently increased resistance in the vasculature with increasing length of UC and long cords are prone to hypercoiling, entanglements, obstructed blood flow, and suboptimal pregnancy outcomes.

Coiling

Ninety five percent of UC demonstrate an inherent, irreducible twist due to spiraling of the arteries around the vein. The underlying basis for this is not understood, but *coiling* may allow the UC to be acutely stretched like a phone cord, utilize the spiraling umbilical arteries to protect the umbilical vein, and employ arterial pulsations as a counter-current peristaltic pump to move oxygenated umbilical venous blood toward the fetus.

Clinical Pearl

Left twisting is more common than right twisting by a 7:1 ratio. Twisting is quantified by the number of diagonal coils per cm [4]. UC with <0.2 coils/cm associate with SUA, trisomies, preterm delivery, and stillbirth. UC with >0.4 coils/cm are more commonly left-twisted, with peripheral placental insertion, delayed villous maturation, fetal heart rate abnormalities, thrombosis, birth asphyxia, and stillbirth (Figure 15.4).

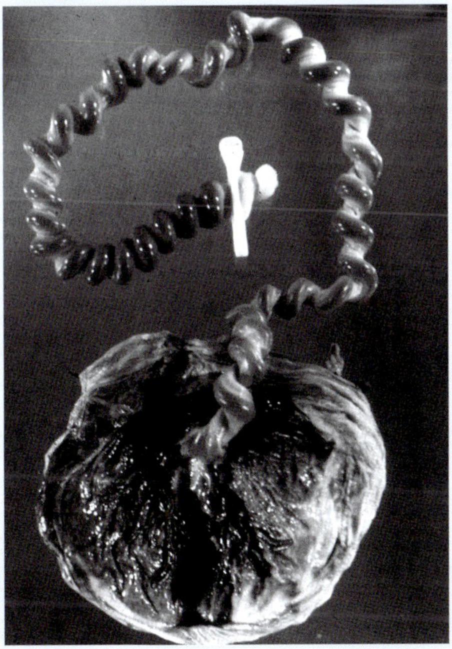

Figure 15.4 Excessive coiling of umbilical cord (see text for details).

Stromal volume

Variations in stromal volume are a function of the composition and hydration of Wharton's jelly. Large UC are observed with diabetes and Beckwith Wiedemann syndrome due to excessive matrix and with hydrops fetalis due to increased extracellular fluid. A thin UC <0.8 cm diameter associates with fetal growth restriction, NICU admission, and perinatal death. Thin UC is usually caused by uteroplacental insufficiency and secondary decreased fetal extracellular fluid.

Strictures

UC strictures may be an isolated finding or the result of a hypercoiled UC. Animal studies have shown that a single, transient compression of the UC in early pregnancy can lead to later stricture. Most strictures occur at the fetal insertion site, a finding that may be explained by physiologic constriction of the umbilical vein near the umbilicus in the second half of gestation. While most strictures are seen in macerated stillbirths, their presence in well-preserved autopsy cases, their association with adjacent thrombosis, fibrosis, and hemosiderin deposits, and their tendency to recur in some families suggest that they are not artifacts of maceration. Twin studies suggest that recurrence does not have an underlying genetic basis [5].

Secondary vascular abnormalities

Fetal growth restriction with abnormal Doppler flow has been associated with a decreased area and increased medial thickness of the umbilical vein and umbilical arteries [6]. Similar changes plus duplication of the elastic lamina are seen in the veins of UC from mothers with preeclampsia and sickle cell trait. Biochemical changes in UC vessels occur with fetal growth restriction where there is increased collagen in the umbilical arteries, with preeclampsia where there is increased collagen along with replacement of hyaluronate with sulfated proteoglycan as well as decreased elastin in the umbilical vein, and with diabetes where there is increased fibronectin and tenascin.

Disruption

Infection and Inflammation

Microorganisms or their soluble products, called PAMPs for pathology-associated molecular products, can enter the UC from either the amniotic fluid or fetal circulation. Different organisms elicit specific fetal inflammatory responses that can be useful in determining the nature and timing of infection. Most placental infections are caused by bacteria ascending from the cervicovaginal region. PAMP and other chemotactic factors produced by these bacteria promote the extravasation of neutrophils, first from the umbilical vein and later from the arteries. Different patterns of gene expression have been described in affected arteries and veins and involvement of the artery has been associated with higher levels of fetal cytokines than vein alone. There is controversy related to what deleterious effects there are on the fetus due to the cytokine response associated with UC inflammation. Neutrophils spread with time into Wharton's jelly, where they form arcs around the UC vessels. Calcification and neovascularization within the arcs indicate prolonged infection and is called *necrotizing funisitis*. Candidal infections form microabscesses on the external surface of the UC, called peripheral funisitis. Syphilis is associated with necrotizing perivenous inflammation. Toxoplasma cysts are commonly observed in Wharton's jelly but elicit no inflammatory response.

Toxic exposures

Alcohol is the only identified teratogen with an acute affect on umbilical blood flow that yields fetal acidosis in an animal model [7]. Umbilical veins in vitro undergo vasospasm, endothelial loss, and degeneration of the elastic lamina when exposed to meconium or medium from group B streptococcal cultures [8]. Structural UC lesions that develop after prolonged exposure to meconium include segmental thinning of the vascular wall, localized or helical ulcerations overlying umbilical arteries, and meconium-induced vascular necrosis. The latter lesion is characterized by widespread apoptosis of vascular smooth muscle cells and is associated with adverse neurologic outcome.

> **Clinical Pearl**
>
> Meconium staining, green discoloration of Wharton's jelly, can be seen in the UC within an hour of passage from the fetus. This may be important when determining the timing of event in cases of fetal meconium aspiration syndrome.

Vascular obstruction

Sudden intrapartum vascular obstruction most commonly occurs with UC prolapse, defined by descent and compression of the UC below the presenting fetal part [4]. Prolapse occurs in 0.14–0.62% of deliveries and has a perinatal mortality rate varying from 36 to 345/1000 births, with a trend toward the lower figure over the past 25 years. Risk factors for prolapse include high vertex, breech presentation, polyhydramnios, low birth weight, and grand multiparity. UC entanglements are the most common cause of intrapartum obstruction. Entanglements can involve any body part, but are most common around the neck (nuchal cord, NC). Overall prevalence of a NC at delivery varies from 15% to 35%. Multiple coils are noted in 0.3–3.8% of deliveries. Type A NC, where the placental end of the cord overlies the fetal end, is easily reduced and relatively innocuous. Type B NC occurs in 0.25% of deliveries and is where the placental aspect passes under the fetal end. Although less frequent, this is more commonly persistent and, when reduced by passage over the fetal head, results in a true knot of the UC. The severity and duration of entanglement is best predicted by secondary findings such as venous dilatation, thrombosis, or compression of the fetal skin. Increased risk for adverse outcomes is controversial and may be masked by low incidence relative to the high overall frequency of entanglements. The role of chronic partial or intermittent UC obstruction in the antepartum period is less well defined [9]. Adverse outcomes have been associated with cord entanglements seen on antenatal ultrasounds. Pressure-related intimal fibrin cushions in large placental veins and numerous small foci of avascular villi are placental findings consistent with chronic, partial, or intermittent obstruction of the UC. Compression-related stasis in the UC is the primary risk factor for fetal thrombotic vasculopathy, a placental lesion strongly associated with cerebral palsy.

Clinical Pearl

Recently defined pathologic criteria implicate significant UC obstruction in 34% of stillbirths at >28 weeks [10].

Thrombi of the UC are relatively uncommon. Umbilical venous thrombi are most frequently seen in association with maternal diabetes. Arterial thrombi are even less common and usually associated with UC malformation, deformation, or both. They may be lethal with SUA or absence of Hyrtl's anastomosis.

Loss of integrity

Complete or partial avulsion of the UC usually occurs in association with abnormal fetal insertions such as omphalocele or gastroschisis or placental insertions such as marginal, membranous, or furcated. Fetal vessels within membranes overlying the cervical os is called a vasa previa and occurs in 1/2,761 deliveries. The vessels within the *vasa previa* may tear with cervical dilatation or membrane rupture and fetal exsanguination can follow. Intrafunicular hemorrhages within the UC may occur antenatally with amniocentesis, umbilical blood sampling, or fetal movement. However, most intrafunicular hemorrhages are artifacts secondary to pulling on the UC after delivery. Noniatrogenic cord hematomas occur in 1/5,500 deliveries and usually involve abnormal vessels. Venous hemorrhages outnumber arterial hemorrhages by a wide margin and usually occur in varicosities called *false knots*, which are present in ≤2% of term placentas. Arterial hemorrhages associate with thrombosis and medial degeneration and may yield dissecting aneurysms. Such aneurysms are most frequent with Trisomy 18.

Teaching Points

1 Thrombi and cytokines generated in the placental circulation may be directly transmitted to the fetal CNS via the umbilical vein, ductus venosus, inferior vena cava, foramen ovale, and carotid arteries.

2 Development of the umbilical circulation is largely independent of the fetus and placenta and under the control of an extraembryonic organizer.

3 Umbilical agenesis is a major cause of spontaneous abortions that present clinically as anembryonic pregnancies.

4 Excessively long umbilical cords have intrinsically reduced vascular resistance and are more prone to hypercoiling, entanglement, and prolapse.

5 Prolonged exposure of the umbilical cord to amniotic fluid meconium can cause ulceration and necrosis of the umbilical cord and its vessels.

References

1. Downs KM (2009) The enigmatic primitive streak: Prevailing notions and challenges concerning the body axis of mammals. *Bioessays* 31(8): 892–902.
2. Blackburn W and Cooley NR (1993) The umbilical cord. In: Stevenson RE, Hall JG, and Goodman RM (eds). *Human Malformations and Related Anomalies.* New York, NY: Oxford University Press.
3. Misra DP, Salafia CM, Miller RK et al. (2009) Nonlinear and gender-specific relationships among placental growth measures and the fetoplacental weight ratio. *Placenta* 30(12): 1052–7.
4. Collins JH, Collins CL, and Collins CC (2010) *Umbilical Cord Accidents 2010.* Available: wwwpregninst-com/UCA_2010pdf. Accessed 29 January 2010.
5. Rodriguez JI, Marino-Enriquez A, Suarez-Aguado J et al. (2008) Umbilical cord stricture is not a genetic anomaly: A study in twins. *Pediatric and Developmental Pathology* 11(5): 363–9.
6. Bruch JF, Sibony O, Benali K et al. (1997) Computerized microscope morphometry of umbilical vessels from pregnancies with intrauterine growth retardation and abnormal umbilical artery Doppler. *Human Pathology* 28(10): 1139–45.
7. Mukherjee AB and Hodgen GD (1982) Maternal ethanol exposure induces transient impairment of umbilical circulation and fetal hypoxia in monkeys. *Science* 218(4573): 700–2.
8. Redline RW (in press) Meconium-associated vascular necrosis. *Pathology Case Reviews.*
9. Redline RW (in press) Fetal thrombotic vasculopathy. *Pathology Case Reviews.*
10. Parast MM, Crum CP, and Boyd TK (2008) Placental histologic criteria for umbilical blood flow restriction in unexplained stillbirth. *Human Pathology* 39(6): 948–53.

16

CHAPTER 16
Ultrasound Imaging and Doppler Studies of the Placenta

Methodius G. Tuuli and Anthony O. Odibo

Division of Maternal-Fetal Medicine and Ultrasound-Genetics, Department of Obstetrics and Gynecology, Washington University in St. Louis, St. Louis, MO, USA

Introduction

Imaging of the placenta is an integral part of the standard obstetric ultrasound examination. The goal is to document placental location, size, texture, and the presence of specific abnormalities that have clinical implications. The uterine and umbilical vessels connect the placenta to the mother and fetus, respectively. Doppler imaging of these vessels reveal parameters that may be of prognostic value. Recent advances in ultrasound technology permit a more accurate delineation of placental volume, structure, vascularization, and blood flow using a combination of power Doppler and 3D ultrasonography. The indices obtained with this technology may further assist in clinical management by predicting risk for adverse pregnancy outcomes.

Two-dimensional imaging

Two-dimensional (2D) real time gray scale ultrasound is the most common modality of placental imaging and displays small differences in acoustical impedance as different shades of gray. This assessment suffices for the detection of most placental abnormalities, but gray scale ultrasound has limitations, which include poor resolution, difficulty assessing nonanteriorly located placentas, and wide variability in the morphology of normal placentas.

Between 5 and 7 weeks' gestation, the gestational sac appears as a diffuse echogenic ring of chorionic tissue. By 8–13 weeks' gestation, a region of focal thickening, representing the chorion frondosum, indicates the site of placentation. For most of the second and early third trimester, the placenta is a uniformly echogenic structure with occasional sonolucencies. Later in the third trimester, the placenta assumes a more heterogeneous texture with multiple sonolucent areas and occasional echogenicities presumed to be calcifications (Figure 16.1).

Location

Documentation of placental location is a requirement in all obstetric ultrasound guidelines. The placenta may be anterior, posterior, lateral, or fundal. By far, the most clinically relevant feature of placental location is the relationship to the lower uterine segment and cervix. Clinical implications of abnormalities of placental location, including previa, accreta, vasa previa, and velamentous cord insertion, are discussed in more detail in Chapter 38. Therefore, we limit the discussion here to pertinent diagnostic considerations.

Placenta previa

A midline longitudinal view of the bladder and lower uterine segment on ultrasound is a good screen for placenta previa. However, the transabdominal approach tends to over-diagnose placentas that are low lying and therefore close to the internal cervical os. Additionally, a full bladder

The Placenta: From Development to Disease, First Edition. Edited by Helen H. Kay, D. Michael Nelson and Yuping Wang.
© 2011 Blackwell Publishing Ltd. Published 2011 by Blackwell Publishing Ltd.

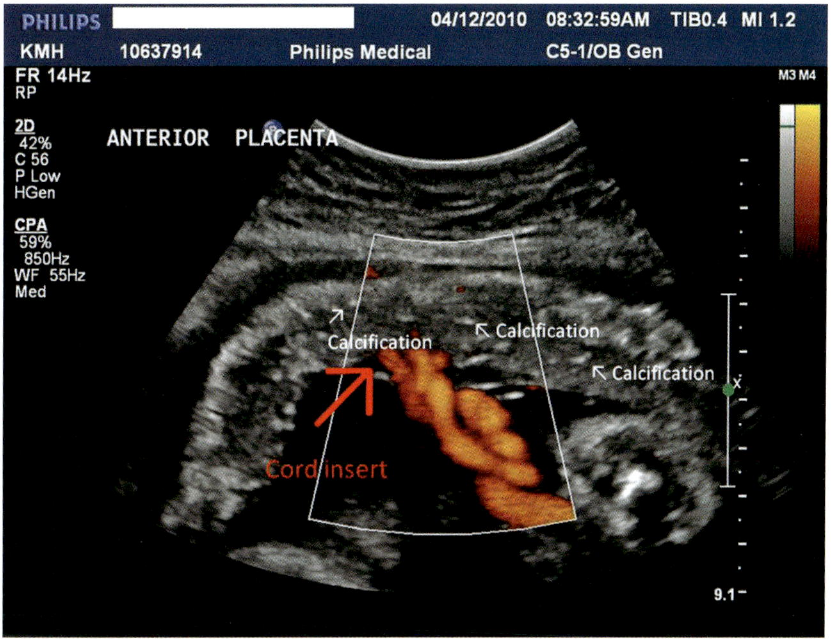

Figure 16.1 Two-dimensional grayscale image of the placenta. Umbilical cord insertion is easily visualized with color Doppler (red arrow). Calcifications are frequent findings in term placentas (white arrows).

and a spontaneous contraction in the lower uterine segment can artificially create the impression of placenta previa. When suspected, a transvaginal ultrasound with the bladder empty is indicated for definitive diagnosis. Current terminology categorizes the placenta as "*previa*" if the edge is within 2 cm of the endocervical os, "*complete previa*" if the placenta covers the os and "*low- lying*" if the edge is >2 cm from the os but in the lower aspect of the uterine cavity.

At least 90% of placentas identified as "low lying" in early pregnancy resolve by term. Of note, the likelihood of persistence to term is related to the gestational age at diagnosis, the degree to which the placenta overlies the cervix and the thickness of the placental edge. When noted early in pregnancy, follow-up examinations are recommended between 28 and 32 weeks' and then at 36 weeks if previa persists. Many previas resolve as differential growth of the uterus and placenta changes the location of the placental edge relative to the cervical os.

Placenta accreta

Placenta accreta is abnormal adherence of the placenta to the myometrium. Placenta *increta* involves invasion of the myometrium while *percreta* involves invasion through the serosal surface of the uterus. Diagnosis is made on ultrasound with reported sensitivities and specificities of up to 80% and 95%, respectively. Ultrasonographic findings suggestive of placenta accreta include placental lacunae, interruptions or bulging of the border between the bladder and myometrium, and lower uterine segment thickness <1 mm. The addition of color-flow and power Doppler to demonstrate turbulent blood flow may improve the sensitivity and specificity of diagnosis. Magnetic resonance imaging (MRI) may be used to confirm or better delineate the presence or extent of accreta. MRI is most useful in the evaluation of posterior placentas, which are often not optimally visualized on ultrasound. However, neither ultrasound nor MRI can absolutely establish the presence or absence of placenta accreta.

Vasa previa

Prenatal diagnosis of vasa previa is crucial, since diagnosis prior to labor improves survival from 44% when not previously diagnosed to 96% [1]. The most common cause is a succenturiate lobe followed by velamentous cord insertion. Diagnosis is accomplished by demonstration of vessels over the endocervix using color Doppler. Although not part of standard obstetric ultrasound guidelines, screening for vasa previa can be performed by identifying the cord insertion in patients at high risk, including those with succenturiate lobes, velamentous insertion, or multifetal pregnancies, the latter especially if conceived through IVF.

> **Clinical Pearl**
>
> Identification of the cord insertion site is recommended in patients at high risk for vasa previa, including those with succenturiate lobes, velamentous insertion, and multiple pregnancies.

Size and shape

Because the placenta is primarily a fetal organ, placental size normally correlates with fetal size and health. Placental size estimates are made using measurements of length, width, thickness, and volume, which are inserted into formulas that incorporate these 2D measurements to yield a 3D estimate. Such methods for volume assessment are complex and have not been widely adopted.

Placentomegaly

Placental thickness correlates with gestational age. Normal growth in thickness is about 1 mm per week and the maximum thickness in millimeters is roughly equal to the gestational age in weeks. Placentomegaly refers to an abnormally thickened placenta. While the specific cutoffs vary, placental thickness >40 mm is considered abnormal. Causes include a normal variant, fetal macrosomia, fetal hydrops of any etiology, maternal medical conditions (e.g., anemia, hypertension, diabetes), placental mosaicism, intrauterine infection (e.g., syphilis, cytomegalovirus), and Beckwith-Wiedemann syndrome. Irrespective of the cause, risk of placental insufficiency is increased when placentomegaly occurs.

Circumvallate placenta

Circumvallate placenta results from attachment of fetal membranes to the fetal surface of the placenta rather than the villous margin. This results in circumferential elevation of the placental margin off the uterine wall, creating a thickened and smaller diameter placental disk. The margins become fibrotic with time and appear as an echogenic rim on ultrasound. This condition is usually benign but may be associated with placental hemorrhage and fetal growth abnormalities if more than two-thirds of the margin is involved.

Battledore placenta

Battledore placenta occurs when the umbilical cord inserts within 2 cm of the placental edge. Color Doppler confirms the cord insertion site and presence of branching vessels within the placenta, distinguishing the battledore placenta from a *velamentous insertion* where the vessels are membranous. A Battledore placenta may be associated with a single umbilical artery in up to 18% of cases and associates with increased morbidity when present with monochorionic twins.

Succenturiate lobe

Succenturiate lobe is an accessory lobe separate from the main placenta that is usually smaller than the primary lobe and that may be located anywhere within the uterus. Gray scale imaging identifies the lobe, while color Doppler identifies communicating vessels. A transvaginal ultrasound with color Doppler is recommended to rule out vasa previa and velamentous cord insertion.

> **Clinical Pearl**
>
> The risk of placental insufficiency is increased when placentomegaly occurs, irrespective of the cause.

Placental texture and structure

In standard gray scale 2D imaging, the normal placenta is relatively homogeneous but areas of differing echogenicity appear as pregnancy progresses. Grannum proposed a *grading system* for the placenta in 1979 [2]. While this system has been largely abandoned, premature placental senescence, indicated by the finding of grade 3 prior to 36 weeks', is seen more commonly in pregnancies with IUGR, maternal hypertension, diabetes, and smoking.

Placental sonolucencies are discrete hypoechoic lesions in the subchorionic region or in the placental parenchyma, where they are surrounded by normal placenta. They usually represent enlarged intervillous vascular spaces, which initially have blood flow as so-called placental lakes, and later contain intervillous thrombi. Placental lakes are identified by the presence of swirling streams of blood on real-time gray scale imaging. Color Doppler, which characterizes direction and velocity of flow as colors and shades, is often negative due to the extremely slow flow. They are seen in 2–18% of pregnancies between 15 and 34 weeks' and are mostly considered normal findings. Placental lakes that occur with a frequency of >3/placenta, or a size >2 cm, associate with IUGR, oligohydramnios, preeclampsia, and unexplained elevated maternal serum alpha fetoprotein. They must be distinguished from more significant placental lesions, including gestational trophoblastic disease, chorioangioma, subchorionic hemorrhage and abruption.

A method for systematic 2D placental ultrasound examination has been described and used in combination with other parameters for screening for adverse pregnancy outcomes [3]. This approach has not been independently validated and is not widely used.

Table 16.1 Definitions of placenta parameters.

Parameter	Definition
Placenta quotient (PQ)	• Ratio of the placental volume to fetal crown–rump length. • Quantifies the size of the placenta in relation to the fetus.
Vascularization index (VI)	• Ratio of color-coded voxels to all voxels within 3D volume expressed as a percentage. • Thought to reflect the number of blood vessels within the volume.
Flow index (VI)	• Power Doppler signal intensity from all color-coded voxels • Thought to reflect intensity of flow at the time of the 3D sweep
Vascularization flow index (VFI)	• Mathematical relationship derivative from VI and FI • Thought to reflect both vascularization and blood flow

3D and power Doppler imaging

Placental size and vascular flow patterns within the villous tree in early pregnancy can now be evaluated. Small placental volume suggests shallow invasive activity of the extravillous trophoblast. Improvements in sonographic imaging provide a tool for estimating placental volume and villus blood flow using 3D scanning techniques [4,5]. Relevant parameters that can be measured include placental volume, placental quotient (PQ), and vascular indices (Table 16.1).

Placental volume is acquired as an image obtained in 3D mode with the volume box adjusted to include the entire placenta. Machine-specific software such as the Virtual Organ Computer-Aided Analysis (VOCAL™) program is then used to calculate the volume (Figure 16.2).

PQ is the ratio of the placental volume to the fetal crown–rump length in the first trimester. This quantifies the size of the placenta in relation to the fetus. Decreased placental volume at 11–14 weeks' gestation has been implicated in the subsequent development of preeclampsia and IUGR. On the other hand, a normal PQ has been reported to have a high negative predictive value, thereby identifying a subgroup at low risk for perinatal complications [6].

Vascular indices

The combination of power Doppler and 3D ultasonography enables the calculation of vascular indices within the placenta from 3D data formed by voxels, the basic information units of volume. Power Doppler depicts the amplitude (power) of Doppler signals rather than frequency shifts and is much better at visualizing small vessels. After acquisition of the 3D image, machine-specific software calculates placental indices (Figure 16.2). The vascularization index (VI) quantifies the number of color-coded voxels to all voxels within the volume expressed as a percentage; flow index (FI) represents the power Doppler signal intensity from all color-coded voxels; vascularization flow index (VFI) is the mathematical relationship derived from VI and FI. These indices reflect the number of blood vessels within the volume (VI), the intensity of flow at the time of the 3D sweep (FI), and both vascularization and blood flow (VFI).

When the entire image of the placenta cannot be obtained in a single sweep, "*sonobiopsy*" has been proposed to obtain a representative sample of the placenta. We recently validated sonobiopsy for obtaining representative vascular indices. Indices obtained using sonobiopsy and whole placental evaluation on the same images were found to be correlated and not significantly different for VI and VFI, but were different for FI [7].

Placental vascular indices have been correlated with gestational age, alterations in fetal growth, amniotic fluid volume, and Doppler parameters of the feto–placental circulation [8]. Reduction in these indices may be an

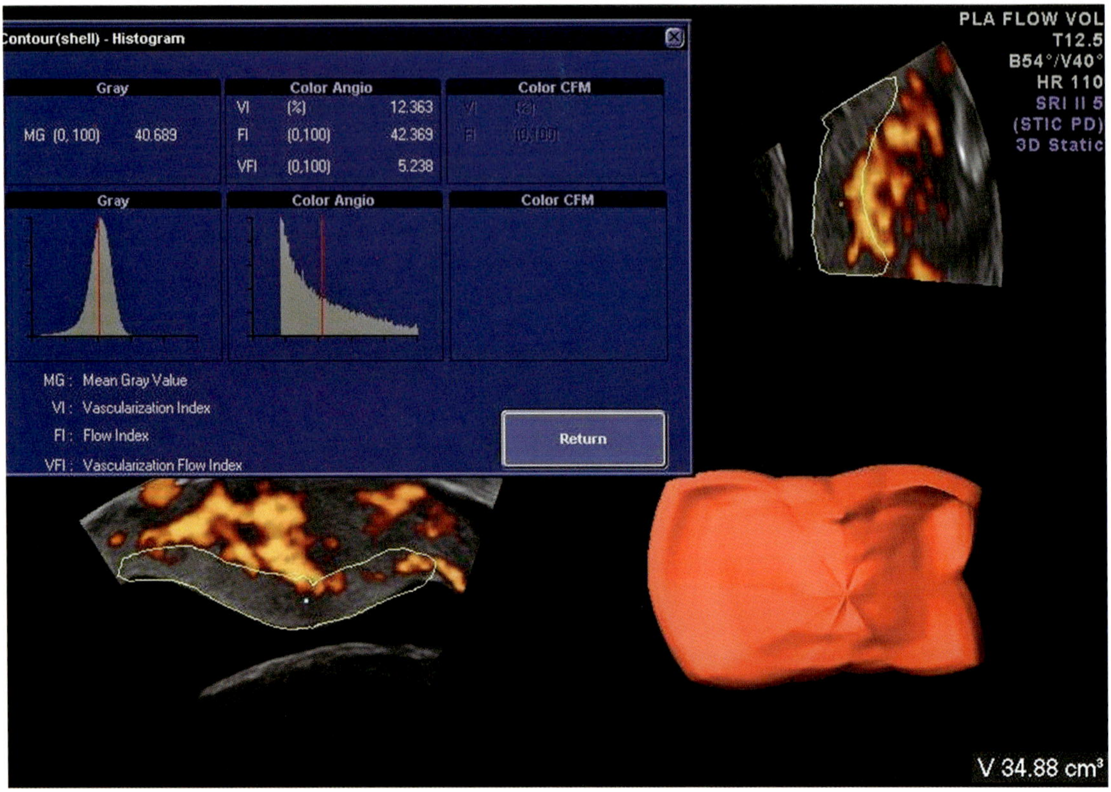

Figure 16.2 Three-dimensional and power Doppler ultrasound of the placenta. The image is obtained by 3D imaging and the placenta outlined in the VOCAL system, which then calculates volume and vascular indices (VI, FI, VFI).

early marker of placental dysfunction. Recently, Rizzo et al. evaluated the relationship between placental vascular indices and the subsequent development of IUGR and adverse pregnancy outcomes in pregnancies with low-pregnancy-associated protein-A. All the 3D indices were significantly lower in those pregnancies with birth weight <10th percentile and umbilical artery pulsatility index (PI) >95th percentile [9].

While this technology shows promise, large-scale studies are needed to validate clinical use. In addition, technical and methodological concerns must be addressed to ensure standardization before application to the general population [10].

Research Spotlight

Sonobiopsy has been validated by obtaining representative placental vascular indices (VI and VFI) [7].

Uterine artery Doppler velocimetry

Doppler ultrasonography provides a noninvasive means of measuring resistance to blood flow in the uterine arteries. Increased uterine artery resistance reflects failure of trophoblastic invasion of the spiral arteries and is associated with the development of preeclampsia and IUGR [11]. The uterine artery is identified with the aid of color Doppler. Pulse-waved Doppler is then used to obtain waveforms from which indices are calculated (Figure 16.3(a)). Relevant indices include the systolic(S) to diastolic (D) velocity ratio (S/D), pulsatility index ($PI = S - D/V_m$, where V_m is the mean velocity throughout the cardiac cycle), resistive index ($RI = S - D/S$), and the presence of early dichotic notching, a characteristic waveform indicating decreased early diastolic flow in the uterine artery compared with later diastolic flow. Increased uterine artery resistance is quantified as PI or RI

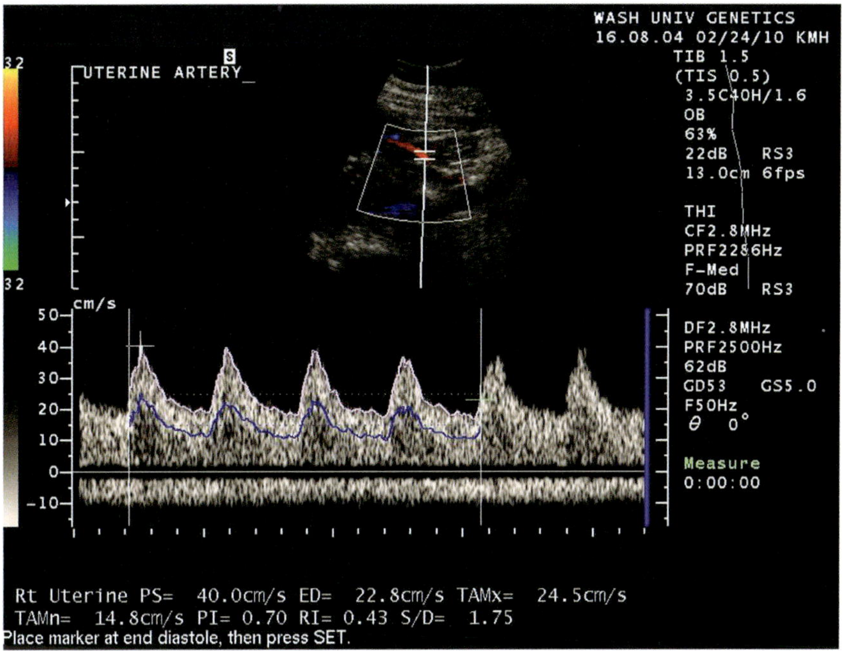

(a)

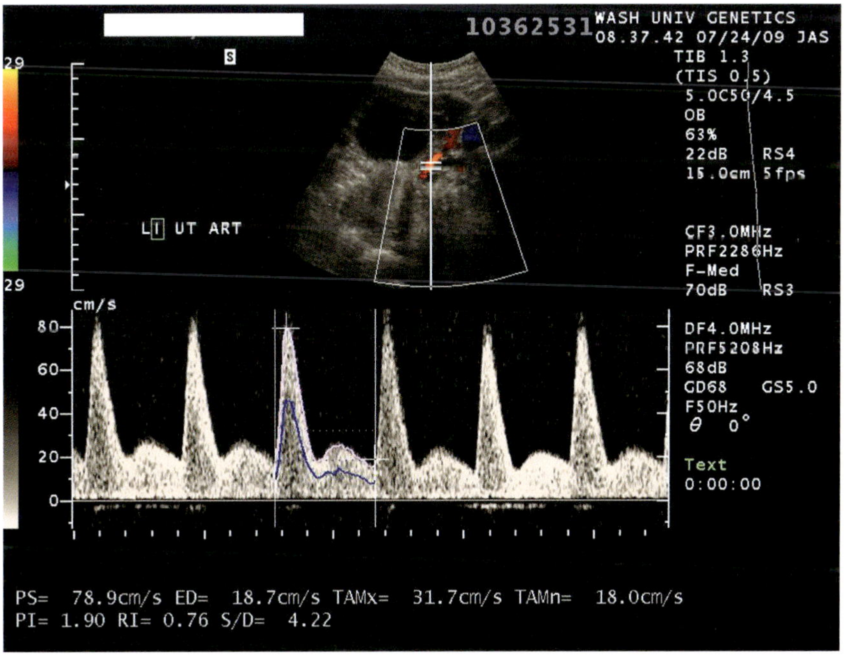

(b)

Figure 16.3 Uterine artery Doppler velocimetry. The uterine artery is identified with the aid of color Doppler and waveforms obtained with pulse wave Doppler. (a) Normal uterine artery Dopplers and normal pulsatility and resistance indices (PI and RI, respectively). (b) Abnormal uterine artery Dopplers with notching and elevated PI and RI.

above a chosen value and/or percentile or the presence of unilateral or bilateral diastolic notching (Figure 16.3(b)).

Abnormal uterine artery Doppler indices in both the first and second trimesters are associated with preeclampsia and IUGR. The most recent meta-analysis of studies using uterine artery Doppler indices to predict preeclampsia and IUGR concluded that (1) predictive accuracy is moderate to minimal in low-risk and minimal in high-risk populations, (2) the best predictor indices are increased PI and the presence of bilateral notching in the second trimester, and (3) the predictive accuracy for early onset preeclampsia is moderate to good, irrespective of the index or combination of indices used [12]. Although uterine artery Doppler velocimetry shows promise for the prediction of early onset preeclampsia and IUGR, gestational age standards for screening are lacking and the criteria for an abnormal test that optimizes sensitivity and positive predictive value are unknown. Therefore, current evidence does not support routine screening.

Research Spotlight

While the value of uterine artery Doppler studies to predict preeclampsia remains limited, increased PI with notching in the second trimester is the best predictor of preeclampsia [12].

Umbilical artery Doppler velocimetry

Umbilical arteries normally have low resistance and high blood flow, which further increases with advancing gestational age as the number of tertiary stem villi increase. Pathological conditions that obliterate muscular arteries in tertiary stem villi result in a progressive decrease in end-diastolic blood flow until absent and reversed diastolic flow occurs (Figure 16.4). Reversed diastolic flow represents the most advanced stage of placental abnormality and occurs when >70% of muscular arteries in tertiary stem villi are obliterated [13].

Doppler sampling of the umbilical arteries can be performed at any segment along the umbilical cord. Most commonly, waveforms are obtained from a free-floating loop of cord. While examinations closer to the placental insertion show more diastolic flow, the differences in indices are generally minor and of little clinical significance. Indices used to quantify increased umbilical artery resistance include the S/D ratio and PI. Values >95th percentile for gestational age are considered abnormal. Of the two indices, PI appears to have greater specificity for adverse perinatal outcomes [14].

Umbilical arterial velocimetry is of considerable value in predicting perinatal outcomes in fetuses with IUGR. Randomized trials demonstrate a decrease in perinatal deaths when umbilical arterial Doppler assessment is used in conjunction with other types of antenatal testing. Such an approach is standard when evaluating fetuses with suspected IUGR. In general, normal indices in a fetus suspected to be small is indicative of a constitutionally small but otherwise normal fetus.

Clinical Pearl

Reversed diastolic flow represents the most advanced stage of placental abnormality and occurs when >70% of placental arteries are obliterated.

Conclusion

In conclusion, careful standard ultrasound imaging of the placenta provides important information for clinical management and measurement of uterine and umbilical artery velocimetry provide noninvasive tools for evaluating placental structure and function. Together with improved measurements of placental volume and vascularization accorded by recent advances in ultrasound technology, placental imaging has potential far beyond the diagnosis of gross abnormalities.

Teaching Points

1. Examination of the placenta should be part of the standard obstetric ultrasound.
2. Suspected placenta previa should be confirmed by transvaginal ultrasound with the bladder empty.
3. The majority of placenta previa diagnosed early in pregnancy resolve by term.
4. 3D ultrasound with power Doppler is superior to 2D ultrasound for assessment of placental volume and vascularization.
5. Umbilical artery Doppler assessment in conjunction with other antenatal testing reduces perinatal mortality and should be part of the evaluation of fetuses with suspected IUGR.

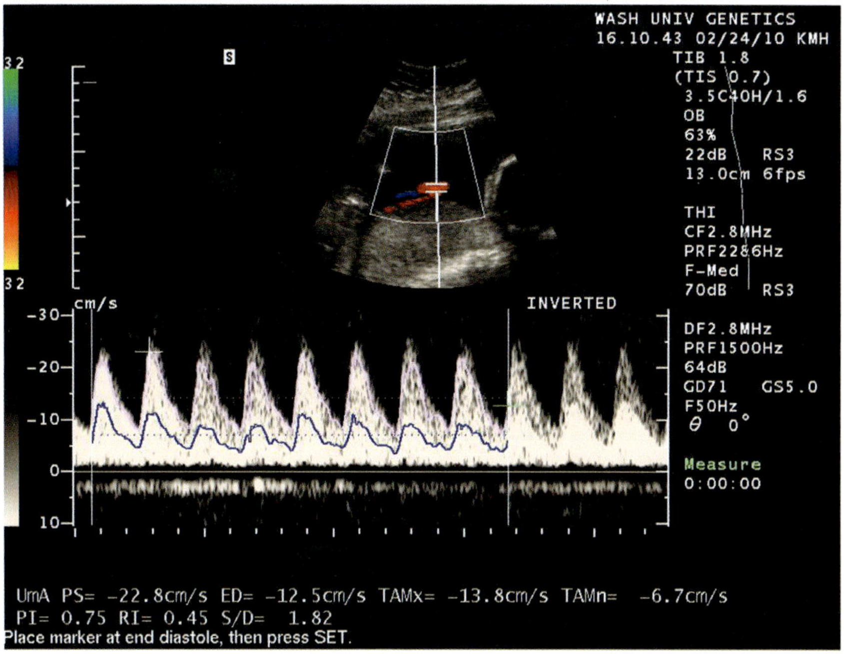

(a)

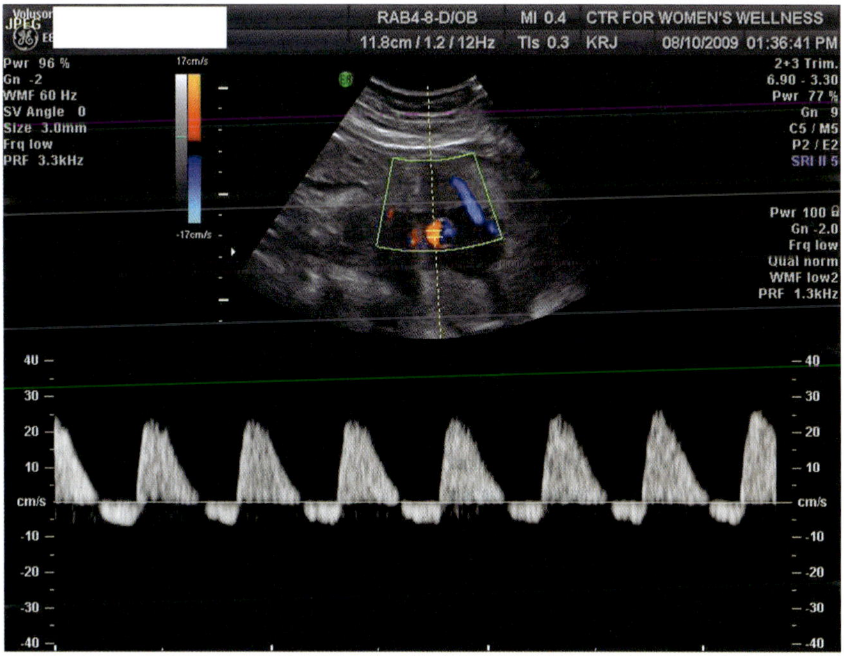

(b)

Figure 16.4 Umbilical artery Doppler velocimetry. Umbilical artery is identified with the aid of color Doppler on a free loop, waveforms obtained with pulse wave Doppler and systolic/diastolic ratio and pulsatility index calculated. (a) Normal umbilical artery Doppler flow with normal pulsatility index and systolic/diastolic ratio. (b) Abnormal umbilical artery Dopplers with reversed diastolic flow.

References

1. Oyelese Y, Catanzarite V, Prefumo F et al. (2004) Vasa previa: The impact of prenatal diagnosis on outcomes. *Obstetrics and Gynecology* 103(5 Pt 1): 937–42.
2. Grannum PA, Berkowitz RL, and Hobbins JC (1979) The ultrasonic changes in the maturing placenta and their relation to fetal pulmonic maturity. *American Journal of Obstetrics and Gynecology* 133(8): 915–22.
3. Viero S, Chaddha V, Alkazaleh F et al. (2004) Prognostic value of placental ultrasound in pregnancies complicated by absent end-diastolic flow velocity in the umbilical arteries. *Placenta* 25(8–9): 735–41.
4. Pretorius DH, Nelson TR, Baergen RN et al. (1998) Imaging of placental vasculature using three-dimensional ultrasound and color power Doppler: A preliminary study. *Ultrasound in Obstetrics and Gynecology* 12(1): 45–9.
5. Konje JC, Huppertz B, Bell SC et al. (2003) 3-dimensional colour power angiography for staging human placental development. *Lancet* 362(9391): 1199–201.
6. Hafner E, Metzenbauer M, Hofinger D et al. (2006) Comparison between three-dimensional placental volume at 12 weeks and uterine artery impedance/notching at 22 weeks in screening for pregnancy-induced hypertension, pre-eclampsia and fetal growth restriction in a low-risk population. *Ultrasound in Obstetrics and Gynecology* 27(6): 652–7.
7. Tuuli MG, Houser M, Odibo L et al. (2010) Validation of placental vascular sonobiopsy for obtaining representative placental vascular indices by three-dimensional power Doppler ultrasonography. *Placenta* 31(3): 192–6.
8. Noguchi J, Hata K, Tanaka H et al. (2009) Placental vascular sonobiopsy using three-dimensional power Doppler ultrasound in normal and growth-restricted fetuses. *Placenta* 30(5): 391–7.
9. Rizzo G, Capponi A, Pietrolucci ME et al. (2009) First-trimester placental volume and vascularization measured by 3-dimensional power Doppler sonography in pregnancies with low serum pregnancy-associated plasma protein a levels. *Journal of Ultrasound in Medicine* 28(12): 1615–22.
10. Raine-Fenning NJ, Nordin NM, Ramnarine KV et al. (2008) Determining the relationship between three-dimensional power Doppler data and true blood flow characteristics: An in-vitro flow phantom experiment. *Ultrasound in Obstetrics and Gynecology* 32(4): 540–50.
11. Toal M, Keating S, Machin G et al. (2008) Determinants of adverse perinatal outcome in high-risk women with abnormal uterine artery Doppler images. *American Journal of Obstetrics and Gynecology* 198(3): 330 e1–7.
12. Cnossen JS, Morris RK, ter Riet G et al. (2008) Use of uterine artery Doppler ultrasonography to predict pre-eclampsia and intrauterine growth restriction: A systematic review and bivariable meta-analysis. *Canadian Medical Association Journal* 178(6): 701–11.
13. Giles WB, Trudinger BJ, and Baird PJ. (1985) Fetal umbilical artery flow velocity waveforms and placental resistance: Pathological correlation. *British Journal of Obstetrics and Gynaecology* 92(1): 31–8.
14. Dicke JM, Huettner P, Yan S et al. (2009) Umbilical artery Doppler indices in small-for-gestational age fetuses: Correlation with adverse outcomes and placental abnormalities. *Journal of Ultrasound in Medicine* 28(12): 1603–10.

17

CHAPTER 17

Magnetic Resonance Imaging (MRI) and Positron Emission Tomography (PET) of the Placenta

Christine H. Comstock[1,2] *and Helen H. Kay*[3]

[1]Department of Obstetrics and Gynecology, Oakland University William Beaumont School of Medicine, MI, USA

[2]Division of Fetal Imaging, William Beaumont Hospital, Royal Oak, MI, USA

[3]Division of Maternal-Fetal Medicine and Ultrasound-Genetics, Department of Obstetrics and Gynecology, Washington University School of Medicine, St. Louis, MO, USA

Introduction

Because of safety, convenience, cost, and accuracy, ultrasound remains the mode of choice in imaging the placenta. However, there are several niches in which MRI has been useful, despite the cost. PET usage in pregnancy is limited by the nuclear reagents employed, but this modality can be helpful in imaging metastases from placental trophoblastic tumors.

Magnetic resonance imaging (MRI)

Technology

MRI is a nonradiation imaging modality that relies on the natural presence of the hydrogen nucleus, i.e., proton or ^{1}H, in water molecules distributed throughout all biologic tissues. Protons have magnetic moment, and when placed within a powerful external magnet, they align within the direction of the magnetic field. An electromagnetic field, in the form of radiofrequency waves, is then applied. The radio signal, in one of a number of patterns and sequences, flips the magnetic spin of the protons based on the energy absorbed, causing a movement of the protons away from the alignment they initially assumed when first oriented by the magnet. When the electromagnetic field is turned off, the flipped protons will return to their baseline, releasing the absorbed energy, which is then detected by scanners. Contrast between structures in the body is provided by the concentration of excited protons in different electromagnetic environments within tissue, e.g., fat versus muscle, by the relaxation times of the nuclei (T1, T2) after the radiofrequency signal is discontinued and by the variations in the patterns and sequences of the radiofrequency perturbations. T1 is known as the spin–lattice relaxation time and T2 as the spin–spin relaxation time. In a T2-weighted image, water and tissue are generally bright and fat is dark. In T1-weighted images, the reverse is seen. The strength of the magnet is measured in Tesla (T), with most clinical magnets in the range of 1.5–3 T. The stronger the magnetic field, the better the signal-to-noise ratio, but the more expensive the magnet.

Safety

MRI has been used since its inception in imaging newborns and children with no negative effects found. The question that remains is how safe this imaging modality

The Placenta: From Development to Disease, First Edition. Edited by Helen H. Kay, D. Michael Nelson and Yuping Wang.
© 2011 Blackwell Publishing Ltd. Published 2011 by Blackwell Publishing Ltd.

is for the developing fetus? The literature to date has suggested the safety of 1.5 T magnets, but not of the 3.0 T magnets. Fortunately, there are no indications for MRI in the first trimester, but MRI has been used in the second and third trimesters when there is a clinical indication. The Safety committee of the Society for Magnetic Resonance Imaging states that MRI procedures are indicated for use in pregnancy when other diagnostic imaging methods are inadequate or when the exam would provide important information that would otherwise require ionizing radiation. The US Food and Drug Administration states that the safety of MRI procedure during pregnancy has not been definitely proved.

Contrast agents for MRI

The most commonly used contrast agent is a solution of Gadolinium (Gd), a highly magnetic rare earth element with atomic number 64. Gadolinium is incorporated into the minerals monazite and bastnasite from which the nontoxic, free element is extracted and then chelated to other compounds. Gadolinium reduces both the T1 and T2 relaxation times of nearby protons. Reduction of T1 times produces a hyperdense signal while reduction of the T2 relaxation time produces a hypointense signal. Gadolinium as a contrast agent can be used to highlight the placenta in relation to the uterus by differentiating chorionic villi and decidua basalis. The placenta enhances before the myometrium after gadolinium is first injected, and the distribution follows the lobular structure of the placenta (Figure 17.1). However, after 45 seconds, the distribution of contrast is homogenous throughout the placenta [1].

The half-life of gadolinium within the amniotic fluid is not known. Gadolinium crosses the placenta, appears rapidly in the fetal bladder, and slows development in rats when given in doses 2.5 times the human dose. Gadolinium is thus classed as a category C drug and therefore should only be used if the benefits outweigh the risks.

Normal placenta on MRI

The placenta lends itself to MRI because it is immobile and contains a large volume of blood. On MRI, the normal placenta is homogenous with low signal intensity on T1-weighted images and high signal intensity on T2-weighted images. Both the longitudinal (T1) and transverse (T2) relaxation times decrease through gestation, a reflection of the changing environment for the protons within the placenta as a result of decreased blood flow and fibrosis. Relaxation times are also depressed in pregnancies complicated by intrauterine growth restriction and preeclampsia. The volume of the placenta can be measured by MRI, but the placentas in IUGR are not distinct as they are in the low range of the normal distribution.

First trimester

Placenta accreta, increta, and percreta are most likely present from the earliest weeks of pregnancy, as many cases associate with massive bleeding following early dilatation and curettage. Magnetic resonance images of an early placenta percreta showed a gestational sac implanted anteriorly on the uterine scar from a cesarean section [2]. A subsequent MRI of this patient showed obliteration of the bladder and uterine walls, and pathology later showed placenta percreta. The MRI appearance above is similar to ultrasound findings in patients with a surgical scar destined to have a placental attachment disorder (PAD) [3]. MRI expense, limited access, and unproven safety limit use in the first trimester. However, MRI identified a growing suprapubic mass as a missed pregnancy (i.e., scar pregnancy) that was lying within a cesarean section scar and not available in the uterine cavity at time of a previous dilation and curettage.

Second and third trimesters

With the rising incidence of cesarean sections, PADs increase morbidity in pregnancy related to scarring of the uterus by cesarean section. Separation of the placenta from the myometrium can be catastrophic in these women, and antenatal identification of PAD changes management. For example, massive blood loss can be avoided by cesarean hysterectomy or by leaving the placenta in place. The diagnosis can usually be made by ultrasound at 18 weeks, if not before. Ultrasound has high sensitivity and specificity for the diagnosis of accreta by imaging irregular vascular lakes. However, MRI may be more reliable in inconclusive cases (Figure 17.2). The problem with MRI is that both placenta and myometrium have high signal intensities. Warshak et al. imaged by ultrasound initially and then by MRI [1] and found ultrasound had a sensitivity of 77% and specificity of 96%. Importantly, MRI correctly ruled out placenta accreta in 14 of 14 cases inconclusive by ultrasound and accurately diagnosed accreta in 23 of 26 cases. MRI was first used without contrast and, if suspicious, then the contrast agent Gadolinium was injected. MRI findings of accreta are similar to those of ultrasound:

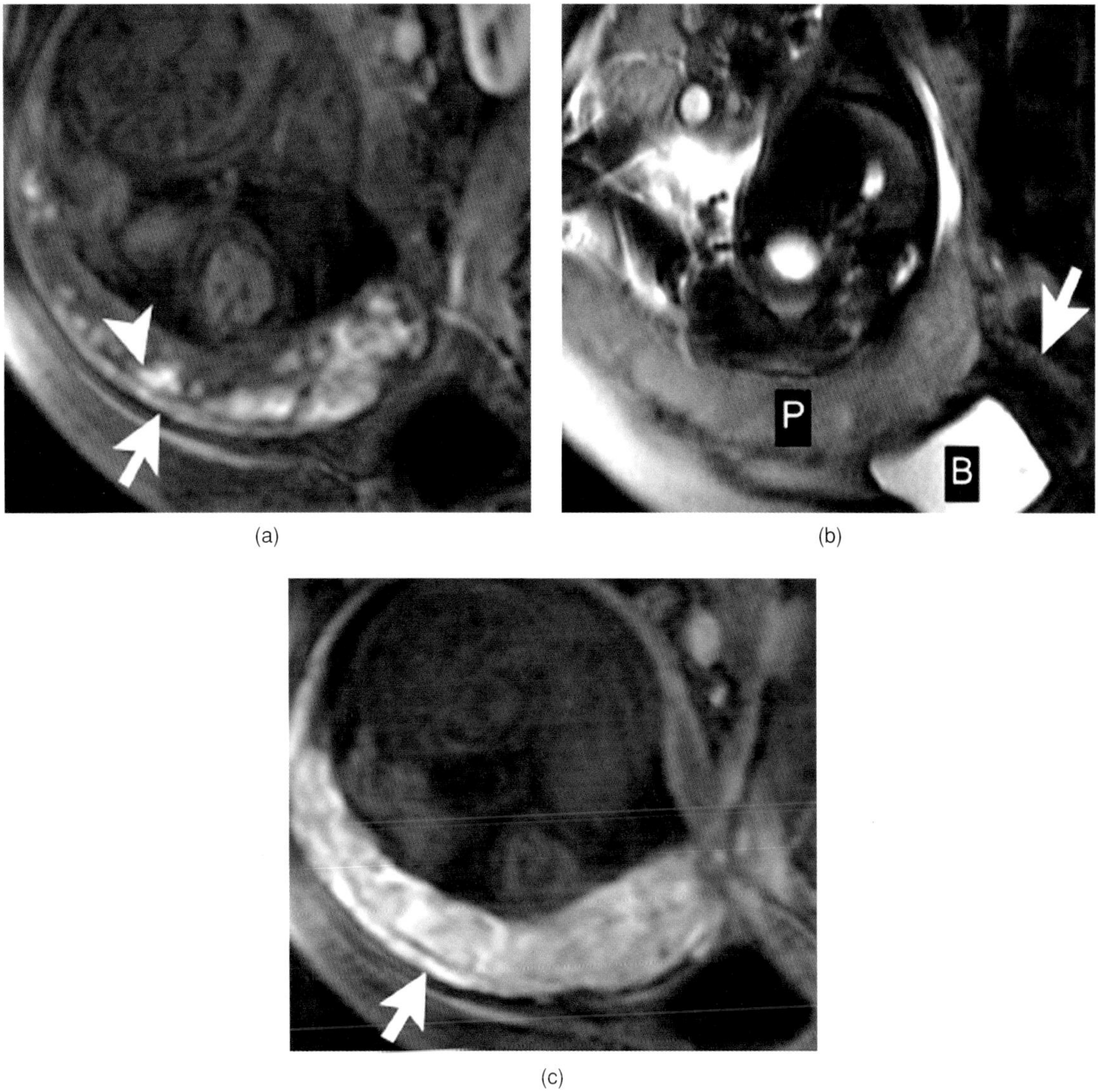

Figure 17.1 MRI scans of the placenta with and without contrast. (a) Myometrium (arrow) and placenta in the early phase after Gadolinium injection showing enhancement only of placental lobules (arrowhead). (b) Without contrast, the normal placenta (P) is very homogeneous. In this T2 image, the bladder (B) appears white. An arrow highlights the cervix. (c) Enhancement during the later phase when Gadolinium has reached the myometrium (arrow). (With permission from Warshak CR et al. (2006) Accuracy of ultrasonography and magnetic resonance imaging in the diagnosis of placenta accreta. *Obstetrics and Gynecology* 108: 573–81.)

thinning of the uterine serosa bladder interface, irregular intraplacental lacunar spaces, and exophytic masses. As in sonography, a partially filled bladder will help in the evaluation of the uterine–vesical interface. The difference in the abilities of the two modalities was insignificant, even with gadolinium. In comparing ultrasound and MRI, Levine et al. found ultrasound to be more sensitive except in a posterior placenta [4]. Masselii et al. found no difference in the value of MRI or ultrasound in making the diagnosis of PAD, but MRI could more reliably distinguish placenta increta and percreta (Figure 17.3) from placenta accreta [5].

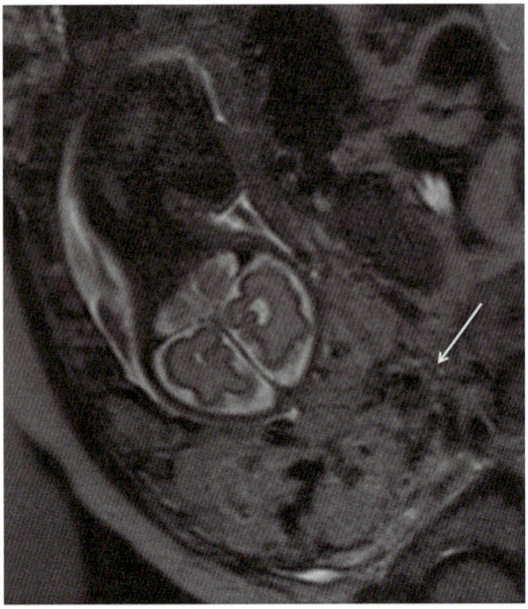

Figure 17.2 Placenta accreta. Note many vascular areas in the placenta (arrow).

Clinical Pearl

Ultrasound is a sensitive diagnostic tool in PADs, but MRI provides better evaluation of the posterior placenta and degree of invasion.

Clinical Pearl

There are no imaging studies that have addressed the antenatal diagnosis of PADs in patients who have not had previous surgery.

Infarcts

T2 and SSFP sequences have high sensitivity in detecting acute ischemic lesions and are optimal for nonhemorrhagic lesions such as infarctions [6]. In 32 cases, MRI detected ischemic infarctions with a specificity of 63%. Infarcts have an increase in central signal intensity with low intensity rims.

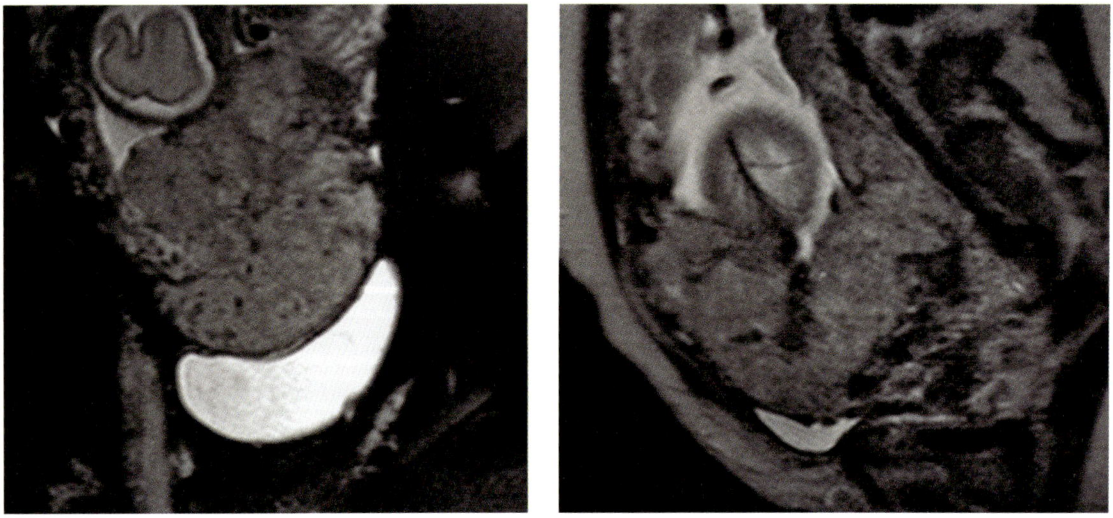

(a) (b)

Figure 17.3 (a) Placenta accreta. Note the smooth upper bladder wall. (b) Placenta percreta. MRI T2 HASTE sequence shows invasion into the bladder wall and many vascular spaces in the placenta. There was invasion into the bladder found at surgery and on pathology examination of the removed uterus.

Abruption

T1 sequences are optimal for large hematomas. In 3 cases of suspected retroplacental hematomas, MRI findings were 100% sensitive and 98% specific. In the 14 patients with subchorionic hematomas, 64% were detected with MRI with a specificity of 100%. Intervillous hemorrhages occurred in 8 cases with sensitivity of 75% and specificity of 97%.

Chorioangioma

Ultrasound is the method of choice for this diagnosis. A placental surface mass with arterial flow is almost always a chorioangioma. However, MRI was occasionally used to confirm the diagnosis. On T1-weighted images, the mass was isodense compared to the normal placenta but had an area of increased signal intensity at the periphery and near the base. On T2-weighted images with fat suppression, the mass showed increased signal intensity with an area of decreased signal near the surface.

Diffusion-weighted imaging (DWI)

DWI is a modification of normal MRI imaging and is used extensively in the evaluation of ischemic strokes. DWI incorporates additional magnetic-field gradients with the conventional spin-echo imaging sequences. DWI shows tissue-specific characteristics based on the specific diffusion motion of water molecules within them. Instead of the normal random Brownian movement of molecules in a glass of water, for example, tissues impede the direction of water diffusion in planes characteristic of that tissue. In axons, water moves along the length of the axon, not out of the axon sheath. Each voxel of information shows the rate of water diffusion, rather than relaxation time (T1, T2). In the case of DWI of the placenta, contrast between the myometrium and placenta is improved. Normal endometrium is very cellular and therefore has a high DWI signal intensity (b value of 0 s/mm^2). The placenta itself has even higher signal intensity than myometrium (b value of 1,000 s/mm^2). DWI can show contrast between the placenta and myometrium and thus can show the thickness of the myometrium and visualize thinning of the myometrium. However, it has not been useful in placenta accreta because in the last trimester the myometrium is normally thin and even more so over a cesarean section scar. Conversely, DWI is useful when *irregular* thinning of the myometrium is seen in placenta increta. It is also useful in detecting small hemorrhagic lesions in the placenta.

The safety of DWI has not been established. It has higher absorption rates and magnetic fields than the common sequences that have been studied.

Positron emission tomography (PET)

Technology

Positron emission tomography displays functional processes in biologic tissue using positron-emitting radionuclides (tracer). These radionuclides are usually isotopes with short half-lives such as carbon-11 (~20 minutes), nitrogen-13 (~10 minutes), oxygen-15 (~2 minutes), and fluorine-18 (~110 minutes) attached to a biologically active compound such as a sugar. After injection, the compound is incorporated into the body. As the radioisotope decays, it emits a positron. When the positron hits an electron, a pair of gamma positrons is created that are detected by the scanner, thus the name "Positron Emission Scanning" or PET. After computerized Fourier transformation, the result can be displayed as a series of 2D or 3D images. PET scanning can thus image metabolism of biologically active compounds that complement CT scanning to show more anatomical detail.

Pharmaceuticals/contrast agents for PET

The most common radiopharmaceutical to date is 18F-fluorodeoxyglucose (18F-FDG), half-life about 2 hours. Because the placenta is a very glycolytic organ, 18F-FDG is highly suitable for uptake and tracing. In primate models, this compound readily crosses the placenta and accumulates in the fetal brain and bladder. The radioactive uptake in the placenta has been calculated as 0.19% of the injected activity (Figure 17.4) [7].

Placental site trophoblastic disease

Because of the ionizing radiation, PET scanning is only used in OB GYN for the management of trophoblastic disease. Elevated human chorionic gonadotropin (hCG) levels indicate the persistence of tumor, but do not localize the lesion. To find metastases, 18-fluorodeoxyglucose is used because trophoblastic disease has a high glycolysis rate and can show metastases within the lung and lymph nodes. In a series of 14 cases of chemotherapy-resistant gestational trophoblastic disease, PET scanning benefited six patients by disclosure of chemotherapy-resistant

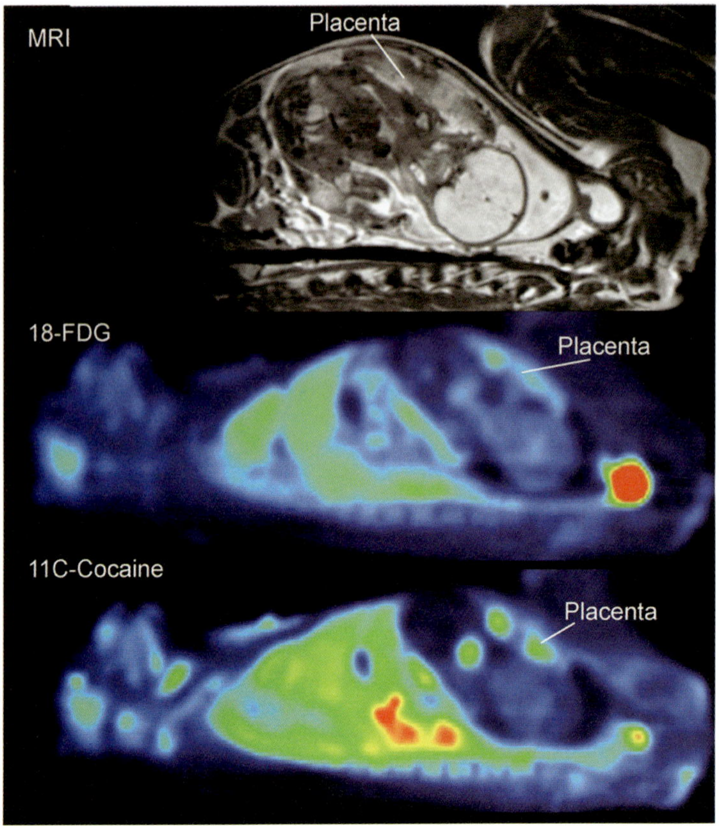

Figure 17.4 PET images of an anesthetized 3rd trimester pregnant *Macaca radiata* (saggital view) and the corresponding T2-weighted MRI image demonstrating the anatomical position of the fetus. The 18-FDG and 11C-Cocaine PET image is derived as a sum of all time frames for the given study. The location of the placenta adjacent to the fetus is indicated on all three multimodality images. It is clear that 11C-Cocaine and its metabolites accumulate in the placenta. (Acknowledgement: Images are courtesy of Dr. Helene Benveniste, Department of Anesthesiology, Stony Brook University, Stony Brook, NY.)

lesions, exclusion of false-positive CT lesions, and confirmation of a complete treatment response or recurrent resistant gestational trophoblastic disease. PET scanning may someday be added to primary staging of high-risk disease. Four potential roles for PET scanning are to discover chemotherapy-resistant lesions not found by CT scans, to rule out false positive lesions found by a CT scan, to define the tumor extent before starting treatment, and to confirm a complete treatment response or recurrent resistant gestational trophoblastic disease.

Research Spotlight

PET scanning is somewhat useful in the management of trophoblastic disease.

Safety

The safety of PET imaging has not been established in humans and most studies to date have been performed in animals. Some rare human reports were of patients who underwent nonplacental imaging for malignant diseases. At present because of requirement for radiopharmaceuticals, PET imaging *in pregnancy* is currently limited to animals.

Future research

PET imaging can trace the metabolic pathway of any compound radiolabeled with a PET isotope injected into a living organism. A case in point is drug metabolism of cocaine [8]. In the placenta, PET imaging is also useful to study the time course of drug uptake from maternal circulation to the placenta and subsequent transport to the fetus. PET can also determine the biologic volume of the placenta based on photon emission from the placenta. The opportunities for PET usage are limitless as long as there are tracers and biologic compounds that contain them.

☞ Teaching Points

1 MRI does not involve ionizing radiation, whereas PET scanning does. Therefore, PET scanning is not utilized in pregnancy unless there are unusual circumstances.

2 The contrast agent Gadolinium is not generally used in the United States in pregnant women due to concern for harm to the fetus. However, there are no data to support significant risk and the agent is now used in Europe in imaging pregnant women.

3 The current best utility of MRI in placental imaging is to detect bladder invasion in PADs.

4 Although not currently used in human studies, PET imaging has a strong future in studies of organ uptake, distribution, kinetics, and metabolism of isotope labeled compounds.

References

1. Warshak CR, Ramez E, Hull AD et al. (2006) Accuracy of ultrasonography and magnetic resonance imaging in the diagnosis of placenta accreta. *Obstetrics and Gynecology* 108: 573–81.
2. Thorp JM, Wells SR, Wiest HH et al. (1998) First-trimester diagnosis of placenta previa percreta by magnetic resonance imaging. *American Journal of Obstetrics and Gynecology* 178: 616–18.
3. Comstock CH, Lee W, Vettraino I et al. (2003) The early sonographic appearance of placenta accreta. *Journal of Ultrasound in Medicine* 22: 19–23.
4. Levine D, Hulka CA, Ludmir J et al. (1997) Placenta accreta: Evaluation with color Doppler US, power Doppler US, and fast MR imaging. *Radiology* 205: 773–6.
5. Masselli G, Brunelli R, Casciani E et al. (2008) Magnetic resonance imaging in the evaluation of placental adhesive disorders: Correlation with color Doppler ultrasound. *European Radiology* 18: 1292–9.
6. Linduska N, Dekan S, Messerschmidt A et al. (2009) Placental pathologies in fetal MRI with pathohistological correlation. *Placenta* 30: 555–9.
7. Zanotti-Fregonara P, Jan S, Champion C et al. (2009) In vivo quantification of 18F-FDG uptake in human placenta during early pregnancy. *Health Physics* 97: 82–5.
8. Benveniste H, Fowler JS, Rooney W et al. (2005) Maternal and fetal 11C-cocaine uptake and kinetics measured in vivo by combined PET and MRI in pregnant nonhuman primates. *The Journal of Nuclear Medicine* 46: 312–20.

18

CHAPTER 18
Chorionic Villus Sampling and Amniocentesis

Marion S. Verp
Departments of Obstetrics and Gynecology, and Human Genetics, The University of Chicago, Chicago, IL, USA

Introduction

Chromosome analysis of tissues derived from the fetus and placenta generally reflect the fetal karyotype. Initial studies demonstrated that fetal sex can be predicted by X-chromatin analysis of cells in the amniotic fluid. Methods for culturing amniocytes were then developed, allowing karyotyping and the first antenatal diagnosis of a chromosome abnormality. Simultaneously, in utero detection of the enzyme abnormality causing galactosemia, based on analysis of amniotic fluid cells, was also reported. Amniocentesis then became a standard method for detection of multiple genetic disorders in the fetus. Chorionic villus sampling was developed in the 1980s, and this approach allowed detection of genetic abnormalities earlier in pregnancy. Importantly, this approach also revealed occasional discrepancies in chromosome number depending on the cell type that was analyzed. This heretofore unrecognized phenomenon in human pregnancy was called placental mosaicism.

Chorionic villus sampling

Technique

Chorionic villus sampling (CVS) is an outpatient procedure performed between 10 and 12 weeks gestation for the diagnosis of fetal chromosomal and genetic disorders. Ultrasound examination is performed prior to the procedure to determine gestational age, viability, number of fetuses, location of the placenta, and cervical–uterine angle. Continuous ultrasound scanning monitors and directs the placement of the catheter or needle.

Tissue sampling is usually via a transcervical or transabdominal approach. Rarely, an approach through the posterior vaginal wall is required. In transcervical CVS, a catheter (diameter 1.9 mm) is passed through the cervix into the uterus. A small amount of placental chorionic villi are aspirated with a 20 mL syringe filled with 2 mL of tissue culture medium or saline (Figure 18.1). The transabdominal approach to CVS requires ultrasound guidance for insertion of an 18- to 20-gauge needle through the maternal abdominal wall into the placenta. Villus tissue is again aspirated into a 20 mL syringe filled with a small amount of culture medium (Figure 18.2). Local anesthesia is usually used at the insertion site.

> **Clinical Pearl**
> A double-needle device that employs a 21.5-gauge needle within a 19.5-gauge needle allows multiple aspirations of villus tissue if necessary without repeated puncture of the uterus.

The sample obtained by either approach is immediately observed under a dissecting microscope or imaged against a light source background to insure the presence of

The Placenta: From Development to Disease, First Edition. Edited by Helen H. Kay, D. Michael Nelson and Yuping Wang.
© 2011 Blackwell Publishing Ltd. Published 2011 by Blackwell Publishing Ltd.

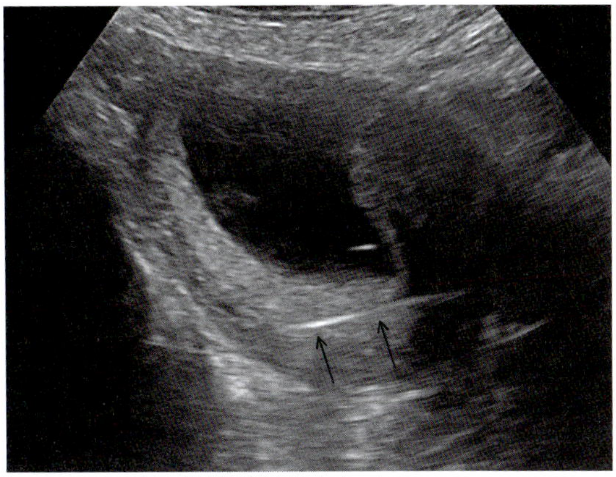

Figure 18.1 Transcervical CVS. Sagittal ultrasound view of uterus, posterior placenta, and sampling catheter (arrows) in the placenta.

adequate villus material for analysis. In general, an aliquot of 10–25 mg of villus tissue is obtained per sampling, and the volume can be determined by comparison with a standardized visual chart. Villi are identified by a characteristic branching morphology (Figure 18.3). Insufficient villi or samples with maternal decidua only require a second attempt to obtain villus tissue.

Chromosomal, biochemical, and DNA analyses can often be done directly on the freshly isolated villus tissue without the need to culture constituent cells, a method known as "direct preps." Trophoblastic tissues at that early gestation contain abundant cytotrophoblasts in metaphase, which allows determination of the chromosomal karyotype within 2 days. This contrasts with amniocytes that require culturing to obtain cells in metaphase, lengthening the time to results to 1–2 weeks. However, direct preps can give false-positive or false-negative results, although less than 1% of the time. Thus, laboratories that do direct preps also culture villi to analyze mesenchymal cells to confirm the initial diagnosis. Fluorescence in situ hybridization (FISH) can also be performed on uncultured chorionic villus cells in interphase, enabling rapid but specific analysis of some chromosome abnormalities and microdeletion syndromes.

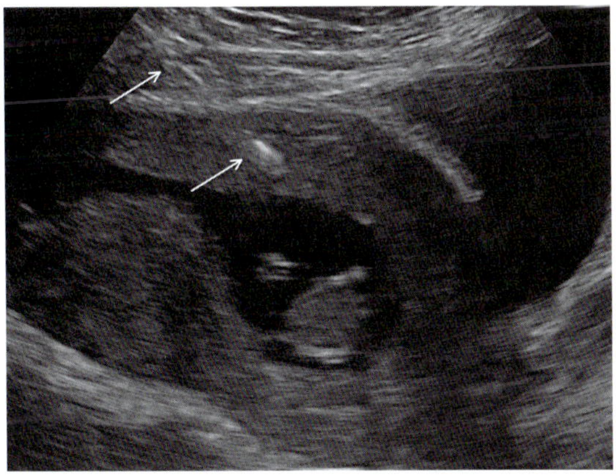

Figure 18.2 Transabdominal CVS. Sagittal ultrasound view of uterus, anterior placenta, and sampling needle in the placenta (arrows).

CVS can be performed on multiple gestations as long as the individual placentas can be distinguished and each sampled separately. This requires confident ultrasound visualization and skilled and accurate catheter or needle placement. Rh immune globulin is given to Rh-negative women after CVS unless the father of the fetus is known to be Rh-negative.

Clinical Pearl

We routinely collect a maternal blood sample from all CVS patients. If the CVS chromosome results are 46,XX, the DNA laboratory compares the blood and villus tissue for polymorphisms unique to the fetus to exclude maternal contamination and misdiagnosis.

Origin of chorionic villus cells

Aspirated chorionic villi (CV) consist of trophoblast and mesodermal cells. The trophoblast lineages differentiate from the trophoectoderm of the blastocyst independent of the inner cell mass that is destined to become the embryo and the extraembryonic mesodermal primordial cells that evolve into the membranes. This independent proliferation of trophoblastic, embryonic, and membrane precursor cells allows aneuploidy to arise from nondisjunction in one of the lines but not the others. Such nondisjunctions yield karyotype abnormalities in the trophoblast, mesenchymal membrane cells, or both that are not present in the embryo. For this reason, an abnormal karyotype from direct metaphase preparations of trophoblast cells is not considered diagnostic until a culture of villi (mesenchymal cells) confirms the abnormality. This discrepancy among cell lines in CVS analyses unveiled the presence of placental mosaicism, a finding not uncommon in pregnancies with intrauterine growth restriction, but

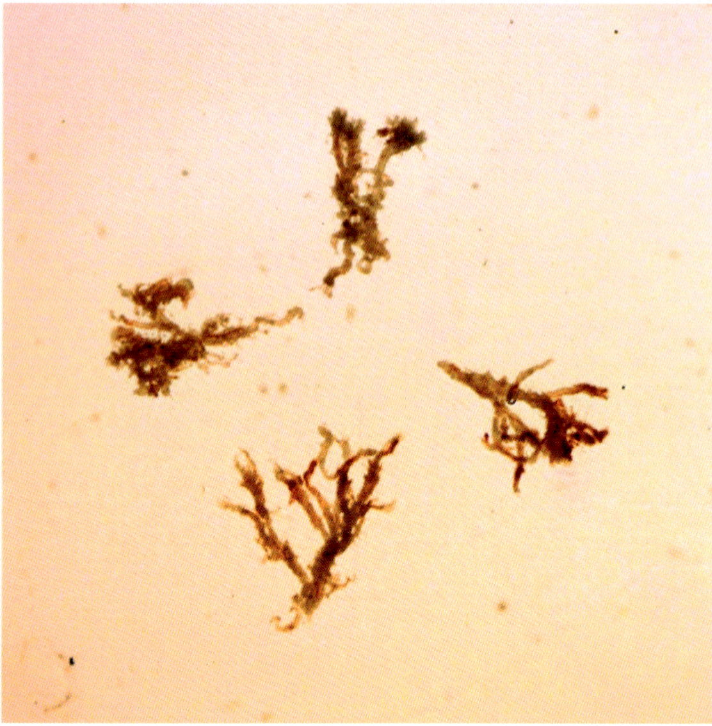

Figure 18.3 Magnified image of chorionic villus fragments obtained from CVS as viewed through a dissecting microscope.

also found in otherwise normal pregnancies. There may also be discrepancies between mesodermal and embryonic karyotypes (see later section on confined placental mosaicism).

Safety

Maternal spotting and bleeding are common (30%) following transcervical CVS but less common after transabdominal CVS. A series of over 4,000 women who underwent transcervical CVS showed no serious maternal complications [1], with serious maternal infections limited to case reports.

Theoretical fetal risks include disruption of the amniotic sac leading to fetal deformation, and intrauterine growth restriction from placental injury. Although one case of a fetus with amniotic band syndrome after CVS has been reported, the overall frequency of congenital defects, premature delivery, placental abruption, placenta previa, and low birth weight is not increased in CVS patients. Thus, there is no evidence of clinically significant placental damage in ongoing pregnancies after CVS.

The fetal loss rate associated with CVS has been investigated in several large studies. Total loss rates from spontaneous abortion, induced abortion, and stillbirth, although generally a little higher in the CVS groups compared to patients having amniocentesis, were frequently not significantly different [1]. More recent studies show a decreasing loss rate from CVS, likely related to operator and sonographer experience [2] (Table 18.1). Randomized comparisons of transcervical and transabdominal CVS by practitioners experienced in both approaches also do not show a significant difference in loss rates. Importantly, an international CVS registry that included thousands of subjects did not support an excess number of infants with limb reduction defects following CVS.

Table 18.1 Pregnancy loss rates after CVS vs. amniocentesis [2].

Year of Procedure	AOR[a]	*P*
1983–87	19.56	<.001
1988–92	5.69	.012
1993–97	3.63	.092
1998–2003	1.03	.968

[a] Adjusted odds ratio.

In summary, the risk of loss associated with CVS either transcervical or transabdominal is probably ≤ 0.5% when performed by experienced individuals.

Amniocentesis

In early gestation, amniotic fluid contains electrolytes present in concentrations similar to those found in maternal serum because the unkeratinized fetal skin allows passage of fluid, urea, creatinine, sodium, and chloride. Amniotic fluid also contains fetal proteins such as alpha-fetoprotein (AFP) as well as cells desquamated from amnion, fetal skin, and the bronchopulmonary, gastrointestinal, and genitourinary tracts. These cells can be cultured for fetal karyotyping.

Research Spotlight

Amniotic fluid contains pluripotent stem cells that can give rise to adipogenic, osteogenic, myogenic, endothelial, neurogenic, and hepatic lineages [3]. Similar stem cell populations are isolated from CVS samples. These stem cells could provide a source for future autologous therapy.

Cell number increases with gestation, although only 35% of cells are viable at 15–17 weeks gestation. A traditional karyotype requires cultivation of viable cells to obtain mitotic figures. Amniotic fluid supernatant or uncultured cells may be sufficient for certain biochemical, DNA, or chromosomal studies such as FISH analysis.

Technique

Amniocentesis is the aspiration of amniotic fluid from the uterus for diagnosis of chromosomal or genetic disorders. This is an outpatient procedure traditionally performed at 15–17 menstrual weeks gestation because at this stage of gestation, approximately 200 mL amniotic fluid is present and the uterus is accessible by a transabdominal approach. The ratio of viable to nonviable cells is greatest at this time, and adequate time is available to complete the diagnosis before fetal viability.

An ultrasound examination is performed immediately before amniocentesis to confirm gestational age, assess position of the placenta, identify the size and location of amniotic fluid pockets, confirm the presence of fetal cardiac activity or fetal movement, and quantify the number of fetuses. Lidocaine may be infiltrated into the subcutaneous tissue, although this is generally unnecessary. A 22-gauge needle is passed transabdominally into the uterus in aseptic fashion, avoiding the placenta if possible. Ultrasound monitoring is continued during needle insertion to direct the course of the needle. Fifteen to 30 mL of amniotic fluid are aspirated into two or three sterile syringes; the amount withdrawn varies with individual laboratory requirements, the indication for the procedure, and gestational age, as less amniotic fluid is removed from earlier gestations (Figure 18.4).

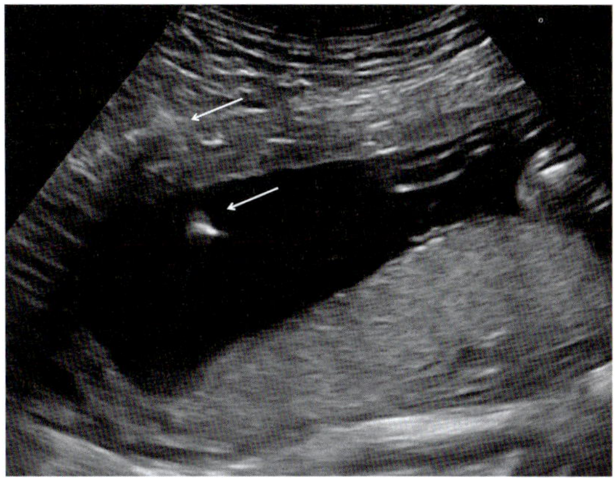

Figure 18.4 Amniocentesis. Transabdominal ultrasound image showing needle track (arrows) and the needle tip in the amniotic fluid sac inserted close to the edge of the placenta.

Clinical Pearl

The initial few milliliters of amniotic fluid should be aspirated into a separate syringe and either discarded or used for AFP analysis. This avoids the possibility of maternal cell contamination (MCC) of the specimen.

Grossly bloody amniotic fluid is aspirated on occasion and microscopic evidence of maternal erythrocytes can be found in most specimens; fortunately, blood usually does not adversely affect amniocyte growth. Gross blood may, however, interfere with biochemical or DNA assays because this reflects MCC. Brown or green fluid is aspirated in ≤5% of second trimester amniocenteses. Usually, such patients have a history of first trimester bleeding and the discoloration results from hemoglobin breakdown products in the amniotic sac. This does not reflect a technical problem and does not prevent amniocyte culture for diagnosis.

In experienced hands, failure to aspirate fluid during an amniocentesis occurs in $\leq$1% of attempts, usually related to uterine contraction, maternal obesity, or early gestational age. Rh immune globulin is indicated in unsensitized Rh negative women undergoing amniocentesis, unless the father of the fetus is known to be Rh negative.

Amniocentesis can be reliably performed on twin gestations by the injection of dilute indigo carmine into the first sac after aspiration of fluid. A second amniocentesis is then performed in the ultrasonographically determined location of the second sac. Aspiration of clear amniotic fluid without a blue-tinge confirms that the second sac has been entered correctly. In the case of a higher order gestation, the same dye can be added to each sac in succession until clear fluid has been aspirated from all sacs.

Safety

Amniocentesis involves risk to both mother and fetus; however, maternal risks are low. In a study conducted by the US National Institute for Child Health and Human Development (NICHD) [1], minor maternal complications such as transient vaginal spotting and minimal amniotic fluid leakage occurred in 2–3% of cases while serious complications such as amnionitis occurred in only 1:1,040 patients.

Potential fetal risks include needle puncture, umbilical cord hematoma and occlusion, placental separation, chorioamnionitis, and premature labor. Reported major injuries have been extremely rare. The issue of increased fetal loss after amniocentesis has been addressed by several large studies that have shown the relative safety of the procedure (Table 18.2). Contemporaneous studies [4,5] have shown no significant difference in loss rate between patients undergoing amniocentesis and controls or compared to the calculated background risk for spontaneous abortion in a large reference population (Table 18.2). One clinical study and several animal studies have suggested that respiratory problems may occur more often in children born after amniocentesis. However, respiratory problems in offspring of women undergoing amniocentesis have not been observed by other investigators. Moreover, long-term follow-up for 5–18 years in children whose mothers had undergone amniocentesis have shown no increase in physical or neurodevelopmental problems. To summarize, the risk of fetal loss associated with amniocentesis is relatively low. In counseling patients, we cite a 0.25% risk of spontaneous abortion secondary to amniocentesis.

Table 18.2 Fetal Loss Rates After Amniocentesis [1,4,5].

	Study Patients	Controls
NICHD[a]	2.8%	2.4%
UK[a]	2.6%	1.1%
Tabor et a1.[a]	1.7%	0.7%
Mazza et al.[b]	0.81%	0.65%
Eddleman et al.[c]	1.0%	0.94%

[a]28 weeks gestation.
[b]Term.
[c]24 weeks gestation.

Early amniocentesis

Some centers offer amniocentesis at 13–14 weeks of gestation. The number of viable amniotic fluid cells increases with gestational age; therefore, the number of culture failures and the time required for culturing prior to harvest is increased at earlier gestational ages. Amniocentesis at earlier gestational ages may result in "tenting" of the membranes due to incomplete fusion of amnion and chorion; this leads to a higher failure rate in obtaining fluid on the first attempt. In addition, the total fetal loss rate (7.6% vs. 5.9%) and the incidence of clubfoot (1.3% vs. 0.1%) are significantly increased following amniocentesis prior to 13 weeks gestation [6]. Therefore, the American College of Obstetricians and Gynecologists and others recommend that amniocentesis not be performed prior to 14 weeks gestation [7].

Indications for cytogenetic studies

Advanced maternal age

Most prenatal diagnoses are performed for cytogenetic analysis. Cytogenetic studies can be performed readily from amniotic fluid cells or cells derived from chorionic villus sampling. Trisomy 21, trisomy 13, trisomy 18, 47,XXX, and 47,XXY all occur more frequently with increasing maternal age. Traditionally, invasive diagnostic testing was offered to women $\geq$35 years of age at delivery. More recently, American authorities have opined that prenatal diagnosis should be available to all women.

Concurrently, first-trimester screening became available and this combined with the availability of second-trimester screening and better quality ultrasound examination to influence women of all ages to choose risk assessment prior to, or instead of, invasive diagnostic testing.

The prevalence of abnormalities in antenatal studies at 16–18 weeks gestation is about 50% higher than that in liveborn infants, and the prevalence of chromosome abnormalities in first-trimester CVS studies is even higher. Discrepancies between the frequency of aneuploidy in liveborns and in first- and second-trimester fetuses are due to the disproportionate number of chromosomally abnormal fetuses that abort spontaneously before birth.

Previous child with chromosome abnormality

The risk for a second offspring with Down syndrome (trisomy 21) or another chromosome abnormality is increased only for women age 29 or younger at the time of the birth of the proband. Recurrence risk after the birth of a child with a chromosome abnormality other than trisomy 21 is 1–2% for the same or a different chromosome abnormality [1].

Parental chromosome rearrangement

A third indication for antenatal cytogenetic studies is the presence of a balanced translocation, inversion, or numerical chromosome abnormality in a parent. The precise recurrence risk depends on the particular chromosome abnormality in question, which parent is the carrier, and the method used to ascertain the abnormality.

Ultrasound abnormalities

Fetuses with structural abnormalities or severe intrauterine growth restriction not infrequently have chromosome abnormalities; therefore, antenatal chromosome testing should be offered to the parents of such fetuses.

Other indications

Mendelian disorders

Diagnosis of a Mendelian single gene disorder is more difficult than a cytogenetic diagnosis. The correct diagnosis of the previously affected child must be assured, and the condition must be associated with a known gene mutation or an abnormal gene product that is expressed in chorionic villi or amniotic fluid cells. If gene expression is key to the diagnosis, sampling cannot be performed prior to the gestational age at which expression of the protein normally occurs. Finally, diagnosis of rare disorders is only available in a limited number of laboratories.

AFP analysis

Assay of AFP can be performed in amniotic fluid but not CVS. AFP is the major serum protein of fetal life and is produced by the fetal liver and intestinal tract. AFP enters the amniotic fluid by fetal renal excretion and by transudation across fetal skin. Elevated levels are found in the presence of open neural tube defects, open anterior abdominal wall defects, and fetal lesions that allow escape of abnormal amounts of the protein into the amniotic fluid, e.g., congenital nephrosis and extensive skin lesions.

Isoimmunization

Serial amniocentesis and determination of bilirubin content in amniotic fluid traditionally have been performed to determine if hemolysis of fetal red blood cells was occurring in women who have Rh antibodies or antibodies to other antigens that are known to result in isoimmunization. However, fetal genotyping to determine fetal Rh status can now be performed on amniotic fluid cells or chorionic villus cells earlier in gestation. This obviates the need for serial amniocentesis in patients with an antigen negative fetus.

Mosaicism (the presence of two or more cell lines)

Maternal cell contamination

In 0.3% of amniocentesis and 2% of cultured CVS specimens, maternal rather than fetal cells are cultured [1]. Almost all cases of 46,XX/46,XY mosaicism in amniotic fluid or CVS cultures are caused by MCC of a sample from a normal male fetus. In addition to creating difficulties in cytogenetic interpretation, MCC may be disastrous if undetected in a sample destined for biochemical or DNA diagnosis. MCC in amniotic fluid is minimized by discarding the first few milliliters of aspirated fluid for cell culture. In CVS, careful separation of villi from decidual tissue in the laboratory is mandatory.

Pseudomosaicism

A potential source of error in interpretation is in vitro origin of chromosomal aberrations. In vitro aberrations arise in all culture systems and should be suspected if many different abnormalities are detected in the same specimen or if an abnormality is detected in only one of several cultures initiated from the same specimen. Cells containing an extra chromosome occur in about 3% of amniotic fluid and CVS specimens. If the aberrant cell(s) are confined to a single clone *(in situ* technique) or culture (flask technique) and multiple other clones or cultures do not contain cells with the identical aberration, the finding is termed *pseudomosaicism* and is without clinical significance in almost all cases.

True mosaicism

In contrast to pseudomosaicism, *true fetal mosaicism* may be present if cells with the same abnormal complement are detected in more than one flask or clone. True fetal mosaicism was found in only 0.25% of cultures in a large multicenter study of cultured amniocytes. When consistent abnormalities were present, 70% of those neonates were subsequently confirmed to be true mosaics. Autosomal mosaicism was more frequently associated with phenotypic anomalies at birth or spontaneous abortion (35%) than was sex chromosome mosaicism (8%) [1].

The finding of true mosaicism in chorionic villi is more common than in amniotic fluid cultures, occurring in about 1% of cases. In most cases, the abnormality has proved to be limited to villi, "confined placental mosaicism [CPM]" and is not present in the fetus; therefore, confirmation with amniocentesis is recommended if the result will determine whether the pregnancy is continued. CPM is usually associated with a normal outcome; however, intrauterine growth restriction is more common in such cases. See Chapter 35 of this text for further details.

Finally, true mosaicism may not be detectable prenatally if the minority cell line is limited to tissues not sampled, e.g., fetal blood, or if the line is of low frequency in the fetus. Despite this potential for error, accuracy of cytogenetic diagnosis is greater than 99%.

☞ Teaching Points

1. Chorionic villus cultures derive from mesenchymal cells that provide more reliable cytogenetic diagnosis than do the trophoblast-derived cells used for "direct" diagnosis.
2. The risk of procedure-associated pregnancy loss with CVS is ≤0.5% in experienced hands.
3. The risk of amniocentesis-associated pregnancy loss is ≤0.3%.
4. Amniocentesis prior to 14 weeks gestation is associated with a higher risk of pregnancy loss and of talipes equinovarus and is contraindicated in routine circumstances.
5. CVS and amniocentesis are both options for prenatal diagnosis of many, but not all, genetic conditions. AFP analysis to determine presence of an open neural tube defect cannot be performed in chorionic villus samples.
6. CPM must be distinguished from true mosaicism to accurately predict neonatal phenotype.

References

1. Verp MS (1992) Prenatal diagnosis of genetic disorders. In: Gleicher N (ed.) *Principles and Practice of Medical Therapy in Pregnancy*. 2nd edn. Norwalk: Appleton & Lange; pp. 159–70.
2. Caughey AB (2006) Chorionic villus sampling compared with amniocentesis and the difference in the rate of pregnancy loss. *Obstetrics and Gynecology* 108: 612–16.
3. De Coppi P, Bartsch G, Jr, Siddiqui MM *et al.* (2007) Isolation of amniotic stem cell lines with potential for therapy. *Nature Biotechnology* 25: 100–6.
4. Mazza V, Pati M, Bertucci E *et al.* (2007) Age-specific risk of fetal loss post second trimester amniocentesis: Analysis of 5043 cases. *Prenatal Diagnosis* 27: 180–3.
5. Eddleman KA, Malone FD, Sullivan L *et al.* (2006) Pregnancy loss rates after midtrimester amniocentesis. *Obstetrics and Gynecology* 108: 1067–72.
6. Canadian Early and Mid-Trimester Amniocentesis Trial (CEMAT) Group (1998) Randomized trial to assess safety and fetal outcome of early and midtrimester amniocentesis. *Lancet* 351: 242–7.
7. American College of Obstetricians and Gynecologists (2007) Invasive prenatal testing for aneuploidy. ACOG Practice Bulletin No. 88. *Obstetrics and Gynecology* 110: 1459–67.

19

CHAPTER 19

Cordocentesis and Fetoscopy

Cristiano Jodicke[1,2] *and Ray Bahado-Singh*[1]

[1]Department of Obstetrics and Gynecology, Wayne State University, Detroit, MI, USA
[2]Perinatology Research Branch, NICHD/NIH/DHHS, Detroit, MI, USA

Cordocentesis

Introduction

Initial attempts at fetal blood sampling involved aspiration of placental blood under ultrasound guidance, placentocentesis. A predictable disadvantage of this procedure was the contamination of the fetal specimen by maternal blood. Placentocentesis was subsequently replaced by fetoscopy. Selective puncture of the umbilical cord or a straight segment of the subchorionic vein close to the placental cord insertion yielded fetal blood of high purity. The procedure, however, required hospitalization of the patient and could be performed only during the second trimester of pregnancy (between 16 and 22 weeks' gestation). In addition, there were associated fetal risks. The improvement of ultrasound imaging permitted direct needle puncture of the umbilical vessels under sonographic guidance or cordocentesis, reducing both fetal risks and maternal blood contamination. Cordocentesis, or percutaneous umbilical fetal blood sampling (PUBS), was first described by Daffos et al. in 1983 and subsequently widely adopted [1]. The frequency of utilization has decreased in current practice for a variety of reasons, which will be discussed below.

Indications

Cordocentesis allows direct access to the fetal circulation and thus expands the prenatal diagnosis and therapeutic options available to the Maternal–Fetal Medicine specialist. The procedure is as an alternative to, or as a confirmatory test for, amniocentesis and chorionic villous sampling (CVS) for obtaining fetal genetic information. This is particularly so in more advanced gestation when rapid results are desired. Over time, however, the use of cordocentesis for the prenatal diagnosis of genetic disorders of the fetus has diminished because of the availability of amniocentesis and CVS, which are less challenging technically and are associated with less fetal and maternal risks. The diagnosis and therapy of disorders such as fetal alloimmune thrombocytopenia and red blood cell alloimmunization remains an important clinical application. The evaluation of fetal hydrops, infections, and less commonly acid–base status in fetal growth restriction remains legitimate clinical indications. Cordocentesis may also be safely performed in multifetal pregnancies for similar indications. Table 19.1 presents the most common indications for cordocentesis.

Weiner et al. [2] in 1987 reported the feasibility of cordocentesis for the direct measurement of fetal hematocrit in anemic disorders such as red cell alloimmunization, parvovirus infection, feto–maternal hemorrhage, and red blood cell sensitization. Fetal transfusion at the same sitting, after rapid hematocrit determination, represented a further therapeutic benefit to this approach. With the advent of Rhesus immune globulin (RhIG), there has been a sharp decline in RBC alloimmunization in pregnancy. In 2000, Mari et al. demonstrated the diagnostic accuracy of Doppler middle cerebral artery (MCA-PS) peak systolic velocity for the prediction of severe fetal anemia [3]. There has thus been a significant shift to noninvasive techniques for the evaluation of fetal anemia.

PUBS for the assessment of fetal acid–base status has never been widely used in the United States because of the

The Placenta: From Development to Disease, First Edition. Edited by Helen H. Kay, D. Michael Nelson and Yuping Wang.
© 2011 Blackwell Publishing Ltd. Published 2011 by Blackwell Publishing Ltd.

Table 19.1 Indications for cordocentesis.

Rapid karyotype
Red blood cell alloimmunization
Featl hemoglobinopathies (thalassemia)
Congenital infection
Nonimmune hydrops
Acid-base status
Twin–twin transfusion syndrome (TTTS)
Neonatal alloimmune thrombocytopenia
Late termination of pregnancy (feticide)

technical difficulties. Further, Manning et al. showed a close relationship between the biophysical profile test and umbilical venous pH values, demonstrating that noninvasive assessment of fetal acid–base status was a clinically acceptable alternative [4].

Technique

The cordocentesis is performed in an outpatient setting after proper counseling and informed consent is obtained. The procedure can be performed as early as 12 weeks of gestation [5], but ideally after 18 weeks because of the small size of the fetal vessels before this gestational age. The procedure is done under continuous ultrasound guidance. The placental cord insertion is the preferred site for puncture because this location is fixed and immobile, rendering it easier target than a free loop of cord. Maternal sedation and analgesia are achieved with morphine and diazepam. Some centers utilize intravenous substances for fetal paralysis, such as pancuronium and vecuronium instead of maternal sedation [6]. We do not utilize either tocolysis or prophylactic antibiotics. The maternal abdomen is prepped and draped in sterile fashion and local anesthesia is generally not performed prior to needle puncture.

Two different techniques are described for performance of cordocentesis, a "free-hand technique" and one utilizing a needle guide. Both techniques may also be combined. We prefer the free-hand technique because this approach does not limit the needle angulation and allows repositioning in case of fetal motion. Regardless of technique, a 22-gauge spinal needle is introduced under ultrasound guidance, with complete visualization of the trajectory of the needle tip and shaft. The length of the needle used depends on the depth of the distance to the cord. The umbilical vein is the preferred target, as opposed to the umbilical artery, in order to avoid the risk of vasospasm and bradycardia, which often complicates puncture of the latter vessel. The umbilical vein is preferentially accessed. A brisk but gentle thrust is required to traverse the vessel wall. The operator senses a "pop" or loss of resistance when the needle successfully traverses the vessel wall and enters the lumen. To verify correct needle placement, a small amount of blood is obtained for a complete blood count to confirm the fetal source. If no blood returns, the needle is withdrawn a few millimeters and rotated. A one mL syringe is used for blood aspiration to avoid excessive suction pressure and vessel collapse. Infusion of a small amount of normal saline yields sonographically observable intravascular turbulence and confirms correct needle placement. At completion of the procedure, the needle is withdrawn under ultrasound visualization. Continued ultrasound observation is warranted post procedure to identify significant bleeding from the puncture site or the development of a cord hematoma. In the Rh-negative woman not previously sensitized, anti-D immunoglobulin is given at the end of the procedure. In all viable gestations, an extended nonstress test of 1–2 hours is warranted to assess for fetal heart rate changes.

Clinical Pearl

The blood sample aspirated must be confirmed to be of fetal origin. The fetal red blood cells (RBCs) are significantly larger than the maternal RBCs, and the mean corpuscular volume of the fetal red cells will reflect this. Later confirmation by Kleihauer–Betke staining and blood typing can be used to confirm that the sample was indeed of fetal origin.

Complications

While a relatively safe procedure in expert hands, cordocentesis should be reserved for specific situations in which the indications and risks are justified. Operator experience, indication for the procedure, technique, and gestational age are important variables implicated in the complication rate. The most common complications after fetal blood sampling are umbilical cord hemorrhage, cord hematoma, fetal bradycardia, infection, abruptio placenta, fetomaternal hemorrhage, preterm labor, premature rupture of membranes, and fetal death (Table 19.2).

The indication for the procedure greatly increases the risk of procedure-related pregnancy loss. Wilson et al. found that the procedure-related pregnancy loss risk in a

Table 19.2 Complications of cordocentesis.

Fetomaternal hemorrhage
Umbilical cord bleeding
Umbilical cord hematoma
Fetal bradycardia
Chorioamnionitis
Abruptio placenta
Fetal death

group with fetal anomalies or intrauterine growth restriction was 3.25%, compared to 1.25% in a group of fetuses with normal growth and anatomy [7].

Gestational age is an important determinant of complications. In a low-risk population, fetal blood sampling performed by an experienced operator carries an approximate 2.2% risk of fetal loss before 28 weeks of gestation and a 1.4% risk after 28 weeks [8]. Orlandi et al. performed 500 cordocentesis between 12 and 21 weeks and noticed that there was no difference in fetal loss rate with advancing gestation until 19–21 weeks, when the risk of fetal loss decreased to 2.5% [5]. As noted previously, delaying to a more advanced gestational age is preferred, provided that the clinical circumstances justify this. The rate for preterm delivery in a low risk population of patients who underwent fetal blood sampling is 5–6% [5,10].

The complication rate is further related to the placental location, and the experience of the operator. Complication rates increase if the procedure lasts more than 10 minutes, involves more than three punctures, or both. Thus, a cordocentesis should not be prolonged beyond 10 minutes and no more than two punctures should be attempted in any one session [9].

Umbilical cord bleeding is the most common complication, but this is generally transient and not associated with fetal losses. Daffos et al. found that bleeding occurred in 41% of sampled cases, but in 80% of these efflux of blood from the punctured vessel lasted <60 seconds [9]. Moreover, Tongsong et al. reported that bleeding from the cord puncture site was observed in 20.2% of the procedures, but only 5.2% persisted longer than one minute.

Clinical Pearl

Amniocentesis, if indicated, should be done prior to the cordocentesis to avoid blood contamination of the amniotic fluid specimen.

Clinical Pearl

Fresh frozen plasma should be available for fetal transfusion at the time of cordocentesis for possible fetal coagulopathies since excessive bleeding has been reported after sampling for this indication.

Cord hematoma is the second most common adverse event associated with PUBS [11]. Jauniaux et al. demonstrated that 17% of umbilical cords examined visually within 48 hours of diagnostic PUBS revealed a small cord hematoma at the puncture site [12]. Feto–maternal hemorrhage reportedly occurs in about 40% of procedures [14]. Sampling sites other than the placental cord insertion reduces the risk of feto–maternal hemorrhage [14].

Fetal bradycardia is a relatively frequent consequence of cordocentesis. Fortunately, the heart rate change is generally a transient event, usually occurs immediately after the procedure attempt and lasts no longer than one minute in the vast majority of cases. Increases in fetal morbidity and mortality can, however, be associated with this complication. Weiner et al. reported that 91.6% of their losses were associated with postprocedure fetal bradycardia [13]. This occurs more frequently when the umbilical artery is punctured instead of the umbilical vein [2].

Clinical Pearl

Cordocentesis should always be performed close to an operating room and with intravenous access in place since an emergency cesarean delivery may be required.

Infection occurs in about 0.5% of cases and this serious complication generally leads to spontaneous abortion or preterm delivery. Abruptio placenta occurs <0.5% and is one of the less common complications of cordocentesis [11].

Conclusion

The decreased demand for cordocentesis in the last decade has resulted in a decline in physician competence in this area. Patients in need for this procedure should be referred to tertiary centers possessing this capability to achieve optimal results.

Fetoscopy

Fetoscopy, a minimal invasive technique, allows access to the intrauterine cavity for diagnostic and therapeutic reasons. Fetoscopy was introduced in the 1970s for fetal blood sampling and transfusion for visualization of malformations, or for fetal biopsies. With the advent of high resolution ultrasound, fetoscopy was practically abandoned. In the last decade, however, fetoscopy has regained a place in fetal therapy. The high maternal morbidity (i.e., preterm labor and premature rupture of membranes) and fetal morbidity (i.e., hypothermia) associated with open fetal surgery has encouraged the development of minimal access fetal surgery techniques. Recent improvements in technology and instrumentation, associated with an increase in accumulated experience, have led to the rapid expansion and evolution of fetoscopy. There has been parallel progress in the design and manufacture of instruments suitable for fetal access.

Indications

Fetoscopy is now utilized for multiple obstetrical and fetal indications [15].

Obstetrical fetoscopy

Obstetrical fetoscopy is the intervention performed to operatively address placental, umbilical cord, and fetal membrane complications. Notably, fetoscopy has been used for the treatment of complications associated with monochorionic pregnancy, amniotic band syndrome, and the placental tumor chorioangioma [16].

Monochorionic pregnancies are associated with a marked increased morbidity and mortality, as compared with dichorionic twins. This increased rate of morbidity and mortality is partially attributed to unbalanced vascular communications present in monochorionic placentas, leading to the development of twin–twin transfusion syndrome (TTTS) and twin–reverse arterial perfusion sequence. Intrauterine death of one fetus in TTTS is associated with death of the co-twin in about 25%, and intracranial lesions at birth in up to 45% of survivors. These complications are usually attributed to an acute hypotensive episode of the normal twin from hemorrhage into the circulation of the co-twin. Because of the high rate of complications overall in monochorionic twins, the early sonographic establishment of placental chorionicity is imperative in all multiple gestations.

TTTS occurs in approximately 15% of monochorionic twins. The abnormal sharing of blood through vascular communications in a monochorionic placenta results in a net transfer of blood from the donor twin to the recipient twin, leading to development of TTTS. The perinatal mortality rate of expectantly managed TTTS pregnancies is high at >90%. Identification and laser coagulation of placental anastomoses for the treatment of TTTS that occurs as a complication of monochorionic twins is a key application of fetoscopy. Endoscopic identification of all vascular anastomoses and laser photocoagulation of communicating placental vessels is now the most common indication for fetoscopy. The objective of laser surgery is to separate the two circulations of the twins completely by occlusion of all chorionic plate vascular anastomoses while preserving placental perfusion. Lasering the arteriovenous anastomoses between donor and recipient twins results in an improved hemodynamic status and decreased likelihood of intrauterine fetal demise of the donor twin. Overall survival of one or both twins after laser therapy approaches 91% with dual survival as high as 72%.

Technique

Fetoscopy is performed under ultrasound guidance. A small trocar is inserted through the abdomen, uterus, and into the amniotic cavity of the recipient fetus. The placental vascular equator is next identified, and the placental vascular communications on the chorionic surface are mapped (Figure 19.1). All visible anastomoses are coagulated with laser (i.e., Nd/YAG or diode laser energy; Figure 19.2). Residual anastomoses may inadvertently be overlooked after laser surgery, leading to the recurrence of TTTS in 14% of cases and twin anemia–polycythemia sequence in 13% of cases post therapy.

Twin reversed arterial perfusion sequence affects approximately 1% of monochorionic twins. In this condition, umbilical arteries from one twin with desaturated blood undergo reversed perfusion to the umbilical arteries and umbilical vein of the other twin. This leads to failure of development of structures such as the head, cranium, heart, thorax, and upper limbs in the recipient. This result occurs as the vessels perfuse the fetal pelvis and lower extremities but have an interrupted communication with the iliac arteries and aorta. The condition is lethal for the acardiac twin and is associated with a poor prognosis in the normal twin, including hydrops, cardiac failure, and fetal death. Fetoscopic cord occlusion by ligation

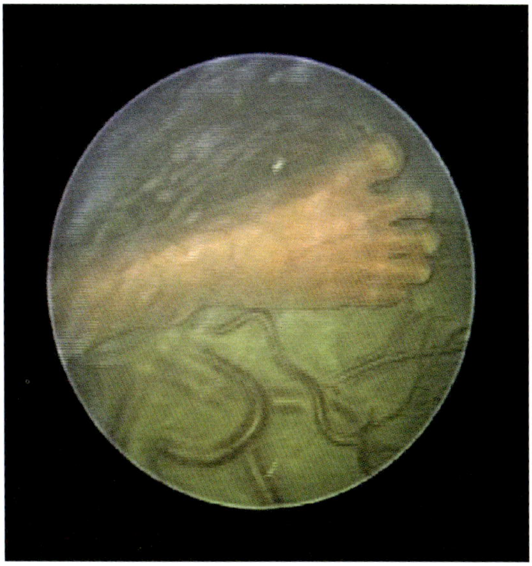

Figure 19.1 Fetal foot and superficial chorionic plate vessels visualized during a fetoscopy procedure. (Courtesy of Drs Anthony Johnson and Kenneth J. Moise Jr. Texas Children's Fetal Center, Baylor College of Medicine, Houston, TX, USA.)

or coagulation of the vascular communications between the two fetuses significantly improves the survival of the normal twin. Cord occlusion may be accomplished using fetoscopic cord ligation, laser photocoagulation, bipolar electrocautery coagulation or intra-fetal radiofrequency

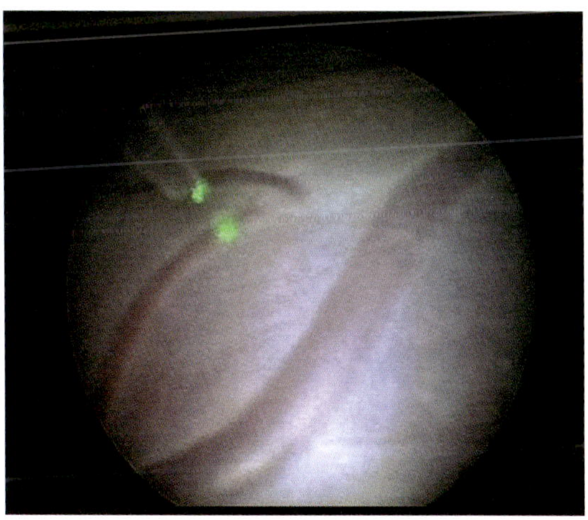

Figure 19.2 Fetoscopic laser coagulation of anastomozing vessels (Courtesy of Drs Anthony Johnson and Kenneth J. Moise Jr. Texas Children's Fetal Center, Baylor College of Medicine, Houston, TX, USA.)

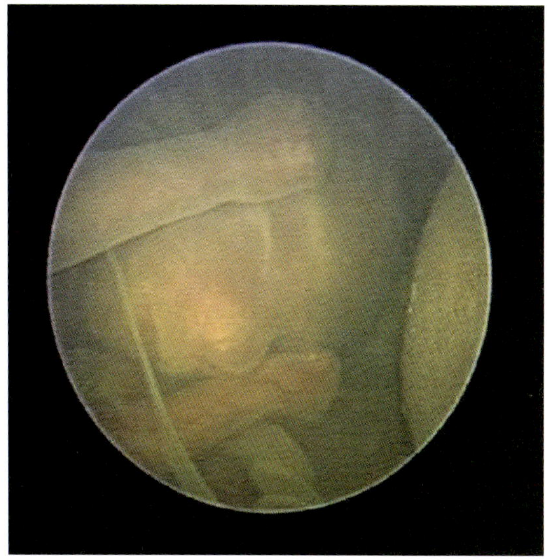

Figure 19.3 Donor face viewed with fetoscopy in a case of twin–twin transfusion syndrome. Note the inter-twin intact septal membrane covering the face. (Courtesy of Drs Anthony Johnson and Kenneth J. Moise Jr. Texas Children's Fetal Center, Baylor College of Medicine, Houston, TX, USA.)

ablation. Bipolar cord coagulation has a fetal survival rate of over 80%. The sac of the acardiac twin when technically feasible should always be the one entered for the occlusion. Complications occur in approximately 40% of cases, and these include fetal loss, rupture of membranes, preterm labor, fetal death or neurologic injury of the co-twin, and inadvertant occlusion of the cord of the normal twin. Bleeding from an incompletely occluded cord and intra-operative exsanguination of the "pump" or donor normal twin may occur with resultant hemorrhage and death.

Amniotic band syndrome is a congenital malformation due to rupture of the amnion and entrapment of fetal structures by amniotic membrane flaps. Consequences include limb amputation and craniofacial, visceral, body wall deformities, and fetal death. Fetoscopy has been performed to release the bands to re-establish perfusion of the affected structures.

Chorioangioma is the most common benign tumor of the placenta. Clinically large chorioangiomas (i.e., >4cm in diameter) are associated with an overall fetal loss rate of approximately 40%. They are also associated with increased fetal morbidity (i.e., polyhydramnios, oligohydramnios, fetal hydrops, cardiomegaly, intrauterine growth retardation, and fetal thrombocytopenia) and maternal complications (i.e., thrombocytopenia, consumptive coagulopathy, preeclampsia, and abruptio placenta). *In utero* devascularization of large chorioangiomas via operative fetoscopy has been done by suture ligation of the arterial supply, bipolar electrocautery, and laser photocoagulation with successful outcomes.

Fetal endoscopy

The fetal endoscopy relates to interventions in the fetus itself. The most common indications for fetal endoscopy are congenital diaphragmatic hernia (CDH), lower urinary tract obstruction, and sacrococcygeal teratoma [16]. The fetoscopic approach to close myelomeningocele was abandoned due to technical complexity and poor results.

Clinical Pearl

Fetal skin and muscle biopsies are also performed under continuous visualization with fetoscopy, although most biopsies are performed with ultrasound needle guidance alone. Muscle biopsies may be used for the diagnosis of Duchenne muscular dystrophy, as an example [16].

Complications

Although the aim of fetoscopy is to decrease or even eliminate the complications created by open fetal surgery, decreasing maternal and fetal morbidity/mortality, complications still exist. Fetoscopy has important technical limitations such as reduced working space, fetal movement, placental localization, and suboptimal fetal position. The most common complications after fetoscopy are bleeding, preterm labor, chorioamniotic separation, and premature rupture of membranes. Although bleeding is not a major concern during fetoscopy, avoiding the placenta and the use of radially expanding trocars has dramatically reduced this risk. The blunt obturator used to expand the sleeve of the radially expanding trocar during its insertion pushes the blood vessels aside and also create tissue compression, decreasing the likelihood of serious vascular injury and bleeding during the trocar placement.

Preterm labor remains one of the main complications related to fetoscopy despite the use of small bore instruments. The use of tocolytics to prevent preterm labor has been disappointing, as several patients still experience this complication despite tocolysis.

Preterm premature rupture of membranes (PPROM) is the most common complication associated with fetoscopy. Despite numerous closure techniques, puncturing the membranes results in local weakness initiating a mechanical and biochemical cascade that results in PPROM. The rate of PPROM is 6–10% of cases in single port procedures and up to 40–60% in multiple port procedures with longer operating times [15].

Conclusion

Progress in ultrasound and instrumentation design along with greater accumulated experience by fetal surgeons have secured a place for fetoscopy in the diagnosis and therapy of fetal disorders. Advances in this field have excited the popular imagination and further developments are eagerly anticipated.

Teaching Points

1. A number of factors affect the risk of complications associated with cordocentesis, including the indication for the procedure, operator experience, number of punctures, and actual procedure performed, namely transfusion vs. blood sampling. These factors should be emphasized in patient counseling.
2. The perinatal mortality is greater than 90% for untreated twin transfusion syndrome. With laser therapy, survival of one or more fetus occurs in 90% of cases with survival of both fetuses approaching 70% in experienced hands.
3. PPROM is the most common complication of fetoscopy. The frequency depends on the number of ports of uterine puncture occurring in 6–10% of cases with single vs. 40–60% when multiple uterine ports are employed.

Reference

1. Daffos F, Capella-Pavlovsky M, and Forestier F (1983) Fetal blood sampling via the umbilical cord using a needle guided by ultrasound. Report of 66 cases. *Prenatal Diagnosis* 3: 271–7.
2. Weiner CP (1987) Cordocentesis for diagnostic indications: Two years' experience. *Obstetrics and Gynecology* 70: 664–8.
3. Mari G, Deter RL, Carpenter RL et al. (2000) Noninvasive diagnosis by Doppler ultrasonography of fetal anemia due

to maternal red-cell alloimmunization. Collaborative Group for Doppler Assessment of the Blood Velocity in Anemic Fetuses. *New England Journal of Medicine* 342: 9–14.

4. Manning FA, Snijders R, Harman CR et al. (1993) Fetal biophysical profile score. VI. Correlation with antepartum umbilical venous fetal pH. *American Journal of Obstetrics and Gynecology* 169: 755–63.
5. Orlandi F, Damiani G, Jakil C et al. (1990) The risks of early cordocentesis (12–21 weeks): Analysis of 500 procedures. *Prenatal Diagnosis* 10: 425–8.
6. Weiner CP and Anderson TL (1989) The acute effect of cordocentesis with or without fetal curarization and of intravascular transfusion upon umbilical artery waveform indices. *Obstetrics and Gynecology* 73: 219–24.
7. Wilson RD, Farquharson DF, Wittmann BK et al. (1994) Cordocentesis: Overall pregnancy loss rate as important as procedure loss rate. *Fetal Diagnosis and Therapy* 9: 142–8.
8. Boulot P, Deschamps F, Lefort G et al. (1990) Pure fetal blood samples obtained by cordocentesis: Technical aspects of 322 cases. *Prenatal Diagnosis* 10: 93–100.
9. Duchatel F, Oury JF, Mennesson B et al. (1993) Complications of diagnostic ultrasound-guided percutaneous umbilical blood sampling: Analysis of a series of 341 cases and review of the literature. *European Journal of Obstetrics and Gynecology and Reproductive Biology* 52: 95–104.
10. Daffos F, Capella-Pavlovsky M, and Forestier F (1985) Fetal blood sampling during pregnancy with use of a needle guided by ultrasound: A study of 606 consecutive cases. *American Journal Obstetrics and Gynecology* 153: 655–60.
11. Ghidini A, Sepulveda W, Lockwood CJ et al. (1993) Complications of fetal blood sampling. *American Journal of Obstetrics and Gynecology* 168: 1339–44.
12. Jauniaux E, Donner C, Simon P et al. (1989) Pathologic aspects of the umbilical cord after percutaneous umbilical blood sampling. *Obstetrics and Gynecology* 73: 215–18.
13. Weiner CP and Okamura K (1996) Diagnostic fetal blood sampling—Technique related losses. *Fetal Diagnosis and Therapy* 11: 169–75.
14. Nicolini U, Kochenour NK, Greco P et al. (1988) Consequences of fetomaternal haemorrhage after intrauterine transfusion. *British Medical Journal* 297: 1379–81.
15. Gratacos E and Deprest J (2000) Current experience with fetoscopy and the Eurofoetus registry for fetoscopic procedures. *European Journal of Obstetrics and Gynecology and Reproductive Biology* 92: 151–9.
16. Crombleholme TM and Johnson MP (2003) Fetoscopic surgery. *Clinical Obstetrics and Gynecology* 46: 76–91.

IV

PART IV

Research Techniques to Study the Placenta

20

CHAPTER 20
Trophoblast Isolation and Culture

Mila Cervar-Zivkovic and Christina Stern
Department of Obstetrics and Gynecology, Medical University of Graz, Graz, Austria

Introduction

Primary human trophoblast culture offers an important tool to investigate normal and abnormal placental function associated with pregnancy maladies. Alternative models are sometimes useful and trophoblast cell lines like the immortalized HTRSV first trimester cells and commercially available choriocarcinoma cell lines, such as BeWo, JAR, and JEG cells, may be selectively used depending on the phenotype of interest. Caution should be used, however, as these lines unlikely reflect in vivo trophoblast function. This is underscored by gene chip analysis and hierarchical clustering, which show large differences among primary trophoblast cells compared to cell lines [1]. Recent models for trophoectoderm differentiation and placental development use cells from the early blastocyst, and these can differentiate into all trophoblast subtypes, including extravillous cells of anchoring cell column, invasive intermediate trophoblast or villous cytotrophoblasts, and syncytiotrophoblasts [2].

Isolation of trophoblast cells

The reagents important for processing are listed in Table 20.1. All steps for trophoblast culture are described in detail here [3] and summarized in Table 20.4.

Term or first trimester placentas are placed on ice as soon as possible and all procedures are performed under sterile conditions (Figure 20.1).

Cell isolation from term placenta requires removal of several millimeters of basal plate surface, and as many grams of villous tissues as possible from multiple healthy appearing cotyledons are separated and rinsed thoroughly in PBS at room temperature. The villous tissue is then gently scraped free from vessels and connective tissue using a blunt edge scalpel. The tissue is washed three times with PBS and stored in Medium 199 supplemented with 1% P/S, pH 7.4, at 4°C for up to 1 hour. About 40–120 g of tissue is commonly obtained. Forty grams of minced and washed tissue is digested in 50 mL of warmed 0.25% trypsin and Dispase Grade II (1:1) with 0.2 mg/mL DNAse I, pH 7.4, and incubated in a shaking water bath at 37°C for 15 minutes. The same procedure is repeated three times. The supernatant after each digestion is collected and portioned in 50 mL conical polystyrene centrifuge tubes, which are subsequently filled with DMEM supplemented with 1% P/S and 10% FCS, gently mixed and centrifuged immediately at 350*g* at 4°C for 10 minutes. After the last step, all tubes from the digestion are filtered through double thickness gauze and the last supernatant is collected. These pellets are soft and the supernatant should be aspirated very carefully.

Pooled pellets are resuspended with 100 mL DMEM, filtered through a double layer of sterile gaze, transferred into multiple 50 mL conical tubes, and centrifuged at 350*g* at 4°C for 10 minutes. These pellets are firmer and require resuspension in 15 mL DMEM by gentle pipetting.

Five milliliters of cell suspension is layered with a Pasteur pipette onto the top of a preformed Percoll-gradient

The Placenta: From Development to Disease, First Edition. Edited by Helen H. Kay, D. Michael Nelson and Yuping Wang.
© 2011 Blackwell Publishing Ltd. Published 2011 by Blackwell Publishing Ltd.

Abbreviation	Full Name	Source
Dispase	Dispase grade II	Gibco/Roche
DNAse	Deoxyribonuclease	Sigma/Roche
DMEM	Dulbecco's modified Eagle medium	Gibco
FCS	Fetal calf serum	Hyclone
HBSS	Hank's balanced salt solution	Gibco
HEPES	Hydroxypiperazineethansulphonic acid	Sigma
Medium 199	Medium 199	Gibco
PBS	Phosphate buffered saline	
P/S	Penicillin/streptomycin 1%	Gibco
Percoll	Percoll solution	Biochrom/Sigma
Trypan blue	Trypan blue	Sigma
Trypsin	Trypsin 0.25 %	Gibco/Sigma
Dynabeads	Dynabeads	Invitrogen
DMSO	Dimethyl sulfoxide	Sigma

Table 20.1 Reagents and antibodies used for trophoblast isolation and culture.

(Table 20.2) and centrifuged at 730*g* at 4°C without braking for 20 minutes. Gradient tubes are handled very carefully and placed into an upright support. The upper layer between 35 and 25 mL marks on the tube is aspirated and discarded with a vacuum connected to a Pasteur pipette. Layers between 25 and 10 mL contain trophoblast cells (density 1.050–1.060 g/mL) and are collected with the Pasteur pipette into two 50 mL polystyrene centrifuge tube, resuspended with DMEM and centrifuged at 350*g* at 4°C with braking after 10 minutes. Supernatant is removed, and pellets are resuspended in 10 mL of DMEM, and cell numbers per volume are determined in a cell counter or with the Bürker-Türk chamber (Figure 20.1).

Cell isolation from first trimester placental tissues proceeds soon after tissue is harvested and transferred into the Medium 199 with 1% P/S. The tissue is washed in PBS, and villous fragments removed (Figure 20.1). The first trimester villous tissue is soft and floats in saline while decidual tissues are firmer and do not float. Villous tissue is again gently scraped free of gross vessels and connective tissue using a blunt scalpel, washed three times with PBS, and incubated in 30 mL of warmed 0.25% trypsin and Dispase Grade II (1:1) with 0.2 mg/mL DNAse I, pH 7.4, in a shaking water bath at 37°C for 15 minutes. This step is repeated twice, all supernatants are collected, decanted through a strainer into conical polystyrene centrifuge tubes filled with fresh DMEM, and centrifuged at 350*g* at 4°C for 7 minutes. Pellets are pooled, washed again, resuspended in 5 mL DMEM with gentle pipetting and loaded onto a Percoll gradient, and centrifuged at 730*g* at 4°C for 20 minutes without braking. The layer at density between 1.050 and 1.060 g/mL is resuspended in DMEM and centrifuged at 350*g* at 4°C for 7 minutes with braking. The supernatant is removed, the pellets are resuspended in 5 mL of DMEM, and cell count is determined.

Research Spotlight

Term placentas provide cytotrophoblast yields of 100–300 million cells (from 150–200 g of tissue), while first trimester preparations commonly provide 10–20 million cells (20–30 g of tissue). This difference results from the limited amount of tissue available from first trimester specimens.

Immunopurification of cytotrophoblasts

Immunomagnetic microspheres coated with antibodies against specific antigens on cell surface are used to deplete cell harvests of nontrophoblastic cells (lymphocytes, leukocytes, macrophages, endothelial cells, fibroblasts, and syncytial fragments) before primary culture (Table 20.3). Syncytial fragments and macrophages do not attach to most growth surfaces after 4 hours and these can be removed by careful, triplicate washing to yield 95–99% pure cytotrophoblasts. Mesenchymal cells commonly contaminate cytotrophoblasts harvested from term placentas, especially if the harvest includes densities outside of 1.050 and 1.060 g/mL on the Percoll gradients. These cells can be eliminated using microspheres coated with

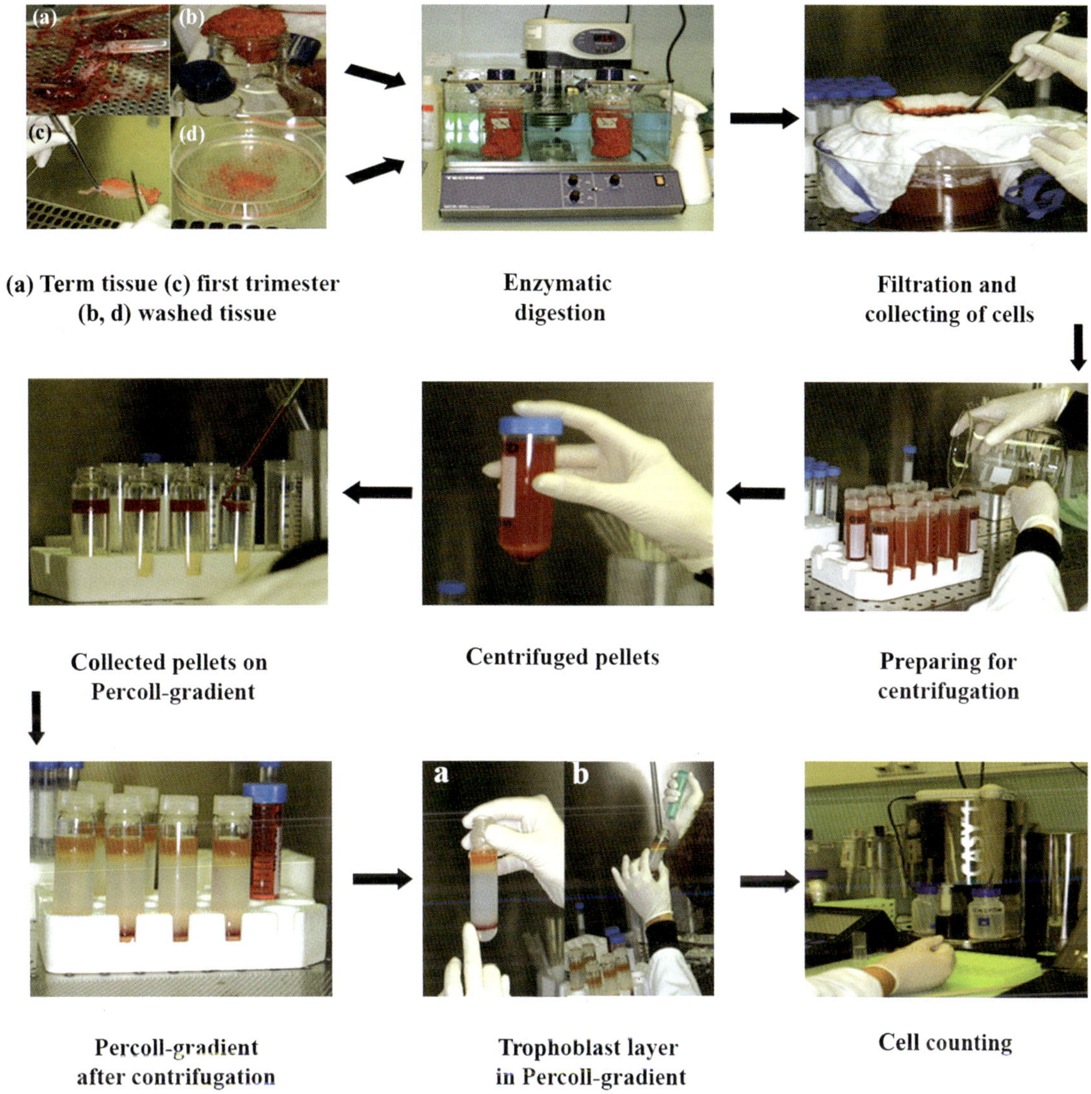

Figure 20.1 Trophoblast cell isolation; main steps.

antibodies to HLA class I antigens, which are present on mesenchymal cells but not villous trophoblasts. However, first trimester cytotrophoblast cell preparations contain about 40% extravillous trophoblast cells that normally express HLA class I antigen. For this reason, microspheres coated with antibodies to CD45RB to detect all cells of myeloid origin and FSA antibodies to detect fibroblasts can be used to reach high purity from first trimester isolates (Table 20.3). Although antibody-coated immunomagnetic microspheres can be used to eliminate virtually all nontrophoblastic cells, the extra cost for this approach and the reduction in cytotrophoblast yield makes this step prohibitive for most purposes. Indeed, a single placental preparation that commonly yields 1.5–3.0 × 10^8 cells costs about 420 US dollars without the microsphere step!

Purification of term cytotrophoblast

Twenty million cells in a 5 mL suspension are mixed with 1 mL Dynabeads (Invitrogen, Dynal coated with

Table 20.2 Preparation of Percoll gradient.

Step	Percoll Solution + 10× HBSS (mL)	1× HBSS (mL)
1	16.8	7.2
2	14.4	9.6
3	12.0	12.0
4	9.6	14.4
5	7.2	16.8
6	4.8	19.2
7	2.4	21.6

Percoll solution + 10× HBSS (1:4) is diluted with ddH2O (1:1) and the gradients are made in advance by gently layering the below Percoll solutions into a 50 mL conical tube starting with solution #1 and ending with solution #7. It is easiest to layer by tilting the tube at a slight angle. Once completed, gradients should remain undisturbed in an upright position until the cells suspension is laid on top before centrifugation.

goat anti-mouse IgG and with 25 μL mouse anti-human HLA class I ABC antigens. After 1 hour of gentle swirling, separation of contaminating cells is done by use of a magnet for 10 minutes. The supernatant, which contains trophoblasts, is transferred to 50 mL tubes, and the tubes are filled with supplemented DMEM and centrifuged at 350*g* for 10 minutes. The pellets are resuspended in 10 mL DMEM by gentle pipetting.

Purification of first trimester cytotrophoblasts

Purification of cytotrophoblasts isolated from first trimester villi is a two-step process: (1) Elimination of CD45RB positive myeloid origin cells. This is achieved by incubation of isolated trophoblasts with 200 μL of Dynabeads coated with antibody against CD45RB. After mixing for 10 minutes (Table 20.3), the Dynabeads and CD45RB positive cells are then separated on a magnet for 4 minutes. This procedure will remove 20–30% of cells of myeloid origin. (2) Elimination of contaminated fibroblasts. The supernatant containing trophoblasts will be incubated with 200 μL anti-fibroblast Dynabeads for 10 minutes (Table 20.3). After separation of Dynabeads on a magnet for 4 minutes, the supernatant that contains pure trophoblasts is then transferred to 50 mL tubes, the tubes are filled with DMEM, and centrifuged at 350*g* at 4°C for 7 minutes. The pellet is resuspended in 5 mL DMEM by gentle pipetting.

Cryopreservation

Trophoblast cells may be preserved for years with reasonable viability as long as general precautions are followed for freezing and thawing.

Freezing of freshly isolated cytotrophoblasts in suspension requires 10% DMSO in DMEM. Two milliliters of final cell suspension (1 million cells/mL) is transferred to cryogenic vials, placed into a cell-freezing container, stored at −80°C overnight, and then in liquid nitrogen for long-term storage.

Thawing requires frozen vials be placed in a water bath at 37°C, agitated gently for <1 minute, transferred to 5 mL prewarmed FCS in 50 mL tube, and centrifuged at

Table 20.3 Antibodies used for immunopurification and characterization. All recommended antibodies are monoclonal mouse anti-human.

Abbreviation	Full Name	Source
CD45RB	Leucocyte common antigen CD45RB antibody	Dako
CD68	Makrophage lysosomal glycoprotein CD68 antibody	Dako
CD14	Makrophage marker CD14 antibody	Becton/Dickinson
CD163	Makrophage markers CD163 antibody	Dako
FSA	Fibroblast specific antibody	Dianova
HLA I	HLA I ABC antibody	Serotec
CK 7	Anti-cytokeratin 7 antibody	Dako
Vimentin	Anti-vimetin antibody	Dako
Desmoplakin	Anti-desmosomal protein antibody	Sigma
CD49f	CD49f VLA6	Dako
CD49a	CD49a alpha 1	Dako
CD49e	CD49e alpha 5	Dako
M30	M30 CytoDEATH antibody	Roche
p85	PARP p85 fragment antibody	Promega
FITC	Fluorescein isothiocyanate antibody	Sigma

290*g* for 7 minutes. Supernatant is decanted and pellets resuspended in 5 mL supplemented DMEM.

Seeding

Isolated cells are plated on growth surfaces at a density of 350,000 cells/cm^2 and in DMEM, containing 10% FCS, 20 mmol/l HEPES (pH 7.4), penicillin (10 U/mL), and streptomycin (10 μg/mL), and cultured at 37°C, in 5% CO_2/95% air. This density optimizes differentiation during culture. After 4 hours, to allow cell attachment, medium and unattached cells are removed. Cultures are washed three times with medium gently pipetted down the side of the culture vessel. Equal gentle care is needed for medium removal. Fresh medium is replaced and experiments begun. If marked reduction in density occurs during longer experiments, results may be inconsistent from one primary culture to another.

Viability

Viability of freshly isolated cells is usually tested by the trypan-blue exclusion. A more dynamic test of viability is difluoroacetate that requires an intact surface membrane and cytoplasmic activity of an esterase.

Characterization

Immunocytochemical staining for selected antigens is the most expeditious approach to characterize primary cell isolates for purity. Fluorescein isothiocyanate (FITC)-conjugated monoclonal antibody against cytokeratin-7 (CK7) is a useful and specific marker for all forms of trophoblast phenotypes (Table 20.1). The initial cell isolate from the Percoll gradient contains a variable number of syncytial fragments that are observed by their immunoreactivity for exteriorized phosphatidylserine (ePS) and placental alkaline phophatase (PLAP). These fragments do not attach to culture surfaces and can be eliminated by washing three times with medium after 4 hours, which allows viable trophoblasts to attach. Monitoring the presence of these fragments in culture by microscopy can be supplemented with assay for human placental lactogen. HPL diminishes within hours in early culture as these fragments disappear.

After first trimester trophoblast isolation, extravillous trophoblast cells with proliferative features express α_6 integrin and can be identified by CD49f VLA6 antibody. Those with an invasive phenotype express α_1 integrin and can be identified by anti-CD49a, while α_5 integrin-expressing cells are immunoreactive for CD49e (Table 20.3) [4]. There are subpopulations of extravillous cytotrophoblast cells, according to their morphologic properties and their expression of HLA-G.

Nontrophoblast cells are also identified by immunocytochemistry, using vimentin for cells of mesenchymal origin, FSA for fibroblasts, common leukocyte antibody CD45RB for cells of myeloid origin, and CD14, CD68, and CD163 for macrophages (Table 20.3) [5].

Trophoblast cell culture

Oxygen content has been shown to play a critical role in trophoblast differentiation and function in culture. The physiologic environment of early trophoblast is hypoxic with a pO_2 of 15–20 mm Hg at eight weeks' gestation rising to a pO_2 of 50 mm Hg by 12 weeks of gestation. The hypoxic environment of very early pregnancy can thus be simulated by 2–3% oxygen. This low level selects the proliferative cytotrophoblast phenotype. A predominantly invasive phenotype develops when cultures contain 8% or 20% oxygen [6]. Trophoblast cells cultured in hypoxic conditions should be plated, incubated, handled, and terminated exclusively in hypoxic chambers to avoid reoxygenation effects that will alter cell response. Term trophoblasts are exposed to 40–60 mm Hg in vivo, and oxygen levels of 5–8% have been proposed for culture that may better reflect that pO_2. Extreme hypoxia of <1 mm Hg in cultures of cytotrophoblasts from term inhibits syncytial formation and enhances apoptosis in vitro.

Differentiation of trophoblast cells in culture

Differentiation of term trophoblast

Cytotrophoblast cells isolated from villous trophoblast of term placenta aggregate soon after plating in culture (Figure 20.2(a)). Numerous genes associated with syncytiotrophoblast differentiation will be upregulated by 4 hours in FCS. After 24 hours in culture, >95% of cells

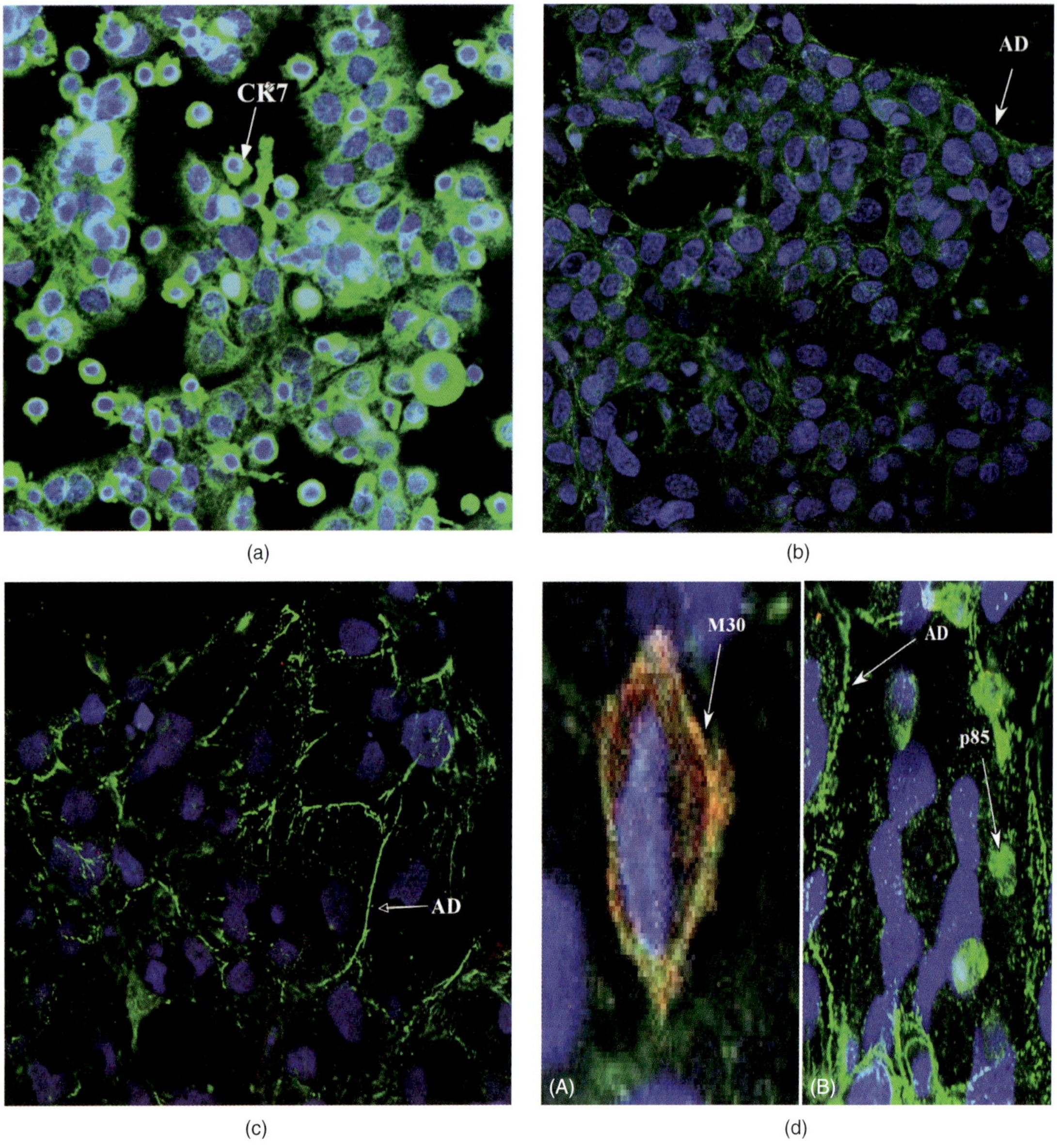

Figure 20.2 (a) Cytotrophoblast cells after 4 hours in culture. Highly purified cytotrophoblast after washing and medium change stained green with FITC-conjugated anti-cytokeratin 7 (CK7) antibodies. Nuclei are stained blue with TO-PRO. Confocal microscopy, magnification 600×. (b) Cytotrophoblast aggregates after 24 hours in culture. Cytotophoblast aggregated in monolayer of mononuclear cells (nuclei are stained blue with TO-PRO), connected with desmosomes stained green by FITC-conjugated anti-desmosomal proteine antibody (AD). Confocal microscopy, magnification 600×. (c) Trophoblast cells after 72 hours in culture. After 72 hours in culture, there are some enlarged new binuclear and trinuclear cells in culture with desmosomes arrays, ending blindly or attached to surrounding cytotrophoblast. Green, staining with FITC conjugated anti-desmosomal proteine antibody (AD); blue, TO-PRO for nuclei. Confocal microscopy, magnification 600×. (d) Cytotrophoblast and syncytiotrophoblast marked for apoptosis. (a) Cytotrophoblast cell after 24 hours in culture. Red, M30, marker for cytoplasmic apoptosis. (b) Syncytiotrophoblast after 72 hours in culture. Green, p85 for apoptotic nuclei and AD for desmosomes. Nuclei are stained blue with TO-PRO.

are mononuclear and in aggregates (Figure 20.2(b)). Cell contact associates with gap junction formation and expression of connexins and these channels allow the exchange of ions and small molecules between the cells. The immunostaining with anti-desmosome antibody or anti-E-cadherin antibody delineates surface membranes and allows identification of syncytium formation, prominent after 72 hours (Figure 20.2(c)). The appearance of syncytiotrophoblast is biochemically characterized by increases in cyclic adenosine monoposphate (cAMP), decreases in basal Ca^{2+}activity, and increased synthesis and expression of trophoblast-specific proteins human chorionic gonadotropin (hCG) and human placental lactogen (hPL), among others.

Differentiation of term cytotrophoblasts can be stimulated by epidermal growth factor (EGF), vascular endothelial growth factor (VEGF), granulocyte macrophage colony-stimulating factor (GM-CSF), whereas hypoxia, endothelin-1, and transforming growth factor ß1 (TGF-ß1) impair this process. These growth factors can be used to modulate the villous trophoblast phenotype for some studies. Apoptotic cell death is apparent in trophoblasts cultured under standard conditions (Figure 20.2(d)) and is generally higher in cytotrophoblasts than in syncytiotrophoblasts [7]. Apoptosis is enhanced by extreme hypoxia, homocysteine, lipid peroxides, thromboxane, and TNF-alpha, but is attenuated by EGF and endothelin-1 [8].

Differentiation of first trimester trophoblast in culture

Trophoblast cells isolated from early pregnancies are about 60% villous and 40% extravillous. They differentiate in culture into syncytiotrophoblast and invasive

Table 20.4 "Step-by-step lab protocol" for trophoblast cell preparation.

Step	Procedure	Short Description
1	Transport	Immediately place placenta on ice
2	Tissue preparation	Remove superficial layer on basal plate, cut about 40 g of placental tissue, rinse and scrape, mince and wash, and store in medium at 4°C to prepare the next steps
3	Digestion	Tissue in 50 mL 0.25% trypsin + dispase II (1:1) with 0.2 mg/mL DNAseI, pH 7.4, at 37°C, for 15 min, repeat twice (first trimester tissue) or thrice (term placental tissue)
4	Centrifugation	Transfer the cell solution into 50 mL tubes, fill up with medium and centrifuge at 1,200 rpm at 4°C for 10 min, collect, wash, and centrifuge all pellets once again
5	Percoll	Resuspend the final pellets in 5 mL of cell suspension and put carefully on the top of Percoll gradient, centrifuge without brake on 2,500 rpm at 4°C for 20 min
6	Centrifugation	Resuspend with medium, centrifuge at 1,200 rpm with brake at 4°C for 10 min, remove supernatants, and resuspend the pellets in10 mL medium
7	Counting	Use Bürker-Türk chamber or automatic cell counter
8	Immunopurification	Use Dynabeads coated with anti-HLA 1 ABC antibodies for term trophoblast and CD45RB antibodies for first trophoblast isolation
9	Freezing	Dilute to the density of 1–10 × 10^6 cells/mL, store aliquots at −80°C overnight, transfer in liquid nitrogen
10	Thawing	Shake frozen vials in water bath at 37°C for max 1 min, transfer in pre-warmed FCS, centrifuge at 1,000 rpm for 7 min, resuspend pellet in DMEM, make all steps quickly
11	Seeding	Cells in the density of 350,000 cells/cm^3, culture in DMEM (10% FCS, 20 mmol/l HEPES, 1% P/S), pH 7.4, at 37°C in 5% CO^2/95% air for 4 hours
12	Medium change	For isolation without immunopurification is the first time after 4 hours in culture, to remove all nonattached cells. All other medium changes are determined by the experiment protocol
13	Cell viability	For viability of fresh isolated cells use Trypan-blue exclusion, for viability of cultured cells biochemical markers and sequential microscopy
14	Characterization	Immunocytochemistry or FACS analysis could be performed after cell labeling with specific antibodies for each cell type
15	Culture protocol	Take enough time for planning and make pilot experiments

trophoblast, respectively. Extravillous trophoblast cells proliferate, migrate, and invade in culture, according to their origin and behavior in anchoring villi, in vivo. Extravillous trophoblast cells derive from cell columns and have different integrin receptors. The gradual switching from the basal lamina receptor $\alpha_6 \beta_4$ in the proximal part of the cell column (40–60% of isolated extravillous cells) to the receptors $\alpha_5 \beta_1$ and $\alpha_1 \beta_1$ (40–50% of isolated extravillous cells) in interstitial trophoblasts in the distal part of the cell column marks the transition from the proliferative to the invasive phenotype of extravillous trophoblast. Trophoblast cells rapidly lose the capacity to proliferate, whereas invasive cells develop strong invasive phenotype in culture. These points must be considered in designing experiments using cultured trophoblasts.

How to use trophoblast culture?

The use of culture depended on the experimental protocol (Step 15, Table 20.4). Experiments aspire to simulate the investigated homeostatic condition or the pathology in vivo. There are endless possibilities to adjust culture conditions, e.g., incubation with serum, and modification of culture medium, oxygen content, growth factors, and cytokines. The key point for designing experiments is to focus on a single independent variable, i.e. what is controlled, so that the dependent variables, i.e. what is measured as biological output, provides insights into trophoblast function. This approach allows hypothesis testing with maximal validity. What is true is that the isolation of primary trophoblasts for culture is an important advance in our understanding of human placental function.

☞ Teaching points

1 Enzymatic digestion, immunopurification, and cryopreservation are critical points in cell isolation because of decreased cell viability and should be performed strictly according to protocol.

2 High purity of term trophoblast cells can be reached by washing for 4 hours in culture medium, whereas first trimester trophoblast cell purity requires additional immunopurification.

3 Trophoblast cells from term placenta have villous phenotype and differentiate in culture into syncytiotrophoblasts, whereas trophoblast cells from early pregnancies are of villous and extravillous phenotype and differentiate in culture into syncytiotrophoblasts and invasive trophoblasts.

References

1. Lash GE, Ansari T, Bischof P et al. (2009) IFPA meeting 2008 workshops report. *Trophoblast Research* 23: S4–14.
2. Douglas GC, VandeVoort CA, Kumar P et al. (2009) Trophoblast stem cells: Models for investigating trophoectoderm differentiation and placental development. *Endocrine Reviews* 30: 228–40.
3. Kliman JH, Nestler JE, Sermasi E et al. (1986) Purification, characterisation, and in vitro differentiation of cytotrophoblasts from human term placentae. *Endocrinology* 118: 1567–82.
4. Cervar M, Puerstner P, Kainer F et al. (1996) Endothelin-1 stimulates the proliferation and invasion of first trimester trophoblast cells in vitro—A possible role in the etiology of pre-eclampsia? *Journal of Investigative Medicine* 44: 447–53.
5. Blaschitz A, Weiss U, Dohr G et al. (2000) Antibody reaction patterns in first trimester placenta: Implications for trophoblast isolation and purity screening. *Placenta* 21: 733–41.
6. Rampersad R and Nelson DM (2007) Trophoblast biology, responses to hypoxia and placental dysfunction in preeclampsia. *Frontiers in Bioscience* 12: 2447–56.
7. Hu C, Smidt SD, Pang L et al. (2006) Enhanced basal apoptosis in cultured term human cytotrophoblasts is associated with a higher expression and physical interaction of p53 and Bak. *Placenta* 27(9–10): 978–83.
8. Nelson DM, Sadovsky Y, Robinson JM et al. (2006) Advanced techniques in placental biology. *Trophoblast Research* 20: S87–90.

21

CHAPTER 21

Isolation and Culture of Human Umbilical Vein Endothelial Cells

Yuping Wang

Departments of Obstetrics and Gynecology, and Molecular and Cellular Physiology, Louisiana State University Health Sciences Center – Shreveport, Shreveport, LA, USA

Introduction

Successful isolation and in vitro culture of endothelial cells (ECs) from umbilical cord vein (HUVECs) was described by Jaffe et al. in 1973 [1]. Weibel-Palade bodies and the expression of von Willebrand factor (vWF) provide the cells with morphological, immunological, and functional markers to identify ECs [1]. HUVECs are continually and widely used as a model system for studying endothelial function. ECs serve to sense and transduce signals within the circulatory vascular system. They maintain the homeostatic balance of vessels through factors that regulate vessel tone, angiogenesis, lipid transport, coagulation, and fibrinolysis. They respond to internal and external stimuli and thereby are targets for drug delivery. Importantly, the integrity of the vascular endothelium also determines the permeability of the vasculature. HUVECs are not only used as a model system to study general properties of human ECs, but also employed as a cell model to study specific pathophysiological conditions that alter endothelial cell function such as atherosclerosis, inflammation, oxidative stress, and vasoconstriction.

This chapter describes the method for isolation and culture of ECs from umbilical cord vein, as originally described by Jaffe et al. [1] and modified by our own experiences. The initial isolates of primary ECs are 95–98% pure, and this consistently rises to >98% after the first passage in culture.

HUVEC isolation and primary culture

Pre-isolation notes

1 Isolation and use of HUVECs must follow Federal and Institutional regulations for handling of human-derived materials [2].

2 All equipment and solutions that contact HUVECs must be sterile.

3 Isolation procedures are performed under a Type II BioSafety hood.

4 Surgical gloves are worn during the entire isolation procedure.

HUVEC isolation

Buffer, medium, and solutions used for HUVECs isolation are listed in Table 21.1 and the procedures for HUVEC isolation are given in Table 21.2.

Umbilical cords used for isolation of HUVECs should be harvested from the placenta as soon as possible after delivery. The cord is preserved in cold phosphate buffered saline (PBS). If the isolation cannot be performed immediately, the cord should be stored at 4°C in a refrigerator. Delayed processing will reduce the yield and viability of HUVECs if isolated the day after delivery.

Before isolation, the cord should be carefully examined to remove areas with needle stick or clamp marks, and then both ends of the cord are cut off, giving the cord with clean transverse ends. Cords with length

The Placenta: From Development to Disease, First Edition. Edited by Helen H. Kay, D. Michael Nelson and Yuping Wang.
© 2011 Blackwell Publishing Ltd. Published 2011 by Blackwell Publishing Ltd.

Table 21.1 Reagents used for HUVEC isolation, subculture, and cryopreservation.

Name	Sources
Phosphate buffered saline (PBS) w/o Ca^{2+} and Mg^{2+}	Sigma/Gibco
Hank's balanced salt solution (HBSS)	Sigma/Gibco
Type II collagenase	Worthington Biochemical Corp.
Fibronectin	Biochemical Technology Inc.
Endothelial cell growth medium (EGM)	Lonza Walkersville, Inc.
Medium 199 (M199)	Sigma/Gibco
Antibiotic-Antimycotic solution	Sigma/Gibco
Trypsin-EDTA	Cellgro
Dimethyl sulfoxide (DMSO)	Sigma
Fetal bovine serum (FBS)	Atlanta Biologicals/Sigma
Penicillin/streptomycin	Sigma/Gibco

The working concentration for Type II collagenase is 400 unit/mL and for fibronectin is 25 μg/mL.

of at least 6 inches (20 cm) yield adequate HUVECs harvest.

To isolate HUVECs, the vein needs to be flushed free of blood before collagenase digestion. This is done by injection of 30–50 mL of cold PBS into the vein with a syringe. For collagenase digestion, clamp one end of the cord with a homeostatic forceps, inject prewarmed (37°C) collagenase solution into the vein from the other end of the cord until the lumen is distended, and clamp that end of the cord with a homeostatic forceps. The concentration of collagenase is 400 unit/mL, which is made up with Hank's balanced salt solution (HBSS). In general, 1.5–2.0 mL of collagenase solution is needed per inch of cord and the cord should be verified with absence of leaks before incubation. For digestion, place the cord with homeostatic forceps into a 37°C prewarmed PBS container and incubate the cord for 10 minutes.

After incubation, remove the cord with homeostatic forceps from the container, lay cord on sterile pad, and gently massage along the cord to assist cell detachment from the vessel wall. To collect released HUVECs, cut one end of the cord at the inner side of the homeostatic forceps and then collect collagenase solution (containing HUVECs) into a 50 mL conical tube. To get maximum HUVECs out of the vein, cut the other end of the cord at the inner side of the homeostatic forceps and flush the vein with 30 mL of HBSS from one end and collect the eluate containing HUVECs into another conical tube.

Repeat above procedures if more than one cord is ready for isolation, and keep the incubation solution (PBS) at 37°C.

To obtain HUVECs, pellet the cells by centrifugation of the collagenase and eluate solution at 250*g* for 5 minutes and carefully remove the supernatant and suspend the cell pellet with 5 mL of endothelial cell growth medium (EGM). Medium 199 supplemented with 20% fetal bovine serum (FBS), and antibiotics is often used for HUVECs culture. For culture, transfer the cell suspension to a fibronectin (25 μg/mL)-coated flask or plate. Isolated cells

Table 21.2 Procedures for HUVECs isolation.

1. Check the cord and cut off needle stick or clamp marks.
2. Flush the vein free from blood with cold PBS with a syringe.
3. Inject prewarmed type II collegenase (37°C) into the vein and incubate the cord at 37°C for 10 min.
4. After incubation, gently massage along the cord to assist cell detachment from the vessel wall.
5. Flush the detached HUVECs out of the vein with cold PBS and collect the eluate into a 50 mL conical tube.
6. Pellet the cells by centrifugation at 250*g* for 5 min.
7. Carefully remove the supernatant and suspend the cell pellet with 5 mL of cell culture medium.
8. Transfer the cell suspension to a fibronectin (25 μg/mL) coated flask or plate.
9. Verify isolated cells under a phase-contrast microscope before placing the flask or plate in an incubator.

should be verified as single cells and cell clusters under a phase-contrast microscope before placing the flask or plate in an incubator at 37°C with 5% CO_2/95% air. The suspension may contain red blood cells but these do not affect cell attachment. Fresh medium should be changed 24 hours after isolation and then every 3 days until cells grow to confluence. To remove red blood cells in the culture, rinse the cells with 5 mL of prewarmed HBSS (37°C) and add 5 mL of fresh cell culture medium. This is done 24 hours after isolation. In general, a successful HUVEC isolation from a 6-inch cord will yield approximately 1–3 $\times$ 10^5 cells, which will grow to confluence in 4–5 days in a T25 flask.

For subculture, upon confluence, trypsin-EDTA solution is used to detach the cells, and cells in 1 T25 flask are usually split in a ratio of 1:3 (e. g., one T25 flask to three T25 flasks or an equivalent area of culture surface), which will reach confluence in 3–4 days.

The cells are a homogeneous population of large, closely in contact, polygonal cells with a centralized nucleus and indistinct cell borders. Confluence is typically achieved in 4–5 days. "Cobblestone" morphology appearance is a typical endothelial characteristic revealed under phase-contrast microscope as shown in Figure 21.1(a, b). In general, the yield of a T25 flask is about 1–1.5 $\times$ 10^6 cells when cells reach confluence.

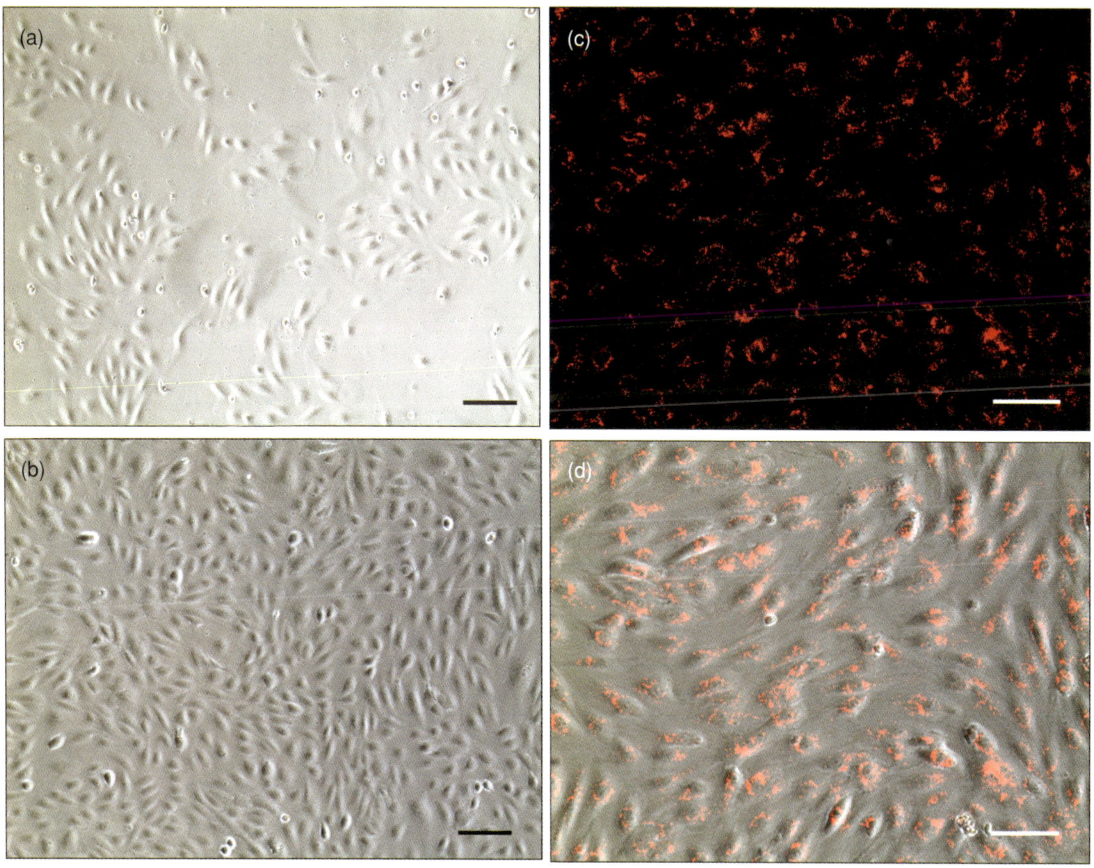

Figure 21.1 HUVECs in culture. (a) 24 hours after isolation. (b) Cells reached confluence. Note the "cobblestone" morphology appearance of ECs revealed under microscope. (c) Cells labeled with Dil-Ac-LDL (red). (d) Phase-contrast image overlapped with (c) (fluorescent). Note the abundance of punctate perinuclear fluorescence indicating Dil-Ac-LDL uptake by ECs in culture. Bar = 100 μm for (a, b) and 50 μm for (c,d), respectively. Positive Dil-Ac-LDL labeling revealed 100% purity of ECs in culture.

Hints and troubleshooting

1 The absence of cells in the eluate from the collagenase treatment of the cord is likely due to a poor collagenase digestion [3]. Try another aliquot of collagenase, freshly made collagenase, or a different lot # of collagenase.
2 Poor fibronectin is likely the problem when abundant cells are present at seeding but they do not adhere after 24 hours [3]. Use freshly prepared fibronectin solution the next time.
3 Smooth muscle cells, fibroblasts, or both may contaminate the preparation. This results from overdigestion of the cord with collagenase or the presence of cord injury from clamps or needles at the time of delivery [3]. Such injury can disrupt the endothelial basement membrane and expose contaminating cells.
4 Cultures that become rapidly senescent or fail to reach confluence after 1 week are usually the result of delayed isolation, bad fibronectin, or contaminating cells.
5 Bacterial or fungal contamination is easily identified by microscopic examination. Disinfect the cultures affected with contamination and discard the flask.
6 Cells should be subcultured for experimental needs or placed in cryostorage once they reach confluence. Confluent cells left for more than 2 days will detach and cease to grow.
7 During subculture, avoid prolonged exposure of cells to trypsin-EDTA solution, which can damage cells and reduce viability.

In most of laboratories, cells in 2–4 passages are used for the designed experiments. Cell growth rate declines with increased passages and thus, usage of cells after passage 5 is not recommended.

We use primary isolates or first passage cells for our experiments, as we test hypotheses that compare and contrast the in vivo behavior of ECs in pregnancy maladies. Primary cell isolates or cells in early passages retain many characteristics of the in vivo phenotype of ECs from placentas in women with clinical conditions, such as diabetes, fetal growth restriction, or preeclampsia. For example, increased expression of endothelial inflammatory adhesion molecules that reflect increased endothelial activation [4], altered endothelial junction protein distribution as an indicator of altered barrier function [5], and reduced endothelial nitric oxide synthase expression as an indicator of endothelial dysfunction [6] have been demonstrated in early passage HUVECs derived from preeclamptic placentas, compared to those from nonhypertensive controls.

Cryopreservation and retrieval of HUVECs

Dimethyl sulfoxide (DMSO) is used as a cryoprotectant reagent for cryopreservation of HUVECs. The cryopreservation solution can be made with either 10% DMSO and 90% FBS (vol/vol) or 10% DMSO plus 90% endothelial growth medium. DMSO is a polar chemical reagent that is widely used as a cryoprotectant in preserving cells in freeze–thaw processes due to its efficiency as a carrier for a wide range of chemicals, its low toxicity, and good miscibility with the test medium. Cells are arrested in G_1 phase in DMSO and reversible after thawing in culture. For HUVEC cryopreservation, trypsin-EDTA is used to detach the cells. The procedures for detaching the cells are the same as for subculture and then pellet the cells by centrifugation at 250*g* for 5 minutes at room temperature. After removing the supernatant, cells are resuspended with cryopreservation solution, mixed well, and aliquoted into 1.5 mL cryogenic vials. The optional cell density for cryopreservation is of 1×10^6 cells/mL. The cryogenic vials should be placed in a Cryo Freezing Container (Nalgene Labware, Rochester, NY) and the container placed into -80°C freezer as soon as possible, leaving the container at -80°C overnight. Cryo Freezing Container containing 100% isopropyl alcohol at -80°C freezer will give a -1°C/minute cooling rate that is required for successful cell cryopreservation and recovery. The cryogenic vials should then be transferred to a liquid nitrogen Cryosystem for long-term preservation.

To retrieve HUVECs from storage, thaw the cryogenic vial in a 37°C water bath for 1 minute, wipe the vial briefly with 70% ethanol, open the vial in a culture hood, and transfer the contents to a 15 or 50 mL conical centrifuge tube that contains 5 mL of culture medium. After centrifugation at 250*g* for 5 minutes at room temperature, discard the supernatant, add 5 mL of fresh cell culture medium, mix well, and transfer the cell suspension to a fibronectin-coated flask or plate.

Research Spotlight

Cryopreserved HUVECs stored in liquid nitrogen are viable for up to 7 years.

Table 21.3 Makers for endothelial cells.

	Makers	Methods	Location
Live cells[a]	Monolayer cobblestone appearance	Phase contrast microscopic examination	
	Dil-Ac-LDL uptake	Cells incubated with Dil-Ac-LDL for 4 hours	Cytosol, Perinuclear
Fixed cells	vW Factor[b]	Stained with fluorescent-labeled antibody	Cytosol (Weibel-Palade bodies)
	Factor VIII-related antigen (F VIII-Rag)	Stained with fluorescent-labeled antibody	Cytosol
	CD31 (PECAM-1)	Stained with fluorescent-labeled antibody	Surface, Junction
	Ulex europaeus agglutinin I (UEAI)[c]	Stained with fluorescent-labeled antibody	Surface, Perinuclear
	VE-cadherin (CD144)[b]	Stained with fluorescent-labeled antibody	Junction

[a]See Figure 21.1.
[b]See Figure 21.2
[c]UEAI gives an even surface staining but no binding to pericellular material without permeabilization. After permeabilization of the cells, UEAI decorates the Golgi apparatus as a juxtanuclear structure.

Phenotypic characterization of ECs

ECs can be identified by their "cobblestone" morphology as revealed under phase-contrast microscope and shown in Figure 21.1(a,b). These cells maintain their ability for uptake of acetylated low-density lipoprotein in culture, as shown in Figure 21.1(c,d). Immunoreactivity for vW Factor, Factor VIII-related antigen, CD31, *Ulex europaeus* agglutinin I, and endothelial junction adhesion protein VE-cadherin are often used as markers for ECs (Table 21.3).

Dil-Ac-LDL uptake—Identification of ECs in culture

ECs have scavenger receptors for acetylated low-density lipoprotein (Ac-LDL). Dil-Ac-LDL, Ac-LDL labeled with 1,1′-dioctadecyl 3,3,3′,3′-tetramethyl-indocarbocyanine perchlorate (Dil), is used to label ECs and thereby identify ECs in culture or for further purification of ECs via fluorescence-activated cell sorting (FACS). Labeling cells with Dil-Ac-LDL has many advantages compared to the other endothelial-associated antigens. The labeling procedure is simple and one step. Once the cells are labeled, the fluorescent probe (Dil) is not removed by trypsin digestion. Labeled cells can be digested and purified by FACS for further purification if contamination of fibroblast cells or vascular smooth muscle cells is a problem, but in general, the isolation can reach >95% purity and further purification is not needed.

The labeling procedure is as follows: (1) after change of fresh EGM in the testing flask, add Dil-Ac-LDL labeling reagent (Biomedical Technologies Inc., Stoughton, MA) at a concentration of 10 μg/mL to the cell culture and incubate at 37°C for 4 hours; (2) remove the medium and wash the cells twice with HBSS, add fresh EGM to the flask, and visualize via fluorescent microscope; (3) positive Dil-Ac-LDL uptake is reflected by an abundance of punctate perinuclear fluorescence, and positive Dil-Ac-LDL uptake should be 100% if all cells are endothelial in origin. Figure 21.1(c) shows an image of positive Dil-Ac-LDL uptake by ECs in culture and Figure 21.1(d) shows the phase-contract image of the same area. Contaminating fibroblasts, smooth muscle cells, or pericytes are not fluorescent as they do not exhibit Dil-Ac-LDL uptake.

Research Spotlight

Labeling cells with Dil-Ac-LDL does not affect endothelial cell viability. It is a reliable method to identify ECs in culture.

Endothelial-specific molecules vWF, CD31, and VE-cadherin

ECs express selective antigen markers such as vWF, CD31, and endothelial junction adhesion protein VE-cadherin. These molecules are often used not only as markers for ECs but also as indicators of endothelial function or integrity. vWF is a glycoprotein that binds to Factor VIII, that is localized to endothelial cell Weibel-Palade bodies, and that plays an important role in anticoagulation. CD31 or PECAM-1 is an endothelial marker involved in interaction with platelets and removal of aged neutrophils from circulation. VE-cadherin is an endothelial specific adhesion molecule at cell junctions. VE-cadherin thereby plays a fundamental role in maintenance of endothelial integrity and barrier function. Reduced VE-cadherin

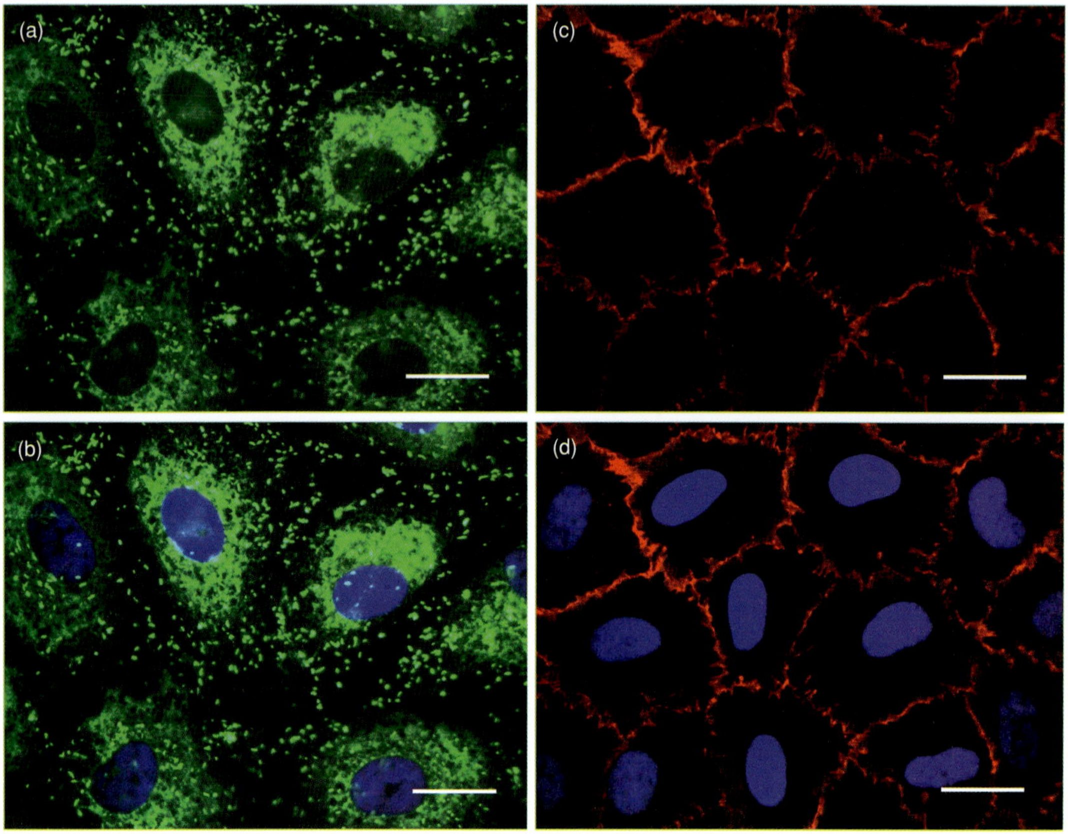

Figure 21.2 Fluorescent staining of HUVECs with antibodies against vW Factor and VE-cadherin. (a) vW Factor staining overlapped with nuclear staining (b). vW Factor is a major component stored within Weibel-Palade bodies of ECs. Note the round, oval, or rod-shaped positive staining of vWF at subcellular (cytosol) component of ECs. (c) VE-cadherin staining overlapped with nuclear staining (d). Note the continuous zigzag pattern of VE-cadherin staining located at cell contact region (junction). Bar = 20 μm.

expression or disorganized junction VE-cadherin distribution reflect altered cell integrity and increased endothelial permeability. Examples of immunofluorescent staining of vWF and VE-cadherin in fixed ECs are shown in Figure 21.2.

Research Spotlight

HUVECs provide an invaluable cell model system to study endothelial function.

After 40 years of use, the advantages of the HUVECs as a model system are apparent: (1) Umbilical veins are the most readily available source of human vascular ECs; (2) The isolation procedure is simple and reproducible; (3) The yield and purity are high; and (4) Cells in early passages maintain features and phenotypes of vascular endothelial function in vivo.

Table 21.4 is a list of examples of a few functional studies in vitro that used HUVECs as a testing model. Indeed, HUVECs have provided a valuable and indispensable model system for the past and current studies of vascular biology and will continually be one for the years to come.

Teaching Points

1 Primary cultures of HUVECs propagate to confluence in 4–5 days when grown in a T25 flask. Cells can then be subcultured at a ratio of 1:3, which then reach confluence in 3–4 days.

Table 21.4 A list of examples of in vitro functional studies with endothelial cells.

Function	Experiments	Application
Activation	Assay for endothelial adhesion molecules[a]	Inflammatory response
Adhesion	Co-culture assay with leukocytes and platelets	Inflammatory response, transmigration
Angiogenesis	Wound-healing assay	Cell–matrix and cell–cell interaction, invasion and migration
	Cells grown on matrix gel	
Barrier function	Endothelial electrical resistance: cells grown on insert	Permeability
	Albumin or horse-radish peroxidase leakage assay	Permeability
	Junction protein expression and distribution[b]	Permeability
Vessel tone	Vasoactivator production and release[c]	Vasoconstriction and vasodilation
	ACE[d] and AT-1[e] expression	
Gene regulation	Gene transfer/over-expression or siRNA transfer	Specific gene or signal pathway regulations
Anticoagulation	Protein expressions such as TM[f], EPCR[g], etc.	Endothelial anticoagulation activity

[a]Endothelial adhesion molecules: P-selectin (CD62P), E-selectin, ICAM-1 (CD54), and VCAM.
[b]Tight junction protein occludin and claudin, and adhesion junction protein VE-cadherin (CD144).
[c]NO, prostacyclin, endothelin-1, angiotensin II, and thromboxane.
[d]Angiotensin-converting enzyme.
[e]Angiotensin II receptor-1.
[f]Thrombomodulin.
[g]Endothelial protein C receptor.

2 HUVECs should not be used beyond passage 5 as phenotypic changes develop.

3 HUVECs are commonly used as a model system to study endothelial function in normal pregnancy and in pregnancy disorders such as IUGR, preeclampsia, and diabetes.

4 For safety reasons, a cord from placenta derived from a pregnancy complicated with infection, STD, HIV, and hepatitis is not recommended for harvesting of HUVECs.

5 There is endothelial diversity among different sites of the vascular tree, i.e., phenotypic differences noted between large vessel and microvascular endothelium [7]. Prior to experimentation, one must verify that the hypothesis testing to be undertaken will be usefully explored by using a HUVEC cell source.

Acknowledgement

This work is supported in part by grants from National Institute of Health, NHLBI (HL65997) and NICHD (HD36822).

References

1. Jaffe EA, Nachman RL, Becker CG et al. (1973) Culture of human endothelial cells derived from umbilical veins. Identification by morphologic and immunologic criteria. *The Journal of Clinical Investigation* 52: 2745–56.
2. Cheung AL (2007) Isolation and culture of human umbilical vein endothelial cells (HUVEC). *Current Protocols in Microbiology* 4: A.4B. 1– 8.
3. Baudin B, Bruneel A, Bosselut N et al. (2007) A protocol for isolation and culture of human umbilical vein endothelial cells. *Nature Protocols* 2: 481–5.
4. Wang Y, Adair CD, Coe L et al. (1998) Activation of endothelial cells in pre-eclampsia: Increased neutrophil–endothelial adhesion correlates with up-regulation of adhesion molecule P-selectin in human umbilical vein endothelial cells isolated from pre-eclampsia. *Journal of the Society for Gynecologic Investigation* 5: 237–43.
5. Wang Y, Gu Y, Granger DN et al. (2002) Endothelial junctional protein redistribution and increased monolayer permeability in HUVECs isolated during pre-eclampsia. *American Journal of Obstetrics and Gynecology* 186: 214–20.
6. Wang Y, Gu Y, Zhang Y et al. (2004) Evidence of endothelial dysfunction in pre-eclampsia: Decreased endothelial nitric oxide synthase expression is associated with increased cell permeability in endothelial cells from pre-eclampsia. *American Journal of Obstetrics and Gynecology* 190: 817–24.
7. Chi JT, Chang HY, Haraldsen G et al. (2003) Endothelial cell diversity revealed by global expression profiling. *Proceedings of National Academy of Sciences USA* 100: 10623–8.

22

CHAPTER 22

Perfusion Technique for Studying the Placenta Cotyledon

Leslie Myatt

Department of Obstetrics and Gynecology, Center for Pregnancy and Newborn Research, University of Texas Health Science Center San Antonio, San Antonio, TX, USA

Introduction

The ready availability of the human placenta following delivery of the fetus offers immense opportunities to study this tissue ex vivo. This approach overcomes the ethical limitations on studying human placental function in vivo. The placenta is usually delivered in an intact manner with good structural integrity suitable for in vitro perfusion studies. Not only is the fetal–placental vasculature intact, allowing it to be cannulated and perfused, but the intervillous space (IVS) can also be accessed and perfused, allowing simultaneous perfusion of both sides of the placental barrier. Indeed, the literature is replete with perfusion studies to examine a variety of placental functions, including nutrient and drug transfer and metabolism, transfer of nanoparticles, antibodies and viruses, synthesis and release of steroid and peptide hormones, growth factors and cytokines, release of trophoblast microparticles, placental metabolism, and vascular reactivity. Additionally, comparison of characteristics of placentae from normal uncomplicated pregnancy with those from pregnancies complicated by various pathologies, e.g., diabetes, preeclampsia, or IUGR, offers additional opportunities to study pathophysiology at the whole tissue systems level in comparison with molecular or cellular approaches, or to serve as an adjunct to such studies.

The major challenges in placental perfusion experiments are maintenance of integrity of the placental barrier and ultrastructure coupled with the ability to maintain or replicate placental metabolism at, or close to, the in vivo situation. Even with many years of experience, these challenges have not been completely overcome. The intact placenta offers the opportunity to perfuse over 500 g of tissue. In the earliest perfusion studies performed in the late 1950s/early 1960s, the whole placenta was perfused but encountered problems due to the inevitable tears in the placenta as the result of delivery. The vast majority of studies now solely perfuse a single intact cotyledon of 10–30 g in weight.

Equipment required for perfusion

Equipment required for perfusion is not particularly sophisticated. The minimum requirements and optional equipment are given in Table 22.1. A placental perfusion laboratory is optimally adjacent to the delivery suite to minimize transport time, to ensure rapid cannulation of the placenta, and to minimize the period of ischemia (see below).

Perfusion technique

The placenta should be collected immediately following delivery and transported to the laboratory. A fetal artery

The Placenta: From Development to Disease, First Edition. Edited by Helen H. Kay, D. Michael Nelson and Yuping Wang.
© 2011 Blackwell Publishing Ltd. Published 2011 by Blackwell Publishing Ltd.

Table 22.1 Required and optional equipment.

Required
2 adjustable speed roller pumps (1–15 mL/min)
Blunt ended cannulae 18G, Butterfly needles 18G)
2 Pressure transducers
2 Oxygenators (bubble or membrane)
2 Perfusate reservoirs (0.5–1.0 L)
Gas tight tygon tubing (ID 1/16 inch)
37°C thermostatically controlled cabinet with heating elements
Plexiglass holding device for placental cotyledon
Gas cylinder with desired gas mixture
Optional
2 perfusate flow meters
Oxygen electrodes and meters
pH electrodes and meters
Injection loops or infusion pumps
Multichannel data collection system
Chart recorders
Fraction collectors

and corresponding vein supplying a single cotyledon are identified, usually near the periphery of the placenta, and cannulated using blunt or bulbous-ended cannulae (20 G). Arteries are easily recognized as they cross over the top of veins. There are several techniques for gaining entry to the vessels, including dissection with fine scissors or the use of a needle cannula. Cannulae should be firmly anchored into the vessels by sutures around the vessels to prevent subsequent dislodging when handling the preparation. A skilled operator can cannulate the fetal–placental circulation in less than 10 minutes. Perfusate flow is started at a low rate (0.5–1 mL/min) as vascular resistance is high after a period of ischemia. The success of cannulation can be quickly assured by perfusate return through the vein. When initially establishing perfusion, care should be taken to avoid high perfusion pressure, particularly when clearing the circuit of blood. Initial flow rate should be low until blood is washed out and the increased vascular tone starts to subside after which time the flow rate can be incrementally increased up to 4 mL/min over a time period of 30–45 minutes. As soon as perfusion is started on the fetal side, the cotyledon perfused can be identified by an area of blanching on the maternal side of the placenta. The IVS supplying the maternal side of the placental barrier is then cannulated with minimum delay. The earliest perfusion studies achieved this by blunt penetration through the basal plate into the IVS. Now commonly two or three cannulas are inserted directly into the IVS through remnants of spiral arteries (identified as dark spots) on the basal plate (Figure 22.1). The effluent from the IVS emerges through venules. A variety of cannulas have been used for the IVS, including 18 G butterfly needles, glass cannulae with barbs, or bulbous-ended cannulae. The major problem is to keep the cannulae inserted while handling the preparation.

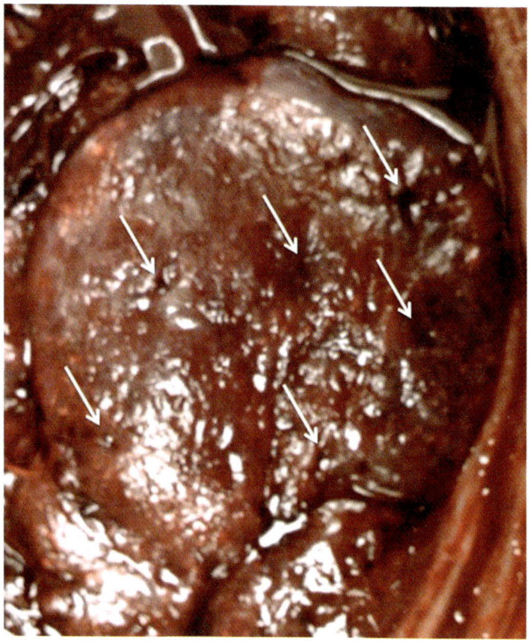

Figure 22.1 Location of spiral arteries in basal plate of cotyledon.

A variety of "home-made" devices have been manufactured, usually of plexiglass, to hold the cotyledon during perfusion. If these are performed with chorionic plate uppermost, the maternal effluent can be collected via gravity into a cone sitting under the basal plate (Figures 22.2 and 22.3). The alternative orientation has the basal plate uppermost but requires a pump to collect the effluent. Commonly, the perfused cotyledon is centrally mounted in a holder and excess nonperfused tissue trimmed away. Perfusate flows are of the order of 4–5 mL/min (fetal) and 10–12 mL/min (maternal) for this weight of tissue to approximate an in vivo flow of 500 mL/min for the whole placenta in vivo. The resulting perfusion pressures are approximately 20–40 mm Hg in each circuit, approximating those in vivo. Perfusion pressure is recorded via transducers placed at the level of the point of inflow in either fetal

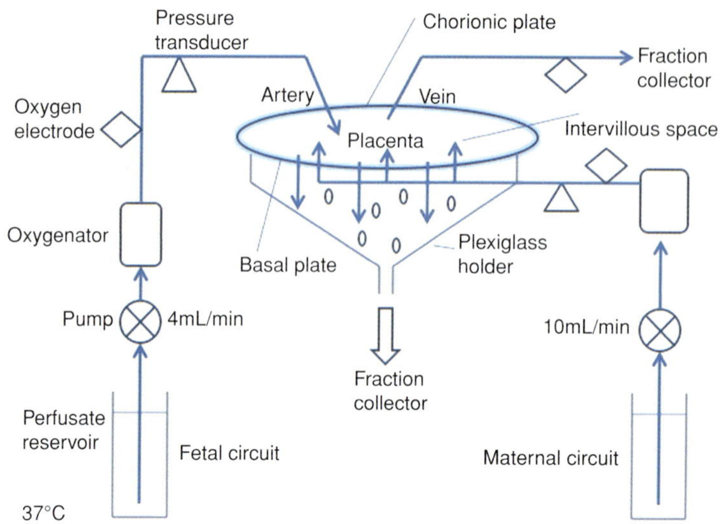

Figure 22.2 Schematic of placental perfusion apparatus.

or maternal circuits. The perfusate flow rates should be adjusted if necessary, both to keep resting perfusion pressures in this range and also approximately equal in both circuits in order to avoid hydrostatic transfer of perfusate due to pressure mismatch. At the end of an experiment, the area perfused can be easily identified by injection of blue dye into the fetal circuit, and it can then be dissected out and weighed. The weight of a single cotyledon can be from 10–30 g tissue. For skilled laboratories, probably about 75% of perfusions begun are successful. The majority of failures are due to cannulation problems, perfusion pressure mismatches, tears, or leaks in the placental barrier.

Research Spotlight

Collection of placentas at elective cesarean section prior to labor avoids exposure of the tissue to oxidative stress associated with labor. If the perfusion laboratory is not adjacent to the delivery room, heparin infused into the chorionic circulation will maintain patency of the vasculature and allow transport to the laboratory.

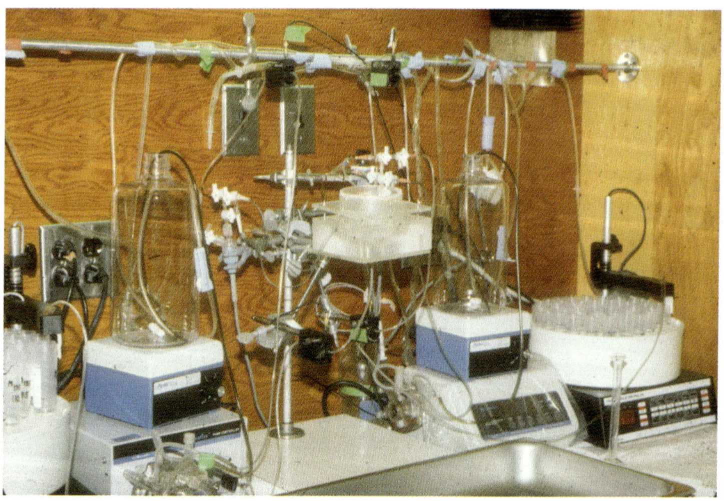

Figure 22.3 Photograph of placental perfusion apparatus.

Composition of perfusate

For isolated tissue bath experiments, oxygenated balanced salt solutions are commonly used. However, the high metabolic capacity and the desire to maintain placental perfusion for protracted periods of time (up to 24 hours) mandates the delivery of nutrients to the placenta. This is commonly done by perfusing with a tissue culture medium (minimum essential medium or medium 199) prewarmed to 37°C before use, containing physiologic concentrations of glucose (4.5 mM), amino acids, co-factors, and buffered with balanced salts (Hank's or Earle's). In addition, perfusion medium usually contains an antibiotic/antimycotic solution and an agent to prevent edema. Oncotic agents include bovine serum albumin, dextran, or the cell impermeant, Polyvinylpyrollidone 40.

Placental oxygenation during perfusion—The conundrum

Oxygen consumption

The placenta is subjected to a period of anoxic ischemia immediately after separation from the uterine wall that lasts until perfusion is re-established. Once perfusion is re-established, oxygen consumption will, however, only reach 20% or less of that in vivo. The placenta has a high rate of oxygen consumption in vivo, with a weight specific consumption of 37 mL/min/kg (1.65 mmoles/min/kg), and a high synthetic rate reaching 29 g protein per day [1]. The proteins synthesized comprise a wide range of structural proteins, enzymes, and peptide hormones, which account for about 30% of oxygen consumed to drive ATP synthesis. These proteins are mainly secreted to the maternal circulation. Indeed, secretion of hPL at term is about 1 g/day. Significant oxygen consumption, about 20% of oxygen consumed, goes into ATP to drive the Na^+-K^+ pump, which maintains the Na^+ gradient for active transport of amino acids and other substances. Under in vitro conditions, oxygen consumption of the placenta is greatly reduced mainly because it does not receive an adequate oxygen supply. The placenta is an oxygen conformer with oxygen uptake in the perfused placenta being directly related to oxygen delivery [2]. The highest values for oxygen supply and consumption are obtained when the placenta is perfused in both circuits with 95% O_2/5% CO_2 in aqueous solution where oxygen concentration is 23 mL/L at 37°C and placental oxygen consumption of 5.3 mL/min/kg is achieved. Maternal and fetal blood, however, contain hemoglobin, which has a high oxygen carrying capacity such that the oxygen capacities are 6.4 and 6.8 mM (150 mL/L) in maternal and fetal blood, respectively. When the placenta is perfused with whole blood or red blood cells suspended in buffer and equilibrated with room air, placental oxygen consumption is much greater than when perfused with a buffered salt solution [2]. Correspondingly, glucose uptake is greater when the placenta is perfused with blood equilibrated with air, compared to a buffered salt solution equilibrated with 95% O_2 [2]. Moreover, conversion to lactate through anaerobic glycolysis is much greater when perfused with buffer. This disparity in oxygen uptake between perfusates of differing oxygen content affects placental metabolism and function and can be evidenced, for example, by measuring hormone secretion.

Oxygenation in vitro

The potential problem this poses in interpretation of experiments does not appear to be fully appreciated and indeed certain recent developments in perfusion conditions have heightened concern. In vivo, the maternal blood entering the IVS has a pO_2 of 90 mm Hg from which oxygen is extracted and transferred to the fetal circulation, which has a pO_2 of 20–30 mm Hg in vivo. Measurements of the pO_2 of mixed intervillous blood yield values of 50–60 mm Hg corresponding to 8–9% O_2. This has led to gradual adoption of use of such gas tensions in trophoblast cell culture experiments as "physiologic." The aqueous media used in both maternal and fetal circuits during perfusion experiments have traditionally been gassed with 95% O_2/5% CO_2, which gives a theoretical pO_2 of 722 mm Hg. In practice, this usually does not exceed 550 mm Hg due to loss of oxygen through the tubing wall. However, this level of oxygenation has been deemed to be hyperoxic, so more recently, the trend has been to utilize oxygenation of perfusate with room air, i.e., 21% O_2, which yields a pO_2 of 160 mm Hg. This has also been coupled with perfusion of the fetal circuit with 95% N_2/5% CO_2 presumably on the basis that in utero oxygen is transferred from the maternal to fetal circuits. While the pO_2 of maternal and fetal perfusates may then approximate those seen in vivo, the oxygen carrying capacity of the aqueous perfusate is much lower than that of maternal and fetal blood. The placental tissue is then subjected to a combination both of anemic hypoxia (lack of hemoglobin) and hypoxemic hypoxia. Even when oxygenated with 95% O_2, the oxygen carrying capacity of an aqueous perfusate is only 1.03 mM and at 21% O_2 would be 224 μM. When perfused with aqueous solution even at a high pO_2, the metabolically active placenta, which uses about 1.65 μmol O_2/g/min in vivo, would be hypoxic and even more so at low pO_2.

Oxygen carriers

This recent move to lower pO_2 may have, therefore, only heightened problems with adequate oxygenation in vitro. The ideal approach may be to add hemoglobin. A limited amount of blood can be collected from the umbilical circulation after delivery for addition to perfusate. As an alternative, some investigators have utilized expired blood bank material. We have attempted to use fluorocarbon [3] to increase the oxygen carrying capacity of perfusate, but fluorocarbons are difficult to put in solution and also permeates the tissue. The recent synthesis of recombinant hemoglobin and encapsulation or crosslinking of this agent would offer an alternative approach to blood. No studies have thus far reported use of recombinant hemoglobin, perhaps due to costs. However, in addition to binding oxygen, hemoglobin also will bind molecules such as nitric oxide, which affects vasoactivity. Oxygenation of the perfusate is simply achieved by bubbling gas through the perfusate warmed to 37°C. More recently, sophisticated membrane oxygenators have been employed. An inline oxygen electrode placed proximal to the point of cannulation of the placenta will give the best measurement of oxygen tension.

Research Spotlight

An important point to remember in perfusion studies is always to use gas tight (tygon) tubing for all perfusion circuits; otherwise, gas inside and outside tubing will rapidly equilibrate and perfusate gas tensions will be less (or more) than predicted.

Assessment of success of perfusion and structural and functional integrity

Multiple parameters have been used to gauge the success of a perfusion and the structural and functional integrity of the placental barrier. Assuming that the equipment is available for immediate measurement, simple criteria of success and adequacy of perfusion include constancy of perfusion pressure throughout an experiment following a 30–45 minutes equilibrium period, limited transfer of perfusate between compartments (less than 4 mL/h transfer in either direction), and constant oxygen consumption, measured as pO_2 in inflow and outflow lines. Post hoc analyses that can be performed to assure the adequacy of perfusion include measurements of glucose consumption, lactate production, hCG or hPL production, and also clearance of antipyrine (mol. wt. 188, a flow limited substrate) added to the maternal circuit. Leakage in the trophoblast barrier can also be studied by transfer of radiolabelled inulin (mol. wt. 5,000). Morphologic examination, including electron microscopic examination of placental structure, will yield details of cellular integrity. Characteristic changes indicating cellular damage would include swelling of mitochondria and endoplasmic reticulum and edematous tissue, with 200–800 nm vacuoles in syncytiotrophoblast, due to fluid shifts [4]. Morphologic changes caused by the anoxic ischemia following delivery can be reversed by oxygenation [5], and then morphology can be preserved even during considerable periods of perfusion, up to 24 hours [6], despite the reduced oxygen consumption relative to that in vivo.

Research Spotlight

Success of perfusion usually can be quickly assessed by the ability to cannulate the chorionic plate vessels and by measurement of perfusate inflow and outflow from the fetal placental circulation

Maintenance of energy metabolism

The placenta has high metabolic activity in vivo, similar to liver and kidney, and higher than the fetus. This implies high oxygen and glucose consumption. At delivery following separation, the placenta is ischemic and will remain so and be subject to progressive injury until perfusion is re-established in vitro in the laboratory. Although cooling of the placenta will slow metabolism and injury, rapid re-establishment of perfusion (most easily performed in the fetal circulation) is desirable in a laboratory adjacent to the labor and delivery area. Measurement of the energy state of a tissue is an indicator of its viability. Placental tissue ATP levels are very sensitive to oxygen deprivation so ATP levels may be adversely affected by labor-associated ischemic events and fall rapidly following separation from the uterine wall. Bloxam et al. [7] measured ATP/ADP ratios and found they fall rapidly following delivery and there is no acceleration of anaerobic glucose metabolism to generate lactate and ATP. The placenta can convert considerable amounts of glucose to lactate, but this will only generate 17% of total energy from glucose; hence, glycolysis is not a major energy source in the placenta. Perfusing the placenta following delivery halts the decline in energy charge and allows the placenta to recover somewhat but not to in vivo levels. The so-called oxygen paradox of the placenta, i.e., a high rate of oxygen consumption in vivo with a resistance to hypoxia in vitro suggests the placenta is resistant to hypoxia, as is the fetus, perhaps as an evolutionary adaptation to withstand the rigors of labor. The placenta can exist with low oxygen by anaerobic glycolyis and by partial metabolic arrest where ATP consumption is reduced but maintained over a long time period [7] as the placenta functions as an oxygen conformer [2].

Research Spotlight

Measurement and constancy of oxygen consumption over several hours gives a real time index of viability and integrity.

Techniques for studying placental transfer, function, and metabolism

There are several techniques that have been described for the study of placental transfer of substances. Substances with a molecular weight less than 1,000 can cross the placenta by diffusion but above that size transport must be via carrier-mediated uptake, either facilitated diffusion or active transport. The simplest method for studying transfer is to place the compound of choice in one circuit (maternal or fetal) and then collect and measure at specified time intervals in the opposite circuit. The major technical decision to make is choice of method to assay the compound. This can be achieved using radiolabel, spectroscopic, or some other analytical technique, e.g., RIA, ELISA, etc. Such experiments are usually performed using re-circulating systems to allow transfer from one circuit to another. The kinetic data that can be derived is, however, limited. More specific data on transport kinetics can be achieved using a single pass paired tracer technique [8]. With this technique, the compound under study, e.g., prostaglandin E2 (mol. wt. 352) labeled with tritium, is used together with a compound of similar molecular size, e.g., sucrose mol. wt. 342 labeled with carbon 14, an extracellular marker that is nonmetabolizable by the placenta. Transfer of the nonmetabolizable substance across the placenta will give an indication of the leakage across the placenta. Any transfer of the test substance beyond this will then be indicative of actual transfer. The use of a single pass paired tracer technique together with infusion of increasing concentrations of the "cold" test compound will provide measurements of uptake kinetics and affinities [8]. In addition, the use of radiolabeled compound can simultaneously allow study of metabolism by the placenta, although other techniques, e.g., mass spectroscopy, can also be used to study metabolism.

There are many studies of placental metabolism and synthetic capacity. Again these may involve single pass or closed recirculating perfusions with measurement of analytes in the collected perfusate. In this manner, we have learnt much concerning synthesis of steroid and peptide hormones and their vectorial secretion to either maternal or fetal sides of the placenta. As there is no innnervation of the fetal–placental circulation and vascular reactivity is regulated by humoral or local agents, the perfusion preparation is well suited to studies of fetal–placental vascular reactivity using agonists and antagonists for a wide range of autocoids. The longevity of the preparation lends itself to generation of dose response curves and use of inhibitors.

Teaching Points

1. Rapid re-establishment of perfusion is necessary to reverse the decline in energy charge but which however does not return to in vivo levels.
2. Consideration of the consequences of anemic and hypoxemic hypoxia needs to be given when choosing perfusate composition and gas tensions.
3. Transport kinetic data can be obtained using single pass paired tracer techniques.

References

1. Carter AM (2000) Placental oxygen consumption. Part I: In vivo studies—A review. *Placenta* 21(Suppl A): S31–7.
2. Schneider H (2000) Placental oxygen consumption. Part II: In vitro studies—A review. *Placenta* 21(Suppl A): S38–44.
3. Mover-Lev H, Dreval D, Zakut H et al. (1996) O_2 consumption in the in vitro fetal side human placenta. *Respiratory Physiology* 106(2): 199–208.
4. Bachmaier N, Linnemann K, May K et al. (2007) Ultrastructure of human placental tissue after 6 h of normoxic and hypoxic dual in vitro placental perfusion. *Placenta* 28(8–9): 861–7.
5. Kaufmann P (1985) Influence of ischemia and artificial perfusion on placental ultrastructure and morphometry. *Contributions to Gynecology and Obstetrics* 13: 18–26.
6. Di Sant'Agnese BA, Demesy-Jensen L, Miller RK et al. (1987) Long-term human placental perfusion—An ultrastructural study. *Trophoblast Research* 2: 549.
7. Bloxam DL (1985) Human placental energy metabolism: Its relevance to in vitro perfusion. *Contributions to Gynecology and Obstetrics* 13: 59–69.
8. Yudilevich DL, Eaton BM, Short AH et al. (1979) Glucose carriers at maternal and fetal sides of the trophoblast in guinea pig placenta. *American Journal of Physiology* 237(5): C205–12.

23

CHAPTER 23

Three-Dimensional Culture Modeling of the Placenta

Douglas A. Kniss[1,2] *and Teng Ma*[3]

[1]Division of Maternal-Fetal Medicine and Biomedical Engineering, Department of Obstetrics and Gynecology, The Ohio State University, Columbus, OH, USA
[2]Laboratory of Perinatal Research, The Ohio State University, Columbus, OH, USA
[3]Department of Chemical and Biomedical Engineering, Florida State University, Tallahassee, FL, USA

History and context

The human placenta regulates maternal-fetal exchange of micro- and macronutrients (i.e., monovalent and multivalent ions, and small molecules such as carbohydrates, amino acids, nucleic acids, and fatty acids), species respiratory gases (oxygen, carbon dioxide, reactive oxygen, and nitrogen species), and xenobiotic agents administered to the mother during gestation. Moreover, the placenta serves important endocrine functions (e.g., secretion of human chorionic gonadotropin, estrogens and progesterone, placental lactogen, to name a few) that sustain pregnancy. Very few other macromolecules easily traverse the syncytiotrophoblast layer of the placenta with the possible exceptions of some viruses (e.g., cytomegalovirus, CMV; human immunodeficiency virus-1, HIV-1, and Rubivirus, rubella). During the development and cellular differentiation of the placenta, trophoblasts become specialized into distinct cellular subsets that form the parenchyma of the mature placenta.

The trophoblast lining the intervillous space at the maternal-fetal interface forms a multinucleated syncytium known as the syncytiotrophoblast, and a subjacent, single layer of mononucleated cells comprise a population of progenitors (stem cells) that give rise to the overlying fused structure as maturation of the placenta proceeds. The syncytiotrophoblast performs the barrier function of the fully functional mature placenta. In contrast, the cellular elements that migrate and invade into the uterus and maternal circulatory system (i.e., uterine spiral arterioles) to establish a low-resistance, high-capacitance circulation that is essential for normal perfusion of the fetus are collectively known as the extravillous trophoblasts.

An intricate balance between proliferative trophoblasts and trophoblasts that differentiate into syncytiotrophoblasts and extravillous trophoblasts is critical for placental function throughout pregnancy. Moreover, the developmental origins hypothesis (see Chapter 1) suggests the placenta provides a window into the prospective health and well-being of the fetus throughout pregnancy and into adulthood. While a discussion of this aspect of placental biology is beyond the scope of this chapter, extensive research carried out over many decades has demonstrated that aberrant trophoblast differentiation can have profound and often devastating consequences on pregnancy outcome. Thus, the isolation, characterization, expansion, and study of primary cultures of trophoblast cells, their precursors, and descendants is an important approach for the study of trophoblast biology and the role trophoblasts play in placental function and pathology [1].

The Placenta: From Development to Disease, First Edition. Edited by Helen H. Kay, D. Michael Nelson and Yuping Wang.
© 2011 Blackwell Publishing Ltd. Published 2011 by Blackwell Publishing Ltd.

Development of 3D culturing methods

Cell culture models of human trophoblast

A variety of preparations has historically been employed for investigation of problems in placental histogenesis and physiology, A complex ex vivo physiological protocol was developed many years ago. This dual-perfusion model has been instrumental for studies of whole-organ physiology of the human placenta [2], such as transport of solutes (ions, glucose and other carbohydrates, amino acids, fatty acids, vitamins and cofactors, and various pharmaceuticals), and respiratory and metabolic gases during an acute timeframe of a few hours.

This elegant experimental method complements whole-animal models and has yielded extensive data about maternal-to-fetal and fetal-to-maternal transfer of nutrients. However, the nature of this complex whole-organ perfusion model makes some intricate cellular and molecular analyses impractical. Thus, reproductive scientists have devised a variety of additional, more reductionist paradigms to assess details of trophoblast development, function, and interactions with other cellular elements of the placenta.

Explant and dispersed trophoblast cultures

Placental explants

The simplest in vitro cultures to prepare, although highly complex in terms of cell composition are *tissue explants*. These ex vivo preparations are established by mechanical dissection of whole-villous fragments that are typically derived from mincing a few cubic millimeters from placental cotyledons, and these are placed on tissue culture plastic or onto matrices (e.g., type I collagen or gelatin or other extracellular matrix (ECM) proteins) in serum-supplemented nutrient media. Explant cultures have been useful for assessing the overall production of bioactive molecules (e.g., cytokines, chemokines, growth factors, hormones, steroids, and arachidonic acid metabolites). The multiple origins of the cells in fragments limits the ability of the model to provide fine details about individual cell populations within the explants. Furthermore, larger tissue fragments are highly susceptible to oxygen deprivation within the core of the explants and often necrosis begins to occur within a short period in vitro. Some investigators have attempted to override this oxygen diffusion limitation by growing explants in 95% O_2 instead of 95% air (approximately 21% O_2), but these may actually elicit hyperoxic injury in delicate tissue fragments.

Thus, in situ studies are needed to correlate macromolecule expression of mRNAs or proteins and function to a particular cell type. These explant cultures are 3D in that they retain the histiotypic organization of normal placental villi. While the villous explant model is a superb, simple method for screening of villi for select functions, newer culture systems have evolved during the past three decades to address the issue of the multiple cell types contained in the Petri dish containing explants.

> **Clinical Pearl**
>
> The human placenta is a highly dynamic organ during mammalian fetal development that originates from mononucleated trophoblasts that progressively differentiate (fuse) into a multinucleated syncytium. The advent of three-dimensional model systems to study the trophoblast will revolutionize our understanding of the nature of human placental development, differentiation, and physiological function.

Dispersed 2D trophoblast cultures

As in other tissues that are cultured in vitro, placental trophoblasts are isolated by a combination of mechanical and chemical dispersions (i.e., trituration and enzyme digestion) and seeded into tissue culture plastic dishes in nutrient media supplemented with fetal bovine serum [3]. The isolated cytotrophoblasts and small intact fragments of syncytiotrophoblast form a monolayer, and during the first few days of culture they fuse into large multinucleated syncytiotrophoblast islands comprising the parenchymal unit of the villous placenta.

In contrast to simple explant methods that require few technical manipulations, enzyme dispersed monolayer trophoblast culture preparations are painstaking and requires multiple washing, enzyme digestion, and centrifugation cycles before a cell population enriched in trophoblasts is obtained. At the end of a long day, the technician is left with an interface of cells within the centrifuge tube that are highly enriched upon assessment of trophoblast markers using antibody-directed flow cytometry, immunocytochemistry, or both. The disadvantage of the prolonged time for processing is offset by the ability to assign specific functions to the dominant trophoblast phenotype isolated, using methods for gene expression and sequencing, antibody-based assays, proteomics, and cellular physiology. A commonly used method carries the eponym the Kliman procedure and yields isolates with enriched villous trophoblast populations, albeit frequently contaminated with fetal endothelial cells and stromal fibroblasts. This method is described in more detail in the chapter on trophoblast cell isolation. Importantly, the revisions such as solid-phase antibody panning methods to remove non-trophoblast elements yield cultures highly enriched in cytokeratin-positive cell types with only a minority of vimentin-positive (fibroblasts) or von Willebrand factor-positive endothelial cells.

Research Spotlight

Cell and tissue cultures of the human placenta have evolved dramatically in the past four decades. Whole-organ perfusion preparations and simple explants cultures have been replaced in many cases by highly enriched trophoblast cultures grown on tissue culture plastic or 3D scaffolds.

3D trophoblast cultures to model in vivo biology

Trophoblasts isolated for growth as explants or in monolayer cultures are ultimately from the trophectoderm that differentiate from the blastocyst into the multiple trophoblast phenotypes that are determined to differentiate and that cannot become any other cell line in the placenta. The many subtypes of trophoblasts are described in detail in the chapter on anatomy of the placenta. Complex modeling systems are required to formulate a multicellular, three-dimensional structure that simulates the anatomical and functional complexity of the human placental villus.

Early attempts to culture human trophoblasts, on both synthetic polymers such as polycarbonate films and naturally derived materials such as amniotic membranes and collagen gels, were aimed to study transplacental transfer when isolating the syncytiotrophoblast layer from the mature placenta seemed too difficult. The two-component culture models now use cells plus underlying matrix composed of biological extracellular matrix proteins or synthetic materials) to mimic the maternal-fetal interface. To construct this in vitro placental model, the matrices must support trophoblast growth, preserve their phenotype, and promote subsequent differentiation into syncytiotrophoblasts, extravillous trophoblasts, or both.

For polymeric scaffolds, important parameters include scaffold surface properties, degradation, pore size, and distribution, as well as their interconnectivity and pore size distribution. The appropriate pore size and pore structure allow cell penetration, adherence to the interior surfaces, and formation of 3D cellular structures, including extracellular components. For example, human mesenchymal stem cells (hMSCs) cultured in fibrous, porous poly(ethylene terephthalate) (PET) scaffolds exhibited markedly different cellular behaviors as compared to the PET films of same surface chemistry. In 3D PET scaffolds, collagen forms highly structured fibrils, similar to their organization in differentiated tissues, but is mainly found in pericellular region in 2D culture (Figure 23.1). The amount of expressed ECM proteins is also upregulated in 3D culture, and the alignment of the ECM fibrils is influenced by the orientation of neighboring fibers of the PET matrix (Figure 23.2). Together, these results suggest that three-dimensionality itself is an important factor contributing to in vitro tissue development and indicate the possibility to direct cells to form the desired tissue architecture by configuring the 3D structure of the scaffold [4].

In contrast to the synthetic polymeric scaffolds, matrices obtained from tissues mimic the natural tissue microenvironment and contain large amounts of growth factors, often including heparin-binding growth factors as well as a 3D network for cell-matrix interactions. These scaffolds approximate the complex 3D architecture of the tissue extracellular environment and can serve as model systems for the delineation of specific pathways associated with cell proliferation, differentiation, metabolism, and solute and water transport. For example, Matrigel™ (a complex extracellular matrix product isolated from a mouse sarcoma) has been used to study trophoblast-endothelium cell interactions and significant changes in endothelial cells' phenotype observed upon differentiation in Matrigel. The model system allows the monitoring of trophoblast migration, and analysis of the factors involved in endothelial-trophoblast interaction. Cell-cell interactions in a physiologically appropriate 3D culture system captures the process of trophoblast invasion and subsequent matrix transformation, unlike other current in vitro culture models or animal systems [5].

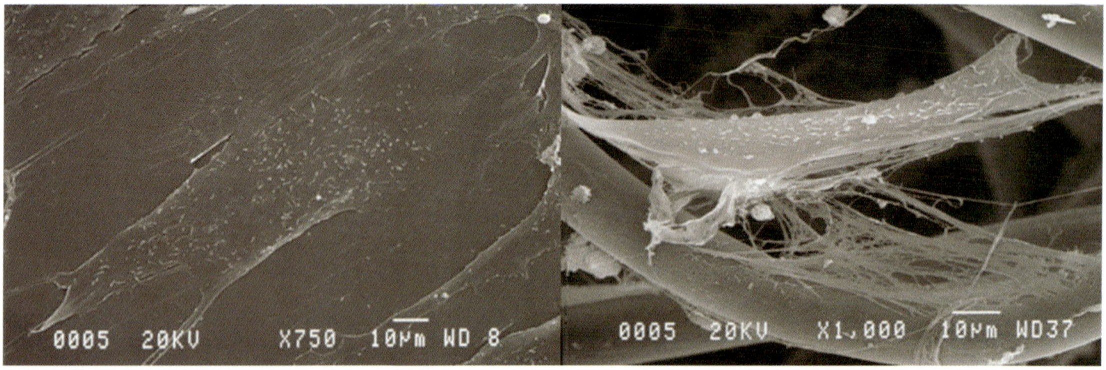

Figure 23.1 Scanning electron micrographs of hMSCs grown (a) on flat cover slips show very little extra-cellular matrix proteins (ECM), but when grown on PET matrices (b) they spread across pore spaces to attach to different fibers and form large amounts of ECM which organize into extensive fibrous networks. (Adapted from Grayson et al, *Biotechnol Prog* 2004, 20: 905–12.)

Progress in biomaterials is rapidly advancing our ability to recreate the cellular microenvironment that enables us to recapitulate the dynamic interactions between cells and their milieu. An emerging technology known as electrospinning can produce micro- and nanofibers from a polymer solution and deposit them as a fibrous mesh. The electrospun fibers can be produced in the length that reflect natural extracellular matrix components, providing 3D ECM matrices with defined composition and structural properties. Consequently, these electrospun fibrous scaffolds can provide tools for study of both biological and structural cues that direct cell-substrate interactions.

Research Spotlight

The various tissue culture preparations described in Chapter 43 each have their own distinct advantages and shortcomings. A thorough consideration of the objectives of a set of experiments is necessary to select the optimal methods of culture for a given hypothesis.

Bioreactors in 3D culture

An outstanding issue in 3D culture system is the spatial heterogeneity induced by high cell density in 3D matrices. In contrast to the 2D surface culture, where each cell has equal access to media, 3D cell organization alters molecular diffusion and generates concentration gradients. The distribution of regulatory macromolecules is especially sensitive to the spatial impediment due to their high molecular weight and low diffusivity. The spatial variation in growth environment can lead to cell heterogeneity that must be fully considered when interpreting culture results. The application of a perfusion bioreactor system

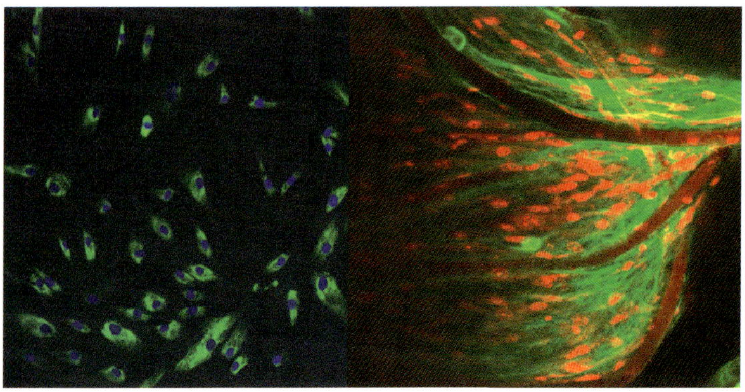

Figure 23.2 Collagen I in cells grown on (a) flat cover slips was seen to be confined to the cytoplasm, but formed extensive fibrils (b) when cells were grown in 3D PET scaffolds. (Adapted from Grayson et al, *Biotechnol Prog* 2004: 20, 905–12.)

is a dynamic culture environment that improves nutrient distribution and mitigates culture heterogeneity. Convective fluid flow imparts physical forces and this is another important component of in vivo tissue environment. An emerging approach in the design and application of perfusion bioreactor system for 3D culture is to replicate the in vivo biomechanical conditions to provide a physiological relevant growth environment. The convergence of 3D matrix technology and biomimetic perfusion bioreactor systems will springboard the century-old in vitro tissue culture technology to a new era [6–9].

Teaching Points

1 Very few organisms, except for some viruses (e.g., rubella, measles virus, HIV-1, and CMV), cross the syncytiotrophoblast barrier in the placenta, a very important organ for fetal development. Thus, the isolation, characterization, expansion, and study of primary cultures of trophoblast cells, their precursors, and descendants is an important approach for the study of trophoblast biology, and the role trophoblasts play in placental function and pathology

2 Synthetic and biomimic polymeric scaffolds prepared by a number of methods (e.g., electrospinning, nonwoven fabric weaving, and salt-leaching) simulate the three-dimensional microenvironment in which trophoblasts can be cultured.

3 Bioreactors add an entirely new dimension to trophoblast cell culture. Cells can be grown in 3D tissue engineering scaffolds and placed into the bioreactor through which culture medium is perfused in an oxygen- and temperature-controlled environment to more faithfully simulate the in vivo milieu.

References

1. Bloxam DL, Bax BE, Bax CMR (1997) Culture of syncytiotrophoblast for the study of human placental transfer. Part II: Production, culture and use of syncytiotrophoblast. *Placenta* 18: 99–108.
2. Myllynen P, Mathiesen L, Weimer M et al. (2010) Preliminary interlaboratory comparison of the *ex vivo* dual human placental perfusion system. *Reprod Toxicol* 30(1): 94–102. PMID: 2043453
3. Kliman HJ, Nestler JE, Sermasi E et al. (1986) Purification, characterization, and in vitro differentiation of cytotrophoblasts from human term placentae. *Endocrinol* 118: 1567–82.
4. Sutherland RM, Durand RE (1976) Radiation response of multicell spheroids–an in vitro tumour model. *Curr Top Radiat Res Q* 11: 87–139.
5. Discher DE, Mooney DJ, Zandstra PW (2009) Growth factors, matrices, and forces combine and control stem cells. *Science* 324: 1673–77.
6. Grayson WL, Ma T, Bunnell B (2004) Human mesenchymal stem cells tissue development in 3D PET matrices. *Biotechnol Prog* 20: 905–12.
7. Aldo PB, Krikun G, Visintin I et al. (2007) A novel three-dimensional in vitro system to study trophoblast–endothelium cell interactions. *Am J Reprod Immunol* 58: 98–110.
8. Zhao F, Grayson WL, Ma T et al. (2009) Perfusion affects the tissue developmental patterns of human mesenchymal stem cells in 3D scaffolds. *J Cell Physiol* 219: 421–29.
9. Grayson WL, Ma T, Bunnell B (2004) Human mesenchymal stem cells tissue development in 3D PET matrices. *Biotechnol Prog* 20: 905–12.

24

CHAPTER 24

The Use of Ultrasound Contrast Agents in Placental Imaging

Jacques S. Abramowicz

Department of Obstetrics and Gynecology, Rush Fetal and Neonatal Medicine Center, Rush University, Chicago, IL, USA

Introduction

Placental examination is a major application of ultrasound in obstetrical practice. Ultrasound imaging is based on two principles of physics: the piezzo-electric effect and the pulse–echo principle. The first one, discovered in 1880 by Jacques and Pierre Curie, states that special crystals, under an electric current, will vibrate and create waves similar to sound waves but far above the audible range (hence ultrasound). These waves can travel through tissues. The pulse–echo principle describes the reaction of these sound waves when they meet the interface between two tissues: they generate echoes that return to the crystal and, by a "reverse piezzo-electric" effect, are transformed back into electronic signals displayable on a monitor, the ultrasound picture. The stronger the interface between two tissues, i.e., the larger the difference in "hardness" between these tissues, the stronger the echoes will be. Therefore, bone appears white, while fluid appears black since no echoes are generated when the ultrasound wave travels through a homogeneous medium. More sound reflectors within a tissue will create more frequent and stronger echoes, both in B-mode or when using Doppler technology. Adding contrast agents to an insonated tissue should therefore permit better visualization due to increased heterogeneity, particularly of cavities and vasculature. Contrast agents have, in fact, been used for many years in radiological procedures, from X-rays to MRI because of the added information they provide. The same concept has led researchers to attempt similar image enhancement in ultrasound [1]. In recent years, these agents have been introduced into clinical medicine and are now routinely used in studying some organs such as the myocardium, liver, kidneys, breast, among others, although in the United States, the use is limited to myocardial imaging. The use of these agents in obstetrics and gynecology is very limited and has not changed over the last 10–15 years [2]. Since these agents greatly improve imaging of vascular beds [3], it is logical that a structure particularly rich in blood vessels, such as the placenta, should lend itself to imaging with these agents. Although this is technically possible, some issues have limited this application in clinical practice.

Historical note

The idea of using contrast enhancement in ultrasound procedures goes back more than 40 years, when Gramiak and Shah, working at the University of Rochester, noticed a strong "cloud of echoes" in the aortic root, with improved delineation, after injecting agitated saline through an intra-aortic catheter. This probably was due to reflection of ultrasound waves from mini bubbles present in the contrast medium or due to the acoustic mismatch between free air microbubbles in the saline and the surrounding

The Placenta: From Development to Disease, First Edition. Edited by Helen H. Kay, D. Michael Nelson and Yuping Wang.
© 2011 Blackwell Publishing Ltd. Published 2011 by Blackwell Publishing Ltd.

blood. Since then, ultrasound contrast agents (UCAs) have rapidly developed, first and mostly in echocardiography for valve detection, improved border delineation, shunt detection, Doppler enhancement as well as myocardial perfusion imaging. Several other medical specialties have adopted these agents for enhanced imaging [4]. A natural development has been in the field of tumor imaging, secondary to the presence of increased, albeit abnormal, vascularization [3]. The most recent advance in this field has been in molecular imaging, a process whereby any imaging modality, such as ultrasound, may be enhanced by the use of specific nanomolecular UCAs [5].

Ultrasound contrast agents

As briefly mentioned in the introduction, all ultrasonographic images depend on echoes being produced by the insonated structures (acoustic backscatter). Introducing solid agents in the insonated area will increase the amount of echo-producing substances, which creates additional echoes. If these are properly processed, they will provide additional information. This may help to determine presence or absence of perfusion, or changes in vascular patterns, and should be important when imaging tiny vessels such as the placental vasculature in which visualization is beyond the normal resolution of gray scale ultrasonography, color imaging, or power Doppler imaging. [6].

UCAs are very small gas-filled bubbles (1–7 μm in diameter compared to a mean diameter of 6–8 μm for red blood cells). These bubbles consist of an external shell made of albumin or phospholipid, which encapsulates the gas core providing stability and protection, allowing for survival once injected into the circulation. Some examples of first-generation UCAs include: Albunex® and Optison® (Mallinckrodt, Inc, St Louis, MO), made of denaturated human serum albumin in the outer shell and air or octafluoropropane internally; Levovist® (Schering AG, Berlin, Germany), made of air covered by a thin layer of palmitic acid in a galactose solution. Newer agents include: Definity® (Lantheus Medical Imaging, N. Billerica, MA), perflutren in a phospholipid blend shell; Sonovue® (Bracco SpA, Milan, Italy), sulfur hexafluoride in a phospholipid shell; and Targestar-P® and Visistar-Integrin® (Targeson, La Jolla, CA), both with perfluorocarbon encapsulated in a lipid shell. The UCA spheres' small size allows them to pass through the smallest capillaries and not be trapped in the lungs. These agents have very high intrinsic ultrasound wave compressibility compared with plasma or tissue, resulting in high echogenicity improving the signal-to-noise ratio and thus spectral, color, and power Doppler signals. The UCAs are generally injected into the vascular system as a bolus or by constant infusion. Major signal enhancement (more than 30 dB) can be obtained with modern equipment, which can even detect a single microbubble. Depending on the specific settings of the ultrasound scanner, the bubbles may be destroyed by the beam or recirculated. New contrast-specific imaging technologies, such as pulse-inversion, have been developed to demonstrate blood flow within capillaries of organ parenchyma (microvasculature). For further technical details, several reviews can be consulted [7].

Identification of small vessels is important in the field of oncology. Tumors are associated with the creation of new vessels known as neoangiogenesis, or new vasculature known as neovascularization. This is common to all malignant tumors as well as some normal physiologic processes such as the involuting corpus luteum and the developing placenta. The new vessels are usually abnormal and irregular in size, branching, and distributed in bizarre directions. These vessels cannot be visualized using conventional ultrasonography, but can be visualized with the addition of a UCA. Additionally, pharmacokinetic studies of UCA absorption and release may be performed to differentiate between benign and malignant lesions. In these studies, the time-intensity curves created demonstrate the degree, speed (slope), and duration of enhancement produced by the UCA and thereby permit characterization of the vasculature. Generally, the time-intensity curves of malignant tumors show steeper rise than benign processes due to the angiogenesis, while time-concentration curves show slower washout [8].

Clinical Pearl

UCAs can help differentiate between benign and malignant lesions by analyzing the pharmacokinetics of the injected agent.

The major applications of UCAs include untargeted and targeted ultrasound imaging. In untargeted imaging, improved organ edge delineation is obtained and blood volume and tissue perfusion can be assessed. In targeted imaging, pathologic processes, such as inflammation or cancer, can be analyzed due to expression of specific receptors such as VCAM-1 (vascular cell adhesion molecule-1) in inflammation and VEGF (vascular endothelial growth factor) in cancer [9]. This is obtained by coating the UCA with specific ligands that bind to these receptors. Although most experience with UCAs to date has focused on imaging tumors, all applications can be theoretically utilized in clinical placental imaging.

Clinical applications of UCA in obstetrics

The indications for the use of UCAs in obstetrics are very limited [2]. In the past, radiologic contrast agents were used to delineate fetal external contour and internal organs by X-ray. The same concept was used by injection of saline into the amniotic sac to improve ultrasonographic visualization in cases of severe oligohydramnios. There are rare reports of UCA usage in clinical obstetrics: one analysis of 30 ectopic pregnancies with demonstration of abnormally located placental blood flow [10], two cases of placenta accreta [11], and one report of 14 complex cases of twin–twin transfusion with direct injection of a UCA into the intrahepatic umbilical vein of one twin to delineate placental vasculature [12]. These are directly related to placental flow and not to placental structure or morphology.

Placental imaging with UCAs

Several adverse obstetrical conditions may be related to defects of placental implantation, permeability, or perfusion. Much of the pathophysiology and the mechanisms for such are incompletely understood. Changes in vasculature may occur well before clinical manifestations become obvious. For example, in the case of preeclampsia, abnormal trophoblastic invasion occurs in the late first trimester and the subsequent deficient blood flow to the intervillous space can lead to placental ischemia and preeclampsia, intrauterine growth restriction, or both. However, the clinical disease may not be diagnosed until the second or third trimesters by current imaging tools. In addition, inflammatory conditions may also be problematic to diagnose, and clinical symptoms may appear late. Placental function cannot, at the moment, be analyzed in vivo. Various noninvasive biophysical and biochemical methods, many described in this book, can assess placental anatomy and function from implantation to term. Most have been used in animal experiments, but not in human clinical interventions. These methods include several conventional X-ray techniques, such as soft tissue placentography, amniography, and retrograde femoral angiography. Also included are computer-assisted tomography (CT scanning), radionuclide scintigraphy, thermography, magnetic resonance imaging (MRI), positron emission tomography (PET), and single-photon emission computed tomography [13].

While placental anatomy can be adequately analyzed with ultrasound imaging, direct assessment of vasculature and perfusion remains difficult. Doppler analysis of uterine and umbilical artery waveform can be helpful in predicting certain conditions or evaluating placental reserve, but these are indirect methods that do not directly assess perfusion or fetomaternal exchanges. Qualification of perfusion with UCAs has been shown in some vascular beds [6]. Color enhancement of placental blood flow has been described in pregnant macaque monkeys with the use of Levovist [14] and Albunex [15], two rather outdated UCAs. Intravillous flow can be demonstrated with injection of UCA into third-trimester pregnant rhesus monkeys [16]. In other experiments using a dually perfused human placenta, improvement in gray-scale imaging (Figure 24.1) and color Doppler (Figure 24.2) was obtained, and spectral Doppler signals were vastly enhanced (Figure 24.3) with the use of the agents Albunex or iodipamide ethyl ester [17]. At the same time, there were no discernible changes in perfusion pressure, flow rate, fetal volume loss, maternal and fetal acid-base balance, or oxygen consumption. Additionally, no morphological damage could be demonstrated by light and electron microscopy. Analysis of metabolic activity of the placenta did not reveal any abnormal changes in glucose utilization, lactate and hormone production, or protein synthesis. These findings testify to the safety of use of certain UCA. Moreover, the UCA (Albunex) allowed for visualization of changes induced by injection of vasoactive substances to the perfused

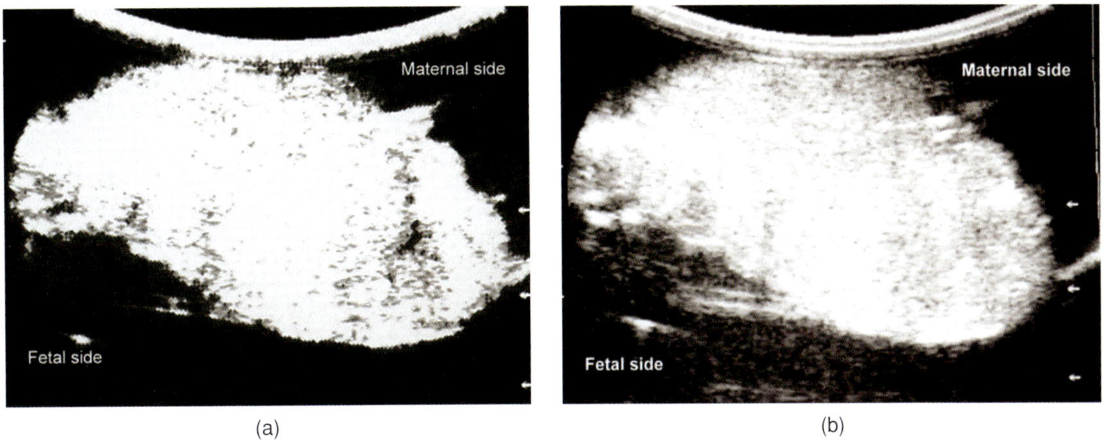

Figure 24.1 Gray-scale B-mode imaging of perfused placental lobule. (a) Native imaging. Some areas appear darker, an indication that no echoes are returning from that area. (b) After infusion of UCA. Echogenicity is increased and the entire field appears echogenic. The UCAs have filled the vasculature and echoes are now obtained from small vessels not previously seen. (Modified from Panigel M, Abramowicz JS, Miller RK (1996) Techniques: biophysical methods for assessment of placental function. In: Rama Sastry BV (ed.) *Placental Pharmacology*. Boca Raton, New York, London, Tokyo: CRC Press; pp. 1–23.)

placenta lobule [18]. After infusion of the UCA, an injection of a potent vasoconstrictor (U46619, a thromboxane agonist), potent vasodilator (nitroglycerin), or both was given. Following the addition of U46619, mean pressures on the fetal side rapidly rose from 23.2 +/− 0.8 to 118 +/− 2. 9 mm Hg (mean +/− standard error of mean; $p \leq 0.001$) and venous flow rates decreased as anticipated. Following that, color Doppler imaging showed flow changing markedly from a pattern of general distribution throughout the lobule to flow localized near the chorionic plate. Color persistence, which was detected with Albunex, was 39.8 +/− 3.4 seconds after U46619 injection

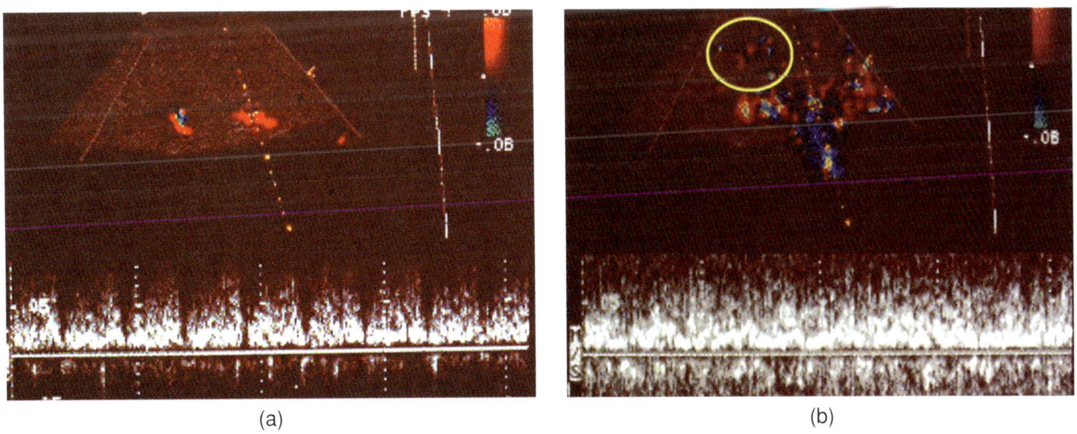

Figure 24.2 Color Doppler of perfused placental lobule. (a) Native imaging. Some color is demonstrated. (b) After infusion with UCA. Substantial increase in color signal is evident. In addition, some areas not previously visualized now show a color signal (yellow circle) secondary to the presence of echo-producing microspheres. The same phenomenon is evident with spectral Doppler, as seen in the lower part of the figure. (From Abramowicz JS (1997) Ultrasound contrast media and their use in obstetrics and gynecology. *Ultrasound Med Biol* 23:1287–98.)

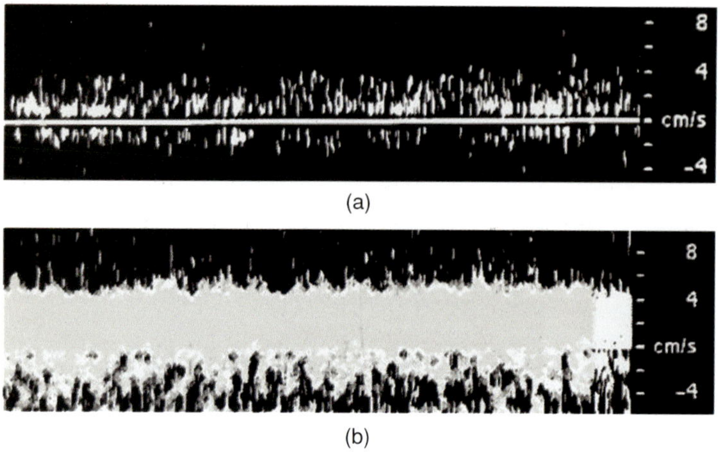

Figure 24.3 Spectral Doppler of perfused placental lobule (digitalized version). (a) Native signal from tubing inserted into lobule, representing umbilical artery. (b) After infusion with UCA, major enhancement in signal secondary to the presence of a large number of reflectors (contrast agent microspheres). (Modified from Panigel M, Abramowicz JS, Miller RK (1996) Techniques: biophysical methods for assessment of placental function. In: Rama Sastry BV (ed.) *Placental Pharmacology*. Boca Raton, New York, London, Tokyo: CRC Press; pp. 1–23.)

and increased to 94.4 +/− 6.5 seconds after nitroglycerin injection, a significant difference ($p \leq 0.001$). Nitroglycerin had no effect when injected alone but when injected after U46619, nitroglycerin returned the "constricted" flow to a "normal" pattern. These experiments may lead to studies of other drugs that modulate placental flow, particularly in cases of suspected placental vascular bed constriction.

Clinical Pearl

Conventional ultrasound demonstrates placental anatomy. Doppler analysis can furnish some information on function. UCAs may be helpful in characterizing early changes, not detectable by traditional imaging.

Safety issues

Research experience in UCA placental imaging is limited. Two major reasons exist. The first is that lung hemorrhages have been described in several neonatal animal species after ultrasound exposure, limiting the overall antenatal imaging experience. This was thought to be due to the UCA's ability to decrease the threshold for cavitation occurring in air bubbles, typically absent in the fetal lung. The gas bodies presumably lead to cavitation-induced hemorrhage. In vitro, the UCA increased hemolysis of fetal red blood cells by ultrasound. [19]. Additionally, premature ventricular contractions have been detected during imaging with UCA. Therefore, the concern is that by introducing a UCA into the insonated tissues, new risks, minimal or nonexistent before the addition of the UCA, may now become an issue [20]. Despite these concerns, several reports demonstrate the relative safety of UCAs, at least in animal experiments [21]. The second major reason, a corollary of the above, is the reticence of manufacturers and researchers to apply for approval for use in obstetrics, although no damage has been reported in the placenta or the fetal heart rate after scanning with UCAs [22]. The main argument is that other imaging modalities have demonstrated transplacental passage of contrast agents, used in radiological procedures other than ultrasound, to the fetus. [23] Although no obvious harmful effects were demonstrated, this is sufficient concern to deter investigations using agents that would have, at best, a very limited use.

Research Spotlight

Some of the harmful bioeffects of ultrasound are thought to be secondary to cavitation occurring in gas bubbles, when present in tissues. UCAs are known to decrease the threshold for cavitation of these bubbles.

Conclusions

UCAs have the potential to revolutionize the field of clinical ultrasound and may already have done so in certain applications [4]. However, at the moment, there are no accepted clinical indications for their use in placental imaging. The potential for improved sonographic analysis of vasculature and perfusion is evident, but unknown risks to the fetus prevent further development at this time. Hopefully, additional research will demonstrate the safety of this approach and allow introduction of these agents into clinical obstetrical imaging practice. This is a process similar to contrast-enhanced MRI and the very appropriate title of a recent article entitled "Placental functional assessment using MRI: mice today, humans tomorrow?" [24] could be modified with the word "MRI" easily substituted for "contrast-enhanced ultrasound."

☞ Teaching Points

1. UCAs are used in clinical fields to enhance gray-scale B-mode imaging as well as Doppler signals.
2. In experimental settings, these agents allow visualization of very small placental blood vessels and enhanced Doppler analysis of flow velocity waveforms in them.
3. Abnormal vascularization may be demonstrated, and this abnormality is partly responsible for several pathological conditions, such as preeclampsia and intrauterine growth restriction.

References

1. Feinstein SB (2004) The powerful microbubble: from bench to bedside, from intravascular indicator to therapeutic delivery system, and beyond. *American journal of physiology* 287(2): H450–7.
2. Abramowicz JS (2005) Ultrasonographic contrast media: has the time come in obstetrics and gynecology? *J Ultrasound Med* 24(4): 517–31.
3. Greis C (2009) Ultrasound contrast agents as markers of vascularity and microcirculation. *Clinical hemorheology and microcirculation* 43(1): 1–9.
4. Madsen HH (2008) Ultrasound contrast: the most important innovation in ultrasound in recent decades. *Acta Radiol* 49(3): 247–8.
5. Lindner JR (2009) Molecular imaging of cardiovascular disease with contrast-enhanced ultrasonography. *Nat Rev Cardiol* 6(7): 475–81.
6. Bruce M, Averkiou M, Tiemann K et al. (2004) Vascular flow and perfusion imaging with ultrasound contrast agents. *Ultrasound Med Biol* 30(6): 735–43.
7. Burns PN, Wilson SR (2006) Microbubble contrast for radiological imaging: 1. Principles. *Ultrasound Q* 22(1): 5–13.
8. Derchi LE, Martinoli C, Pretolesi F et al. (1999) Quantitative analysis of contrast enhancement. *Eur Radiol* 9 (Suppl. 3): S372–6.
9. Willmann JK, Lutz AM, Paulmurugan R et al. (2008) Dual-targeted contrast agent for US assessment of tumor angiogenesis in vivo. *Radiology* 248(3): 936–44.
10. Orden MR, Gudmundsson S, Helin HL et al. (1999) Intravascular contrast agent in the ultrasonography of ectopic pregnancy. *Ultrasound Obstet Gynecol* 14(5): 348–52.
11. Kirkinen P, Helin-Martikainen HL, Vanninen R et al. (1998) Placenta accreta: imaging by gray-scale and contrast-enhanced color doppler sonography and magnetic resonance imaging. *J Clin Ultrasound* 26(2): 90–4.
12. Denbow ML, Welsh AW, Taylor MJ et al. (2000) Twin fetuses: intravascular microbubble US contrast agent administration–early experience. *Radiology* 214(3): 724–8.
13. Panigel M, Abramowicz JS, Miller RK (1996) Techniques: biophysical methods for assessment of placental function. In: Rama Sastry BV (ed.) *Placental Pharmacology*. Boca Raton, New York, London, Tokyo: CRC Press; pp. 1–23.
14. Schmiedl UP, Komarniski K, Winter TC et al. (1998) Assessment of fetal and placental blood flow in primates using contrast enhanced ultrasonography. *J Ultrasound Med* 17(2): 75–80; discussion 1–2.
15. Simpson NA, Nimrod C, De Vermette R et al. (1998) Sonographic evaluation of intervillous flow in early pregnancy: use of echo-enhancement agents. *Ultrasound Obstet Gynecol* 11(3): 204–8.
16. Ragavendra N, Tarantal AF (2001) Intervillous blood flow in the third trimester gravid rhesus monkey (Macaca mulatta): use of sonographic contrast agent and harmonic imaging. *Placenta* 22(2–3): 200–5.
17. Abramowicz JS, Miller RK, Parker KJ et al. (1994) Enhancement of doppler signal in the placental perfusion model by injection of a contrast medium. *J Maternal Fetal Invest* 4: 59.
18. Abramowicz JS, Phillips DB, Jessee LN et al. (1999) Sonographic investigation of flow patterns in the perfused human placenta and their modulation by vasoactive agents with enhanced visualization by the ultrasound contrast agent albunex. *J Clin Ultrasound* 27(9): 513–22.
19. Miller MW, Brayman AA, Sherman TA et al. (2001) Comparative sensitivity of human fetal and adult erythrocytes to hemolysis by pulsed 1 MHz ultrasound. *Ultrasound Med Biol* 27(3): 419–25.
20. Barnett SB, Duck F, Ziskin M (2007) Recommendations on the safe use of ultrasound contrast agents. *Ultrasound Med Biol* 33(2): 173–4.
21. Hua X, Zhu LP, Li R et al. (2009) Effects of diagnostic contrast-enhanced ultrasound on permeability of placental barrier: a primary study. *Placenta* 30(9): 780–4.

22. Orden MR, Leinonen M, Kirkinen P (2000) Contrast-enhanced ultrasonography of uteroplacental circulation does not evoke harmful CTG changes or perinatal events. *Fetal Diagn Ther* 15(3): 139–45.
23. Hill BJ, Saigal G, Patel S et al. (2007) Transplacental passage of non-ionic contrast agents resulting in fetal bowel opacification: a mimic of pneumoperitoneum in the newborn. *Pediatr Radiol* 37(4): 396–8.
24. Salomon LJ, Siauve N, Taillieu F et al. (2005) [Placental functional assessment using MRI: mice today, humans tomorrow?]. *J Gynecol Obstet Biol Reprod (Paris)* 34(7 Pt 1): 666–73.

25

CHAPTER 25
Microscopy and the Placenta

William E. Ackerman IV[1], *Toshihiro Takizawa*[2], *and John M. Robinson*[3]

[1]Department of Obstetrics and Gynecology, Ohio State University, Columbus, OH, USA
[2]Department of Molecular Medicine and Anatomy, Nippon Medical School, Tokyo, Japan
[3]Department of Physiology and Cell Biology, Ohio State University, Columbus, OH, USA

Introduction to microscopy

Microscopy has been crucial for the advancement of biomedical science. While microscopy can encompass several different imaging modalities, optical and electron microscopy (EM) are the most commonly used. Since this chapter deals with affinity labeling methods (i.e., the detection of specific biomolecules using antibodies or nucleic acid probes), we will restrict our discussion to the types of microscopy relevant to these applications (see overview in Table 25.1) and examples in (Figure 25.1).

Optical microscopy

The optical (light) microscope is capable of several types of imaging that include brightfield, phase contrast, differential interference contrast, dark field, polarization, and fluorescence. Among these, familiarity with brightfield and fluorescence are most important when considering affinity labeling applications.

Brightfield microscopy (BFM)

BFM, the simplest of optical microscopy techniques, utilizes broad spectrum white light that is transmitted through the sample. This light is focused on the specimen using a series of optical lenses and transmitted to a detection system (the eyes or a camera). Since biological specimens have intrinsically low contrast in BFM, staining procedures are required to permit the identification of tissue structures. In conventional histological preparations the most commonly used stain is the combination of hematoxylin and eosin (H & E), although a number of other dyes with varying degrees of labeling specificity may be applied.

Fluorescence microscopy (FM)

Fluorescence is a property of certain substances in which light at different and usually longer wavelength is emitted, following the absorption of light at a specific excitation wavelength. This phenomenon is frequently exploited for microscopic visualization. Like BFM, FM utilizes optical lenses to focus and collect light, but in contrast to BFM, fluorescence microscopes generally have optical elements that select for narrow bands of the light spectrum. Sets of these optical elements (excitation filters, emission filters, and dichroic mirrors) must be optimized to match the spectral characteristics of individual reporter dyes or fluorophores. When coupled with high-sensitivity detectors, such as charge-coupled devices (CCD), fluorescence microscopes become sensitive analytical devices.

Transmission electron microscopy (EM)

For routine light microscopy, the wavelength of visible light limits the resolution to ~0.2 μm, although highly specialized equipment may exceed this resolution limit. Improvements in resolution are typically achieved by moving from light to EM. In EM instruments, small

The Placenta: From Development to Disease, First Edition. Edited by Helen H. Kay, D. Michael Nelson and Yuping Wang.
© 2011 Blackwell Publishing Ltd. Published 2011 by Blackwell Publishing Ltd.

Table 25.1 Overview of the types of microscopy used frequently to study the placenta.

	Optical Microscopy		
	BFM	**FM**	**EM**
Advantages	Widely accessible due to simplicity of setup	Images can be improved using confocal microscopy or deconvolution algorithms	High resolution
Disadvantages	• Low optical resolution • Use of diffusible chromogenic dyes for IHC may confound subcellular localization	• Requires specialized equipment (now widely available) • Tissue context can be obscured since only fluorophores are visible	• EM equipment is expensive to purchase and maintain • Immuno-EM or CLEM can be technically challenging
Typical Sample Preservation	Chemical fixation (formaldehyde, formalin[a]) or cryopreservation[b]	Cryopreservation[b], with or without chemical fixation (formaldehyde)	• Chemical fixation (glutaraldyhyde for conventional EM) • Formaldehyde (for immuno-EM[c])
Embedding	• Paraffin (conventional histology, IHC, some ISH) • Aqueous cryoprotective medium (for cryopreserved specimens)	Aqueous cryoprotective medium (IHC, fluorescent dyes)	Plastic resin (conventional EM) or 2.3 M sucrose with gelatin encapsulation[c] (immuno-EM)
Sections	5–6 μm thick[d]	5–6 μm thick[d]	50–100 nm thick[e]
Contrast Agents (stains, counterstains)	Histological stains (e.g., H & E)	Fluorescent stains (e.g., DAPI[e])	Solutions containing heavy metals (e.g., lead citrate, uranyl acetate)
Immunolabeling Reporters	Chromogenic substrates, some particulate probes	Fluorophores, quantum dots, or bifunctional conjugates (for CLEM)	Particulate probes or bifunctional conjugates (for CLEM)

BFM, brightfield microscopy; FM, fluorescence microscopy; EM, transmission electron microscopy; IHC, immunohistochemistry; H & E, hematoxylin and eosin staining; CLEM, correlative light and electron microscopy.

[a]Formalin typically refers to commercially prepared formaldehyde solution that contains methanol as a stabilizing agent. In many research laboratories, formaldehyde solutions are prepared freshly using paraformaldehyde (PFA, a powder of polymerized formaldehyde).

[b]For affinity labeling using BFM, formalin-fixed paraffin-embedded specimens are commonly used, although cryopreserved samples may be desired when examining for certain contents (e.g., lipids) that may be lost during paraffin embedding. For IHC using FM, cryopreserved samples are favored, sometimes preceded by chemical crosslinking to improve morphology.

[c]For immuno-EM, samples are typically fixed with formaldehyde (sometimes including a low concentration of glutaraldehyde), encapsulated in a gelatin matrix, infused with sucrose (a cryoprotectant) and then mounted on specimen pins and cooled in liquid nitrogen for cryoultramicrotomy.

[d]A microtome is used to section formalin-fixed paraffin-embedded specimens, while a cryomicrotome (cryostat) is used for cryopreserved specimens.

[e]An ultramicrotome is used to section specimens embedded in plastic for conventional EM, while a cryoultramicrotome is used to produce ultrathin cryosections for immuno-EM.

[f]4′,6-diamidino-2-phenylindole (DAPI) is a fluorescent stain that binds strongly to DNA and is widely used in FM to stain nuclei.

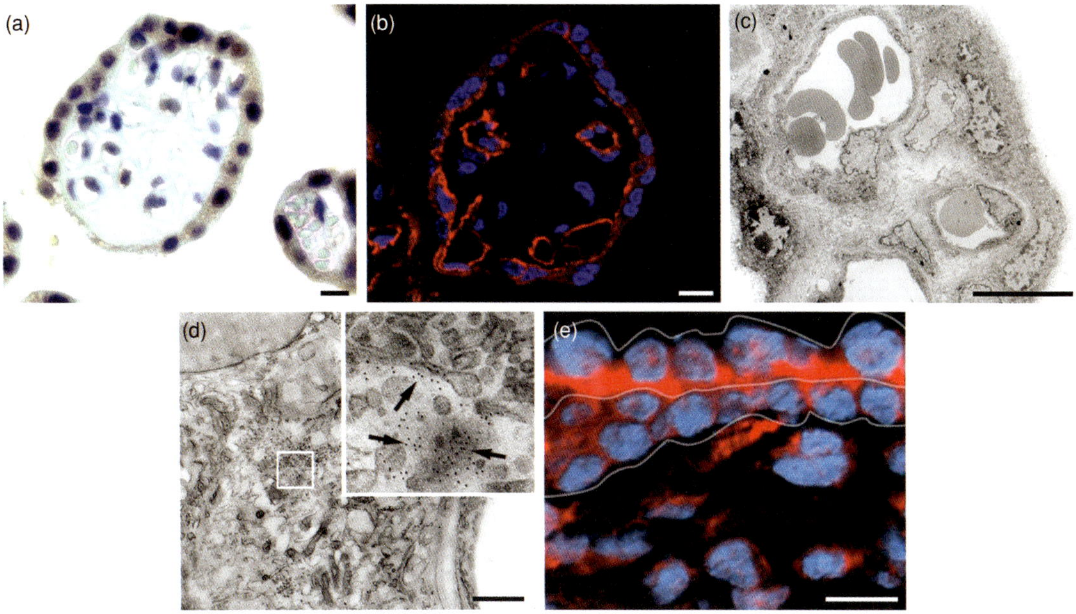

Figure 25.1 Representative micrographs demonstrating the application of microscopy for the study of placental biology. (a) Brightfield image of villous structures in which IHC was performed to detect a nuclear protein. A chromogenic reporter (3,3′-diaminobenzidine tetrahydrochloride, DAB) was used to detect bound antibodies (brown color), and the specimen was counterstained with Mayer's hematoxylin (blue color) to provide contrast. (b) FM was used to visualize fluorophore-conjugated antibodies bound to a protein target (red color) in an intermediate villous. Nuclei were stained using DAPI (4′,6-diamidino-2-phenylindole), which yields blue fluorescence. (c) Transmission electron micrograph stained with heavy metals to reveal details of the cellular composition of a placental villous. Even at this magnification, structures that could not be resolved using optical microscopy are apparent. (d) Immuno-EM in which colloidal gold reporters (arrows in inset) were used to identify the subcellular localization of a placental protein. (e) In vivo localization of a microRNA (red) in the human placenta using RNA ISH. All bars denote 10 μm except panel D, which is 1 μm. (Panel D used with permission from Takizawa T, Robinson JM. *J Nippon Med Sch* 2004; 71(5): 306–7.)

wavelength electron beams rather than photons are used to generate images, and magnets rather than glass lenses are used to provide focus. While the most advanced electron microscopes can achieve atomic resolution in ideal specimens, in routine biological EM, the practical resolution limit is ~2 nm. Since biological specimens are essentially "transparent" to electrons, contrast must be provided using stains comprised of electron-dense heavy metals (e.g., lead citrate, uranyl acetate).

Sample preparation

Several steps are required before a tissue sample, such as placenta, is ready for affinity labeling. In practice, the methods of sample preparation for BFM, FM, and EM applications can differ markedly. As such, attention must be given to the level of resolution desired when planning a study.

Sample preservation

When collecting specimens, timely processing is essential. For example, delivery of the placenta removes this organ from its blood supply, initiating the process of ischemia. To avoid structural and metabolic artifacts resulting from hypoxia, research specimens must be captured in a state that closely resembles the tissue in utero. To this end, a constellation of methods for sample preservation have been developed. For most affinity labeling applications, the placenta should be preserved not more than 20 minutes following its delivery.

The major methods for tissue preservation (fixation) are physical (typically, rapid freezing) and chemical. A goal common to all methods of preservation is stabilization of tissue, which protects specimens from further degradative damage.

> **Clinical Pearl**
>
> Preservation alters native tissue morphology, and artifacts relating to preservation may be introduced. At times, these artifacts can be misinterpreted when scrutinized by microscopy, as is illustrated by the infamous example of "Hydatoxi lualba." In this instance, a certain fixation procedure resulted in the appearance of wormlike microscopic structures in placental samples that, for a short period, were thought to be related to preeclampsia. These structures were ultimately identified as artifactual [1].

Cryopreservation

Cryopreservation (cryofixation) refers to preservation of tissue by rapid cooling to low subzero temperatures (from −80°C to −196°C). In routine practice, small pieces of fresh tissue are placed in a cryoprotective embedding medium and cooled using dry ice or ultra-cool isopentane [2]. Although samples can be cryofixed in the absence of cryoprotective media, this practice is discouraged, since tissue morphology may be heavily distorted due to freezing artifacts. Additionally, unfixed tissue is prone to loss during downstream processing, and chemical fixation of a specimen prior to cryopreservation is advantageous.

Chemical fixation

Chemical fixatives may be classified as: (1) denaturing or (2) crosslinking; however, some fixatives combine both denaturing and crosslinking components. Most denaturing (precipitating) fixatives are organic solvents, such as alcohols or acetone, which reduce the solubility of proteins and dehydrate the tissue. The use of denaturing fixation has fallen out of favor, owing largely to poor morphological preservation and problems with protein retention.

Crosslinking fixatives react covalently with proteins and lipids and, in effect, lock these molecules in place. Formaldehyde is the preferred fixative for optical microscopy, while that for EM is glutaraldehyde, although some fixation protocols call for a combination of both. In standard practice, small samples of tissue a few millimeter in shortest diameter are immersed in a solution containing the crosslinking fixative, a buffer adjusted to physiological pH, and solutes to maintain osmolarity [2]. Attention must be given to the amount of time that a tissue remains in fixative, since extensive crosslinking may impair affinity labeling, while inadequate fixation may lead to morphological denigration and loss of material during subsequent processing.

Both formaldehyde and glutaraldehyde are well-suited for the maintenance of tissue morphology and integrity during embedding, and may be used for long-term storage. Although glutaraldehyde is considered to give better morphological preservation than formaldehyde, this aldehyde limits the diffusion of antibodies into tissues and generates autofluorescence reducing the ability to distinguish fluorophores. For this reason, formaldehyde fixation is more appropriate for most affinity labeling and FM applications, provided that the extent of fixation is optimized.

> **Clinical Pearl**
>
> Choosing an optimal method of preservation requires careful consideration of the intended research goals, as fixation may limit downstream applications. In general there is a trade-off between the preservation of morphology and how amenable the fixed tissue will be to affinity labeling. Greater flexibility in subsequent affinity labeling procedures is achieved when samples are preserved using multiple formats.

Embedding and sectioning

Preserved tissue must be sectioned into slices that are 5–6 μm thick for optical microscopy and 50–100 nm thick for EM. The sections are mounted on a solid support for processing, using a microscope slide or EM grid. To stabilize a tissue for sectioning, the specimen is embedded using a liquid material that can be solidified. There are a number of aqueous embedding materials that can be used to either infiltrate or encapsulate a specimen directly, such as agar, gelatin, glycol, or optimum cutting temperature compound (OCT). Hydrophobic embedding materials (e.g., paraffin wax, plastic resins), on the other hand, require that the tissue first be dehydrated, cleared, and then infiltrated with the embedding material gradually.

To produce frozen sections, fresh or fixed specimens are typically embedded in a water-based medium (such as OCT or a similar product) that hardens during freezing, and sections are cut at a low temperature using a cryostat (cryomicrotome), yielding relatively thick tissue slices for use in optical microscopy. If subjected to specialized processing, specimens can be used to generate ultrathin cryosections (using a cryoultramicrotome) for use in immune-EM. For standard histological sectioning for use with BFM, fixed samples are first dehydrated using a series of ethanol solutions of progressively increasing concentrations, then immersed in hydrophobic clearing agent (such as xylene or toluene) to remove the alcohol, and finally infiltrated with molten paraffin wax, which solidifies when cooled. For EM, tissues must be embedded in a hard plastic matrix such (epoxy or acrylic resin), which allows for very thin sections to be cut using an ultramicrotome. In a typical scenario, fixed samples are first dehydrated through graded ethanol and propylene oxide solutions, then gradually infiltrated with epoxy resin, which is hardened (cured) by heating.

Affinity labeling

Antibody-based (Immunolabeling)

Immunohistochemistry (IHC) and immunocytochemistry (ICC) refer to a collection of techniques designed to use antibodies to determine the spatial distribution of antigens in tissues and cells, respectively. The beginning of this large collection of methods can be traced to the seminal work of Albert Coons (1941) who used fluorophore-conjugated antibodies for FM [3]. However, many years passed before this approach was in widespread usage, which required a number of technical advances to spur the field along. Today, IHC and ICC methods are highly refined and indispensable in many laboratories. Indeed, IHC has become an important tool for diagnosis and prognosis in histopathology.

The labeling procedures used in IHC and ICC can be: (1) direct, in which the detecting (primary) antibody is directly labeled with a reporter; or (2) indirect, in which the detecting antibody is unlabeled, but a secondary or tertiary reagent (e.g., another type antibody that detects the primary antibody) is itself labeled with a reporter. The indirect labeling method is more often employed in practice, since it is more practical and less expensive to conjugate reporters to secondary (or tertiary) reagents that may then be used to label a variety of detecting antibodies. In addition, signal amplification is achieved because more reporter molecules can bind to a given primary antibody using indirect labeling.

There are a number of practical issues to consider when working with antibodies. Antibodies are subject to breakdown and degradation leading to loss of function. Care should be taken to store antibodies in optimal conditions. Antibodies in solution should be frozen for long-term storage (e.g., −80°C) and freeze-thaw cycles should be avoided. When antibodies are stored in a nonfrozen state, 4°C is preferred, and a microbicidal agent (e.g., sodium azide) should be included.

> **Clinical Pearl**
>
> When considering IHC and ICC procedures, antibody specificity is of paramount importance. Antibodies can be notoriously fickle and may produce deceptive or erroneous results. Experience makes it clear to practitioners working with commercial antibodies that they often fail to perform as advertised [2,4]. Stringent and cautious interpretation, guided by the use of appropriate controls, is invariably warranted.

Reporter systems

The binding of an antibody to its antigen in tissue sections is not visible in the light or electron microscope without some sort of reporter (Table 25.2). The most commonly used reporters can be classified into three groups: (1) those that yield a colored product (chromogenic); (2) those that produce a fluorescent signal (fluorophores and quantum dots); and (3) particulate probes (colloidal gold particles and metal-cluster compounds).

Immunolabeling

In routine practice, a sectioned tissue on a solid support is first treated with a blocking reagent to reduce nonspecific binding to the detecting antibody, then is exposed to detecting antibodies, then is washed thoroughly, and either mounted (in direct immunolabeling) or exposed to secondary and/or tertiary reagents (in indirect immunolabeling) prior to mounting [2]. Often, a contrast dye (e.g., Mayer's hematoxylin for BFM or DAPI for FM) is added to provide context when viewing. Unlike when working with cells in vitro, a step to permeabilize the specimen is usually unnecessary since the antigens are already exposed in sectioned tissues.

Antigen retrieval

There are numerous instances in which the level of labeling achieved in IHC or ICC falls below expectation, despite the known presence of an antigen based on other tests. This problem is often related to overfixation, which

Table 25.2 Summary of reporter systems used in IHC and ICC and the modes of detection employed.

Reporter System (Examples)	LM Detection	EM Detection
Chromogens[a]		
• 3,3′-diaminobenzidine (DAB)	+ (BFM)	+[b]
• Tetrazolium dyes	+ (BFM)	–
Fluorophores		
• Numerous different fluorescent dyes are available	+ (FM)	+ (Under special circumstances)[c]
Particulate probes		
• Colloidal gold	+ (BFM)[d]	+
• Metal-cluster compounds	+ (BFM)[d]	+[d]
• FluoroNanogold	+ (FM)	+[d]
• Quantum dots	+ (FM)	+

BFM, brightfield microscopy; FM, fluorescence microscopy.
[a]It should be pointed out that the chromogenic substrates used frequently in brightfield IHC are diffusible. As such, antigen localization is less precise than when a fluorophore-conjugated antibody is used for localization in FM.
[b]Reacting the 3,3′-diaminobenzidine precipitate with OsO_4 can generate an electron-dense reaction product.
[c]Coupling fluorophores to photooxidation of 3,3′-diaminobenzidine and subsequent treatment with OsO_4 generate an electron-dense reaction product. This works with certain fluorophores, but not all.
[d]Autometallography, the process of increasing the size of the gold signal by deposition of a second metal (generally silver, in a process often referred to as silver enhancement). This process renders the normally invisible gold visible for light microscopic examination. Additionally, silver enhancement is generally required to visualize very small gold-cluster compounds and FluoroNanogold by EM.

may impair antigen-antibody interactions. To ameliorate this problem, a great number of experimental methods for antigen retrieval (AR or epitope retrieval) have been devised; however, there is not a single AR method that works equally well in all instances. The major methodological approaches for AR can be classified into two groups:

1 *Thermal methods.* The problem of over-fixation is most pronounced in formalin-fixed, paraffin-embedded tissues used for IHC with BFM. Most methods for AR in such specimens incorporate some form of thermal treatment [5,6]. The methods used for heating samples include microwave ovens, water baths, pressure cookers, and autoclaves. However the method of heating the tissue is less important than the amount of heat energy applied to the sample [5]. Heat alone is not the only consideration; the AR buffer solution is also important. A number of studies have endeavored to find the "best" AR buffer solution [6]. While there is no AR buffer that has been endorsed for all AR applications, citrate buffers at pH 6.0 are used widely, although citraconic anhydride buffers may be substituted.

2 *Chemical methods.* Although heat-based AR is common when working with formalin-fixed paraffin-embedded samples, there may be instances where heat treatment is undesirable (e.g., when antigenicity is lost due to heating). Proteolytic enzyme treatment of sections using trypsin, pepsin, pronase, papain, bromelain, proteinase K, or collagenase has been effective for AR in some cases. When using proteolytic enzymes, care should be taken to avoid overdigestion, as this may lead to antigen extraction and compromised tissue architecture. Certain chaotropic agents that denature proteins have also been used in AR. Sodium dodecyl sulfate (SDS) has been shown to be useful for AR in several instances [7]. Other chemicals used successfully in AR include urea, guanidine hydrochloride, and formic acid [5].

Immunoelectron microscopy (immuno-EM)

EM can be used to study the detailed localization of specific proteins within the ultrastructural (subcellular) context of tissues. Immunolabeling of EM specimens generally requires that appropriately fixed tissues be processed with a specialized cryoultramicrotome, yielding ultrathin (50–100 nm) sections. While powerful for localizing antigens in the ultrastructural context, immuno-EM can be technically challenging, expensive, and often requires rigorous optimization during fixation and processing.

Correlative microscopy

Correlative microscopy examines multiple structures by two or more imaging modalities. The most important type is correlative light and electron microscopy (CLEM) in which the light microscopy component is usually FM. While application of this technique is not trivial, the method allows a labeled structure to be viewed both in broad tissue context as well as in fine ultrastructural detail. For CLEM, the bifunctional reporter FluoroNanogold is used, which incorporates a fluorophore and a gold-cluster compound that can be visualized following silver enhancement. The use of CLEM in research applications is on the ascendance with new developments in methodology presented by several laboratories. A more detailed account of CLEM is beyond the scope of this chapter, and the interested reader is referred to recent review articles [8,9].

Nucleotide-based (in situ hybridization)

RNA in situ hybridization (RNA ISH)

In addition to proteins, cellular expression patterns of genes or other RNA transcripts can be determined. RNA ISH is a powerful technique that enables the study of RNA localization (e.g., mRNA and microRNA) in the complex structure of the placenta. Using RNA ISH, spatial-temporal patterns of placental gene expression may be studied as a function of development or in the context of gestational diseases (e.g., preeclampsia).

The principle of RNA ISH is to hybridize reporter-conjugated nucleotide probes with complementary single-stranded RNA sequences on tissue sections. Successful RNA ISH depends upon: (a) optimal tissue preparation; (b) the type of nucleotide probe used for RNA detection; and (c) hybridization and posthybridization conditions.

Fixation for RNA ISH must be optimized so as to preserve target RNA while retaining morphological detail in tissue sections. Formaldehyde fixation similar to that used for IHC is commonly employed, although other fixatives (e.g., HOPE fixative) and/or cryopreservation may be substituted. Often, following fixation, limited enzymatic digestion (e.g., proteinase K treatment) is necessary for optimal labeling.

Probes that can be used for mRNA ISH include DNA, RNA, and oligonucleotides. In general, antisense RNA probes (copy RNA [cRNA] probes or riboprobes) offer better sensitivity and specificity than DNA probes. Although probes labeled with radioisotopes (e.g., ^{3}H, ^{32}P, ^{35}S) must be detected using autoradiography, those with nonradioisotope labels (e.g., biotin or digoxigenin) may be detected using enzyme or fluorophore-conjugated secondary reagents such as antibodies and avidin-streptavidin. In the latter case, reporter chromogens compatible with BFM or FM fluorophores enable visualization in a manner similar to IHC. To detect microRNA species by ISH, the use of locked nucleic acid (LNA) modified DNA probes is typically required. LNA is a conformationally restricted nucleic acid analogue that is incorporated into a probe to enable high-affinity hybridization of short RNA targets.

For successful RNA ISH, there are many critical parameters that must be considered when performing the hybridization and post-hybridization steps, including optimization of hybridization temperature (typically between 55°C and 62°C); the composition of the hybridization buffer (recipes vary, although the inclusion of dextran sulfate is important to increase the binding of probe to target mRNA); posthybridization washing conditions (these must be chosen to reduce background labeling without loss of the ISH signal); and RNase digestion after the hybridization (RNA–RNA hybrids, but not nonspecifically bound RNA probes, are resistant to RNase and treatment reduces background staining.).

There are many reviews and published protocols for ISH; for further details pertaining to the design and execution of ISH, the reader is referred to other resources (e.g., *Current Protocols in Molecular Biology* or [10]).

DNA in situ hybridization (DNA ISH)

DNA ISH is commonly employed in clinical cytogenetics to investigate abnormalities of chromosome number and structure. There are three major categories of DNA probes that are used: (1) whole chromosome probes (chromosome "paints"); (2) satellite (repeat) sequence probes (e.g., centromeric and telomeric probes); and (3) unique sequence probes. In fluorescent ISH (FISH), DNA probes can be labeled directly with fluorescent reporters, or with molecular tags (e.g., biotin or digoxigenin) that may be coupled indirectly to fluorophores using an intervening molecule. Although DNA ISH probes are most often detected using FM, fluorescent reporters may not be desirable (e.g., when an autofluorescent tissue sample is to be studied). DNA probes may instead be labeled with BFM-compatible reporters in a process termed chromogenic ISH (CISH).

In the context of perinatal biology, DNA ISH is frequently used as an adjunct to classical cytogenetics for prenatal diagnosis. FISH (or CISH) may also be used to distinguish male embryonic cells from maternal cells in research and clinical diagnostics.

☞ Teaching Points

1. Affinity labeling refers to the identification of specific biomolecules in cells using probes. Affinity labeling allows one to determine the expression and distribution of proteins and nucleic acids within tissues such as the placenta.
2. Immunolabeling refers to the use of antibodies to detect protein antigens within cells (ICC) or tissues (IHC), while ISH refers to the use of nucleic acid probes to detect specific DNA or RNA sequences. These techniques are used widely in biomedical research and clinical practice.

3 Preparative procedures can dramatically affect the results of affinity labeling. Methods for tissue preservation, such as chemical fixation or freezing, should be tailored to the intended downstream labeling applications, and tissue should be collected in a manner that closely approximates the native state in vivo.

4 In general, there is a trade-off between morphological preservation and how amenable a tissue will be to affinity labeling. Prolonged chemical fixation tends to minimize architectural distortion, but may impair the interaction between a given probe and its target.

5 With any affinity labeling procedure, the specificity of labeling must be evaluated cautiously. The interpretation of a result must be weighed against available biomedical literature, the results of appropriate positive and negative controls, and if possible, the results of a second probe directed against the same target.

References

1. Polderman AM, van der Knaap AM, Wortel HJ et al. (1984) 'Hydatoxi lualba', an artefact. *Eur J Obstet Gynecol Reprod Biol* 17(4): 301–4.
2. Burry RW (2010) *Immunocytochemistry: A Practical Guide for Biomedical Research.* 1st edn. New York: Springer.
3. Coons AH, Creech HJ, Jones RN (1941) Immunological properties of an antibody containing a fluorescent group. *Proc Soc Exp Biol* 47: 200–2.
4. Saper CB (2009) A guide to the perplexed on the specificity of antibodies. *J Histochem Cytochem* 57(1): 1–5.
5. Yamashita S (2007) Heat-induced antigen retrieval: mechanisms and application to histochemistry. *Prog Histochem Cytochem* 41(3): 141–200.
6. D'Amico F, Skarmoutsou E, Stivala F (2009) State of the art in antigen retrieval for immunohistochemistry. *J Immunol Methods* 341(1–2): 1–18.
7. Robinson JM, Vandre DD (2001) Antigen retrieval in cells and tissues: enhancement with sodium dodecyl sulfate. *Histochem Cell Biol* 116(2): 119–30.
8. Mironov AA, Beznoussenko GV (2009) Correlative microscopy: a potent tool for the study of rare or unique cellular and tissue events. *J Microsc* 235(3): 308–21.
9. Robinson JM, Takizawa T (2009) Correlative fluorescence and electron microscopy in tissues: immunocytochemistry. *J Microsc* 235(3): 259–72.
10. Koji T (ed.) (2000) *Springer Lab Manuals: Molecular Histochemical Techniques.* Tokyo: Springer.

26

CHAPTER 26

Proteomics and the Placenta

Gregory E. Rice

Center for Clinical Research, University of Queensland, Royal Brisbane and Women's Hospital Campus, Brisbane, QLD, Australia

Introduction

The objective of this brief commentary is to address the question "*how proteomics may contribute to developing new insights into placentology.*" The answer is simple though its application is challenging. The proteome is the manifestation of the conditional expression of the genome. Proteomics, thus, is about defining the regional and temporal protein (and peptide) expression that characterizes a given phenotype and how changes in protein expression impact the structure and function of the organism. The contribution of proteomics to all fields of biology, therefore, is in defining the conditional expression of the genome. This chapter is both selective and subjective in highlighting proteomic approaches that may be of most relevance to placentology and in the selection of heuristic vignettes. Contemporary information and complementary reviews of proteomics and its application are noted [1–3].

During ontogeny (and the life of the placenta) the genome remains relatively stable. Its transcriptome (i.e., the RNA species elaborated), the protein products formed by the translation of coding-RNA, and the subsequent post-translational modification of these proteins vary in response to developmental and environmental challenges. This *conditional expression* of the genome is not only determined by conventional transcriptional regulation (e.g., the binding of specific protein transcription factors to consensus sequences within DNA that initiate gene transcription) but also by epigenetic modification of the DNA bases (e.g., the addition of a methyl group to cytosine) and by modification of the structure of chromatin (e.g., acetylation of lysine residues of histone proteins) that regulates the accessibility of DNA and thus its transcription.

In recent years, it has been recognized that the complexity of the mammalian transcriptome and its functional expression as proteins far exceeds previous expectations. It is now estimated that only ~1.2% of the human genome contains protein-coding information. The expression of these ~21,000 genes, the elaboration of ~10^5 transcripts (via alternative splicing, alternate promoters, and RNA editing) and the post-translational modification account for the more than 10^6 proteins comprising the human proteome. It has been estimated that up to 100 different proteins may be derived from the expression of a single gene. An informed understanding of the ontogeny, life, and death of the placenta, therefore, will include not only genomic and transcriptomic analysis but also information as to how global protein expression changes. This is the bailiwick of proteomics—defining the conditional expression of the genome. The application of proteomic technologies to placentology affords further understanding of key processes in placental development and function, including implantation, placentation, adaptation to fetal metabolic requirements, labor, and placental detachment.

The objectives of proteomics, however, extend beyond the mapping of the protein complement of a target. Proteomics needs to be considered in the context of its contribution to the healthcare system.

Two forces are driving the healthcare system: (1) technological development (including proteomics in its

The Placenta: From Development to Disease, First Edition. Edited by Helen H. Kay, D. Michael Nelson and Yuping Wang.
© 2011 Blackwell Publishing Ltd. Published 2011 by Blackwell Publishing Ltd.

various manifestations); (2) information management systems. The former allows the acquisition of extensive multivariate biological and clinical data that define a given clinical circumstance. The latter increases the capacity to ascribe such data to an individual during their life course. The expectation is that we are moving from the episodic, reactionary medicine of today (i.e., symptom-based treatment) to personalized medicine, where defining predisposition to disease and risk assessment will allow the implementation of more efficacious preventative strategies and treatment regimens. Proteomics can contribute to the evolving healthcare system by providing a better understanding of biology, by defining risk, by enabling earlier diagnosis, and by monitoring treatment responses (Figure 26.1).

Current proteomic technologies provide an opportunity to develop multivariate classification models for the assignment of disease risk. Such models may be of utility in the early identification of asymptomatic women at risk for developing pregnancy complications (e.g., gestational diabetes, preeclampsia, and intrauterine growth restriction).

Proteomics overview

Proteomics is the systematic, reproducible, differential, and/or quantitative characterization of the peptide or protein complement under a defined biological state(s). In particular, its raison d'être is to elucidate networks and pathways that ensure coordinated and appropriate development of biologic organisms and to maintain homoeostasis in response to physiological or pathological challenges. Proteomic technology also delivers information sufficient to provide reliable expectations on how systems will behave under defined conditions. The practice of proteomic technology has undergone rapid development over the past decade. The objective has been to expand the scope of biological studies from a reductionist biochemical approach to a proteome-wide approach. The reality is perhaps that a more comprehensive analysis of targeted subpopulations of proteins is now considered.

There are three approaches to the application of proteomics: (i) *cartographic or expression proteomics*—the definition of normal expression profiles of proteins and peptides, how they are modified and processed [4];

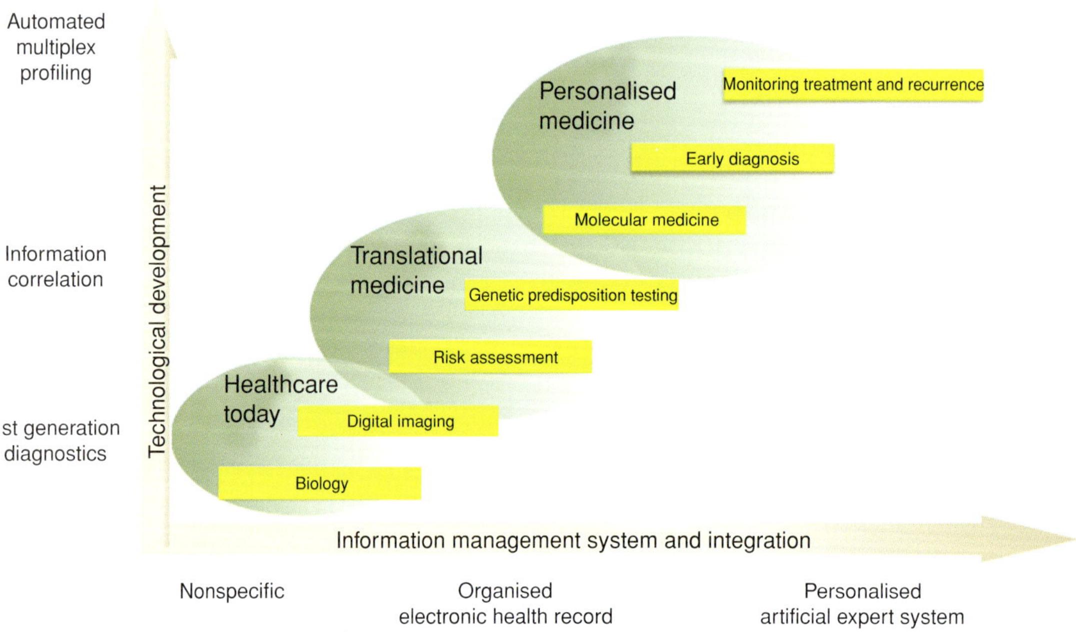

Figure 26.1 The evolving healthcare system. The role of proteomics in the evolution of the healthcare systems may be in the provision of multianalyte protein and peptide profiles that facilitate risk assessment, earlier diagnosis, and more effective treatment response monitoring. (Modified from "*Personalized Healthcare 2010,*" *IBM Business Consulting Services.*)

(ii) *comparative profiling*—in which protein expression profiles from different physiologic and/or pathologic states are compared for the purpose of identifying condition- or treatment-associated changes [5]; (iii) *targeted profiling*—in which specific known subsets of proteins are monitored [6].

Common to the successful application of all approaches are four key processes: (i) reduction in the heterogeneity of samples for analysis; (ii) decrease in the complexity of the targeted protein complement; (iii) isolation and display of the proteins within the targeted proteome; and (iv) quantitation and comparison of expression (Figure 26.2).

As with all analytical techniques, sample heterogeneity (e.g., variation from individual patients, sample collection, and processing) needs to be minimized. This is particularly relevant to the collection of the placenta and membranes where the time from delivery to stabilization of tissue proteins may vary considerably between individual patients, clinical diagnoses, and mode of delivery. Similarly, the collection and processing of blood can dramatically alter the peptide profile (e.g., clotting, temperature, and time taken to process samples).

A reduction in sample complexity and targeting a subfraction of the proteome for analysis is requisite since no currently available platform affords proteome-wide display. Figure 26.2 panel 1 depicts several approaches that have been successfully utilized to reduce sample complexity and allow the display or profiling of a targeted subproteome.

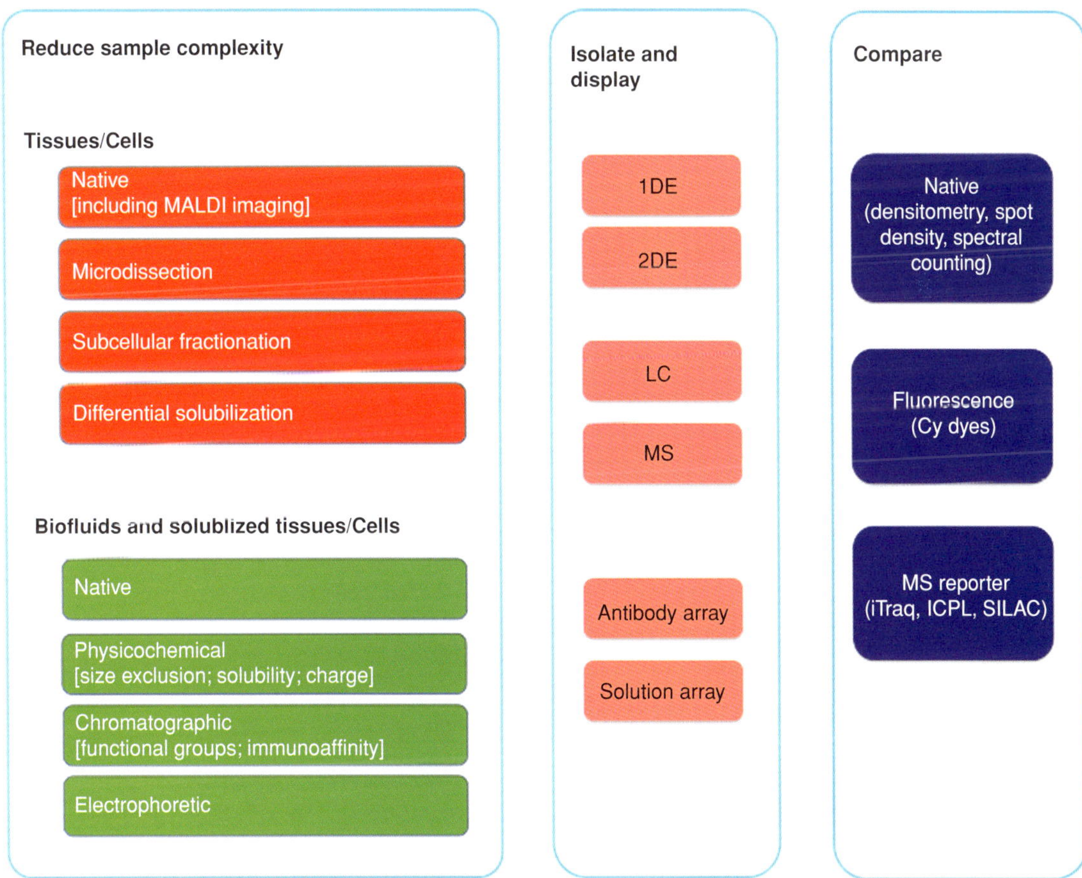

Figure 26.2 Processes that are common to the successful application of proteomic technologies are reduction in sample heterogeneity and complexity; isolation and display the target subproteome; and use of a reporter endpoint to allow comparison and/or quantitation.

Such approaches include direct mass spectrometry (MS) profiling of small molecules (including peptides) using matrix-assisted laser desorption ionization (MALDI) imaging of frozen targeted tissue sections (e.g., placental villi). MALDI imaging is a MS-based technique that allows two-dimensional profiling of peptides, proteins, and molecules within intact tissues. Complexity is reduced in that (i) specific regions within the tissue are targeted, thus allowing the characterization of regional variation in expression; and (ii) by altering preanalytical sample processing, different subfractions of the proteome may be targeted. This approach has been used to characterize protein and peptide expression at the time of implantation [7] and more recently to compare phospholipid expression between terminal and stem villi of human term placenta [8].

Microdissection of placental tissue prior to proteomic analysis reduces sample complexity by specifically targeting a population of cells rather than whole tissue. Laser-assisted cell sampling has been used to isolate trophoblast cells for MS and 2 dimensional gel electrophoresis (2DE) profiling studies.

The isolation of subcellular compartments (e.g., cell membrane, mitochondrial, or microsomal fractions) and the partitioning of proteins based upon their solubility, hydrophilicity, mass, charge, and ligand binding affinity have all been employed to reduce sample complexity.

Research Spotlight

Recently, Robinson and colleagues [9] used an affinity capture, solid-phase approach (colloidal silica) to isolate villous membrane proteins and greatly enrich the fraction. Using routine gel-based two-dimensional displays, they identified a group of proteins not previously identified (including dysferlin) and are now elucidating the role of these proteins in placental function.

Protein isolation by progressive or differential solubilization of tissue is a well-established methodology for reducing sample complexity and targeting protein populations on the basis of solubility and hydrophilicity. In particular, these approaches are useful in analysis of cell membrane proteins. These approaches have not been fully exploited in placentology. Centlow et al. [10] recently reported the efficacy of different extraction buffers and protein precipitation methods in isolating placental proteins for analysis from normal and preeclamptic placentae.

The primary objective of targeting a subproteome is to enhance the display and resolution of proteins (Figure 26.2 Panel 2) using, for example, 1 and 2 dimensional gel electrophoresis (1DE, 2DE) and liquid chromatography (LC). Subsequently, identification of the proteins can be performed by MS and immunospecific methodologies by antibody arrays or protein solution arrays. Finally, protein quantitation can be done by densitometry, spectral counting, and fluorescent or mass tag reports (Figure 26.2 Panel 3).

Analytical platforms

There is no ideal proteomic platform. Each has its own strengths and limitations and ultimately its suitability to any given application. The principal features that prescribe analytical utility include the capacity to resolve protein species, quantify protein expression, and characterize post-translational modifications (PTMs). Table 26.1 summarizes some of the currently available analytical approaches for displaying and resolving peptides and proteins and their respective advantages and disadvantages.

Gel-based approaches

The gel-based platforms such as 1D and 2D polyacrylamide gel electrophoresis and fluorescence 2D difference gel electrophoresis—2D DIGE- have been used in both expression and comparative studies to define placental protein expression and disease-associated or treatment-induced changes (e.g., preeclampsia [11]). The advantage of these approaches resides in the ability to identify PTMs. The limitation of gel-based systems is their relatively low throughput, the necessity for sample processing and fractionation prior to display and limited mass range (~10–200 kDa). In addition, procedural protein losses and the overall experimental variation in estimating endpoints by 2D PAGE may be considerable. Procedural losses of radiolabeled proteins during 2DE PAGE display have been reported to be as high as 80%, but this can vary depending on the starting protein load. As with any other technique, variation is apportioned between technical replication, both within assay and between assay, and biologic variation (i.e., sample-to-sample). Estimates of

Table 26.1

Property	2DE	DIGE	MuDPIT	Isotope Tagging	SELDI	ClinProt	Protein Array	Solution Array
Separation	Eectrophoresis IEF/PAGE	Eectrophoresis IEF/PAGE	LC/LC of peptide	LC/LC of peptide	Affinity binding	Affinity binding	Affinity binding	Affinity binding
Quantitation	Densitometry	Fluorescence Cy dyes	None	Relative difference	Comparison of MS peaks	Comparison of MS peaks	Densitometry/ Fluorescence	Fluorescence
Identification	PMF	PMF	MS/MS	MS/MS	Orthogonal	MS/MS	Specific affinity binding	Specific affinity binding
Number of Peptide	100s	100	100–1000	100–1000	100	100	100	10–100
Hydrophobic	Moderate	Moderate	Moderate/ Good	Moderate	Moderate	Moderate	Moderate	Moderate
Low Abundance	Marginal	Marginal-moderate	Moderate	Moderate	Marginal-moderate	Moderate	Moderate-good	Good
PTM	Good	Good	Nil	Nil	Poor	Poor	Moderate	Moderate
Noncandidate	Yes	Yes	Yes	Yes	Yes	Yes	No	No
Pros	Intact proteins Id of isoforms	Better quantitation Reduced workflow	High resolution MS/MS ID	High resolution Better coverage	Affinity capture	Affinity capture MS/MS protein ID	High throughput Rapid screening	High throughput Quantitation Rapid screening
Cons	Low sensitivity Spot matching Low number of proteins	Low number of proteins	Lack of quantitation	Loss of structural and isoform information	Difficult to ID Matrix-derived noise Low mass Accuracy	Peak intensity delivered to MS/MS	Specificity of antigen/ antibody binding	Fewer analytes Candidate-based

the variation attributable to technical replication average 25–40%. Biological variation has been estimated to be between 24% and 70% [12].

Some of the limitations of gel based approaches have been overcome with the development of difference gel electrophoresis. This minimal labeling approach using fluorescent cyanine dyes increases throughput by reducing sample processing and both gel-to-gel and analytical variation by combining case and control samples into a single processing step, and by the use of an internal standard for normalization of data across gels. DIGE also delivers useful relative quantification of protein expression profiles where the dyes are purported to have subnanogram sensitivity and a linear response to protein concentrations of over five orders of magnitude. The dyes are also compatible with mass spectrometric analysis. With respect to analyzing the plasma proteome, DIGE is still limited by the compositional complexity of plasma and similarly benefits from sample fractionation and the removal of high-abundance proteins.

Nongel-based approaches

Nongel-based proteomic approaches include: mass spectrometry-based profiling- both top-down (the isolation and analysis of intact proteins and the PTMs) and bottom-up (the generation, isolation, and analysis of proteolytic fragments) strategies; and candidate-based techniques such as antibody and protein arrays.

Mass spectrometry-based approaches

Of the mass spectrometry-based approaches currently available including MudPit, Stable Isotope Coding, SELDI, and ClinProt (see Table 26.1), stable isotope coding (Isotope tagging) is becoming the method of choice

Research Spotlight

An advantage of using DIGE to display proteins in two dimensions is that by combining treatment and control samples technical and biological variation is reduced. Figure 26.3 depicts placental proteins, from rats fed either a normal diet or high-fat diet, labeled with cy3 (red) and cy5 (green) dye, respectively. The labeled samples have been combined, run on a single first strip, and then resolved in the second dimension. The images depict the fluorescence of the protein spots that are equally expressed in treatment and control placentae (yellow), overexpressed (green) or repressed (red) in the treatment placentae.

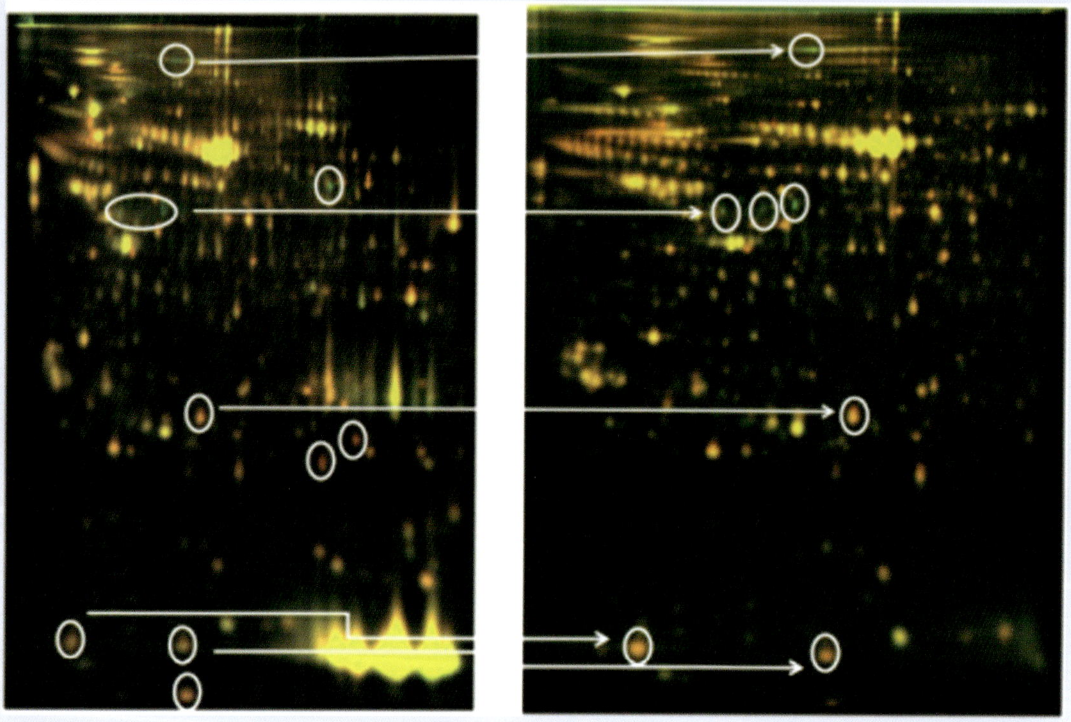

Figure 26.3 2D DIGE of placental proteins from rats fed a normal diet or a high-fat diet. The left panel displays placental proteins (50 μg protein) focused on a pH 3–11 first dimension strip. The right panel displays the same placental proteins focused on a pH 4–7 strip to improve the resolution of spots of interest. Connecting arrows indicate the same protein spots on each gel image. Proteins were resolved in the second dimension on 12.5 SDS gels.

for quantitative proteomics. Isotope coding has the advantages of being more sensitive and reproducible than gel-based methods. These approaches utilize either a mass tag coding strategy (e.g., ICPL isotope coded protein labeling, ICAT isotope coded affinity tag) or iTRAQ (isobaric tag for relative and absolute quantitation) that allow pooling of samples to reduce technical variation or a label-free approach that provides relative quantitative profiling across parallel independent MS analyses.

The underlying principle of isotope-coding approaches involves uniquely labeling individual sample proteomes with molecular tags of different mass (e.g., stable isotopes such as H^3/H^4, O^{18}/O^{16}, N^{15}/N^{14}, ICPL, and ICAT) or with tags of the same mass (i.e., isobaric, iTRAQ), but containing different isotope-encoded reporter ions. As each sample proteome is differentially labeled they can be pooled, processed, and displayed together. Using mass-coded approaches (i.e., ICPL and ICAT), each peptide will be present as a suite of ion peaks separated by the specific mass of its unique tag; thus, allowing comparison of expression between samples. With isobaric strategies (i.e., iTRAQ), differentially-labeled peptides appear as a single peak in MS mode, but when subjected to MS/MS analysis release, tag-specific reporter ions are generated, thus allowing comparison of expression between samples.

A workflow for isotope-coding analysis is presented in Figure 26.4 and depicts a triplex experiment in which three separate samples (S1–S3) are simultaneously analyzed. For iTRAQ experiments, samples are individually digested and the peptides labeled with isobaric tags. The samples are then pooled and complexity reduced at the peptide level (e.g., LC or Off-Gel fractionation) prior to quantification and identification. For ICPL experiments, samples are individually labeled with different mass tags and then pooled. The protein complexity of the pooled sample is reduced (e.g., 1D, 2D, Off-Gel fractionation, or liquid chromatography) and then digested. The complexity of the resultant peptides may be further reduced (e.g., LC or Off-Gel fractionation) prior to quantification and identification.

Label-free mass spectrometry-based proteomic approaches have some efficiencies in sample preparation and cost; however, samples must be processed and analyzed separately. Comparison of protein expression profiles between samples is based upon two metrics: ion peak intensities in LC/MS profiles and spectral counting of identified proteins after MS/MS analysis [13].

In addition to its analytical applications, MS affords opportunities to identify signature profiles contained within biological samples for the purpose of classification. The

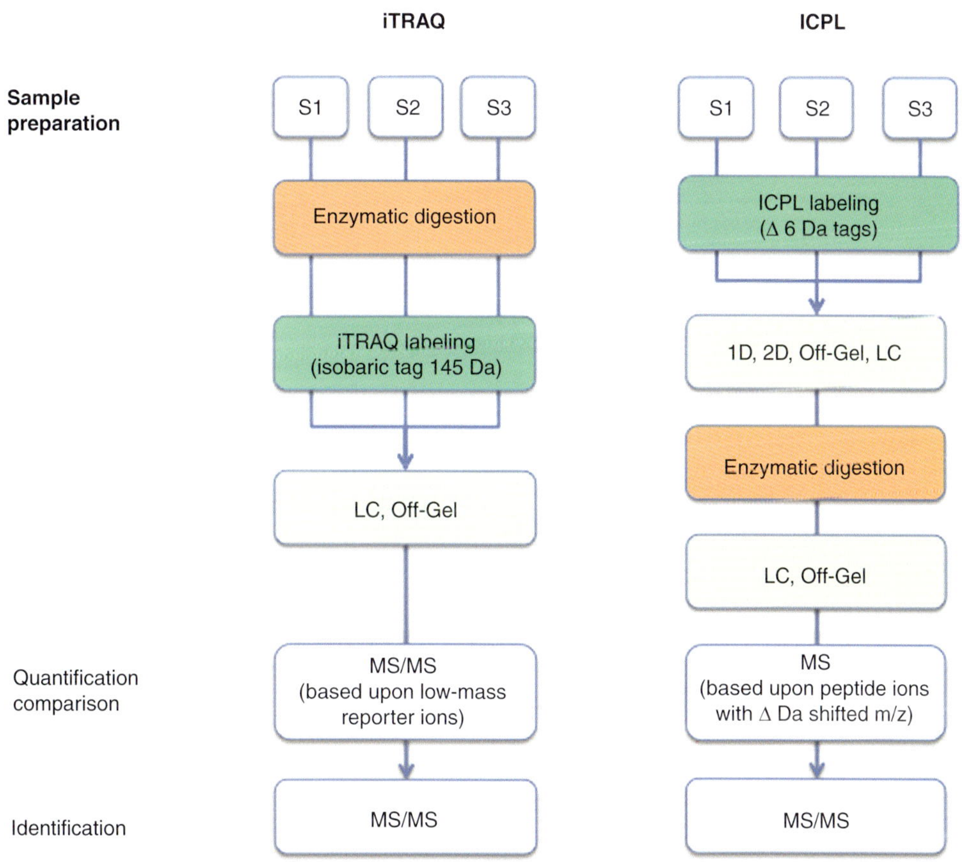

Figure 26.4 Comparison of protein coding workflows for iTRAQ and ICPL analysis.

application of MS is a burgeoning area within the domain of diagnostic and predictive medicine. This approach now affords the opportunity to develop disease-specific patterns or profiles based upon the presence of specific peptides in a patient sample. MS-based protein profiling relies on the presence and spatial relationships between peptide peaks to facilitate the classification of biological samples into different categories (e.g., normal and disease). Based upon the analysis of a training sample set (e.g., disease-free patients), pattern recognition software and multivariate modeling are employed to build peptide profiles or motifs that characterize a disease-free condition. Once established, such reference profiles may be used as a template to detect variance and thus deliver a diagnosis or predictive capacity.

Research Spotlight

To date, few studies have utilized nongel, mass spectrometry-based approaches to explore nongel placental proteomics. One recent study [14] used iTRAQ to identify changes in the placental secretome in response to hypoxia (1% vs. 6% oxygen). Using this approach, 45 differentially expressed proteins were identified in placenta-conditioned media. It is anticipated that the application of quantitative mass spectrometry-based approaches will continue to provide cognitive rich information within the field of placentology in the years to come.

Candidate-based approaches

Protein and antibody arrays represent examples of nongel based, candidate or targeted proteomic approaches. In the case of protein chip arrays, a known array of proteins is immobilized on a surface and binding partners present in the samples (e.g., protein, oligonucleotides, or antibodies) are captured and quantified using an appropriate reporter (e.g., fluorescent or chemiluminescent labels). Alternatively, solid-phase, ligand-specific antibodies may be immobilized on surfaces to facilitate the quantification of known ligands (e.g., antibody array and protein solution array). The advantages of these approaches include: rapid, high throughput screening of known targets and quantitative endpoints. Multiplex protein solution array is one application that represents a generation of antibody-based detection technology that allows the simultaneous quantification of multiple analytes in a single small volume sample [6]. Multiplex protein solution array has a number of advantages over current analyte quantification technologies, including: measurement of many biomarkers (up to 100 different analytes) in a single 50–100 μl sample; wider operational dynamic range; and increased sensitivity and specificity derived from multivariate modeling of combinations of biomarker analytes. This system utilizes a sandwich ELISA-like protocol, in which capture antibodies are coupled to spectrally distinct polystyrene beads (5–6 μm diameter), and biotinylated sandwich antibody and streptavidin-phycoerytherin (PE) fluorophore are used as a reporter complex. Assays are conducted in 96-well filter-bottom plates and beads are manipulated by vacuum filtration. Bead identity and analyte-specific fluorescence are assessed using a flow cytometer. Solution array offers excellent reproducibility (CV $<10\%$) and analyte quantitation, and has the capacity to multiplex up to 100 different analytes in small sample volumes (e.g., 20–50 μl plasma).

Solution array now provides a pathway for the rapid translation of proteomic data obtained from any platform (discovery or candidate-based) into applications of predictive utility. The technology builds upon well-established and conventional immunoassay principles, is independent of the dynamic range effects that limits other proteomic platforms, and is of suitable sensitivity. Candidate-based arrays are being increasingly utilized in the field of placentology for screening purposes and for elucidating signal transduction pathways.

Conclusions

Platform technologies evolve and enhance capacities during the product cycle and proteomics is no exception. While, in general, placentologists acknowledge the utility of proteomic technologies to contribute to developing novel insights, the application of new technologies and the delivery of outcomes remains modest. In particular, the application of quantitative proteomics and peptidomes are underrepresented within the discipline. The current generation of proteomic technologies affords opportunity to define aspects of the conditional expression of the genome and as such deliver better understanding of the functional relationships between environment, genome, and phenotype—both physiological and pathological.

Research Spotlight

Candidate-based profiling of blood-borne biomarkers may be of utility in identifying lead candidates for developing early pregnancy screening tests for gestational diabetes. For example, Georgiou et al. [6] measured multiple plasma biomarkers at 11 weeks' gestation in women who subsequently experienced normal pregnancy outcomes ($n = 14$) and women who subsequently developed gestational diabetes ($n = 14$). Of the biomarkers considered, receiver operator characteristic curves (ROC) for three biomarkers (adiponectin, insulin, and blood glucose) are presented together with a ROC based on the predicted posterior probability values (ppv) generated by a classification model that combined information from all three biomarkers (Figure 26.5). The model outperformed individual biomarkers based upon the area under the ROC (model = 0.94; adiponectin = 0.867; insulin = 0.872; and glucose = 0.827). This simple example demonstrates the putative benefit of a multimarker approach for improving diagnostic efficiency.

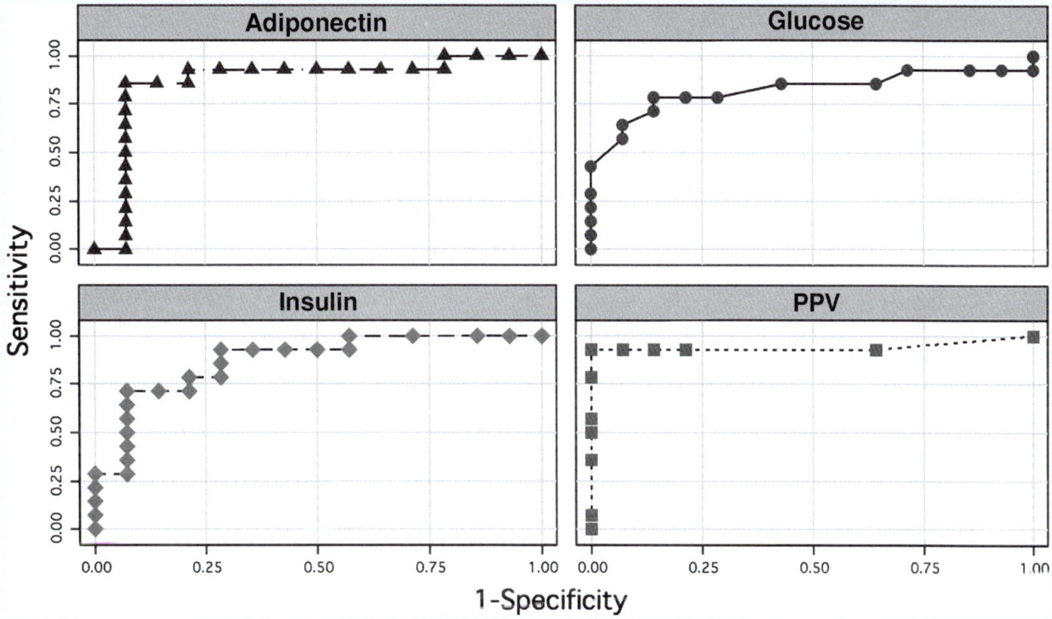

Figure 26.5 A comparison of ROC curves of the performance of individual biomarkers (adiponectin, glucose, and insulin) and a combined model (ppv) to correctly classify women who subsequently developed gestational diabetes.

Teaching Points

1 Proteomics is still best used as a reductive scientific approach. Targeting the smallest component of the proteome that will rigorously test your hypothesis is the most effective strategy. Invest the time and effort in preanalytical fractionation (e.g., laser dissection, subcellular fractionation, or enrichment based upon functional groups).

2 Sample integrity and quality is crucial. The goal standard is inactivation of endogenous proteases as the sample is collected.

3 Establish the effects and variability of processing (e.g., time and temperature) on sample stability and experimental endpoint reporters. If possible, consider a sample pooling approach to reduce biological and technical variance. When assigning significance to the data, account for the false discovery rate.

4 Know the limitations of the proteomic approach you are using. Each approach has strengths and weaknesses, therefore, balance them against what you are trying to achieve.

5 Multivariate modeling, of informative biomarkers, to deliver improved classification (diagnostics) efficiency represents an approach of considerable utility.

References

1. Yan W, Aebersold R, Raines EW (2009) Evolution of organelle-associated protein profiling. *J Proteomics* 72(1): 4–11.
2. Pan S, Abersold R, Chen R et al. (2009) Mass spectrometry based targeted protein quantification: methods and applications. *J Proteome Res* 8(2): 787–97.
3. Vaudel M, Sickmann A, and Martens L. (2010) Peptide and protein quantification: a map of the minefield. *Proteomics* 10(4): 650–70.
4. Di Quinzio MK, Oliva K, Holdsworth SJ et al. (2007) Proteomic analysis and characterisation of human cervico-vaginal fluid proteins. *Aust N Z J Obstet Gynaecol* 47(1): 9–15.
5. Webster RP, Pitzer BA, Roberts VHZ et al. (2007) Differences in the proteome profile in placenta from normal term and preeclamptic preterm pregnancies. *Proteomics Clin Appl* 1(5): 446–56.
6. Georgiou HM, Lappas M, Georgiou GM et al. (2008) Screening for biomarkers predictive of gestational diabetes mellitus. *Acta Diabetol* 45(3): 157–65.
7. Burnum KE, Frappier SL, and Caprioli RM (2008) Matrix-assisted laser desorption/ionization imaging mass spectrometry for the investigation of proteins and peptides. *Annu Rev Anal Chem* 1: 689–705.
8. Kobayashi Y, Hayasaka T, Setou M et al. (2010) Comparison of phospholipid molecule species between terminal and stem villi of human term placenta by imagin mass spectometry. *Placenta* 31: 245–8.
9. Robinson JM, Tewari AK, Kniss DA et al. (2009) Isolation of highly enriched apical plasma membranes of the placental syncytiotrophoblast. *Anal Biochem* 387(1): 87–94.
10. Centlow M, Hansson SR, and Welinder C (2010) Differential proteome analysis of the preeclamptic placenta using optimized protein extraction. *J Biomed Biotechnol*, 2010:458748.
11. Gharesi-Fard B, Zolghadri J, and Kamali-Sarvestani E. (2010) Proteome Differences of Placenta Between Pre-Eclampsia and Normal Pregnancy. *Placenta* 31(2): 121–5.
12. Molloy MP, Brzezinski EE, Hang J et al. (2003) Overcoming technical variation and biological variation in quantitative proteomics. *Proteomics* 3(10): 1912–9.
13. Zhu W, Smith JW, and Haung CM (2010) Mass spectrometry-based label free quantitative proteomics. *J Biomed Biotechnol* 2010:840518.
14. Blankley RT, Robinson NJ, Aplin JD et al. (2010) A gel-free quantitative proteomics analysis of factors released from hypoxic-conditioned placentae. *Reprod Sci* 17(3): 247–57.

27

CHAPTER 27

Stable Isotope Methodologies for the Study of Transport and Metabolism In Vivo

Irene Cetin and Chiara Mandò

Department of Clinical Sciences, Hospital Luigi Sacco and Center for Fetal Research Giorgio Pardi, University of Milan, Grassi, Milan, Italy

Introduction

Stable isotopes are naturally occurring elements with the same number of protons but with different numbers of neutrons to yield different molecular weights. Generally, a single isotopic form is dominant and is distinguished by mass spectrometry. Importantly, molecules with stable isotopes are chemically indistinguishable from each other in metabolic pathways. Stable isotopes have very long half-lives compared to the Earth age, so they are not considered biologically dangerous. Therefore, they are particularly suited for studies of placental transport and metabolism and for investigations of fetal metabolism. A molecule of interest, such as an amino acid, can be tagged with a stable isotope, so that labeled and unlabeled forms of the same compound can be identified by a change in molecular weight. Commonly used stable isotopes are carbon, nitrogen, oxygen, and hydrogen (Table 27.1). The molecule of interest can be uniformly labeled (UL), or labeled with only one specific atom.

Models to study placental metabolism and transport

Amino acids, glucose, and fatty acids are the most important nutrients for fetal growth, where they are utilized for tissue growth and serve as sources of energy from oxidation. The metabolism and transport across the placenta for these nutrients is crucial to our understanding of nutrient partitioning between the mother and the fetus.

A simple way to study the supply of nutrients to the fetus is to measure substrate concentrations in the fetal blood and compare these with the maternal circulation. However, nutrient concentrations measured in the two circulations may not reflect transfer from the mother to the fetus since the placenta metabolizes substrates [1].

Animal models allow dissection of substrate metabolism in multiple compartments. The chronically catheterized pregnant sheep is often used for the investigation of placental and fetal metabolism in vivo. This model allows simultaneous sampling of maternal and fetal nutrient levels so that placental and fetal uptake and turnover can be calculated. Such measurements can also determine rates of metabolism in specific organs including the fetal liver, brain, and muscle.

The dually perfused placenta is a useful in vitro model that allows investigation of both transport and metabolism by creating gradients in the maternal-to-fetal and fetal-to-maternal directions [2]. Together with results from chronically catheterized pregnant sheep, these studies show that the placenta regulates the composition of nutrients carried to the fetus. Notably,

The Placenta: From Development to Disease, First Edition. Edited by Helen H. Kay, D. Michael Nelson and Yuping Wang.
© 2011 Blackwell Publishing Ltd. Published 2011 by Blackwell Publishing Ltd.

Table 27.1 Average natural abundances of the stable isotopes of major elements of interest in placental studies.

Element	Isotope	Abundance (%)
Carbon	^{12}C	98.89
	^{14}C	1.11
Nitrogen	^{14}N	99.63
	^{15}N	0.37
Oxygen	^{16}O	99.76
	^{17}O	0.037
	^{18}O	0.204
Hydrogen	^{1}H	99.985
	^{2}H	0.015

placental interconversion of glutamate and glutamine occurs, and there is preferential maternal to fetal transfer of glucose.

Although helpful for understanding metabolic pathways, these models do not reflect the fetal-placental unit as part of the mother-placenta-fetus three-compartment model. In contrast, stable-isotope methodologies allow comprehensive studies of pregnant women in vivo to be done, so that the rates and kinetics of nutrient consumption by the mother, placenta, and fetus can be determined. Technical difficulties and ethical issues do not allow chronic catheterization of maternal and fetal vessels in human pregnancies. Stable isotopes are a safe research approach that allows collection of in vivo data to complement data obtained in vitro and from animal models.

Stable isotope studies in human pregnancies

Stable isotope studies in human pregnancies require infusion of tracers into the mother and collection of one and, at the most, two fetal samples per subject. The transplacental passage of nutrients, and nutrient metabolism by the fetus and placenta, are estimated by comparing the enrichment of labeled compounds in the fetal circulation, the maternal circulation, or both at the time of cesarean delivery or fetal blood sampling. Blood flow and umbilical veno-arterial nutrient differences can be obtained at the time of cesarean section. Results obtained at one time point, especially at or near term, may not reflect the intrauterine environment steady state at other gestations. Maternal stable isotope infusions, prior to in utero fetal blood sampling, allows measurements of tracers in the fetal circulation at other gestational ages and without the stress of labor. Only umbilical venous samples are obtainable; therefore, measurements of fetal metabolites represent the combination of fetal plus placental metabolism in addition to placental permeability factors.

Non-steady-state or steady-state kinetics

Two different kinetic models have been developed to study transport and metabolism (Figure 27.1):

a nonsteady-state kinetics by maternal bolus infusion to study unidirectional fluxes;

b steady-state kinetics by maternal bolus, followed by a continuous infusion to study placental permeability together with fetoplacental metabolism.

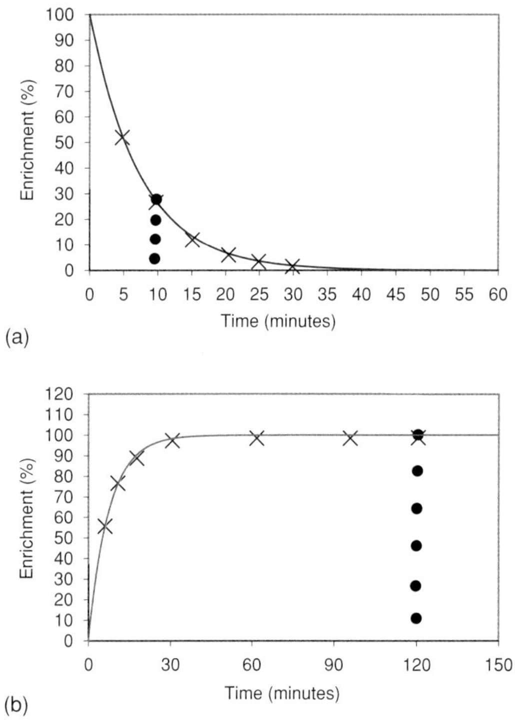

Figure 27.1 Kinetic models for placental stable isotopes studies. (a) Maternal bolus infusion. (b) Maternal primed continuous infusion. ×, maternal sampling; •, fetal sampling.

> **Research Spotlight**
>
> Bolus studies are most impacted by transport. In contrast, steady-state protocols determine the effects of transport combined with placental and fetal metabolism. Estimates of amino acid transport are affected by both metabolism and protein turnover during steady-state conditions.

Planning a study with stable isotopes

Stable isotope studies must be planned to determine the molecule for study, the atom labeled, and position within the molecule for the atom labeled. For example, we may decide to use an essential amino acid, like leucine, if we plan to study protein catabolism, while we would use albumin to study protein synthesis. The position and the atom labeled, e.g., a carbon or hydrogen, are important if we plan to assess the conversion of an amino acid, such as serine to glycine. Moreover, we may label a nitrogen atom to investigate nitrogen metabolism. Proton labeling is useful to study hydrolization reactions and energy requirements. Importantly, labeled atoms that are lost by oxidation are not useful for calculation of a disposal rate for a molecule of interest. The position of the atom labeled is most important when the goal is to determine the metabolic fate of a particular molecule.

The route of administration and consequent blood sampling must be planned carefully. Most molecules are administered by intravenous maternal infusion. In such cases, timing of specimen retrieval is crucial to plot a maternal curve of enrichment, and maternal samples need to be obtained at short intervals, which may be on the order of minutes. In contrast, if we plan a primed continuous infusion, samples are taken after steady state is reached, usually after 30 minutes of infusion, and every 15–30 minutes thereafter. Lipid molecules must be given to the mother orally, and the appearance of the tracer in the maternal circulation depends on gastrointestinal absorption, which requires more time to reach the steady state. If such a study is performed prior to a cesarean section, the tracer needs to be given to the mother several hours before surgery, and maternal samples must be taken every 30–60 minutes.

Blood analysis of stable isotope enrichments

Molecules with stable isotope tracers can only be measured by mass spectrometry due to change in their molecular weight from the more abundant naturally occurring molecule, the tracee. The results are reported as a ratio between the labeled tracer and the tracee, after subtracting the natural abundance for the molecule of interest calculated from the zero time sample. The ratio is multiplied by 100 to yield a percentage, and the result is called Atom Percent (At%). As an example, the enrichment for stable isotopes involving ^{13}C is $[^{13}C]/[^{12}C + ^{13}C + ^{14}C] \times 100$. For the At%^{13}C calculation, the amount of naturally present ^{14}C is usually treated as negligible and the sum of ^{12}C and ^{13}C is taken to be total C. Medical tracer

> **Research Spotlight**
>
> Labeling with stable isotopes allows investigation of the conversion of a specific molecule to another metabolic product. For example, we may calculate the conversion of serine to glycine by labeling one of the carbon atoms in positions 1 or 2, because the 3rd carbon atom is lost and made available into the one-carbon atom pool (Figure 27.2).

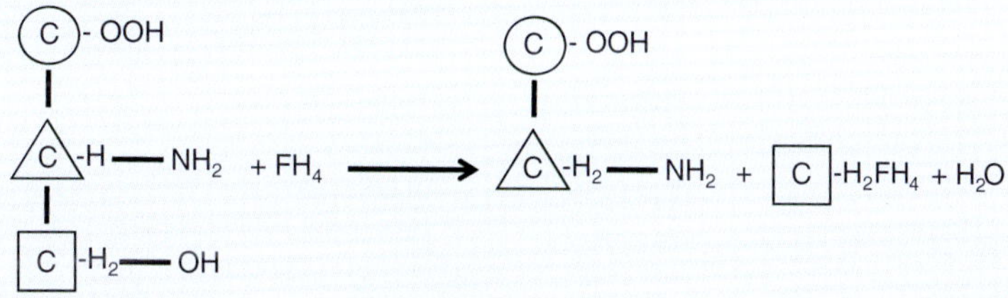

Figure 27.2 Conversion of serine to glycine. C1 (circle) and C2 (triangle) can be labeled to evaluate serine to glycine conversion. C3 (square) is lost into the one-carbon atom pool.

studies of human physiology are most often reported in units of atom percent excess (APE), which is the level of isotopic abundance above a background reading, which is usually considered zero. The background reading in At% is subtracted from the experimental value to give the APE. The absolute concentration of tracer is calculated by multiplying the APE (also called enrichments) by the concentration of the molecule of interest in plasma.

Research Spotlight

A sample must be obtained prior to the administration of the stable isotope solution, and patient weights should be recorded before the beginning of the study. This allows turnover rates to be calculated on a per kg basis.

Amino acids and proteins

The nonsteady state approach has been used to study placental transfer of nonessential and essential amino acids. The possibility of nonessential amino acid production within the fetoplacental compartment has been investigated using ^{13}C-labeled amino acid bolus infusions before cordocentesis. Fetal enrichment of nonessential amino acids, such as glycine and proline, is much lower than maternal enrichment, suggesting they are produced in significant amounts in the fetal placental unit. The essential amino acids leucine and lysine, though, are rapidly transferred from the maternal to the fetal circulation [1]. When all essential amino acids are ^{13}C-labeled and simultaneously infused as a bolus to the mother, striking differences are observed in their in vivo transport. Leucine, isoleucine, methionine, and phenylalanine cross the placenta rapidly with no significant differences among them, while threonine, histidine, tryptophan, lysine, and valine are transported more slowly than the other amino acids. Basic amino acids exit the trophoblast with more difficulty. Therefore, significant differences are observed between essential and nonessential amino acids, confirming that the human placenta modifies and possibly regulates the fetal supply of amino acids.

Rennie and colleagues [3] were the first to quantify the metabolic pathways of leucine and phenylalanine in the human fetus, using a continuous L-[1-^{13}C]-leucine and L-[^{15}N]-phenylalanine infusion model, prior to cesarean section. Umbilical blood flow was measured with a flow probe acutely in the exteriorized fetus, demonstrating that two-thirds of the net leucine uptake was used for protein deposition and one-third was oxidized. Tyrosine production from phenylalanine was also measured in the fetal compartment.

The normal steady-state fetal/maternal plasma enrichment ratios for leucine were also measured in pregnancies in the third trimester. The mother was primed with a constant infusion of L-[1-^{13}C]-leucine, and umbilical venous samples were taken by cordocentesis under ultrasonic guidance [4]. The fetal/maternal enrichment ratios for leucine in normal pregnancies were approximately 20% higher in this cordocentesis study, as compared to ratios reported at cesarean delivery. This difference was attributed to the stress of cesarean delivery and the time required to obtain flow measurements from an exteriorized fetus, compared to the steady state situation of cordocentesis.

In order to evaluate whether steady state is also achieved in the fetal circulation, an approach utilizing multiple infusion start times for two stable isotopes of leucine was applied to assess equilibration times for isotopic studies when a single fetal blood sample is available [5]. Two infusates, one containing L-[1-^{13}C]-leucine and the other L-[5,5,5-D^3]-leucine, were given as a primed constant infusion in the maternal circulation prior to fetal blood sampling by cordocentesis. The data showed that leucine steady state was achieved in both the maternal and fetal circulations 20 minutes after the start of the primed continuous infusion.

Measuring synthesis rates of specific proteins can also provide organ-specific information. Albumin concentrations reflect nutritional status, and rates of albumin synthesis are a measure of liver activity. A multiple tracer infusion protocol is used to estimate albumin synthesis over time in fetuses from different gestational ages in a single sample taken from the umbilical cord at birth [6]. Albumin synthesis rates are higher in preterm fetuses at delivery than in term fetuses, and this should be taken into account in order to meet requirements to sustain albumin synthesis rates after delivery.

Research Spotlight

We can measure two enrichments in one fetal sample when a molecule is labeled with different stable isotopes, such as ^{13}C and ^{15}N, and infused at different start times. This approach allows us to evaluate if the tracer is at steady state in the fetoplacental compartment.

Glucose

Stable isotope methodologies also allow the study of glucose metabolism in the maternal-placental-fetal unit, where a gradient is the driving force for glucose transport. In sheep, a significant amount of glucose taken up by the placenta is not transported to the fetus but is used in placental metabolism, predominantly for oxidative processes. Glucose utilization in human pregnancies is measured by steady state infusion of ^{13}C-glucose into the maternal circulation. Data from this approach show that glucose utilization depends both on maternal glucose levels and on conceptus mass. Thus, glucose utilization decreases in pregnancies complicated by intrauterine growth restriction (IUGR) and increases in multifetal pregnancies.

Whether there is glucogenesis in the fetoplacental unit during intrauterine life is controversial. Significant and similar glucose dilutions were noted in the umbilical vein and umbilical artery compared to the maternal levels, after continuous intravenous infusion of the stable isotope 6,6-(2)H(2)-glucose into the maternal circulation during elective caesarean section. This result suggests that the human placenta at term can produce glucose. However, no dilution of maternally infused UL-^{13}C-glucose was observed in fetal blood obtained by cordocentesis from IUGR pregnancies [7], implying that the above-noted glucose dilution may relate to the stress of cesarean section.

Fatty acids

Fatty acid transport and metabolism in the fetoplacental unit has been extensively studied in the last few years. Higher concentrations of total fatty acids in maternal plasma, compared to cord plasma, create a gradient driving fatty acid flux from the mother to the fetus. The observed percentages of long-chain polyunsaturated fatty acid (LC-PUFA) derivatives, such as arachidonic acid (ARA) and docosahexaenoic acid (DHA), are higher in cord plasma compared with maternal plasma. Notably, these LC-PUFAs are very important for brain tissue accretion and membrane fluidity, and the enrichment of LC-PUFA during intrauterine life has been called "biomagnification." Because of the limited fetal capacity to synthesize LC-PUFA, biomagnification of ARA and DHA in fetal plasma is likely due to specific placental mechanisms. Placental preferential transfer of DHA, and then ARA, ALA (α-linoleic acid), and LA (linolenic acid) into the fetal circulation has been demonstrated by in vivo stable isotope experiments using ^{13}C-labeled fatty acids that are given orally to mothers prior to cesarean delivery [8].

Research Spotlight

Stable isotope studies used to investigate placental incorporation and release of fatty acids show a preferential rate of transfer into the fetal circulation.

Studies in pregnancies with placental insufficiency

Stable isotope methodologies are used for the study of placental transport and metabolism in pregnancies affected by placental insufficiency. This placental phenotype associates with reduced nutrient supply, leading to restricted fetal growth and a sequence of fetal metabolic and cardiovascular adaptations that predispose to hypoxia and organ damage [1].

Alterations in placental transfer and metabolism of amino acids are a characteristic feature of IUGR, independent of changes in oxygenation and acid–base status. Decreased umbilical venous amino acid concentrations are present in IUGR, and a reduction in the activity of placental amino acid transport systems has been demonstrated by in vitro studies of the microvillous trophoblast membrane [2].

These findings have been confirmed by stable isotope studies performed with both the steady state and the bolus approach. The fetal–maternal enrichment ratio for leucine is indicative of protein catabolism when the isotope-labeled essential amino acid ^{13}C-leucine is used as a continuous maternal tracer infusion. Importantly, this value is significantly increased in IUGR compared to normal pregnancies [4]. Moreover, the fetal–maternal ratio progressively decreases with increasing degrees of clinical severity of IUGR, as defined by fetal arterial Doppler velocimetry and fetal heart rate patterns. The difference in leucine enrichment may be due to an increase in protein breakdown that dilutes the fetal plasma enrichment, may be the result of a decrease in the transplacental transfer rate, or may be a combination of these. The fetal–maternal enrichment ratio in IUGR pregnancies was approximately one-half the ratio of normal pregnancies for the essential amino acids leucine and phenylalanine, but similar ratios were observed for nonessential amino acids glycine and proline, when studied by maternal single bolus infusion. These results suggest that slower placental transport rates of essential amino acids can be responsible for the lower tracer appearance in the fetal plasma.

Glucose is transported across the placenta by facilitated glucose transporters belonging to the glucose transporters (GLUT) family, so glucose flux is dependent on the maternal–fetal glucose gradient. Placental transport of glucose is unaffected in most IUGR, but this gradient is increased in severe IUGR fetuses, as defined by altered Doppler velocimetry of the umbilical artery and fetal heart rate. Studies infusing labeled glucose into IUGR fetuses prior to cordocentesis have failed to show any significant dilution of the tracer in the fetal circulation, suggesting that there is no compensatory glucogenesis in the IUGR fetus [7].

Research Spotlight

Stable isotopes infused in IUGR pregnancies allow us to investigate differences in fetal metabolism. Sampling both umbilical vein and artery determines if there is dilution from newly produced compounds in the fetal compartment.

Finally, red blood cells labeled with the nonradioactive stable isotope of chromium have also been used to demonstrate reduced blood volume in preeclamptic patients compared with nonproteinuric gestational hypertensive and normotensive patients. Blood volume was reduced and distribution altered in women with preeclampsia, but both parameters were normal in those with gestational hypertension.

Teaching Points

1 Stable isotopes provide unique tools for the study of placental metabolism and transport. They complement cross-sectional analyses of maternal–fetal concentrations, placental in vitro models, biomolecular placental analyses of nutrient transporters and enzymes, and studies performed in pregnant animals.

2 Stable isotope studies provide information about nutrient transfer rates across the placenta, and allow comparisons among transfer rates for different compounds.

3 Placental metabolic conversions can be studied by infusing a molecule of interest, and then measuring the enrichment of the metabolic derivatives in plasma. In these studies, attention needs to be paid to the position of isotope-labeling within the molecule of interest.

Acknowledgment

This chapter is dedicated to the memory of Giorgio Pardi, an outstanding teacher and an enthusiastic scientist.

References

1. Cetin I (2001) Amino acid interconversions in the fetal-placental unit: the animal model and human studies in vivo [Review]. *Pediatric Research* 49(2): 148–54.
2. Cetin I and Alvino G (2009) Intrauterine growth restriction: implications for placental metabolism and transport. A review. *Placenta* 30(Suppl A): S77–82.
3. Chien PF, Smith K, Watt PW et al. (1993) Protein turnover in the human fetus studied at term using stable isotope tracer amino acids. *American Journal of Physiology* 265: E31–35.
4. Marconi AM, Paolini CL, Stramare L et al. (1999) The steady state maternal–fetal leucine enrichments in normal and fetal growth restricted pregnancies. *Pediatric Research* 46: 114–19.
5. Paolini CL, Marconi AM, Pike AW et al. (2001) A multiple infusion start time (MIST) protocol for stable isotope studies of fetal blood. *Placenta* 22(2–3): 171–76.
6. Van Den Akker CH, Schierbeek H, Rietveld T et al. (2008) Human fetal albumin synthesis rates during different periods of gestation. *American Journal of Clinical Nutrition* 88: 997–1003.
7. Marconi AM, Cetin I, Davoli E et al. (1993) An evaluation of fetal glucogenesis in intrauterine growth-retarded pregnancies. *Metabolism* 42: 860–64.
8. Larqué E, Demmelmair H, Berger B et al. (2003). In vivo investigation of the placental transfer of ^{13}C-labeled fatty acids in humans. *Journal of Lipid Research* 44(1): 49.

V

PART V

Medical Diseases and Complications

28

CHAPTER 28

The Role of the Placenta in Autoimmune Disease and Early Pregnancy Loss

Daniel L. Jackson and Danny J. Schust

Department of Obstetrics, Gynecology, and Women's Health, Missouri Center for Reproductive Medicine and Fertility, University of Missouri-Columbia, Columbia, MO, USA

Introduction

Autoimmune disease and pregnancy—a reciprocal relationship

The placenta is the maternal-fetal interface and induces a complex interaction with the maternal immune system. Proper regulation of the maternal immune response to the placenta is essential for a healthy pregnancy to develop and thrive. Autoimmune disorders result from aberrant immune responses to self or cross-reactive antigens. Women of reproductive age have a substantial prevalence of autoimmune diseases, and these diseases can predispose to adverse pregnancy outcomes. The purpose of this chapter is to discuss the effects of the placenta on selected autoimmune diseases, as well as the effects of autoimmune diseases on the course of pregnancy.

The effects of placental steroids on maternal systemic immunity and autoimmune disease progression

Investigation on the role of sex steroids in general immune responsivity and in autoimmune disease is an evolving field. T helper cell type 1 (Th1)-mediated autoimmune diseases, such as rheumatoid arthritis (RA) and multiple sclerosis (MS), often improve during pregnancy. T helper cell type 2 (Th2)-mediated disorders such as systemic lupus erythematosus (SLE), however, frequently worsen during pregnancy. These differences are attributed to fluctuations in local and systemic maternal estrogen and progesterone levels during pregnancy. The role of estrogen in this process is better defined than that of progesterone. In general, estrogen stimulates humoral (Th2) immune responses and progesterone (along with androgens and glucocorticoids) is typically immunosuppressive. However, the relationship of the sex hormones with individual autoimmune diseases is often unclear.

Multiple sclerosis

Multiple Sclerosis is commonly diagnosed among women of reproductive age and is a Th1-mediated immune disorder that often ameliorates during pregnancy. While the fluctuating levels of estrogen seen outside of pregnancy stimulate both Th1 and Th2 immune responses, the elevated and sustained levels produced by the placenta during gestation shift the natural balance of the immune system towards Th2- and away from Th1-mediated immunity [1]. This change in maternal physiology reduces the severity of MS during pregnancy. On-going research is attempting to translate this phenomenon into clinical treatments for MS. Estrogen has long been known

The Placenta: From Development to Disease, First Edition. Edited by Helen H. Kay, D. Michael Nelson and Yuping Wang.
© 2011 Blackwell Publishing Ltd. Published 2011 by Blackwell Publishing Ltd.

to exert antiinflammatory effects in the central nervous system (CNS). Estrogen receptor agonists reduce the amount of CNS axon demyelination in animal models for MS, and this outcome is independent of estrogen's antiinflammatory properties [2]. Clinical trials are underway to evaluate the efficacy of estrogen as a treatment for MS.

> **Research Spotlight**
>
> Mechanisms for inflammation-independent effects of estrogen on the course of MS have been recently described. Estrogen receptor α (ERα) agonists decrease inflammation and disease severity in animal models. Estrogen receptor β (ERβ) agonists decrease disease severity, but have little effect on inflammation. Proneoplastic effects of estrogen in the breast and uterus are ERα-mediated, making ERβ agonists attractive candidates for MS therapy [2].

Rheumatoid arthritis

Similar to multiple sclerosis, symptomatic RA generally improves during pregnancy; however, this improvement is often temporary, with the disease returning to baseline following delivery. The pathophysiology of these changes is ill-defined. Placental production of estrogen and progesterone metabolites dictate the cytokine constituents present in the synovial fluid of patients with RA. In particular, proinflammatory Th1 cytokines, such as TNF-alpha, IL-1, and IL-6, stimulate peripheral aromatase and lead to conversion of peripheral androgen precursors (e.g., dehydroepiandrosterone (DHEA)) to estrogen. This results in lower androgen concentrations and higher estrogen concentrations in blood, synovial fluid, and saliva. These elevated estrogen levels in the synovial fluid of RA patients are linked to proinflammatory changes via activation of the NFκB pathway [3]. These data clearly demonstrate that a Th1-mediated pathway involving the metabolism of sex steroids is intimately involved in the inflammatory process, but apparently contradict the observation of clinical remissions of RA during pregnancy. The latter observation appears to be the result of the sustained and elevated levels of progesterone characteristic of human pregnancy. Progesterone decreases tumor necrosis factor (TNF) alpha production and stimulate IL-10 production. This suppresses the Th1 arm of the immune system and favors Th2 immune responses [1], presenting a mechanism for pregnancy-associated suppression of RA activity. While the levels of proinflammatory estrogen derivatives are quite elevated during pregnancy, progesterone-mediated immune alterations typically dominate the estrogen-mediated changes (Figure 28.1).

Systemic lupus erythematosus (SLE)

The effects of pregnancy on the activity of SLE are complex. As a general rule, SLE that is uncontrolled prior to the pregnancy often worsens during pregnancy due to increased Th2-type immune activity. Progesterone produced by the corpus luteum leads to differentiation of naïve T helper (Th0) lymphocytes into Th2 lymphocytes, which in turn produce IL-4, IL-6, and IL-10. These cytokines are also produced by the placenta and are essential to the immunologically privileged microenvironment at the maternal-fetal interface needed for placental survival and function [1]. In nonpregnant patients with SLE, many of these same cytokines have been implicated in pathological downstream signaling that correlates with disease activity. Increased peripheral IL-10 levels have been found

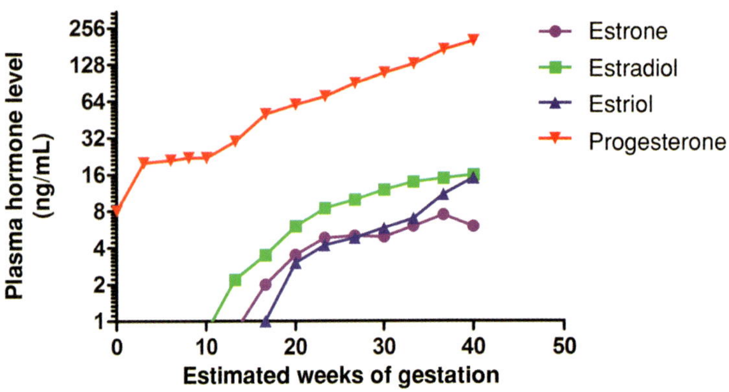

Figure 28.1 Relative levels of estrogens and progesterone during human gestation.

in SLE patients, and elevated IL-10 levels are associated with increased disease activity and elevated levels of anti-DNA antibodies [1]. In pregnant patients without autoimmune disease, the systemic immune effects of the pregnancy-associated Th1/Th2 shift are usually clinically irrelevant. However, in women with SLE the effects of pregnancy may be quite significant.

The high and sustained levels of progesterone characteristic of early pregnancy activate the humoral immune system, and this correlates with increased SLE disease activity. IL-10 promotes beneficial humoral responses that should benefit the course of SLE, but IL-10 levels in SLE remain constant during pregnancy. However, the high-circulating estrogen levels in the latter part of pregnancy stimulate Th1 immunity and augment Th2-type immune responses. Together, these worsen SLE symptoms [1]. Interestingly, pregnancies in SLE patients are also characterized by lower circulating levels of progesterone and estrogen during the third trimester when compared to unaffected pregnancies. Placental damage from the immune injury of SLE may decrease placental steroid hormone synthesis in the third trimester, and this effect decreases severity of SLE in late compared with earlier pregnancy [1].

Clinical Pearl

Testing for circulating autoantibodies (i.e., antinuclear antibodies) is central to diagnosing SLE. Of particular importance in pregnancy are anti-double stranded DNA (anti-dsDNA) antibodies. Their presence is associated with a higher likelihood of lupus flares and preterm delivery among pregnant women. Screening for anti-Ro and anti-La antibodies is relevant to neonatal outcomes.

Cross-reactive autoantibodies, placental function, and autoimmune disease

Some autoimmune diseases result from the development of autoantibodies against placental antigens that then find a target elsewhere in the maternal system. An example of this is pemphigoid gestationis (PG). Human skin and the human placenta both express collagen type XVII. Aberrant expression of major histocompatibility complex class II on the placental surface can lead to maternal development of antibodies to collagen XVII. These antibodies can target the basement membrane of the skin and cause subepidermal bullae that first form microscopically, but then evolve into large, tense blisters on the skin (Figure 28.2) [4]. Adverse pregnancy outcomes, including low birth weight, preterm birth, and small for gestational age (SGA) babies, are more common among women with early-onset PG. Skin lesions accompanying PG typically resolve after delivery, but return if the patient again becomes pregnant.

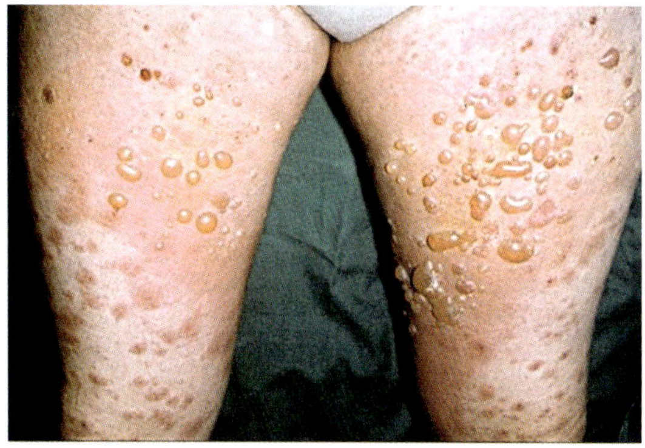

Figure 28.2 Women with PG develop large, tense blisters on their trunks and extremities secondary to cross-reactive tTG antigens in the placenta and epidermal basement membrane. (Reproduced with permission from Semkova K and Black M (2009) Pemphigoid gestationis: current insights into pathogenesis and treatment. *Eur J Obstet Gynecol Reprod Biol* 145: 138–44.)

RA has a relationship with placental antigens, although one not as clear as that for PG. Anti-Sa antibodies are highly specific for RA, but are present in only 40% of patients [5]. The Sa antigen was originally isolated from the placenta and is also expressed on the RA pannus in inflamed joints. There is no association among Sa antigen expression, anti-Sa antibody production, RA disease activity, or pregnancy outcomes. The Sa antigen has been proposed as a target for therapeutic intervention in patients with RA [5].

Clinical Pearl

Some of the newest and most widely used medications among the expanding pharmacologic treatments for RA are disease-modifying antirheumatic drugs (DMARDs). These medications have half-lives of 2 weeks or more and are teratogenic. If patients become pregnant while on these medicines, the drugs should be stopped and elimination protocols using binding resins should be considered.

Systemic disease cross-reactive antigens that affect placental function and pregnancy outcomes

Many autoimmune diseases alter placental function, a fact not surprising given the checks and balances that govern the immunologically privileged maternal-placental interface. Indeed, many autoimmune diseases are associated with poor pregnancy outcomes, and their presence often requires expert consultation with a maternal-fetal medicine specialist.

Systemic lupus erythematosus

SLE is a disease process characterized by the production of antibodies that can cause damage to almost any tissue in the affected patient. Commonly targeted organs include the kidneys, skin, joints, and heart. Notably, recurrent fetal loss can be seen when SLE is associated with the antiphospholipid antibody syndrome (APS), a topic detailed later in this chapter.

> **Clinical Pearl**
>
> Of patients with primary APS, over 10% will eventually be diagnosed with another autoimmune disease, while 30% of patients with SLE will develop secondary APS. The most common of these secondary autoimmune diseases are SLE and mixed connective tissue disorders (MCTD).

Maternal IgG autoantibodies specific to SLE, particularly anti-SS-A/Ro and anti-SS-B/La, cross the placenta and can lead to neonatal lupus. Neonatal lupus, like its adult counterpart, can affect a variety of fetal systems. Neonates can present with a photosensitive rash, liver failure, dysfunction of the biliary tract (cholestasis), thrombocytopenia or pancytopenia, and cardiac dysfunction. A particularly devastating manifestation of neonatal lupus is fetal congenital heart block secondary to maternal antibody-mediated damage to the fetal cardiac conduction system. Although the exact mechanisms are only partially defined, anti-SS-A/Ro and SS-B/La antigens have long been associated with fetal congenital heart block. Recent research has suggested that anti-SS-A/Ro antibodies bind to the Ro antigen in fetal cardiac conductive tissue within the AV node, leading to calcium-mediated cellular apoptosis [6]. Others have suggested that anti-SS-A/Ro and anti-SS-B/La antibodies bind directly to apoptotic cells in the developing fetal heart and inhibit the normal clearance of these apoptotic cells [7]. This leads to increased fibroblast infiltration and subsequent damage to fetal conductive tissue. Finally, while the involvement of maternal autoantibodies is necessary for the development of fetal heart block, environmental and fetal genetic factors also are involved [7].

Celiac disease

Celiac disease results from aberrant autoimmune recognition of antigenic targets in host intestinal villi, resulting in immune destruction of the mucosal surface of the gastrointestinal tract and impaired nutrient absorption. Many of the effects of celiac disease can be ameliorated by dietary alterations that prohibit the ingestion of gluten-containing foods. Celiac disease is also associated with adverse pregnancy outcomes, including intrauterine growth restriction (IUGR), recurrent pregnancy loss, and stillbirth [8]. Poor maternal nutrition and subsequent fetal nutrient deprivation contributes to suboptimal fetal growth in women with celiac disease. Poor pregnancy outcome in these patients also result from autoimmune effects. The most significant target antigen in the small intestines of patients with celiac disease is tissue transglutaminase (tTG). This antigen is also present on the syncytial surface of the placenta, and binding of serum celiac disease IgA antibodies to placental tTG sites inhibits placental tTG activity [8]. The role of autoimmunity and inflammation in adverse pregnancy outcomes among women with celiac disease can be correlated with abnormalities in their placentas (Figure 28.3). The placentas of women with celiac disease who are noncompliant with dietary restrictions exhibit increased apoptosis in extravillous cytotrophoblast cells. Interestingly, the resulting babies display decreased birth weight when compared with controls without celiac disease and from women with celiac disease who were compliant with a gluten-free diet. The increase in placental apoptosis among noncompliant patients was associated with elevated expression of the apoptotic protein Fas-L, the same apoptotic pathway identified to cause destruction in the flattened regions of the intestinal mucosa of patients with celiac disease. (Figure 28.3; [9]). In summary, maternal anti-tTG IgA antibodies in patients with celiac disease inhibit placental function without crossing the placenta and EVT cells at the maternal-fetal interface in pregnant women with celiac disease are subject to the same inflammatory and

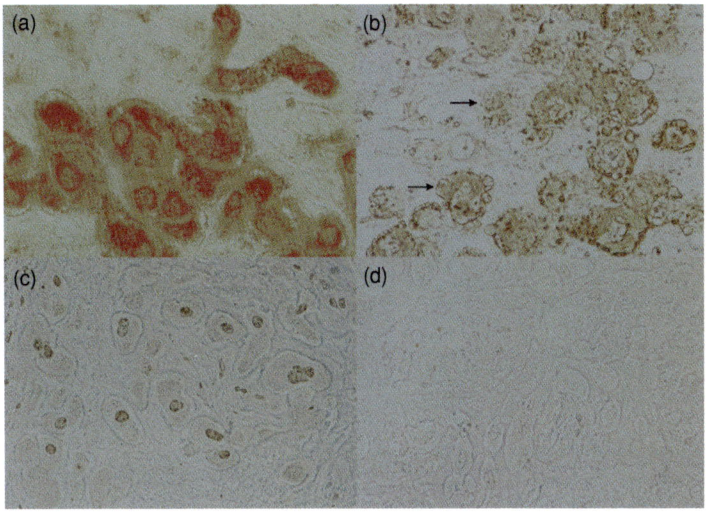

Figure 28.3 Extravillous trophoblast (EVT) from the placentas of women with celiac disease who were compliant with a gluten-free diet, showing peripherally located Fas-L (b) (arrow) and low EVT apoptosis rates (d). These findings are in contrast to increased apoptosis (c) and strong Fas-L expression (a) in EVT from noncompliant women (60×, phase contrast). (Reproduced with permission from Hadziselimovic F, Geneto R, and Buser M (2007) Celiac disease, pregnancy, small for gestational age: role of extravillous trophoblast. *Fetal Pediatr Pathol* 26: 125–34.)

apoptotic pathways that damage the patient's intestinal mucosa.

The antiphospholipid syndrome (APS)

The APS is an autoimmune disorder that results in a hypercoagulable state in small blood vessels. Hypercoagulability is secondary to the presence of autoantibodies against phospholipid-binding proteins. Several specific antibodies have been identified in this syndrome, including anticardiolipin antibodies, anti-β_2 glycoprotein 1 (α-β_2GP1) antibodies, and the lupus anticoagulant. In fact, the diagnostic criteria for the APS have recently been expanded to include each of these tests (Table 28.1). APS is frequently diagnosed following recurrent pregnancy loss (RPL) in the first or second trimesters.

> **Clinical Pearl**
>
> The American Society for Reproductive Medicine recommends consideration of an evaluation for RPL, including an evaluation for APS, after two spontaneous clinical losses prior to 20 weeks of gestation. All investigators agree this evaluation must be instituted after three or more losses.

Table 28.1 Diagnostic criteria for the APS.

Clinical criteria (one or more of the following):

1 One or more confirmed episodes of venous, arterial, or small vessel thrombosis
2 Three or more consecutive spontaneous abortions before 10 weeks' gestation with exclusion of maternal anatomic and hormonal abnormalities and exclusion of paternal and maternal chromosomal abnormalities
3 One or more unexplained deaths of a morphologically normal fetus at or beyond 10 weeks of gestation (normal fetal morphology documented by ultrasound or direct examination of the fetus)
4 One or more premature births of a morphologically normal neonate at or before 34 weeks of gestation due to severe preeclampsia or placental insufficiency

Laboratory criteria (testing for each of these markers must be positive on two or more occasions with evaluations performed twelve or more weeks apart):

1 Positive plasma levels of the lupus anticoagulant,
2 Anticardiolipin antibodies (ACA) of the IgG or IgM isotype at medium to high levels, or
3 Anti-β_2 glycoprotein 1 antibodies of the IgG or IgM isotype in titers greater than the 99th percentile.

Source: Miyakis S et al. 2006 Feb; 4(2): 295–306.
International consensus statement on an update of the classification criteria for definite antiphospholipid syndrome (APS).

Mechanistically, APS is perhaps the best understood disorder in which autoimmune disease alters placental function and one of the few that exhibit histopathologic findings in the placenta. Initial clinical research into APS suggested that thrombosis alone was the cause of RPL. Locatelli et al. [10], studied the histopathology of placentas from patients with APS and SLE and compared them to controls. They found an increased number of small vessel thromboses and thrombosis-related lesions in the placentas of women with these autoimmune disorders and concluded that this explained autoimmune disease-associated adverse pregnancy outcomes, such as pregnancy loss, IUGR, and preeclampsia. This pathophysiologic mechanism was further supported by the fact that use of the anticoagulants, heparin, and aspirin, during pregnancy dramatically increased live birth rates among pregnant women with APS. Despite this seemingly straightforward cause-and-effect relationship, recent research indicates that nonthrombotic factors are also involved among affected women. In fact, some studies have suggested a rather limited role for placental thrombosis in adverse pregnancy outcomes, noting that there does not appear to be a clear correlation between the two among APS patients [11].

Clinical Pearl

Spontaneous fetal aneuploidy is the most common reason for a single spontaneous pregnancy loss at less than 12 weeks of gestation. When recurrent fetal loss occurs, testing for paternal karyotypic abnormalities, maternal anatomic and hormonal abnormalities, and maternal hypercoagulable disorders, including APS and, occasionally, select heritable thrombophilias is indicated.

APS has dramatic effects on the developing placenta by interfering with syncytiotrophoblast development and causing trophoblast apoptosis. The villous trophoblast surface membrane express phosphatidylserine and other phospholipids that can bind β_2 glycoprotein-1. Beta$_2$GP1 on the trophoblast cell membrane binds antiphospholipid antibodies, which impairs placental development [11]. This, in turn, leads to the release of a host of proinflammatory cytokines (IL-8, MCP-1, GRO-alpha, and IL-1beta) via activation of a signaling pathway involving toll-like receptor 4/myeloid differentiation primary response gene 88 (TLR 4/MyD88). Interestingly, high concentrations of heparin attenuate the inflammatory responses that promote apoptosis [12]. Separate from its anticoagulant effects, this antiinflammatory role of heparin is likely important for improvement of pregnancy outcomes among pregnant women with APS. An association between thrombosis-independent impaired trophoblast invasion and APS-associated early pregnancy loss has also been described [13].

Conclusions

Interactions between the placenta and maternal autoimmune disease are complex and incompletely understood. The high prevalence of autoimmune disease among women of reproductive age and the associated impact on pregnancy outcomes makes this an active area of research. Enhanced understanding of the effects of placental sex hormones on disease activity and progression in MS has led to the development of new and exciting therapies. Among patients with APS, pregnancy-related research has led to treatments that may improve poor placentation and certainly result in improved pregnancy outcomes. Importantly, the relationship between the placenta and autoimmune disease remains incompletely defined. Given the importance of this clinical problem, investigations into placental function and autoimmune disease should offer many research opportunities over the next several decades.

Teaching Points

1. Pregnancy has global effects on the immune system and autoimmune diseases. Th1-mediated autoimmune diseases, such as RA and MS that are typically suppressed by estrogen, improve during pregnancy while Th2-mediated autoimmune diseases such as SLE that are typically enhanced by progesterone, generally worsen during pregnancy.
2. Estrogen exerts antiinflammatory effects in the CNS and estrogen receptor ligands offer promising novel candidates for the treatment of MS.
3. PG is caused by the development of unique maternal antibodies against placental collagen XVII that cross-react with collagen XVII in maternal skin.
4. In some women with SLE, maternal anti-Ro and anti-La IgG autoantibodies can cross the placenta, damage the developing fetal cardiac conduction system and cause fetal congenital heart block.

5 Cross-reactive autoantibodies in pregnant women with celiac disease can cause placental dysfunction and apoptosis via the same pathways that damage the maternal gastrointestinal tract.

6 The APS is associated with fetal loss, IUGR, and preeclampsia secondary to autoantibody-mediated trophoblast apoptosis and inflammation. Treatment with heparin improves pregnancy outcomes by decreasing this inflammation and apoptosis. The role of placental thrombosis in APS-related adverse pregnancy outcomes is controversial.

References

1. Doria A, Iaccarino L, Sarzi-Puttini P et al. (2006) Estrogens in pregnancy and systemic lupus erythematosus. *Ann N Y Acad Sci* 1069: 247–56.
2. Tiwari-Woodruff S, Morales LB, Lee R et al. (2007) Differential neuroprotective and antiinflammatory effects of estrogen receptor (ER)alpha and ERbeta ligand treatment. *Proc Natl Acad Sci U S A* 104: 14813–8.
3. Cutolo M, Capellino S, Sulli A et al. (2006) Estrogens and autoimmune diseases. *Ann N Y Acad Sci* 1089: 538–47.
4. Semkova K and Black M (2009) Pemphigoid gestationis: current insights into pathogenesis and treatment. *Eur J Obstet Gynecol Reprod Biol* 145: 138–44.
5. Vossenaar ER, Despres N, Lapointe E et al. (2004) Rheumatoid arthritis specific anti-Sa antibodies target citrullinated vimentin. *Arthritis Res Ther* 6: R142–50.
6. Molad Y (2006) Systemic lupus erythematosus and pregnancy. *Curr Opin Obstet Gynecol* 18: 613–7.
7. Buyon JP, Clancy RM, and Friedman DM (2009) Autoimmune associated congenital heart block: integration of clinical and research clues in the management of the maternal/foetal dyad at risk. *J Intern Med* 265: 653–62.
8. Anjum N, Baker PN, Robinson NJ et al. (2009) Maternal celiac disease autoantibodies bind directly to syncytiotrophoblast and inhibit placental tissue transglutaminase activity. *Reprod Biol Endocrinol* 7: 16.
9. Hadziselimovic F, Geneto R, and Buser M (2007) Celiac disease, pregnancy, small for gestational age: role of extravillous trophoblast. *Fetal Pediatr Pathol* 26: 125–34.
10. Locatelli A, Patane L, Ghidini A et al. (2002) Pathology findings in preterm placentas of women with autoantibodies: a case-control study. *J Matern Fetal Neonatal Med* 11: 339–44.
11. Di Simone N, Luigi MP, Marco D et al. (2007) Pregnancies complicated with antiphospholipid syndrome: the pathogenic mechanism of antiphospholipid antibodies: a review of the literature. *Ann N Y Acad Sci* 1108: 505–14.
12. Mulla MJ, Brosens JJ, Chamley LW et al. (2009) Antiphospholipid antibodies induce a pro-inflammatory response in first trimester trophoblast via the TLR4/MyD88 pathway. *Am J Reprod Immunol* 62: 96–111.
13. Sebire NJ, Fox H, Backos M et al. (2002) Defective endovascular trophoblast invasion in primary antiphospholipid antibody syndrome-associated early pregnancy failure. *Hum Reprod* 17: 1067–71.

29

CHAPTER 29

The Placenta in Preterm Prelabor Rupture of Membranes and Preterm Labor

Chong Jai Kim[1,2], *Roberto Romero*[1,3], *and Sonia S. Hassan*[1,4]

[1]Perinatology Research Branch, NICHD, NIH, DHHS, Bethesda, MD, USA/Detroit, MI, USA
[2]Department of Pathology, Wayne State University School of Medicine, Detroit, MI, USA
[3]Center for Molecular Medicine and Genetics, Wayne State University School of Medicine, Detroit, MI, USA
[4]Department of Obstetrics and Gynecology, Wayne State University School of Medicine/Hutzel Women's Hospital, Detroit, MI, USA

Introduction

Preterm birth is defined as a delivery before 37 weeks gestation and is a leading cause of neonatal morbidity and mortality worldwide. Preterm birth is categorized as "spontaneous" when the delivery is a consequence of preterm prelabor rupture of membranes or preterm labor and "indicated" when the fetus is iatrogenically delivered due to maternal or fetal indications such as preeclampsia or intrauterine growth restriction. Preterm birth is classified as "late" when it occurs between 34 and 36 6/7 weeks of gestation. Late preterm birth accounts for 71% of all preterm deliveries. Moderate prematurity is defined as delivery at 32–33 weeks', severe prematurity at 28–31 weeks', and extreme prematurity at <28 weeks' [1]. Gestational age at delivery is an important predictor of perinatal morbidity and mortality, and pathologic lesions appear to have a different frequency in these subgroups.

Preterm prelabor rupture of membranes (PROM) and preterm labor

The frequency of microbial invasion of the amniotic cavity (MIAC), defined as a positive amniotic fluid culture obtained by amniocentesis, is high in patients with preterm labor with intact membranes and preterm PROM depends upon the clinical presentation and gestational age (Table 29.1). In patients with preterm labor and intact membranes, the rate of positive amniotic fluid cultures is 12.8% [2]. However, among those patients who have preterm labor with intact membranes and deliver a preterm neonate, the frequency is 22%. Among women with preterm PROM, the rate of positive amniotic fluid cultures at admission is 32.4% [2]; however, at the time of the onset of labor, as many as 75% of patients will have MIAC [3], suggesting that microbial invasion occurs during the latency period. Patients with MIAC are more

The Placenta: From Development to Disease, First Edition. Edited by Helen H. Kay, D. Michael Nelson and Yuping Wang.
© 2011 Blackwell Publishing Ltd. Published 2011 by Blackwell Publishing Ltd.

Table 29.1 Frequency of MIAC by clinical presentation.

Clinical Presentation	Frequency (%)
Preterm labor with intact membranes[2]	12.8
Preterm labor with intact membranes and preterm delivery[2]	22
Preterm prelabor rupture of membranes[2]	32.4
Preterm prelabor rupture of membranes in labor[3]	75
Cervical dilatation in the midtrimester[26]	51
Sonographic short cervix[27]	9

likely to deliver preterm, have spontaneous rupture of membranes, develop clinical chorioamnionitis, and have adverse perinatal outcome than are patients with preterm labor or preterm PROM with sterile amniotic fluid. In general, it has been estimated that one in every four preterm deliveries occurs to a mother with microbial invasion of the amniotic cavity; these infections are largely subclinical and are due to microorganisms normally present in the lower genital tract.

Risk factors

The risk factors for preterm labor and preterm PROM include: a sonographic short cervix, previous history of preterm labor or preterm PROM, African-American race, and low maternal body mass index. The reader is referred to a comprehensive review of preterm PROM for an extensive discussion of the risk factors of this condition [4]. Similarly, the etiology of recurrent preterm birth has been recently reviewed by our group [5].

During pregnancy, the chorioamniotic membranes fuse with the decidua. In preparation for delivery, biochemical and cellular events that allow separation of the membranes from the uterine wall take place. We have coined the term "decidual/membrane activation" to refer to a complex set of anatomic and biochemical events resulting in the separation of the lower pole of the membranes from the decidua of the lower uterine segment and, eventually, to spontaneous rupture of membranes and delivery of the placenta. Untimely activation of this mechanism leads to preterm PROM, which accounts for 40% of all preterm deliveries.

Pathophysiology

Placental lesions commonly found in preterm PROM and preterm labor strongly suggest that these disorders represent diverse pathological conditions (syndromes). However, there is no known placental lesion that is pathognomonic of or unique to each phenotype.

Microbial invasion of the amniotic cavity (MIAC) is a well-known and established cause of preterm PROM and preterm labor. Establishment of intra-amniotic infection elicits robust intra-amniotic inflammation characterized by elevated amniotic fluid concentrations of cytokines, neutrophil chemokines (IL-1β, IL-6, TNFα, IL-8, CXCL6, etc.), and amniotic fluid white blood cell count [6,7]. As a consequence, there is extensive amniotropic infiltration (chemotaxis) of maternal neutrophils into the chorioamniotic membranes, this being the most characteristic feature of acute chorioamnionitis (Figure 29.1). Fetal neutrophils also show chemotactic response, and chorionic vasculitis/funisitis is a fetal component of acute histologic inflammation (Figure 29.1). Interestingly, despite extensive maternal neutrophilic infiltration into the chorioamniotic membranes, the majority of the neutrophils in the amniotic fluid is of fetal origin [8].

We have characterized the "Fetal Inflammatory Response Syndrome (FIRS)" as a condition that is operationally defined by an elevation in the plasma concentration of interleukin-6 (fetal plasma or umbilical cord plasma). This condition is frequently observed in patients with preterm labor and intact membranes and preterm PROM and is a risk factor for impending preterm delivery, perinatal morbidity, and long-term handicap (e.g., chronic lung disease and cerebral palsy). Fetuses with FIRS frequently present with microbial invasion of the amniotic cavity, which elicits an intra-amniotic inflammatory response (IL-1β, IL-6, IL-8, TNFα, and multiple chemokines) by engaging pattern recognition receptors (such as Toll-like receptors). Inflammatory mediators eventually lead to increased production of cyclooxygenase-2 (prostaglandin endoperoxide synthase 2) and the production of prostaglandins [prostaglandin E_2 (PGE_2), and prostaglandin $F_{2\alpha}$ ($PGF_{2\alpha}$)] by gestational tissues such as the myometrium and chorioamniotic membranes. Therefore, preterm labor and delivery due to MIAC is also characterized by elevated concentrations of amniotic fluid PGE_2 and $PGF_{2\alpha}$. This is in stark contrast to preterm labor and delivery in the absence of intra-amniotic infection. The histologic hallmarks of FIRS are funisitis and chorionic vasculitis [9].

Chronic chorioamnionitis is characterized by amniotropic infiltration of T lymphocytes into the chorioamniotic membranes (Figure 29.2) [10,11]. This lesion is

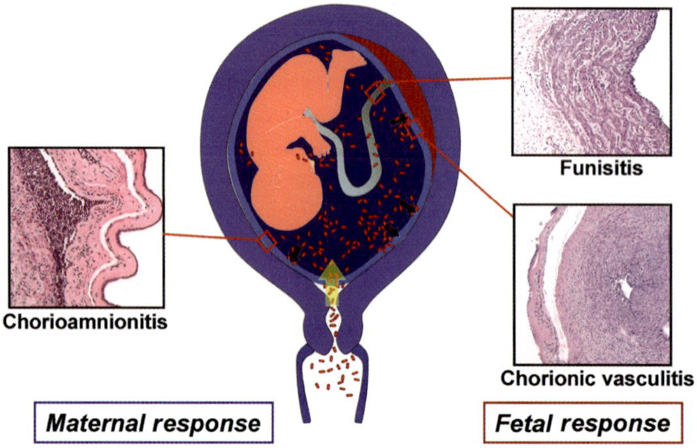

Figure 29.1 Maternal and fetal inflammatory responses to microbial invasion of the amniotic cavity. Acute chorioamnionitis involving extraplacental chorioamniotic membranes represents maternal neutrophilic inflammatory response, while acute funisitis (umbilical vasculitis) and chorionic vasculitis are characterized by fetal neutrophilic reaction.

found in 39% and 34% of preterm PROM and preterm labor cases, respectively, which is higher than that of normal-term placentas (term not in labor, 19%; term in labor, 8%; $P < 0.05$ each) [12]. Importantly, this lesion is associated with increased amniotic fluid concentration of the T cell chemokine CXCL10 (also known as IP-10). In addition, the chorioamniotic membranes of patients with chronic chorioamnionitis overexpress mRNA for CXCL9, CXCL10, and CXCL11, all of which are T cell chemokines. These features and their frequent association with "villitis of unknown etiology" strongly suggest that chronic chorioamnionitis is a manifestation of maternal allograft rejection and graft-versus-host disease [10,11,13]. It is very likely that increased amniotic fluid T cell chemokines (CXCL9, CXCL10, CXCL11), which are produced by the chorioamniotic membranes, induce amniotropic migration of CXCR3 positive T cells. It is noteworthy that CXCL9, CXCL10, and CXCL11 have anti-angiogenic properties.

Acute chorioamnionitis is the most frequent placental lesion among preterm PROM and preterm labor cases before 28 weeks of gestation [14]. In contrast, we have found that chronic chorioamnionitis is more common in late-preterm birth [12]. These findings strongly suggest that acute chorioamnionitis and chronic chorioamnionitis represent major, but separate and distinct, pathologic processes responsible for early- and late-preterm births, respectively.

Another set of lesions observed in preterm PROM and preterm labor are the findings consistent with maternal vascular underperfusion due to superficial implantation of the placenta. We have found placental histological changes consistent with maternal vascular underperfusion in 10% and 16% of preterm PROM and preterm labor cases [12]. This is also quite consistent with our previous observations that 1) the mean number of the spiral arteries with failure of physiologic transformation of the myometrial segment was significantly higher in patients

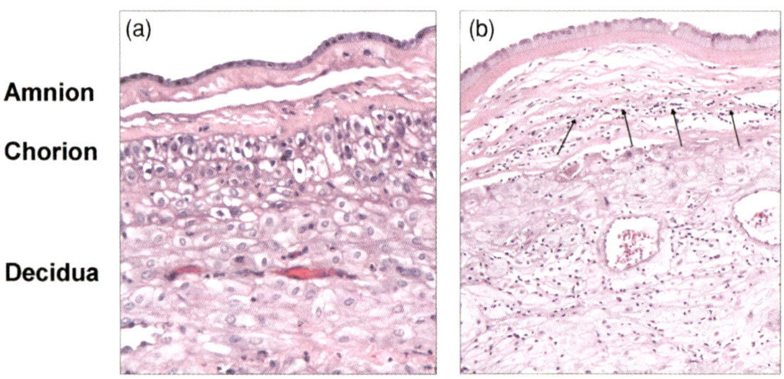

Figure 29.2 Histological characteristics of chronic chorioamnionitis. (a) Normal chorioamniotic membranes composed of amnion, chorion, and decidua. (b) A case of chronic chorioamnionitis showing extensive infiltration of maternal T cells into the chorioamniotic connective tissue (arrows).

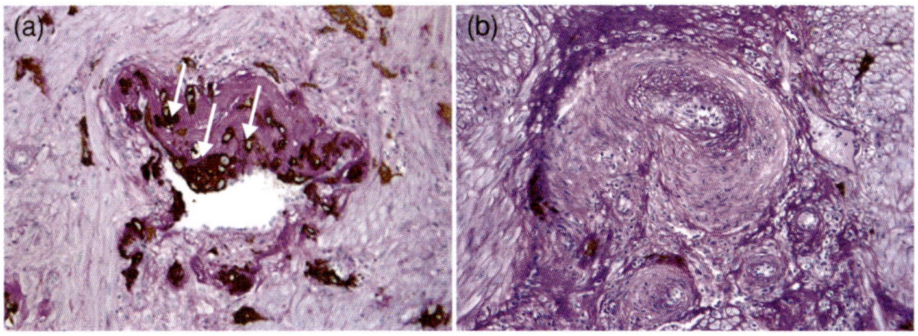

Figure 29.3 Spiral arteries in the placental bed. Periodic acid-Schiff (PAS) staining and immunostaining for cytokeratin-7 was done to label fibrinoids and trophoblasts, respectively. (a) A spiral artery that has undergone physiologic transformation by mural invasion of cytokeratin-7 (+) trophoblasts (arrows). (b) Placental bed biopsy obtained from a patient after preterm labor at 33 weeks gestation. The spiral artery was not transformed and thus retains its intact muscle layer.

with preterm PROM than in normal pregnant women at term ($P = 0.006$) [15] and 2) the mean percentage of spiral arteries with failure of physiologic transformation in the myometrium was significantly higher in patients with preterm labor in normal pregnant women at term ($P = 0.0004$) (Figure 29.3) [16].

Research Spotlight

While the pathophysiology of preterm PROM and preterm labor due to intra-amniotic infection is relatively well-characterized, the molecular mechanisms responsible for chronic chorioamnionitis and maternal vascular underperfusion leading to preterm delivery require further investigation. Since chronic chorioamnionitis is a common pathological lesion in spontaneous preterm birth, it is important to determine whether the derangement in intra-amniotic T cell chemokine concentrations is a central pathology of chronic chorioamnionitis or a consequence of other fundamental changes affecting chemokine concentrations.

Incidence

Preterm birth (delivery <37 weeks) affects 12% of pregnant women [17], and approximately 500,000 preterm neonates are born yearly in the United States. Preterm PROM accounts for 1/3 of all preterm deliveries [1].

Diagnosis

The diagnosis of preterm labor is made in a patient with regular uterine contractions and documented cervical change (i.e., sonographic cervical length or Bishop score). Preterm PROM is confirmed by the presence of a positive nitrazine and ferning test of the pooled amniotic fluid from the vagina of a woman presenting with the symptoms of "leakage" of fluid. In cases in which the nitrazine and ferning tests are equivocal, a transabdominal injection of dye into the amniotic cavity may be used for confirmation of the diagnosis of PROM. A tampon in the vagina can document the subsequent dye leakage in cases of PROM. For a full description the reader is referred to a chapter on preterm PROM by our group [4].

Clinical Pearl

Efforts should be made to determine the cause of preterm labor/preterm prelabor rupture of membranes. The pathological processes implicated in the preterm parturition syndrome include intrauterine infection, uterine ischemia, uterine overdistension, abnormal allogenic recognition, allergic-like reaction, cervical disease, and endocrine disorders. It is important to try to ascertain the mechanism of disease, because this may have implications for future pregnancies. For example, women with intra-amniotic infection tend to have it in future pregnancies.

Clinical Management

In addition to obtaining a careful history and performing a physical examination, providers should order the following studies: (1) examination of cervico-vaginal fluid for *Neisseria gonorrhoeae*, *Chlamydia trachomatis*, bacterial vaginosis; (2) urine culture and sensitivity; (3) urine drug screen; and (4) amniocentesis to rule out intra-amniotic infection/inflammation. For a full discussion of the clinical management of preterm labor with intact membranes and preterm PROM the reader is referred to chapters by our group [4,18].

The emerging picture is that spontaneous preterm labor and preterm PROM are syndromes. Multiple pathological processes may lead to cervical ripening, myometrial and membrane/decidual activation. The clinical presentation will depend on the differential effect and timing of the insults on the various components of the common terminal pathway of parturition. This view of spontaneous preterm labor and preterm parturition has considerable implications for the understanding of the cellular and biochemical mechanisms responsible for the initiation of parturition, as well as the diagnosis, treatment, and prevention of preterm birth. Since spontaneous preterm labor is a heterogeneous condition, it is unlikely that the same treatment will prevent all cases of preterm birth. We consider tocolysis to be a treatment for only one of the manifestations of activation of the common pathway of parturition (i.e., uterine contractility), but not necessarily for the underlying pathological process responsible for this activation. Tocolysis is capable of prolonging pregnancy for up to seven days [19]. This period of time may be helpful to administer steroids, accomplish maternal transfer to a tertiary care center, and institute other measures which may help improve pregnancy outcome (i.e., antibiotic administration to patients with asymptomatic bacteriuria or other infection-related conditions). However, patients with fetuses who present with an episode of preterm labor which apparently responds to tocolysis and deliver at term, are more likely to be small for gestational age (SGA). This suggests that even a single episode of preterm labor that resolves increases the risk of adverse pregnancy outcome [20].

Complications

Preterm birth is the leading identifiable cause of neurologic handicap (e.g., cerebral palsy) and the cost of prematurity to the United States alone is estimated to be $26 billion per year [21]. The most advanced and serious stage of ascending intrauterine infection is fetal infection. The overall mortality rate of neonates with congenital neonatal sepsis ranges between 25% and 90% [22–25]. For further details the reader is referred to recent reviews [18].

Teaching Points

1. Preterm labor and preterm PROM are syndromes with multiple etiologies.
2. The main placental lesions associated with spontaneous preterm birth are: 1) chronic chorioamnionitis; 2) acute chorioamnionitis (including funisitis and chorionic vasculitis); and 3) lesions associated with underperfusion.
3. The frequency of microbial invasion of the amniotic cavity, defined as a positive amniotic fluid culture in fluid obtained by amniocentesis, is high in patients with preterm labor with intact membranes and preterm PROM and depends upon the clinical presentation and gestational age.
4. One in every four preterm deliveries occurs to a mother with microbial invasion of the amniotic cavity.
5. The "FIRS" is a condition which is defined by an elevation in the plasma concentration of interleukin-6 (fetal plasma or umbilical cord plasma). This condition, frequently observed in patients with preterm labor and intact membranes and preterm PROM, is a risk factor for impending preterm delivery, perinatal morbidity, and long-term handicap.
6. Acute chorioamnionitis is the most frequent placental lesion among preterm PROM and preterm labor cases before 28 weeks of gestation [14]; chronic chorioamnionitis is more common in late preterm birth.

References

1. Goldenberg RL, Culhane JF, Iams JD et al. (2008) Epidemiology and causes of preterm birth. *Lancet* 371(9606): 75–84.
2. Goncalves LF, Chaiworapongsa T, and Romero R (2002) Intrauterine infection and prematurity. *Ment Retard Dev Disabil Res Rev* 8(1): 3–13.
3. Romero R, Quintero R, Oyarzun E et al. (1988) Intraamniotic infection and the onset of labor in preterm premature rupture of the membranes. *Am J Obstet Gynecol* 159(3): 661–6.
4. Santolaya-Forgas J, Romero R, Espinoza J et al. (2007) Prelabor rupture of membranes. In: Reece EA, Hobbins JC (eds.) *Clinical Obstetrics: The Fetus and Mother.* 3rd edn. Malden: Blackwell; pp. 1130–888.
5. Mazaki-Tovi S, Romero R, Kusanovic JP et al. (2007) Recurrent preterm birth. *Semin Perinatol* 31(3): 142–58.
6. Yoon BH, Romero R, Park JS et al. (1998) Microbial invasion of the amniotic cavity with Ureaplasma urealyticum is associated with a robust host response in fetal, amniotic, and maternal compartments. *Am J Obstet Gynecol* 179(5): 1254–60.
7. Mittal P, Romero R, Kusanovic JP et al. (2008) CXCL6 (granulocyte chemotactic protein-2): a novel chemokine involved in the innate immune response of the amniotic cavity. *Am J Reprod Immunol* 60(3): 246–57.
8. Sampson JE, Theve RP, Blatman RN et al. (1997). Fetal origin of amniotic fluid polymorphonuclear leukocytes. *Am J Obstet Gynecol* 176(1 Pt 1): 77–81.

9. Pacora P, Chaiworapongsa T, Maymon E et al. (2002) Funisitis and chorionic vasculitis: the histological counterpart of the fetal inflammatory response syndrome. *J Matern Fetal Neonatal Med* 11(1): 18–25.
10. Gersell DJ, Phillips NJ, and Beckerman K (1991) Chronic chorioamnionitis: a clinicopathologic study of 17 cases. *Int J Gynecol Pathol* 10(3): 217–29.
11. Jacques SM and Qureshi F (1998) Chronic chorioamnionitis: a clinicopathologic and immunohistochemical study. *Hum Pathol* 29(12): 1457–61.
12. Kim CJ, Romero R, Kusanovic JP et al. (2010) The frequency, clinical significance, and pathological features of chronic chorioamnionitis: a lesion associated with spontaneous preterm birth. *Mod Pathol* 23(7): 1000–11.
13. Kim MJ, Romero R, Kim CJ et al. (2009) Villitis of unknown etiology is associated with a distinct pattern of chemokine up-regulation in the feto-maternal and placental compartments: implications for conjoint maternal allograft rejection and maternal anti-fetal graft-versus-host disease. *J Immunol* 182(6): 3919–27.
14. McElrath TF, Hecht JL, Dammann O et al. (2008) Pregnancy disorders that lead to delivery before the 28th week of gestation: an epidemiologic approach to classification. *Am J Epidemiol* 168(9): 980–9.
15. Kim YM, Chaiworapongsa T, Gomez R et al. (2002) Failure of physiologic transformation of the spiral arteries in the placental bed in preterm premature rupture of membranes. *Am J Obstet Gynecol* 187(5): 1137–42.
16. Kim YM, Bujold E, Chaiworapongsa T et al. (2003) Failure of physiologic transformation of the spiral arteries in patients with preterm labor and intact membranes. *Am J Obstet Gynecol* 189(4): 1063–9.
17. Hamilton ER, Martin JA, Ventura SJ, United States Department of Health and Human Services, Centers for Disease Control and Prevention, National Center for Health Statistics, and National Vital Statistics System (2010) Births: Preliminary Data for 2008: National Center for Health Statistics; 2010 April 6. *National Vital Statistics Reports* 58(16).
18. Iams JD and Romero R (2007) Preterm birth. In: Gabbe SG, Niebyl JR, Simpson JL, (eds.) *Obstetrics: Normal and Problem Pregnancies.* 5th edn. Philadelphia: Churchill Livingston; pp. 668–712.
19. Romero R, Sibai BM, Sanchez-Ramos L et al. (2000) An oxytocin receptor antagonist (atosiban) in the treatment of preterm labor: a randomized, double-blind, placebo-controlled trial with tocolytic rescue. *Am J Obstet Gynecol* 182(5): 1173–83.
20. Espinoza J, Kusanovic JP, Kim CJ et al. (2007) An episode of preterm labor is a risk factor for the birth of a small-for-gestational-age neonate. *Am J Obstet Gynecol* 196(6): 574 e1–5; discussion e5–6.
21. Institute of Medicine of the Academies (2007) *Preterm Birth Causes, Consequences, and Prevention, Committee on Understanding Premature Birth and Assuring Healthy Outcomes, Board on Health Sciences Policy.* Washington, DC: The National Academies Press; 398–429.
22. Boyer KM, Gadzala CA, Kelly PD et al. (1983) Selective intrapartum chemoprophylaxis of neonatal group B streptococcal early-onset disease. III. Interruption of mother-to-infant transmission. *J Infect Dis* 148(5): 810–6.
23. Placzek MM and Whitelaw A (1983) Early and late neonatal septicaemia. *Arch Dis Child* 58(9): 728–31.
24. Ohlsson A and Vearncombe M (1987) Congenital and nosocomial sepsis in infants born in a regional perinatal unit: cause, outcome, and white blood cell response. *Am J Obstet Gynecol* 156(2): 407–13.
25. Gerdes JS (1991) Clinicopathologic approach to the diagnosis of neonatal sepsis. *Clin Perinatol* 18(2): 361–81.
26. Romero R, Gonzalez R, Sepulveda W, et al. (1992) Infection and labor. VIII. Microbial invasion of the amniotic cavity in patients with suspected cervical incompetence: prevalence and clinical significance. *Am J Obstet Gynecol* 167: 1086–91.
27. Hassan S, Romero R, Hendler I, et al. (2006) A sonographic short cervix as the only clinical manifestation of intra-amniotic infection. *J Perinat Med* 34(1): 13–9.

30

CHAPTER 30
Diabetes and the Placenta

Ursula Hiden[1], *Julia Froehlich*[1,2], *and Gernot Desoye*[1]

[1]Department of Obstetrics and Gynecology, Medical University of Graz, Graz, Austria
[2]Institute of Histology, Embryology and Cell Biology, Medical University of Graz, Graz, Austria

Introduction

In general, the placenta is the organ accounting for the transfer of almost all nutrients and gases between mother and fetus. Thus, the placenta fulfils a fundamental role sustaining adequate fetal growth, and it has been implicated in aberrant fetal growth such as it may be associated with maternal pregestational and gestational diabetes. Both are characterized by changes in hormones, growth factors, and nutrients in the maternal but also in the fetal circulation, which may affect placental development. Indeed, various morphological and functional placental changes can be observed in those pregnancies. They depend on the period in gestation when the diabetic insult occurs.

The clinical problem and potential consequences for the placenta

Diabetes in pregnancy includes gestational diabetes mellitus (GDM), type 1 and type 2 diabetes mellitus (T1D, T2D), and these maladies have become more prevalent with the rise of maternal obesity in the Western world. Complicating this is lack of a uniform definition for GDM as well as profound ethnic differences for carbohydrate intolerance in women. These combine to yield a wide range of 3% to 20% for the prevalence of diabetes in pregnancy depending on the population studied. The increase in diabetic pregnancy prevalence not only carries increased short-term maternal and fetal risks, but also predisposes both individuals to a higher risk for development of obesity, T2D, or both. This results in an enormous burden on the public health care systems to care for the population who develops diabetes and obesity. A recent analysis calculated average costs of $3,305 US for a GDM mother on top of the costs for normal pregnancy care and $209 US for the newborn in its first year of life.

The classical fetal phenotype in GDM is macrosomic, which is commonly defined by a birth weight above 4,000 grams as this raises clinical suspicion for delivery complications. Macrosomia implies a growth pattern that is disproportionate for size. Therefore, a better characterization of this overgrowth fetal phenotype should quantify areas of excessive fetal fat accumulation irrespective of the absolute birth weight and fat-free mass.

> **Clinical Pearl**
>
> The fetal phenotype in GDM pregnancies is characterized by excessive fetal fat accumulation irrespective of the absolute birth weight or birth weight centile.

Elevated levels of fetal insulin with potent lipogenic and mitogenic effects on the adipocyte are the basic principle underlying the increased fat accumulation. Concentrations of glucose, amino acids, and lipids rise in both the maternal and fetal circulations and insulin secretion is induced leading to excess growth.

Owing to its position at the interface between mother and fetus, the placenta is exposed to nutrient concentration changes in both compartments. Villi transport maternal fuels and oxygen to the fetus and synthesize a

The Placenta: From Development to Disease, First Edition. Edited by Helen H. Kay, D. Michael Nelson and Yuping Wang.
© 2011 Blackwell Publishing Ltd. Published 2011 by Blackwell Publishing Ltd.

variety of hormones and growth factors. Therefore, structural and functional changes of the placenta will have an impact on fetal development. Advances in the management of diabetic pregnancies normalize many, but not all of the histopathological characteristics of the placenta in diabetes, e.g., increase in weight and surface area, hypervascularization and edema. Progress in molecular analysis and imaging techniques should clarify the more subtle changes in structure that have been identified.

The maternal and fetal environment in diabetes

The hyperglycemia, proinflammatory nature of diabetes will lead to changes of substrates, growth factors, cytokines, and hormones in both the maternal and fetal environments. These changes include altered levels of insulin, insulin-like growth factors 1 and 2 (IGF1 and 2), fibroblast growth factor-2 (FGF-2), vascular endothelial growth factor (VEGF), tumor necrosis factor-alpha (TNF-alpha), and leptin. TNF-alpha is a cytokine with antiangiogenic and invasion-inhibiting properties, whereas insulin, IGFs, FGF-2, VEGF, and leptin stimulate mitogenic, angiogenic, and invasive processes [1,2].

Trophoblast invasion, placental angiogenesis, and placental vascularization are crucial events in placental development as described in detail in Chapter 5 of this book. Pregestational diabetes (PGD) such as T1D and T2D affects pregnancy from blastocyst development, to trophectoderm implantation and overt placentation. GDM clinically manifests in the second trimester so that the maternal and fetal hyperinsulinemia and dysregulated substrate availability are commonly described to affect placental growth and function in the second half of pregnancy. However, altered levels of maternal insulin, IGF1, and leptin are apparent by the 13th week of gestation, and TNF-alpha is markedly increased by midpregnancy in women who subsequently develop GDM. These newly described changes in early pregnancy physiology are surprising as the gestational age between 12–16 weeks commonly shows enhanced insulin sensitivity, an environment that is in sharp contrast with the progressive increase in the insulin-resistant environment that causes GDM in mid- and late pregnancy.

While the maternal diabetic environment differs between GDM and PGD for a given gestational age, the hyperglycemic fetal environment arising from the mother is independent of the type of maternal diabetes (Table 30.1). For instance, maternal IGF1 is higher in GDM than in nondiabetic controls, whereas IGF1 is reduced in PGD. Maternal leptin is higher in GDM, but normal in PGD and nondiabetic women, even after correction for BMI. In contrast, leptin levels in the fetus are elevated and reflect excess fetal adiposity, regardless of the type of maternal diabetes [2].

Collectively, the above indicates that the maternal metabolic environment depends on the type of diabetes while the fetal environment is characterized by hyperglycemic-induced hyperinsulinemia irregardless of the type of maternal diabetes.

Table 30.1 Changes in levels of insulin, IGF1, IGF2, FGF-2, VEGF, TNF-alpha, and leptin in the maternal and fetal circulation as a consequence of gestational (GDM) or pregestational diabetes (PGD) in early pregnancy and at term.

	Maternal Circulation				Fetal Circulation			
	Early Pregnancy		Term		Early Pregnancy		Term	
	Subsq GDM	PGD	GDM	PGD	Subsq GDM	PGD	GDM	PGD
Insulin	↑ (wk 13)		↑	↑ (IT)	↑ (wk 15)		↑	↑
IGF1	↓ (wk 13)	↓	↑	↓			↑ (corr. with BW)	↑ (corr. with BW)
IGF2			NC	NC			↑	↑
VEGFA			↑					↓
FGF-2			↑	↑			↑	↑
Leptin	↑ (wk 13)		↑	NC	↑ (wk 15)		↑	↑
TNFA	↑ (wk 14–20)		↑				↓ (M)	

NC: no change; IT: insulin treatment; BW: birth weight; M: macrosomia; wk: gestational week.
Differences in GDM versus PGD are marked in gray. If not indicated otherwise, early pregnancy refers to the first trimester.

Clinical Pearl

Cord blood insulin levels are an indicator of maternal metabolic control.

Research Spotlight

Fetal hyperinsulinism is a key feature of GDM. It results from increased maternal-to-fetal flux of glucose and overstimulation of the fetal pancreas.

Oxidative and nitrative stress of the placenta in diabetes

Pregnancy is a state of oxidative and nitrative stress resulting from generation of reactive oxygen and nitrogen species. The most common reactive species include superoxide, hydrogen peroxide, hydroxyl, nitric oxide, and nitrogen dioxide.

Reactive oxygen species (ROS) influence placental development as second messengers in cellular signaling to control cell fate. Excessive free radicals can act on protein, lipids, and DNA to yield massive cell death and tissue damage. There are many enzymatic and nonenzymatic antioxidants to avoid such damage in the human placenta. Key among these are mitochondrial manganese and cytosolic copper-zinc superoxide dismutases, catalase, glutathione peroxidase/reductase, reduced glutathione, vitamin C and vitamin E. Under normal conditions these defense systems have the capacity to induce conversion of ROS to water and molecular oxygen. This conversion prevents ROS overproduction as a consequence of increased metabolic activity of placental mitochondria throughout gestation. Pregnancy pathologies, such as early pregnancy failure, preeclampsia and diabetes mellitus, are often associated with an imbalance between ROS formation and the antioxidant defense mechanisms of a cell or tissue [3].

Alterations in antioxidant defense systems and marker of oxidative stress in PGD mellitus

High glucose concentrations yield excess ROS, especially superoxide. ROS derive from enhanced mitochondrial electron transport chain flow, nonenzymatic protein glycosylation, glucose auto-oxidation, and changes in cellular redox potential. Hyperglycemia-induced oxidative bursts also result in an enhanced production of ketone bodies, reduced concentrations of nicotinamide adenine dinucleotide phosphate (NADPH) and glutathione. Diabetic patients generally have impaired antioxidant defense systems and enzyme activities. For instance catalase and glutathione peroxidase are decreased, and increased oxidative stress could induce trophoblast apoptosis.

Animal models, like the Cohen diabetes-sensitive rats, provide *in vivo* data that maternal hyperglycemia induces embryonic oxidative stress. Nitroxide radicals effective antioxidants that protect rat embryos from oxidative stress-mediated diabetic damage, glutathione peroxidase, and superoxide dismutase are significantly reduced in T1D, whereas malondialdehyde from lipid peroxidation is produced in excess. High concentrations of nitrates and nitrites in placental tissue reflect nitrative stress in patients with preexisting diabetes. Plasma levels of nonenzymatic antioxidants, like vitamin E, are significantly lowered in pregnant women with PGD, compared to controls [3].

Clinical Pearl

Oxidative and nitrative stress markers are increased in GDM and T2D in the maternal circulation.

Research Spotlight

The placenta shows signs of oxidative and nitrative stress because of an imbalance in stressors over defense systems

Antioxidant defense systems in GDM

Diabetic women show increased levels of catalase and glutathione reductase in placental tissue but no differences in glutathione peroxidase and superoxide dismutase, compared to nondiabetic patients. The tissues studied were also less responsive to exogenous oxidative stress, compared to nondiabetic pregnant women. There is less catalase in cord blood, maternal plasma, and placental tissue of GDM women and a decrease of glutathione peroxidase activity but only in placental tissue. Superoxide dismutase was enhanced in cord plasma, but not in maternal plasma and placental tissue. Activation of xanthine oxidase (main free radical-producing enzyme in living cells) and formation of malondialdehyde were highly enhanced in maternal blood, cord blood and placental tissue. Placental explants of GDM mothers exhibited decreased nuclear factor-κB DNA-binding activity and showed no changes in 8-isoprostane (marker for oxidative stress) release in

Table 30.2 Alterations in antioxidant defence systems and marker of oxidative or nitrative stress in pregestational and gestational diabetes mellitus.

	Pregestational Diabetes Mellitus	Gestational Diabetes Mellitus
Antioxidants		
Superoxide dismutase	↓	=/↓
Catalase		↑/↓
Glutathione peroxidase	↓	=/↓
Glutathione reductase		↑
Vitamin E	=/↓	=/↓
Glutathione	↑	↑
Markers of oxidative and nitrative stess		
Malondialdehyde	↑	↑
Thiobarbituric acid-reactive substances		↑
8-isoprostane		=/↑
Xanthine oxidase		↑
Nitrites/Nitrates	↑	

↓ ↑ = Denotes either a decrease, an increase, or no change vs. nondiabetics.

response to oxidative stress. However, also an enhanced placental release of 8-isoprostane in GDM women was reported. Elevation of nitrative stress was shown in blood samples, placental and umbilical cord tissue of GDM pregnancies. Data are summarized in Table 30.2.

These data indicate that oxidative and nitrative stress is present in normal pregnancies, but it is even more pronounced in PGD and GDM pregnancies, resulting from impaired antioxidant defense mechanisms. The considerable variation in findings may reflect differences in oxidative stress associated with the wide range of metabolic control achieved and the inflammatory pro-oxidative environment associated with varying degrees of maternal obesity.

The human placenta in diabetes

The placental responses to the diabetic environment depend foremost on the time of onset and duration of exposure to hyperglycemia. Severity of diabetes, treatment modality, maternal metabolic status, and maternal body weight have lesser but important effects. T1D and T2D in the first trimester may influence trophoblast proliferation, differentiation, and invasion to affect placental development throughout pregnancy. GDM manifests in the second half of gestation but influences villous maturation, vascularization, and branching along with metabolism and transport. Importantly, levels of insulin, IGF1, VEGF, FGF-2, leptin, and TNF-alpha are abnormal as early as the 13th week of gestation in women destined to become GDM. Moreover, insulin and leptin levels in the fetal compartment are elevated by the 15th week of gestation, even before the clinical onset of GDM. Therefore, changes in placental development, function, or both may occur before the clinical manifestation of GDM (Figure 30.1). Indeed, placental morphology at term in GDM is not dissimilar from that in PGD pregnancies. The multicenter HAPO study showed a continuum between maternal glycemia and fetal outcome, and we speculate that placental changes are also on a continuum rather than showing dichotomous outcomes. Here we distinguish among the periods in gestation in the summary analyses of the effects of diabetes on the placenta [2,4].

First trimester of gestation

PGD is associated with a higher risk for missed abortions in the first trimester, which intuitively suggest failure of trophoblast invasion. However, there is sparse literature about early placental changes in diabetes but in rodents, diabetes alters placental ECM composition during placentation that could impact early basal plate development. Human T1D associates with altered levels of matrix-metalloproteinase MT1-MMP, a central molecule for tissue remodeling during the invasive process [5].

Placental changes in the third trimester of a diabetic pregnancy are likely to have their origin from in early pregnancy. Shallow trophoblast invasion in early pregnancy yields reduced uteroplacental blood flow and predisposes to preeclampsia, intrauterine growth restriction, or both. Notably, the incidence of developing preeclampsia in diabetic pregnancy increases directly with the first trimester maternal HbA1c levels T1D pregnancies. Additionally, T1D is associated with a lower than expected fetal crown-rump length at week 12, and because there is a close relationship between fetal and placental weight, one might conclude that impaired trophoblast growth may also yield a smaller than expected placenta. This hypothesis is indirectly supported by lower maternal levels of

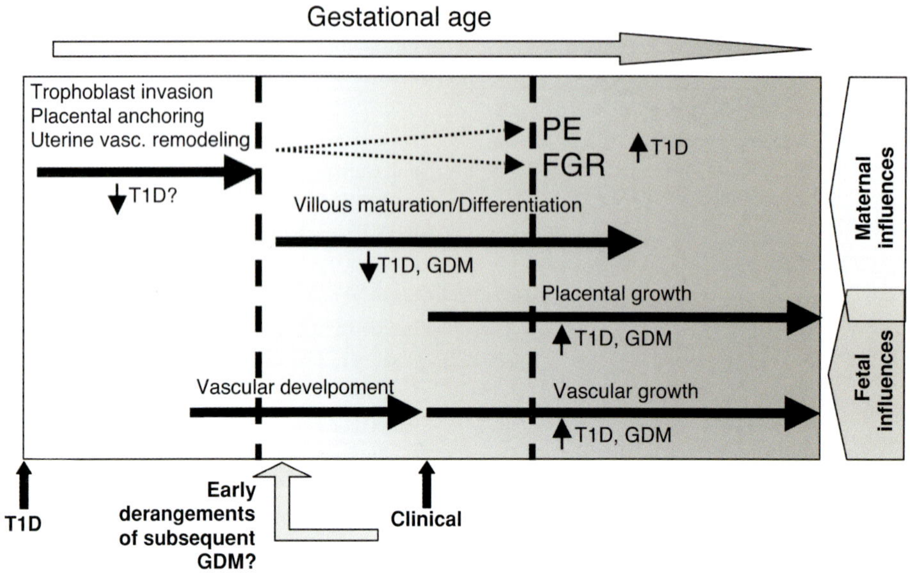

Figure 30.1 Effects of maternal diabetes on the placenta depend on the developmental processes taking place during the insult. PGD may affect trophoblast invasion early in pregnancy, leading to an increased risk for early pregnancy loss, later preeclampsia (PE) or fetal growth restriction (FGR). GDM manifests in the second trimester. Because endocrine changes can be observed before the onset of GDM, an effect of GDM on processes earlier in gestation may be hypothesized. Both GDM and PGD may affect villous maturation as well as vascular and placental growth. Because trophoblasts are in direct contact with maternal blood, the maternal diabetic environment will alter processes that involve trophoblast function. In contrast, the placental vasculature is in direct contact with fetal blood and, hence, fetal derangements resulting from maternal diabetes will mainly affect the placental vasculature.

hPL in first trimester T1D, as the hPL protein hormone is secreted proportional to placental weight.

Third trimester of gestation

Placental structure

Placental morphological changes resulting from T1D and T2D resemble changes also observed in GDM, and all placental phenotypes reflect the quality of glycemic control. The placental morphological characteristics of GDM, T1D, and T2D will thus be discussed in one section. Placental changes in diabetes that can be observed in a cross section of placental villi are schematically shown in Figure 30.2.

Excess placental weight in diabetes correlates with antenatal glucose control. The increase in tissue mass results from overproduction of extracellular matrix and heightened interstitial edema. Furthermore, fibrinoid necrosis is observed more frequently. Villous immaturity and cytotrophoblasts that are more apparent by histology, for any given gestational age are typical in the diabetic placenta. The etiology of this cytotropholast prominence is unclear, but may relate to cytotrophoblast hyperproliferation or to reduced cytotrophoblast fusion to form syncytiotrophoblast. This stated, the concept of villous immaturity in diabetes was challenged recently (Desoye and Kaufmann). Villi in diabetes often exhibit more capillary cross sections, diffuse capillary distribution, and a random arrangement of stem vessels. These findings clearly differentiate them from immature villi that are characterized by less capillaries per section, subtrophoblastic capillary distribution, and central location of stem vessels. Basement membranes of the syncytiotrophoblast and endothelium are thickened in PGD and GDM, and this likely reduces villous diffusion capacity for oxygen [6].

Hypervascularization of the villi is also a common finding [6]. In T1D this is secondary to the enhanced longitudinal growth, whereas in GDM vascular branching is increased. The underlying mechanism for stimulation of branching or non-branching angiogenesis is unknown. The enlargement of the vascular surface and also placental

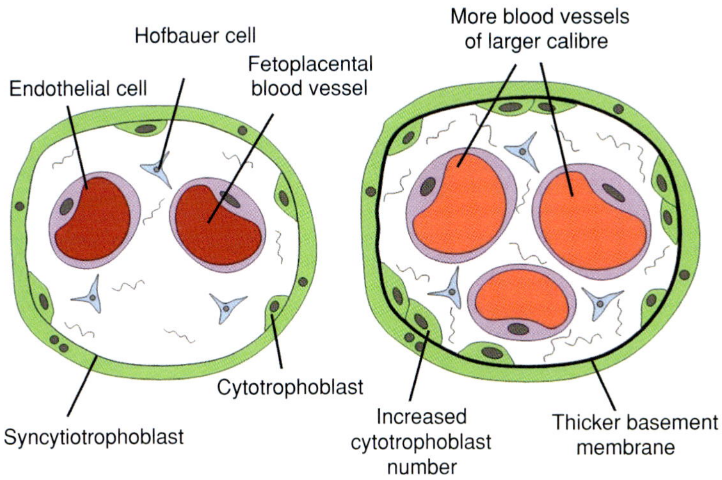

Figure 30.2 Characteristic changes associated with maternal diabetes in placental villi at term of gestation. The scheme depicts a cross-section of a placental villus from normal (left) and diabetic (right) pregnancy. The placenta in diabetes is characterized by increased surface area, thickening of the trophoblast basement membrane, increased number of cytotrophoblasts as well as an increased number (hypervascularization) and calibre of blood vessels embedded in a stroma with more extracellular matrix proteins. Furthermore, fetal hypoxia (indicated by light red colouring of vessel lumen) is a common feature in diabetes as suggested by higher levels of cord blood erythropoietin.

surface area of exchange may by counterintuitive in a situation of maternal nutritional oversupply. However, this may reflect a response to inadequate oxygen supply to the fetus where fetal hypoxia is reflected by polycythemia and elevated cord blood erythropoietin levels. Elevated maternal HbA1c levels with higher oxygen affinity, reduced uteroplacental blood flow, and a longer maternal-to-fetal diffusion distance may diminish oxygen supply. At the same time fetal hyperinsulinemia stimulates aerobic metabolism, thus increasing oxygen demand. Low-fetal-oxygen levels may induce placental expression of proangiogenic factors, such as FGF-2 and VEGF. In PGD as well as GDM, the expansion of the vascular tree is also paralleled by an increase in capillary volume and diameter. This dilatation of the placental capillaries may again result from fetal hypoxia, because low oxygen is known to upregulate eNOS expression via hypoxia inducible factor responsive elements (HRE) enabling the production of higher levels of the vasodilator NO. This hypothesis is further supported by the finding that placental eNOS expression is elevated in diabetes. The scheme in Figure 30.3 shows our current working model of the causes of fetal hypoxia in diabetes and its consequences for placental morphology.

Clinical Pearl

As a consequence of maternal and placental changes in diabetes, oxygen transport is reduced. At the same time fetal hyperinsulinemia stimulates aerobic metabolism, thus increasing oxygen demand. The overall effect is fetal hypoxia.

Research Spotlight

Placental hypervascularization is the result of fetal hypoxia.

Placental function

Diabetes induced structural changes in the placenta increases its expression of transferrin receptors, modifying them to sustain the increased fetal iron demand by stimulated haemoglobin synthesis in order to compensate for impaired oxygen supply.

The collective and current concepts for transplacental glucose transport in diabetes is that transport is unchanged in diabetes and the increased glucose flux is a result of the steeper concentration gradient (details discussed in the chapter by N. Illsley). Maternal, placental, and fetal concentrations of amino acids are elevated in diabetes, but the data are too sparse to allow sensible conclusions on amino acid transport processes [7,8].

Research Spotlight

Transplacental glucose transport is unaltered in GDM. Increased glucose flux is the result of steeper concentration gradients.

Recently, transport and metabolism of lipids has received interest, first because of the role of fatty acids and lipids in enhanced fetal adiposity and to the putative programming of adult atherosclerosis by intrauterine hypercholesterolemia associated with obesity and

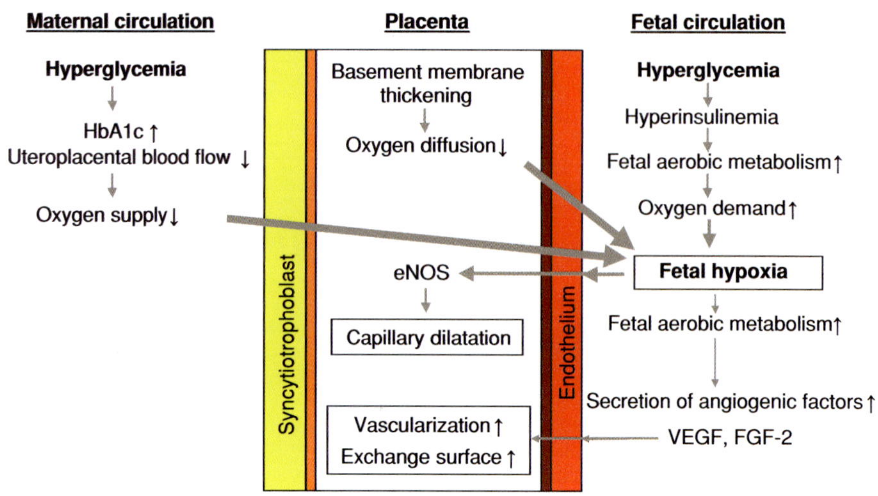

Figure 30.3 Causes for fetal hypoxia and consequences for placental morphology such as enlargement of vascular surface and capillary dilatation. Elevated maternal HbA1c and reduced uterine blood flow impairs oxygen supply to the fetus. There is further hindrance to oxygen delivery from basement membrane thickening in the placenta. Hyperglycemia resulting in hyperinsulinemia in the fetus increase fetal oxygen demand. The imbalance in oxygen supply and demand results in fetal hypoxia that stimulates the expression and secretion of angiogenic factors causing placental hypervascularization. Hypoxia further stimulates eNOS expression ultimately resulting in placental capillary dilatation.

diabetes (details will be discussed in the chapter by Y. Sadovsky).

The placenta is capable of nutrient storage, and elevated levels of placental glycogen, triglycerides, and phospholipids in both T1D and GDM are a common feature. Glycogen is predominantly stored in or around the fetoplacental vessels suggesting a source for the glucose originating from the fetal circulation. Placental glycogen stores may serve as a buffer for excess fetal glucose, but the buffer capacity is lower than that for fetal heart and skeletal muscle. However, the diabetic placenta appears to be the only fetal tissue with the capacity to increase its glycogen depots. At present, it appears more likely that placental glycogen serves as energy stores for local demands.

The placenta stores more lipids in diabetic pregnancy compared with nondiabetic, and the lipid composition is changed in these two phenotypes. T1D is associated with higher placental levels of linoleate, whereas GDM results in enhanced arachidonic and docosahexaenoic acids levels. Microarray analysis of placental tissue from normal, GDM, and T1D pregnancies revealed that, in GDM with maternal obesity, differentially expressed genes involved in metabolic functions are mainly related to lipid pathways. In contrast, metabolism-related genes altered in T1D are more involved in glycosylation and acetylation pathways. This supports the hypothesis that placental lipid accumulation may be a contributing factor towards excess fetal adiposity.

> **Research Spotlight**
>
> Higher placental glycogen and lipid content reflects higher nutrient availability in diabetic pregnancy that ultimately leads to fetal macrosomia.

Metabolic pathways contribute to the formation of NADPH, such as pentose phosphate shunt enzymes and NADP-malate-dehydrogenase. The placental requirements for this cofactor are higher in diabetic pregnancies because of increased activity of the processes listed in Table 30.3.

Uteroplacental and fetoplacental blood flow

Proper placental transport critically depends on adequate uteroplacental and fetoplacental blood flow. Flow-limited transport (oxygen, carbon dioxide, glucose) directly depends on blood flow to the exchange surfaces and can be compromised if either maternal or fetal circulations are suboptimal. Uteroplacental blood flow depends

Table 30.3 NADPH-dependent processes that may be activated in diabetes.

- Fatty acid synthesis
- Reduction of GSSG (GPx)
- Hydroxylation reactions (monooxygenases)
  Cholesterol biosynthesis
  Steroid biosynthesis
  Collagen biosynthesis
  Detoxification reactions

on opening and remodeling of the maternal spiral arteries into low-resistance vessels by invasive trophoblasts. Any impairment in this process may lead to reduced maternal blood flow into the intervillous space. Although indirect evidence exists that trophoblast invasion is reduced in maternal T1D, direct evidence is missing. About one-third of T1D pregnancies are associated with changes in decidual arteries ranging from mild modifications such as thickening or hyalinization of the arterial wall to severe changes including fibrinoid necrosis, thrombosis, or acute atherosis. Blood flow velocity, as measured by Doppler, may be altered in maternal T1D and in GDM depending on the degree of departure form normoglycemia. *Ex vivo* experiments clearly show a tolerance of the fetoplacental vasculature for some degree of hyperglycemia. In some cases of T1D, increased vascular impedance was found, most likely as a consequence of narrowing of placental bed arterioles from acute atherosis. There may be other factors contributing to reduced uteroplacental blood flow either singly or in combination [7] (Table 30.4).

As a consequence of changes in the placental vasculature, fetoplacental blood flow may be compromised. Various studies report controversial results on uterine and umbilical blood flow, which may depend on the type, duration, and severity of maternal diabetes but also on the particular setup of the measurements. Umbilical artery blood flow may be decreased, particularly when maternal HbA1c levels are high. This is different in GDM where changes in uterine and umbilical artery vascular impedance do not correlate with HbA1c but with fetal macrosomia.

Table 30.4 Reasons for reduced uteroplacental blood flow in diabetes.

- Inadequate opening of spiral arteries
- Narrowing of placental bed arterioles (acute atherosis)
- Reduction in intervillous space volume because of villus edema and more bulbous villi
- Hyperglycemia-induced reduction in trophoblast estradiol synthesis, a vasodilator
- Imbalance in local prostacyclin and thromboxane production in favour of the vasoconstrictor thromboxane

Clinical Pearl

Low glycemia control of the mother may result in reduced uteroplacental blood flow.

The human placenta in obesity

Diabetes and obesity are both associated with inflammation. The placenta is capable of producing and releasing virtually all known cytokines. In early gestation these cytokines are involved in establishing pregnancy, but their role at the end of pregnancy is less defined. Placental expression of several cytokines is elevated in obesity thereby contributing to the already existing proinflammatory environment. Placental cytokines may underlie the presence of a higher number of placental macrophages. The placenta is also under more nitrative, but less oxidative stress, in this condition. The expression of insulin signaling molecules is altered in obesity in a fashion that represents an intermediate stage between a normal and a deranged expression in GDM [4].

The scarcity of information to date highlights the importance of further studies into the effect of maternal obesity, without other pregnancy pathology, on placental histology and function. Since obesity in pregnancy is becoming a research focus of increasing interest, abnormalities in the placenta and their effect on the fetus are likely to be discovered. It is important, though, to understand that any study on obesity will have overlap with results from T2D and GDM. Therefore, information obtained on T2D and GDM will have significance for obesity pathophysiology and vice versa.

Teaching Points

1 The fetus in diabetic pregnancies is characterized by excessive fat accumulation irregardless of the absolute birth weight or birth weight centile.

2 The distinct placental changes associated with diabetes mellitus depend on the gestational period during which the diabetic insult occurs, and, thus, on the type of diabetes.

3 Early placental development may be altered by insulin and TNF-alpha-induced changes in matrix-metalloproteinases that degrade extracellular matrix.

4 The placenta is often heavier in women with diabetes with an increase in maternal, i.e., syncytiotrophoblast and fetal, i.e., endothelial surface area.

5 Hypervascularization of placental villi is the most prominent morphological change; it is the collective result of fetal hypoxia.

6 The oxidative and nitrative stress of a normal pregnancy is exacerbated in maternal diabetes.

7 Glucose from the maternal-to-fetal circulation is unaltered in GDM. The higher flux results from the steeper maternal-to-fetal concentration gradient. Amino acid transport may be altered.

References

1. Desoye G and Hauguel-de Mouzon S (2007) The human placenta in gestational diabetes mellitus. The insulin and cytokine network. *Diabetes Care* 30(Suppl. 2): S120–6.
2. Hiden U and Desoye G (2010) The human placenta in diabetes. In: McCance DR, Sacks DA, Maresh JG (eds.) *A Practical Manual of Diabetes in Pregnancy.* 1st edn. Oxford: Wiley-Blackwell; pp. 26–33.
3. Desoye G and Kaufmann P (2006) The human placenta in diabetes. In: Porta M, Matschinsky FM (eds.) *Diabetology of Pregnancy.* Basel: Karger; pp. 94–109.
4. Hiden U and Desoye G (2010) Insulin and the placenta in GDM. In: Kim C, Ferrara A (eds.) *Diabetes During and After Pregnancy.* 1st edn. New York: Springer; pp. 97–111.
5. Hiden U, Glitzner E, Hartmann M, et al. (2009) Insulin and the IGF system in the human placenta of normal and diabetic pregnancies. *J Anat* 215(1): 60–8.
6. Desoye G and Myatt L (2004) The placenta. In: Reece EA, Coustan DR, Gabbe SG, (eds.) *Diabetes in Women: Adolescence, Pregnancy and Menopause.* Philadelphia: Lippincott, Williams & Williams; pp. 147–57.
7. Desoye G and Hauguel-de Mouzon S (2003) The placenta in diabetic pregnancy. In: Hod M, et al. (eds.) *Textbook of Diabetes in Pregnancy.* London: Martin Dunitz; pp. 126–47.
8. Desoye G and Shafrir E (2008) The placenta in diabetic pregnancy: Placental transfer of nutrients. In: Hod M et al. (eds.) *Textbook of Diabetes in Pregnancy.* London: Informa Healthcare; pp. 47–56.

31

CHAPTER 31

Placental Origins of Intrauterine Growth Restriction

Ian P. Crocker

Maternal and Fetal Health Research Centre, School of Biomedicine, University of Manchester, St. Mary's Hospital, Manchester, UK

Introduction

Intrauterine growth restriction (IUGR), or fetal growth restriction (FGR), is a serious complication of human pregnancy. Conceptualized as a fetus failing to achieve its genetically pre-determined growth potential, IUGR contrasts with the diagnosis of small for gestational age (SGA), which reflects newborn birth weights below the 10th percentile for an uncomplicated obstetric population. IUGR affects 3–10% of first time births, and contributes to one-third of all ante-partum deaths, a tenfold increase in perinatal mortality, and severe neurodevelopmental disabilities. IUGR may also portend health complications in adult life, increasing the risk of hypertension, cardiovascular disease, and diabetes. These are chronic conditions attributed to "fetal programming," the concept that fetal responses to undernutrition, placental insufficiency, or both in utero, become permanent adaptations that predispose to adult diseases [1].

Clinical Pearl

IUGR is typically defined as fetal estimated weight <10th percentile for gestational age. However, clinically asymmetric fetal estimated weight <3rd percentile is a better predictor for perinatal morbidity.

Indirect placental origins of IUGR

Fetal growth and development, and placental structure and function, are a result of the dynamic integration of cell proliferation, differentiation and migration. There are numerous perturbations that modulate these processes including hormones, growth factors, extracellular matrix proteins, cell surface receptors, post-receptor signaling pathways, cell cycle control proteins, and apoptosis. The variables affecting these processes can be conveniently subdivided into genetic effects and environmental cues.

The genetic abnormalities that contribute to IUGR include the following: (1) imbalances of chromosome numbers, such as triplody, (2) confined mosaicism and uniparental disomy, karyotypic abnormalities of extra-embryonic tissues, and (3) syndromic disorders such as single gene mutations or partial chromosomal deletions, such as Cornelia de Lang syndrome.

Environmental cues hypothesized to influence fetal growth include infection, drugs and lifestyle factors. Of these, transplacental infection is uncommon, but maternal viremia (with cytomegalovirus) can lead to IUGR, fetal anomalies, or both, depending on gestational age with onset of infection. Doppler velocimetry may reveal umbilical artery waveforms consistent with abnormal placental development, as viral infections are potentially damaging to the placental capillary endothelium.

The Placenta: From Development to Disease, First Edition. Edited by Helen H. Kay, D. Michael Nelson and Yuping Wang.
© 2011 Blackwell Publishing Ltd. Published 2011 by Blackwell Publishing Ltd.

Drugs, such as opiates, cocaine, and antihypertensive medications, alter maternal and fetal physiology to restrict fetal growth. Although the influence of mild to moderate alcohol consumption on fetal growth is debated, alcohol is a teratogen, with extreme cases eliciting fetal alcohol syndrome and associated IUGR. Cigarette smoking at a population level is by far the single most important factor unequivocally linked to impoverished fetal growth. The effects of smoking are mediated through nicotine-induced secretion of vasconstrictive catecholamines and through the adverse impact of carbon monoxide (CO) and other toxins on oxygen transport and oxidative metabolism. Adaptive responses to smoking by the placenta include exaggerated angiogenesis and excessive apoptosis.

Direct placental-dependent origins of IUGR

Clinical signals—ultrasound

IUGR can be distinguished from SGA by evaluation of a combination of factors including prior history, serum biochemical markers such as low PAPP-A, raised inhibin, elevated alpha-fetoprotein and sonographic examination, monitoring fetal weight, disproportionate asymmetric growth (increased head to abdominal circumference ratio), reductions in amniotic fluid volume and abnormal Doppler waveforms in the umbilical artery, ductus venosus and middle cerebral artery.

In pregnancies complicated by severe IUGR, Doppler flow velocity waveforms for umbilical arteries are usually aberrant. In normal pregnancy, forward flow in these arteries is sustained throughout the cardiac cycle. Conversely, feto-placental flow indices in IUGR are higher than normal, detectable by measuring the increase in pulsatility index (PI) that progresses to absent or reversed end diastolic flow (EDF). Such circumstances associate with fetal hypoxia, acidosis, or both and may prompt consideration for early delivery. Increased uterine artery flow resistance manifests as raised PI or resistance index (RI) between 20–24 weeks' gestation, with or without the persistence of a "notched" waveform beyond 24 weeks. These findings are indicative of utero-placental vascular disease and have a positive predictive value of 30% for IUGR.

Reversed flow in the ductus venosus or changes in the cerebral circulation are particularly ominous signs. Increased diastolic blood flow to the fetal brain by Doppler assessment of the middle cerebral artery is considered a "brain sparing effect" and is demonstrated by a low PI. A loss of this effect can be critical to the survival of the overstressed fetus and may portend fetal death.

Other more direct ultrasound assessments of the human placenta have been undertaken. With standard B-mode sonography the placenta appears relatively homogenous, with areas of differing echogenicity with advancing gestation. In early studies, increased echogenicity and cotyledonary segmentation were used to grade placental maturity (Grannum grade) with early maturation considered indicative of IUGR; nevertheless this classification was never widely adopted. Careful ultrasound examination of the human placenta can suggest histopathological changes, such as infarctions, acute atherosis and fibrin deposition. A recent and more reliable sonographic indicator of IUGR is a measurement of placental depth greater than 4 cm, which may reflect compensatory growth by a stressed placenta.

Clinical signals—magnetic resonance imaging (MRI)

Although ultrasound is the preferred tool for antenatal monitoring, MRI is a powerful developing technology that allows quantitative analysis of several indices that relate tissue structure and function. MRI provides quantified volume assessments of the placenta and insights into equivocal ultrasound evidence of placental accreta, increta, or percreta. Pioneering studies, using relatively low field strengths (0.5 T), suggest that MRI relaxation times (T1 and T2) may reflect placental composition, and even distinguish IUGR from a normally growing fetus [2]. The less established techniques of arterial spin labeling (ASL) and intravoxel incoherent motion (IVIM) support an association between growth restriction and aberrant feto-maternal blood flow, but these data are preliminary and require confirmation by imaging at greater electromagnetic field strengths.

Research Spotlight

Uterine and umbilical artery Dopplers currently reflect integrated flow to the entire utero-placenta, while MRI can measure localized flow within the placenta per se.

Placental pathophysiology

Gross placental abnormalities and lesions

IUGR is generally related to a decrease in placental weight and a reduction in functional placental units. These placentas are often greater in thickness, as described above, and have a predisposition for abnormally eccentric cord insertion. Sonographic examination may reveal "placental lakes" or a "jelly-like placenta" in severe cases of IUGR, described by areas of hypoechogenicity, pathologically confirmed as ischemic thrombotic lesions, and a presumed result of spiral artery occlusions and decidual vasculopathy (Figure 31.1). Less common lesions include chronic villitis and hemorrhagic endovasculitis. The placenta has a significant reserve capacity and multiplicity or accumulation of utero-placental lesions and villus injury, and both, are necessary to yield clinically apparent placental dysfunction.

Oxygen and placental development

A key aspect of successful placentation is the invasion of extravillous trophoblasts and transformation of the decidual and intramyometrial portions of uterine spiral arteries. In cases of IUGR, reductions in utero-placental blood flow and alterations in intervillous hemodynamics result from retained spiral arteriole contractility, as a result of inadequate remodeling by trophoblasts. The absence of optimal utero-placental blood flow through these unmodified vessels suggests that hypoxia, re-oxygenation, oxidative stress, or a combination of these, are potential etiologies for IUGR.

The aberrant blood flow, which accompanies these pathologies, is often evident in preeclampsia and is coined "utero-placental hypoxia." This situation has similarities with "pre-placental hypoxia" from other sources such as maternal anemia or pregnancies at high altitude. In such cases, local reductions in oxygen delivery to the villi increase angiogenesis and stimulate trophoblast proliferation to produce highly vascularized terminal villi with restricted intervillous space (Figure 31.2). This is seen in milder cases of IUGR where there is preserved umbilical end-diastolic flow. In contrast, more severe IUGR with absent end-diastolic umbilical artery flow is due to a failure of oxygen transport from the intervillous space to umbilical vein. This restriction in the feto-placental circulation, termed "post-placental hypoxia," also leads to fetal compromise. Whether the villi exposed to these conditions are actually hyperoxic is controversial, but what is known is that there is a reduction in cytotrophoblast proliferation, increased deposition of stromal extracellular matrix, greater signs of nuclear senescence and predominance of non-branching angiogenesis. These changes are reflected by an exaggerated intervillous space and largely unbranched, longer, and filiform intermediate and terminal villi, yielding an increase in capillary mediated vascular impedance. Other histological evidence of maladaptation includes stem artery wall thickening, medial hyperplasia, and luminal obstructions due to stem vessel vasoconstrictions. These features are typical in severe IUGR and may advance to tissue sclerosis and obliteration of distal villi, contributing to reversed end diastolic umbilical artery flow and reflecting a local physiological response to inadequate feto-placental perfusions.

Trophoblast turnover

Apoptosis is a proposed part of (1) normal syncytiotrophoblast formation that occurs through differentiation and fusion of cytotrophoblast cells, and (2) villous trophoblast turnover, described as the extrusion and liberation of aged trophoblast material into the intervillous space and maternal circulation. The incidence of apoptosis in the villous placenta increases as pregnancy progresses and is further exaggerated in IUGR, evident by increases in nuclear condensation, DNA degradation, histologic prominence of syncytial knots, and expression of regulators of apoptosis including p53 and caspase-3. Enhanced apoptosis may result from (1) aberrant utero-placental conditions, as extremes of oxygen and oxidative stress can influence villous trophoblast turnover in vitro, or (2) heightened susceptibility to apoptosis, associated with inherent differences in intracellular apoptotic regulators. Regardless of this, excessive tissue injury is apparent in IUGR on an ultrastructural level, as evident by discontinuities in syncytium and marked fibrin containing fibrinoid deposition on the trophoblastic basement membrane. Such injuries are often not accompanied by compensatory increases in cytotrophoblast proliferation and differentiation. Although the outcome of the effects of these changes are controversial, imbalances in the villous trophoblast life cycle could conceivably reduce the functional capacity of syncytiotrophoblasts in IUGR and limit the ability of the villi to mediate nutrient transport and secretory functions [3].

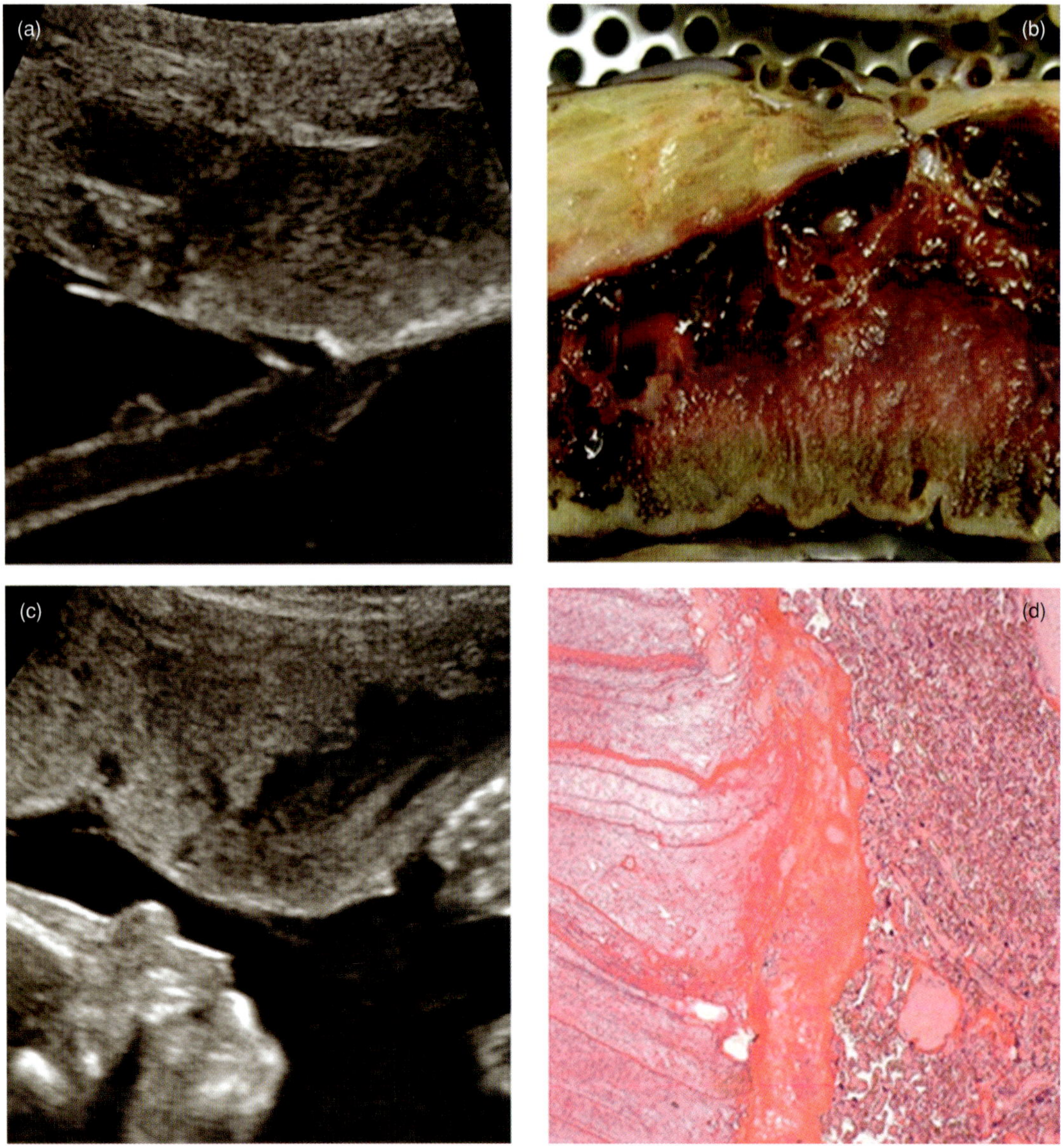

Figure 31.1 Sonographic appearances of gross placental lesions. Thickened "jelly-like" placenta with patchy areas of hypoechogenicity (a) and associated subchorionic thrombus (b). Echolucent "placental lakes" (c) representing areas of intervillous thrombi (d). (Reproduced by permission of BMJ Publishing Group Ltd. From Sebire NJ and Sepulveda W (2008) Correlation of placental pathology with prenatal ultrasound findings. *J Clin Pathol* 61(12): 1276–84.)

Similarities and differences with preeclampsia

IUGR may be superimposed by preeclampsia, a condition diagnosed when new hypertension and proteinuria occur after 20 weeks of pregnancy. Both conditions are thought to originate from failed trophoblast transformation of uterine spiral arteries and therefore, both represent a response by the placenta, the mother, or a combination of these, to utero-placental malperfusion. The presence or absence of preeclampsia does not greatly influence villus

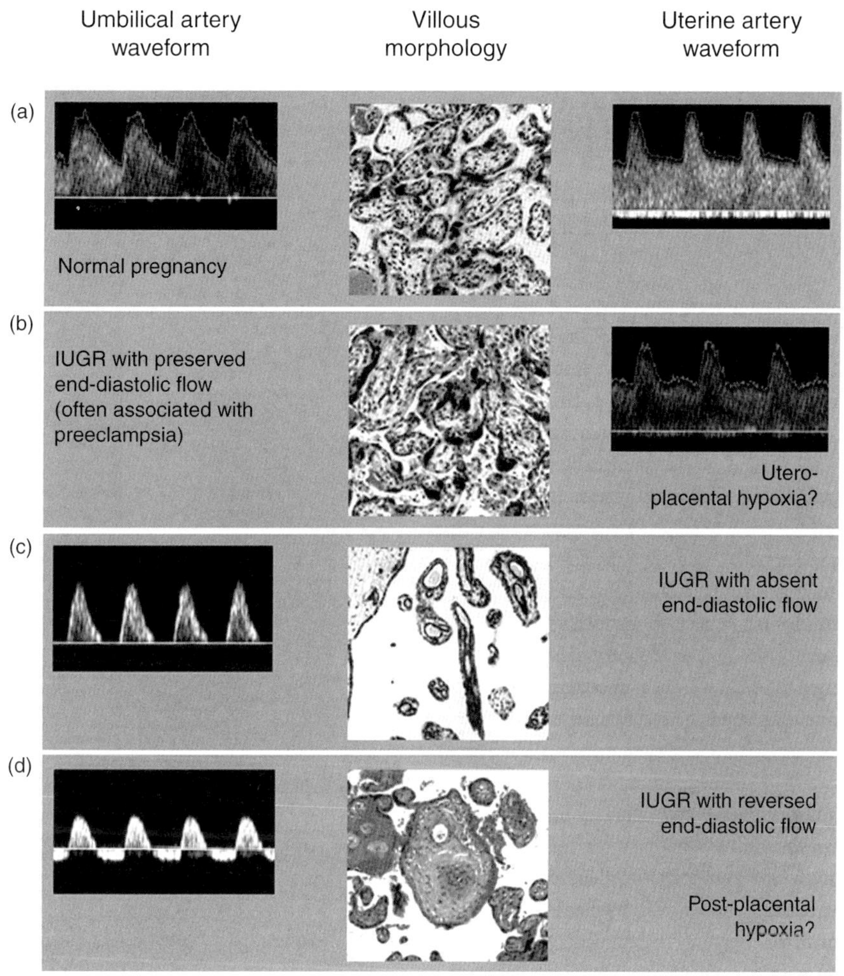

Figure 31.2 The relationship between umbilical and uterine artery Doppler flow velocities and villous placental morphology. (a) Normal umbilical and uterine waveforms corresponding to highly branched villi. (b) IUGR with abnormal uterine waveforms with pre-diastolic notch, suggestive of increased resistance and utero-placental hypoxia/oxidative stress, with compensatory villous branching and restricted intervillous space. (c) IUGR with umbilical artery Doppler with absent end-diastolic component, corresponding to increased placental resistance and post-placental hypoxia associated with unbranched and filiform villi. (d) IUGR with reversed end-diastolic umbilical flow, common with severe growth restriction and fetal hypoxia—associated histology showing fibrin-type fibrinoid deposition and stem vessel vasoconstriction. (Villous placental images reproduced with permission from Mayhew TM, Charnock-Jones DS, and Kaufmann P (2004) Aspects of human fetoplacental vasculogenesis and angiogenesis. III. Changes in complicated pregnancies. *Placenta* 25(2–3): 127–39.)

maturation or capillary formation, suggesting that clinical presentations of preeclampsia are due, in part, to differences in the maternal susceptibility to agents emanating from a stressed placenta. Maternal serum soluble fms-like tyrosine kinase 1 (sFLT-1) and a soluble TGF-beta co-receptor called endoglin are two factors raised in response to placental ischaemia that appear characteristic of the preeclamptic phenotype. A further suggestion is that preeclampsia, but not IUGR, is associated with aponecrosis of trophoblast, a more pathogenic form of cell death whereby trophoblast material is inappropriately packaged for release into the maternal circulation [4]. Supporting evidence in preeclampsia comes from a greater presence of syncytiotrophoblast-derived micro-fragments and fetal-derived cell-free DNA in maternal serum, and these, among other factors, may provoke an excessive maternal inflammatory response and vascular endothelial dysfunction [5].

> **Clinical Pearl**
>
> Although ultrastructural lesions can be identified post-delivery, gross placental lesions are uncommon. An exaggerated placental depth of >4 cm by ultrasound is a more reliable indicator of IUGR.

Growth factors and glucocorticoids

Insulin-like growth factor (IGF) axis

Although the overall control of fetal growth depends upon the interplay among fetal, placental and maternal factors, a family of polypeptides known as the insulin-like growth factors (IGF-I and IGF-II) and their cell surface receptors (IGF-R1 and IGF-R2) have emerged as critical regulators. Human mutations in the genes for IGF-I or IGF-R1 result in severe IUGR, but the majority of growth defects are not inherited. There is a direct correlation between fetal development and reduced IGF, and this is also evident in mice, where ablation of IGF-I and IGF-II genes, or elimination of IGF-R1, results in growth restriction and predisposes to perinatal lethality. In vitro studies have shown that IGFs-I and II stimulate placental cell proliferation, survival, and differentiated function. They also modulate fetal growth through improvements in nutrient transfer. Therefore, subtle alterations in the IGF axis may contribute to the placental-basis for fetal growth restriction [6].

Epidermal growth factor (EGF)

Many factors of decidual and placental origin including transforming growth factors (TGF-alpha and TGF-beta), fibroblast growth factor (FGF-acidic and FGF-basic) and associated proteins, such as endoglin, decorin, heparin sulphate proteoglycan, hematopoietic colony stimulating factor, human chorionic gonadotrophin, activin and inhibin, are implicated in trophoblast invasion and their interaction with the maternal decidua and myometrium. EGF influences placental development. EGF is present in high concentrations in maternal and fetal serum, and is produced by the placenta. This growth factor inhibits tumor necrosis factor-alpha (TNF-alpha) and hypoxia-induced apoptosis through phosphatidylinositol 3-kinase/protein kinase B survival pathways and enhances formation of syncytiotrophoblast. Altered expression of the EGF receptor (EGFR) in late gestation associates with IUGR, with alterations in tyrosine kinase activity, and with reduced auto-phosphorylation. These changes may contribute to deficits in syncytiotrophoblast metabolism and endocrine function.

Angiogenic growth factors and receptors

A number of angiogenic growth factors and their receptors have been identified in the human placenta: basic fibroblast growth factor (bFGF), hepatocyte growth factor, placenta growth factor (PlGF), vascular endothelial growth factor (VEGF) and angiopoietins (Ang) 1 and 2. VEGF-A, PlGF and their receptors are the most studied angiogenic growth factors. The primary receptors for VEGF-A are VEGFR-1 and VEGFR-2, whereas PlGF exerts its angiogenic effects solely through VEGFR-1. High levels of VEGF-A and VEGFR-2 coincide with vasculogenesis and branching angiogenesis during early placentation, and high concentrations of PlGF, Ang1, and Ang2 contribute to the non-branching phenotype of blood vessels in the second trimester. The expression of these major angiogenic factors is regulated by oxygen, with VEGF and VEGF receptors up-regulated by low oxygen, while PlGF is stimulated by elevated oxygen tensions. The molecular dysregulation of placental angiogenesis in IUGR is unclear.

Placental 11β-hydroxysteroid dehydrogenase

Glucocorticoids, such as cortisol, provide key signals for differentiation of fetal organs, in part due to their effects on IGF production. However, an excess of maternal cortisol can limit placental and fetal growth. The syncytiotrophoblast expresses high levels of 11β-HSD2, an intracellular enzyme that converts active cortisol to inactive cortisone. In IUGR, placental expression of 11β-HSD2 is reduced and cortisol–cortisone conversion is impaired. Maternal administration of glucocorticoids is widely considered to decrease neonatal morbidity and mortality for premature fetuses where delivery is anticipated, but more recent evidence shows divergent outcomes in these pregnancies. Certainly, an excess of cortisol associates with fetal programming that predisposes to sub-optimal metabolic and neuroendocrine development.

Research Spotlight

Animal models null for placental-specific transcripts of growth factor genes (e.g., *eNOS* and *Igf2* knockout mice) show placental changes that precede a decline in fetal growth, similar to IUGR in humans.

Placental nutrient delivery and transport

Idiopathic IUGR is generally attributed to aberrant trophoblast transformation of uterine spiral arteries that predispose to reductions in utero- and feto-placental blood flow, fetal hypoxemia, hypercapnia, acidosis and reduced umbilical concentrations of certain nutrients. Nevertheless, this sequence is overly simplistic as there are now an abundance of descriptive data to indicate that placental transport capacity in IUGR pregnancies results from alterations in plasma membrane transport systems [7].

Amino acids

In humans and animal models, IUGR is typified by a decrease in activity of placental amino acid transporters. Of these transporters, System A is crucial in mediating uptake of neutral amino acids across the syncytiotrophoblast. There is a direct relationship between birth weight and syncytiotrophoblast microvillous membrane System A activity in normal pregnancy. In IUGR pregnancies, this activity is reduced proportional to the severity of growth restriction. Other transporters of amino acids, such as taurine, leucine, and lysine, are also decreased in the placentas from IUGR cases. These in vitro findings coincide with in vivo studies using stable isotopes, which have confirmed inadequate placental amino acid transfer.

Protons

Protons are densely charged, hydrophilic, and do not readily cross plasma membranes. Placental ion transport either correlates with fetal growth or is regulated in a compensatory manner. The placental expression and activity of Na^+/K^+ ATPase and Na^+/H^+ exchanger (NHE) are down-regulated in IUGR proportional to growth restriction. These transporters are important for pH regulation, vectorial Na^+ flux, and amino acid uptake. Interestingly, the Ca^{2+} ATPase pump is up-regulated in the villous trophoblast basal plasma membrane in IUGR, possibly representing a compensatory response to increased fetal demand.

Glucose

Glucose is a primary energy source for the fetus and glucose transfer from the maternal circulation by the placenta constitutes the main fetal supply. Glucose transfer by the paracellular diffusion route is complemented by Glucose transporter-1 (GLUT-1) and Glucose transporter-3 (GLUT-3) from the facilitated glucose transport family of proteins. Collected cord blood at delivery shows that plasma glucose concentrations in IUGR fetuses are significantly reduced, particularly in cases with absent end-diastolic flow velocities. This and other findings suggest that utero-placental and feto-placental blood flow plays an important role in determining the net transfer of glucose. Currently, no significant differences in GLUT expression or glucose transporter activities have been established in the placenta in cases of IUGR.

Oxygen and carbon dioxide (CO_2)

Oxygen readily diffuses across the placenta and exchange is primarily limited by the rate of supply from maternal blood flow and removal by fetal blood flow. Uterine O_2 content in pregnancies with IUGR is higher and the coefficient of O_2 extraction is reduced. This suggests that impairments in the feto-placental circulation are more important in oxygenation of the fetus than uterine blood flow per se. This principle also applies to the transplacental transfer of CO_2, where fetal hypercapnia occurs as a consequence of reduced clearance of flow-limited gas.

Placental phenotypes of intrauterine growth

A range of placental phenotypes associate with fetal growth patterns (Figure 31.3). One phenotype is a normal sized placenta of typical thickness, with normal cord insertion and villous histology, and with adequate fetal and maternal blood flow and transport functionality. This phenotype underpins a fetus of normal size, appropriately grown to meet its genetic potential. A second phenotype is a placenta with moderately abnormal features, for example, with lesions or aberrant blood flow, but with compensatory changes in transporters, morphology, or both that optimize exchange to retain adequate function.

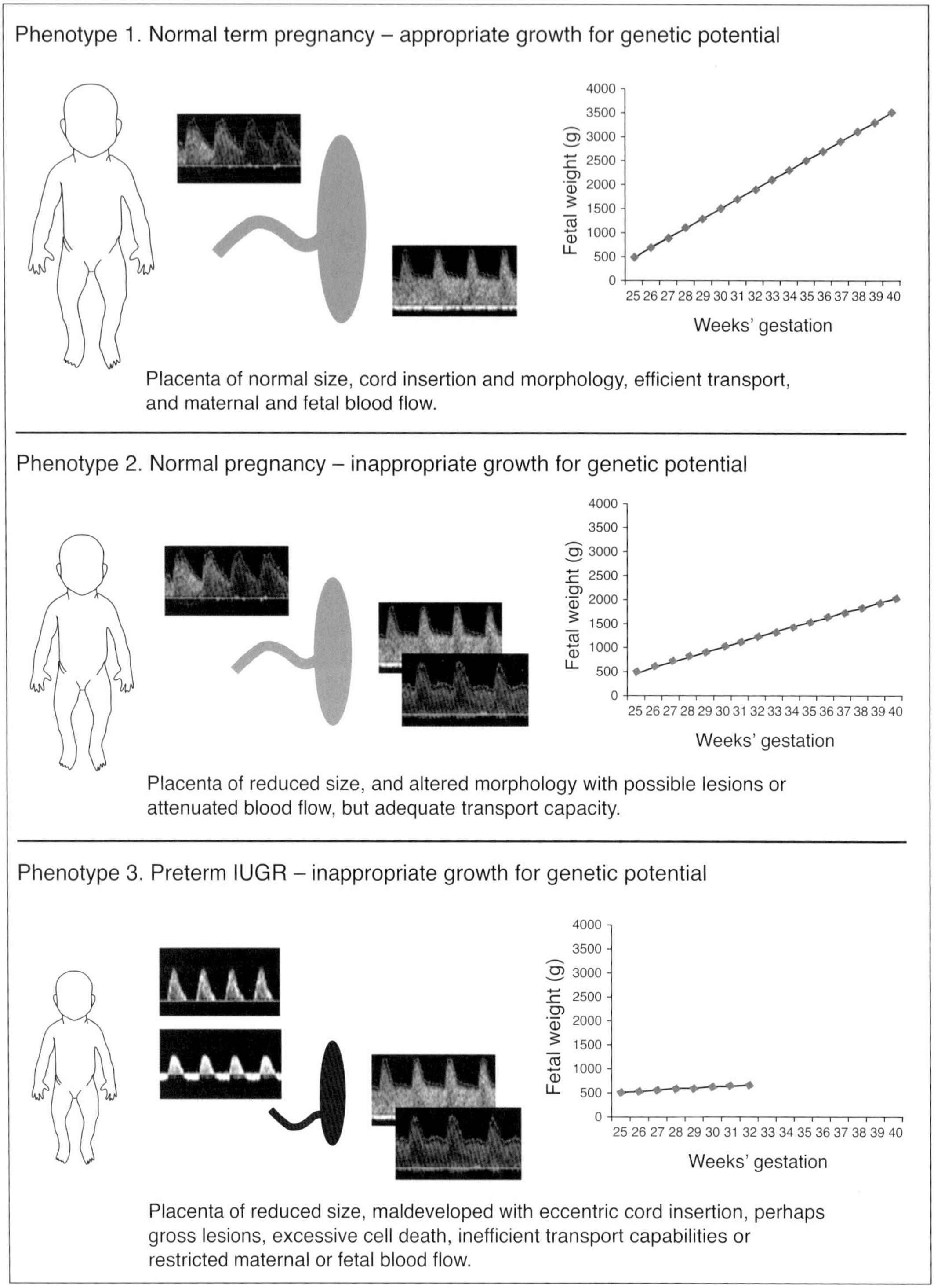

Figure 31.3 Placental phenotypes for normal pregnancies and IUGR.

This placenta yields a fetus with either normal growth parameters or small for gestational age, both of which have failed to attain their full genetic growth potential. Maternal blood flow may be restricted and preeclampsia may evolve with this second phenotype, but these changes will fail to affect the functional reserve of the placenta, not greatly limiting in utero growth. A third placental phenotype is one of villous malformation, eccentric cord insertion, compensatory increases in thickness, with evidence of subchorial thrombosis, aberrant transporter activities, excessive trophoblast cell death, and frequently aberrant umbilical artery resistances and fetal Doppler velocity waveforms. Although the placenta in these cases may adapt to disturbances in both supply and demand, compensatory changes are inadequate to sustain normal fetal development and IUGR with indicated iatrogenic prematurity results.

Future possibilities

The prediction of placental phenotypes in utero is in its infancy, but emerging non-invasive technologies, such as placental power ultrasound and MRI, are promising methodologies. Greater specificity in diagnosis of IUGR is essential to identify pregnancies truly at risk and those that would benefit from the development of in utero therapies. Importantly, improvements in placental phenotyping will disentangle ambiguities in the diagnosis of IUGR and allow targeted interventions to improve neonatal and perinatal sequelae.

☞ Teaching points

1. IUGR and SGA are not synonymous.
2. The etiology of idiopathic IUGR is unclear, but involves impaired placental perfusion.
3. The placenta has significant reserve capacity and compensatory mechanisms sparing fetal growth until severe placental dysfunction eventually yields IUGR.
4. Ultrasound and MRI hold potential to distinguish the placental phenotypes associated with growth restriction.

References

1. Godfrey KM and Barker DJ (2001) Fetal programming and adult health. *Public Health Nutr* 4: 611–24.
2. Gowland P (2005) Placental MRI. *Semin Fetal Neonatal Med* 10: 485–90.
3. Scifres CM and Nelson DM (2009) Intrauterine growth restriction, human placental development and trophoblast cell death. *J Physiol* 587: 3453–8.
4. Huppertz B, Kadyrov M, and Kingdom JC (2006) Apoptosis and its role in the trophoblast. *Am J Obstet Gynecol* 195: 29–39.
5. Redman CW and Sargent IL (2000) Placental debris, oxidative stress and pre eclampsia. *Placenta* 21: 597 602.
6. Randhawa RS (2008) The insulin-like growth factor system and fetal growth restriction. *Pediatr Endocrinol Rev* 6: 235–40.
7. Cetin I and Alvino G (2009) Intrauterine growth restriction: implications for placental metabolism and transport. A review. *Placenta* 30(Suppl A): S77–82.

32

CHAPTER 32
The Placenta in Preeclampsia

Fiona Lyall
Institute of Medical Genetics, University of Glasgow, Yorkhill Hospital, Glasgow, UK

Introduction

The placenta plays an important role in the pathophysiology of preeclampsia. An inability to remodel maternal spiral arteries and subsequent suboptimal placental blood flow is the first problem. The placenta also produces factors that perpetuate the compromised blood flow and enhance placental damage. More recently, placental angiogenic markers have become of interest for clinical prediction of the preeclamptic syndrome, as well as to distinguish among the phenotypes of preeclampsia.

Failed trophoblast invasion and placental abnormalities in preeclampsia

The demonstration of reduced maternal blood flow in the placenta of pregnancies complicated by preeclampsia provided the rationale for performing histological work in the placental bed to identify a cause for underperfusion. Histopathological analyses show spiral arteries in decidua and myometrium in normal pregnancy undergo "physiological change" [1]. The endothelium and smooth muscle of the vessels are replaced with a fibrinoid matrix and invasive trophoblast cells. This physiological change results in a substantial dilatation of the vessels, a loss of most of the response to vasoactive agents, and formation of a high capacitance-low resistance system to provide nutrients and oxygen to the growing placenta and developing fetus. In some publications, authors write that at term trophoblast replace the spiral artery endothelium and assume endothelial properties. However, this is not the case. Although the endothelium is lost early in the arteriole remodeling, the final stages of physiological change involve repair of the maternal endothelium. Histological findings at term indicate that trophoblast do not line vessels and do not express endothelial cell adhesion molecules. Endothelial adhesion molecules are only expressed on endothelial cells at term, further negating the role of trophoblasts in this regard [2].

There are two temporal and spatial pathways of trophoblast invasion known as the *endovascular route* and the *interstitial route*. In the endovascular route, trophoblasts enter the spiral artery lumina. In the interstitial route, trophoblasts move forward around the arteries. Trophoblast invasion is often described to occur in two waves with a month's interval between the invasive trophoblast populations. There is very little evidence or rationale to support this contention. One of the key features of preeclampsia is restricted invasion of spiral arteries in the placental bed, with endovascular trophoblast invasion limited to the decidual vessels. About half to two-thirds of myometrial vessels do not undergo physiological change (Figure 32.1). A misconception in the literature is that preeclampsia is associated with failure of all trophoblast invasion. In fact, the interstitial route of invasiveness into the inner third of the myometrium often proceeds normally (Figure 32.1), refuting the concept that all invasion is restricted.

Blood flow patterns have been measured using Doppler imaging in individual spiral arteries at 17–20 weeks of gestation to show that resistance and pulsatility indices are normally low, as would be expected from arteries that have

The Placenta: From Development to Disease, First Edition. Edited by Helen H. Kay, D. Michael Nelson and Yuping Wang.
© 2011 Blackwell Publishing Ltd. Published 2011 by Blackwell Publishing Ltd.

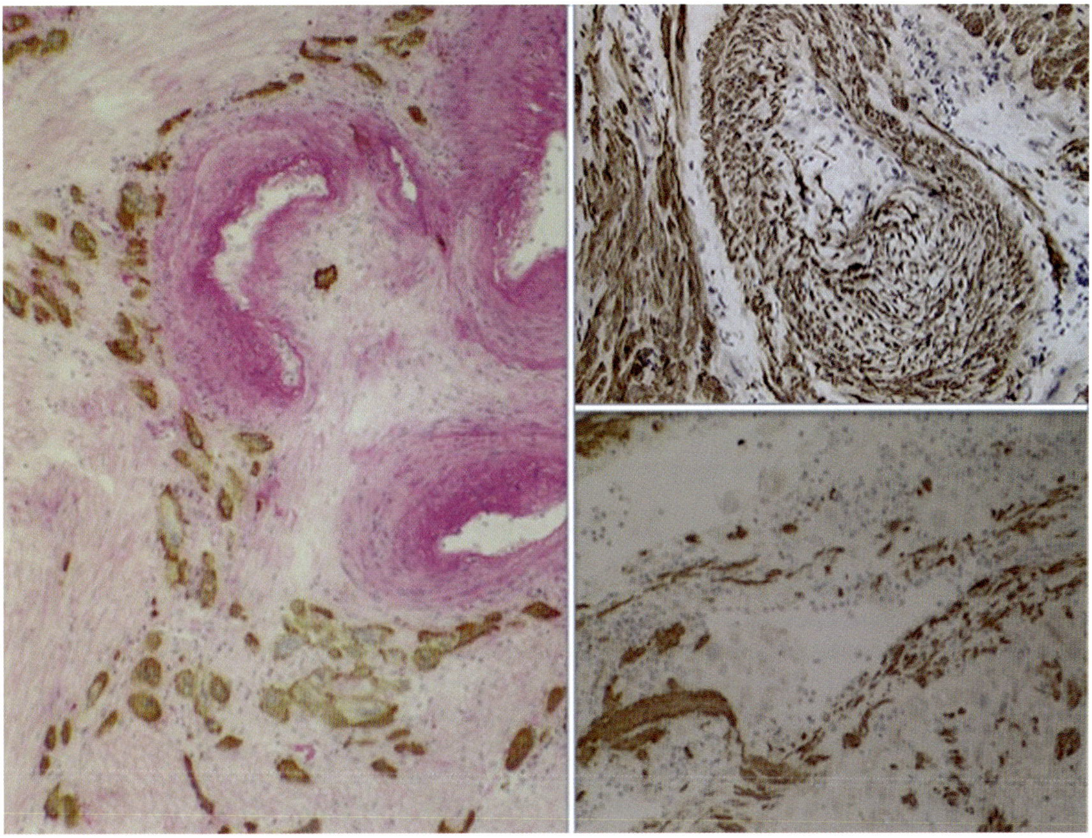

Figure 32.1 Spiral artery changes in preeclampsia. Left panel shows a spiral artery within the myometrium taken from a pregnancy complicated by preeclampsia in the third trimester. The vessel has not undergone physiological change. Despite the absence of endovascular trophoblast, abundant interstitial trophoblast can be seen around the vessel (stained with anticytokeratin antibody). The upper right panel shows a similar nontransformed myometrial spiral artery from a preeclampsia case (muscle wall and surrounding myometrium stained with antidesmin antibody. The lower right panel shows a partially transformed spiral artery. Since some muscle remains, this vessel may retain some contractile ability. Intermittent contractions from this type of vessel may result in an ischemic-reperfusion injury to the placenta.

undergone physiological change. In contrast, women with preeclampsia in the third trimester show high impedance to flow in the spiral arteries. This supports the hypothesis that defects in the maternal spiral arteries underlie reduced utero-placental blood flow in preeclampsia.

Myometrial vessels may also be partially transformed (Figure 32.1). The walls of these vessels may contract intermittently, to yield bursts of blood flow and ischemic–reperfusion insults to the placenta, a feature of preeclampsia [3].

Failure of spiral artery changes in preeclampsia has been proposed to cause altered flow to the placenta, the ensuing oxidative stress, and the associated release of endothelial damaging factors into the maternal circulation. Such factors released from the placenta into the maternal circulation have been evaluated as biomarkers to predict preeclampsia. These are discussed later in this chapter.

Clinical Pearl

There are multiple clinical phenotypes for women with the diagnosis of preeclampsia when based on the commonly used definition of new onset hypertension and proteinuria. These phenotypes likely have different etiologies even though they express similar pathophysiology.

Placental pathology and apoptosis

The principal changes in the placenta in preeclampsia are decidual arteriolopathy, infarcts in the central area, abruptio placentae, Tenney–Parker changes, and impaired growth [4]. Tenney–Parker changes refer to the increased surface budding of the placental syncytium that is characteristic of preeclampsia. They include mushroom-like protrusions containing normal nuclei and tangential sections of syncytial bridges, the latter being sectional artifacts. The sprouting is thought to be an adaptive change to altered maternal blood flow, oxygen content of the intervillous space, or both. Another phenotype of syncytial knots purportedly removes old syncytial nuclei as part of the normal turnover of syncytiotrophoblast. Knot-like apoptotic shedding may be one way of syncytiotrophoblast turnover and involves the apoptotic pathway. Aponecrotic knots resemble apoptotic knots but show edematous changes, plasma membrane defects, and incomplete apoptotic substrate cleavage. They are increased in preeclampsia. In necrotic shedding, parts of the syncytium undergo necrosis to release material that can induce an inflammatory response in the mother's systemic circulation. Total placental volume, total villous volume, and quantifiable cytotrophoblast parameters are generally not altered in preeclampsia, unless associated with fetal growth restriction. However, the relative proportion of mature intermediate villi, and terminal villi, with syncytial knots exhibiting apoptotic nuclei associated with preeclampsia is increased in all cases, irrespective of the presence or absence of fetal growth restriction.

> **Clinical Pearl**
>
> The placentae of women who develop preeclampsia at less than 32 weeks' gestation are usually small with abundant histopathology. The women who develop preeclampsia near or at term commonly have large placentas with more subtle pathology. These observations suggest the etiologies are different in the two groups.

Microparticles and syncytiotrophoblast membrane microparticles

One of the hallmarks of preeclampsia is an excessive systemic maternal inflammatory response. Cytokines and antiangiogenic factors released from the placenta are possible triggers. So-called "placental debris" made up of trophoblast cells and cellular fragments, including multinucleated syncytial knots described above, are possible triggers. Microparticles are membrane-bound vesicles shed into the circulation and derived from trophoblast cell activation, apoptosis, or necrosis. Microparticle production may normally function as a means of tissue to tissue signaling, but they are increased by stimuli such as cell activation, oxidative stress, and hypoxia. Microparticles derived from the synctiotrophoblast are known as syncytiotrophoblast microparticles or STBMs. STBMs are shed from the syncytiotrophoblasts, to be released into the intervillous space and ultimately passing to the systemic circulation to contact the maternal endothelium and leukocytes. The concentration of STBMs is increased in the circulation of women with early-onset preeclampsia. In vitro studies support the idea that microparticles modulate endothelial dysfunction. Plasma from preeclamptic patients contains placental microparticles to expose soluble fms-like tyrosine kinase (sFlt-1), which may influence angiogenesis. In vitro STBMs can activate peripheral blood monocytes with increased production of pro-inflammatory cytokines IL-8, IL-6, and IL-1β [5].

Placental blood flow and oxidative stress

Increased blood flow is achieved in both maternal and fetal circulations of the placenta by alteration of vascular anatomy, changes in vascular resistance, and variations in perfusion pressure. The maternal and fetal cardiovascular systems also have profound effects on placental perfusion. Vascular tone in the placenta is controlled by humoral factors, paracrine effects, and autocrine mechanisms [6]. Although increased impedance to fetal-placental flow is seen in preeclampsia, the source of this altered vascular reactivity is unknown, although production of the potent vasodilator prostacyclin is reduced.

Placenta endothelial cells express *eNOS*, which is responsible for nitric oxide (NO) release and vasodilatation. Studies on the perfused placenta have shown that NO contributes to basal tone of the placenta and attenuates the effects of vasoconstrictors. Both *eNOS* expression on villous endothelial cells and placental production of NO metabolites are increased in preeclampsia. This may be an adaptive response to the increased resistance. Placental syncytiotrophoblast also expresses *eNOS*, and the NO produced may affect platelet and leukocyte adhesion in the maternal intervillous space and have autocrine effects on other trophoblast and villous core components. An altered distribution of *eNOS* noted in syncytiotrophoblast in preeclampsia may well have pathological consequences.

Normal pregnancy is a state of oxidative stress due to the considerable metabolic activity of the placenta and the generation of reactive oxygen species, such as superoxide. This stress is further increased in preeclampsia due to increases in reactive oxygen species and consumption of antioxidant defenses. Although NO is scavenged by superoxide, the half-life of NO can be prolonged by the presence of superoxide dismutase which inactivates superoxide. The balance between superoxide and NO is thus important in determining the availability of NO, and this balance is disturbed in the placenta in preeclampsia.

NO and superoxide can also combine to form peroxynitrite, a potent pro-oxidant. Peroxynitrite is very unstable and hard to measure, but formation of nitrotyrosine by protein nitration is an indirect marker of peroxynitrite formation. Nitrotyrosine residues in the vascular endothelium and smooth muscle are more prominent in the placenta in preeclampsia when compared to normotensive pregnancies. Peroxynitrite treatment of the placental vasculature from normal placenta in vitro alters vascular reactivity to resemble the placental response in preeclampsia.

In preeclampsia, the placenta also experiences endoplasmic reticulum (ER) stress [3]. Activation of ER stress markers Gp96 and Grp78 are linked to peroxyntitrite production. The target for ER stress is primarily the syncytiotrophoblast, where there are adverse effects on protein synthesis.

The mitochondria are a major source of increased oxidative stress in preeclampsia. Superoxide, oxidative stress, and lipid peroxidation are increased in the placenta from preeclamptic pregnancy and are associated with an increase in the number of mitochondria, in mitochondrial enzyme activity and in the susceptibility of mitochondria to oxidation. Consequently, mitochondrial dysfunction caused by peroxynitrite contributes to altered energy metabolism and to the increased apoptosis noted in the syncytiotrophoblast in preeclampsia.

Carbon monoxide (CO) is produced by the hemeoxygenase (HO) enzymes, and like NO, CO causes vasodilatation. HO consists of two isoenzymes, HO-1 and HO-2. CO likely contributes to the maintenance of basal tone in the placenta, as inhibition of HO increases resistance in vitro in the perfused placenta. HO-2 expression is significantly reduced in villous endothelial cells in preeclampsia and this could have deleterious effects on blood flow to the fetus.

Research Spotlight

There is much debate about the level of oxygen in the intervillous space and villous tissues in women with preeclampsia. Hypoxia, ischemia with re-oxygenation, mechanical damage, or other factors may collectively contribute to placental injury in this condition. More research is needed to assess the placental pO_2 and oxygen concentrations present in vivo in women who manifest signs and symptoms of preeclampsia.

Placental derived factors and prediction of preeclampsia

Vascular endothelial growth factor (VEGF) and placenta growth factor (PlGF) are both angiogenic mediators produced by trophoblast. The VEGF receptor-1 (VEGFR-1), known as sFlt-1, is released from the placenta into the maternal circulation to bind both VEGF and PlGF. This reduces free VEGF and PlGF, and abdicates the protective effects of these growth factors on the maternal endothelium. Over a decade ago, VEGF serum concentrations were found to be lower in pregnant compared to nonpregnant women and were further reduced in preeclampsia [7]. The return to nonpregnant concentrations postpartum led the authors to propose that the reduction in VEGF was due to increased production of sFlt-1 from the placenta. sFlt-1 concentrations are indeed increased in established preeclampsia and, more importantly, as early as 5–8 weeks prior to the onset of clinical symptoms. The severity of preeclampsia is also correlated with concentrations of sFlt-1. Serum PlGF levels at 21 to 32 weeks of gestation are lower in preeclampsia that develops at less than 37 weeks, in severe preeclampsia, and in preeclampsia with a small-for-gestational-age infant. Urinary levels of PlGF are also significantly lower in women who develop preeclampsia in the late second trimester. Abnormal uterine arterial flow and low serum PlGF in the second trimester has been strongly associated with both early-onset and severe preeclampsia. The placenta produces several isoforms of sFlt-1. One of these isoforms, sFlt-1–14, is the primary isoform produced by the placenta in preeclampsia. Placental syncytial knots, induced by placental hypoxia, are a major source of sFlt-1–14. What causes increased sFlt-1 release is not known but may be linked to the transcription factor, hypoxia-inducible factor 1 (HIF-1alpha). HIF-1alpha levels are increased in placentas from cases of preeclampsia and HIF-1alpha regulates both *VEGF* and *Flt-1* gene transcription.

> **Research Spotlight**
>
> Serum levels of sFlt-1 and PlGF have 96% sensitivity, and 96% and 95% specificity, respectively, in the prediction of preeclampsia. Moreover, the ratio of sFlt-1/PlGF provides even a better test to aid in the diagnosis of preeclampsia with a 3% false positive rate. Although promising, none of these analyses are yet used in general clinical management of obstetric populations.

Soluble endoglin

Soluble endoglin (sEng) is a cell surface co-receptor for transforming growth factor-β (TGF-β) that is expressed on endothelial cells and trophoblast and up-regulated in placentae from cases of preeclampsia. Circulating sEng concentrations are increased in preeclampsia. sEng disrupts formation of endothelial tubes in vitro and induces vascular permeability and hypertension in vivo. Soluble endoglin concentrations rise approximately 2–3 months before the onset of preeclampsia. sEng levels are markedly elevated in women with pre-term preeclampsia or preeclampsia and a small-for-gestational-age infant. Endoglin and sFlt-1 may synergize and contribute to the syndrome of preeclampsia.

Pregnancy-associated plasma protein A (PAPP-A)

PAPP-A produced by trophoblast in early gestation modulates the activity of insulin-like growth factors (IGFs) and likely plays a role in implantation. PAPP-A concentrations are increased in maternal serum in preeclampsia. Indeed, low first trimester or second trimester PAPP-A levels are predictive of preeclampsia and also associate with other complications of pregnancy. Current studies are combining measurements of placental-derived factors with clinical parameters such as mean arterial pressure and uterine artery pulsatility index in an attempt to increase the sensitivity in the prediction of preeclampsia.

Inhibin A and activin A

Inhibin A and activin A are members of the TGF-β family. They are produced mainly by the placenta and maternal serum concentration increase in the third trimester. Maternal serum concentrations of inhibin A, activin A, or both, are elevated in women with preeclampsia indicating trophoblast dysfunction. They are elevated in the first and second trimester in women who develop preeclampsia. However, these proteins are not good predictors for preeclampsia as the sensitivities for disease are too low to be clinically useful.

Placental protein 13 (PP13)

PP13 is expressed exclusively in the placenta. It has been implicated in implantation and maternal vascular remodeling. In preeclampsia, PP13 is increased in maternal serum despite reduced placental expression. This could be due to increased syncytiotrophoblast membrane PP13 shedding into the maternal circulation. Low concentrations of maternal PP13 in the first trimester predict preeclampsia and this is generally a better predictor of early onset and severe preeclampsia than mild preeclampsia. Combined PP13 and uterine artery Doppler PI (pulsatility index) improve prediction.

Corticotrophin-releasing hormone (CRH)

CRH is synthesized by trophoblast and serum concentrations are increased in preeclampsia. This is associated with an increase in CRH binding protein, which negate the effects of CRH. Fetal, but not maternal, CRH can be stimulated by cortisol. Therefore, increased CRH release may be due to fetal cortisol release.

Human chorionic gonadotrophin (hCG)

hCG is secreted from differentiated trophoblast so alterations in plasma concentrations will reflect trophoblast dysfunction or alterations in trophoblast differentiation. Increases in maternal plasma hCG have been reported as early as 17 weeks of gestation in women who subsequently develop preeclampsia.

Research Spotlight

A cassette of proteins are dysregulated in women with preeclampsia, including VEGF, PIGF, sFlt, endoglin, hCG, PAPP-A, and inhibin to name a few. Research into mechanisms by which these proteins contribute to the pathophysiology may also yield a signature set of proteins that, when measured prospectively, predict risk and thereby allow interventions before clinical manifestations evolve [8].

The placental renin–angiotensin system

Placental proteases control fetal and maternal blood pressure by regulating the concentration of vasoactive peptides in the placenta. Angiotensinase A activity, which converts angiotensin II (Ang II) to Ang III, is abundant in syncytial microvilli. Because angiotensin and vasopressin play a role in normal and aberrant fetal–placental circulation in preeclampsia, the clearance of these peptides in the placenta is important in controlling fetal blood pressure. Pregnancy is associated with a refractory response to Ang II. However, women with preeclampsia are more sensitive to the pressor effect of Ang II and this is thought to be due to decreased degradation of angiotensin II by placental angiotensinase. Angiotensin 1–7 oppose the effects of Ang II, in part by stimulating the release of NO and prostacyclin (PGI_2). The placenta is also a rich source of the endopeptidase which converts AngI/AngII to Ang 1–7 and expression is increased in preeclampsia. Perhaps this

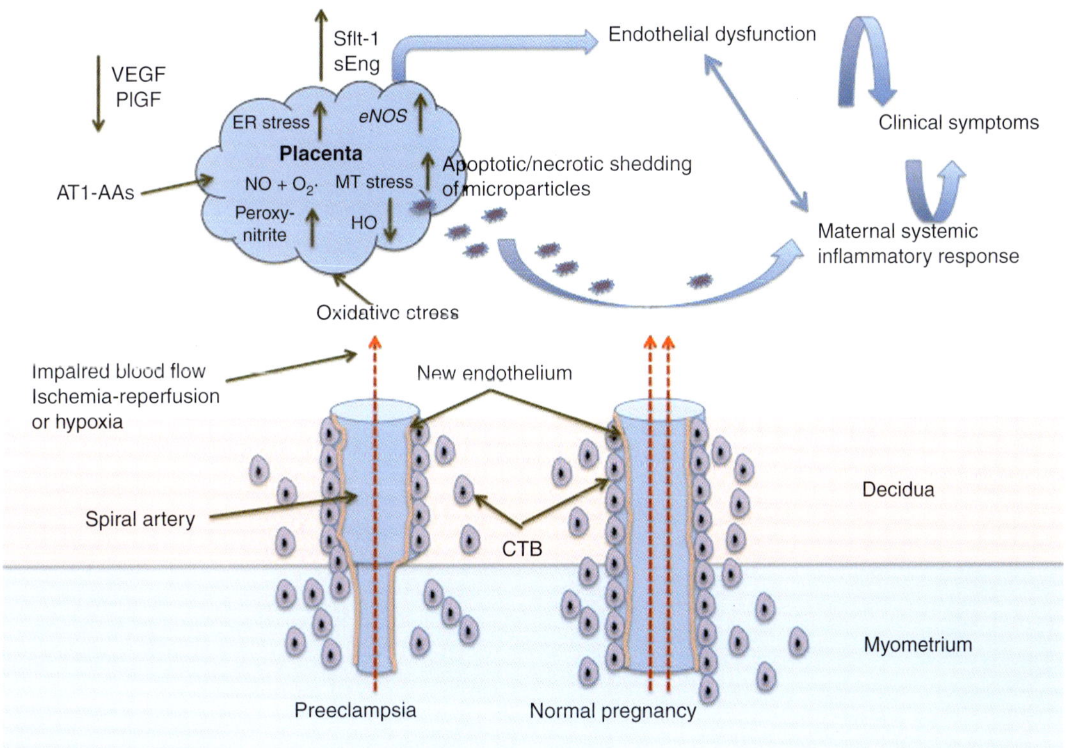

Figure 32.2 Schematic representation of the stages of preeclampsia. See text for full explanation. In stage one, myometrial segments of maternal spiral arteries do not undergo physiological change. Cytotrophoblast only migrate through the lumen of decidual segments. Note that interstitial invasion proceeds normally. At term, a new endothelium lies over the endovascular trophoblast. In stage two, the placenta is exposed to oxidative stress due to abnormal blood flow from the spiral artery. This, is turn, leads to both placenta damage resulting in the release of numerous damaging factors into the maternal endothelium and clinical symptoms as well as possible compensatory responses such as increased *eNOS*. CTB, cytotrophoblast; MT, mitochondria; ER, Endoplasmic reticulum; AT1-AAs, Angiotensin II autoantibodies.

is to counterbalance the effects of endothelial dysfunction. There are conflicting reports on the expression of components of the renin–angiotensin system in the placenta in preeclampsia. Women with preeclampsia have stimulatory autoantibodies to the angiotensin II, type 1 (AT1) receptor. These autoantibodies can activate AT1 receptors on many cell types leading to oxidative stress, increased production of pro-inflammatory mediators and inactivation of NO.

Placental-derived adipocytokines in preeclampsia

Insulin resistance is increased in pregnancy and further increased in preeclampsia. This is attributed to placental hormones and increased maternal adiposity. Adipocytokines, including leptin, adiponectin, TNF-alpha, Interleukin 6, resistin, visfatin, and apelin, are produced within the intrauterine environment. Placental expression, or secretion, or both, of adipocytokines in preeclampsia is controversial and levels do not correlate with maternal circulating concentrations. Further research is required due to their importance in metabolic control.

Summary

It is clear that the placenta plays a key role in preeclampsia by releasing damaging factors into the maternal circulation leading to maternal symptoms. The injury apparent in the placenta appears, at least in part, secondary to failed conversion of spiral arteries which limits normal maternal blood flow (Figure 32.2).

☞ Teaching Points

1. Failure to transform the myometrial segments of spiral arteries is associated with reduced blood flow to the placenta and is believed to be the primary pathophysiologic misstep leading to preeclampsia.
2. The endovascular pathway of trophoblast invasion in early pregnancy is impaired in preeclampsia. There is, however, abundant interstitial trophoblast invasion.
3. Failed spiral artery transformation is often linked to the ensuing oxidative stress in the placenta. Placental injury associates with release into the maternal circulation of endothelial damaging factors, such as syncytiotrophoblast microparticles and angiogenic factors that yield a maternal inflammatory response.
4. The expressions of *eNOS* and HO are altered in the placenta in preeclampsia. Since endothelial cells produce NO and CO, respectively, altered expression could have adverse effects on placental function.
5. Placental derived factors such as sFlt-1 and PlGF are being used as predictors of preeclampsia.

References

1. Pijnenborg R, Verycruysse L, Hanssens M et al. (2007) Trophoblast invasion in pre-eclampsia and other pregnancy disorders. In: Lyall F and Belfort M (eds.) *Pre-eclampsia. Etiology and Clinical Practice.* Cambridge: Cambridge University Press.
2. Lyall F (2007) Development of the utero-placental circulation: purported mechanisms for cytotrophoblast invasion in normal pregnancy and pre-eclampsia In: Lyall F and Belfort M (eds.) *Pre-eclampsia. Etiology and Clinical Practice.* Cambridge: Cambridge University Press.
3. Burton GJ, Jauniaux E, and Charnock-Jones SD (2010) The influence of the intrauterine environment on human placental development. *Int J Dev Biol* 54: 303–12.
4. Kaufmann P and Huppertz B (2007) Tenney–Parker changes and apoptotic versus necrotic shedding of trophoblast in normal pregnancy and pre-eclampsia. In: Lyall F and Belfort M (eds.) *Pre-eclampsia. Etiology and Clinical Practice.* Cambridge: Cambridge University Press.
5. Messerli M, May K, Hansson SR et al. (2010) Feto-maternal interactions in pregnancies: placental microparticles activate peripheral blood monocytes. *Placenta* 31: 106–112.
6. Lyall F (2003) Development of the utero-placental circulation: the role of carbon monoxide and nitric oxide in trophoblast invasion and spiral artery transformation. *Microscopy Res Technique* 60: 402–11.
7. Lyall F, Greer IA, Boswell F et al. (1997) Suppression of serum vascular endothelial growth factor immuoreactivity in normal pregnancy and pre-eclampsia. *Brit J Obstet Gynaecol* 104: 223–8.
8. Sunderji S, Gaziano E, Wothe D et al. (2010) Automated assays for sVEGF R1 and PlGF as an aid in the diagnosis of preterm preeclampsia : a prospective clinical study. *Am J Obstet Gynecol* 202: 40e1–7.

CHAPTER 33

Thrombophilia and the Placenta

Christina S. Han[1] *and Michael J. Paidas*[2]

[1]Department of Obstetrics, Gynecology and Reproductive Sciences, Yale University School of Medicine, New Haven, CT, USA

[2]Division of Maternal-Fetal Medicine and Ultrasound-Genetics, Department of Obstetrics, Gynecology and Reproductive Sciences, Yale University School of Medicine, New Haven, CT, USA

Introduction

Thrombophilia refers to defects of the coagulation system that predispose to thromboembolic events in the venous and arterial systems. Thrombophilia in pregnancy can be divided into two general categories—acquired and inheritable—with two primary obstetrical sequelae—venous thromboembolism (VTE) and adverse pregnancy outcomes. Extensive literature exists on the association of thrombophilias with these sequelae in the gravid patient, the fetus, and the placenta.

Inheritable thrombophilia include high and moderate-risk mutations such as antithrombin (AT) deficiency, factor V Leiden (FVL) homozygosity, prothrombin *G20210A* gene (PG) mutation homozygosity, and FVL/PG compound heterozygosity that interfere with the anticoagulant checks and balances in normal patients (Figure 33.1). Although a strong association exists between some inheritable thrombophilias and VTE, the association between inheritable thrombophilia and adverse pregnancy outcomes remains highly controversial because of the paucity of well-designed large prospective cohort studies. To date, no association has been definitively identified between inherited thrombophilias and specific abnormal placental pathology. Acquired thrombophilia, also known as antiphospholipid antibody syndrome (APAS), is an autoimmune disorder of coagulation. Unlike inheritable thrombophilias, APAS has been well described in association with adverse pregnancy outcomes and abnormal placental findings. This chapter presents a brief overview of the vast topic of thrombophilia, reviews the associated placental pathology and histology, and discusses the treatment options for thrombophilia in pregnancy.

Inheritable thrombophilia

Inheritable polymorphisms studied in pregnancy include FVL, PG, Methyltetrahydrofolate reductase (MTHFR), AT, plasminogen activator inhibitor-1 (PAI-1), protein S, protein C, and protein Z. Each mutation carries a different thrombogenic potential, with AT deficiency, FVL homozygosity, and PG mutation homozygosity being the most thrombogenic. FVL/PG compound heterozygosity is a moderate-risk polymorphism, while low-risk mutations include FVL heterozygosity, PG heterozygosity, protein C deficiency, and protein S deficiency.

Multiple small case-control and cohort studies utilizing heterogeneous populations associate thrombophilia with adverse pregnancy outcomes. However, these reports are fraught with contradictory results and subject to reporting bias. A definitive causal relationship therefore cannot be made between inherited thrombophilias and adverse pregnancy outcomes.

Clinical Pearl

Inherited thrombophilia testing in women who have experienced adverse pregnancy outcomes is not recommended because of insufficient causal association.

The Placenta: From Development to Disease, First Edition. Edited by Helen H. Kay, D. Michael Nelson and Yuping Wang.
© 2011 Blackwell Publishing Ltd. Published 2011 by Blackwell Publishing Ltd.

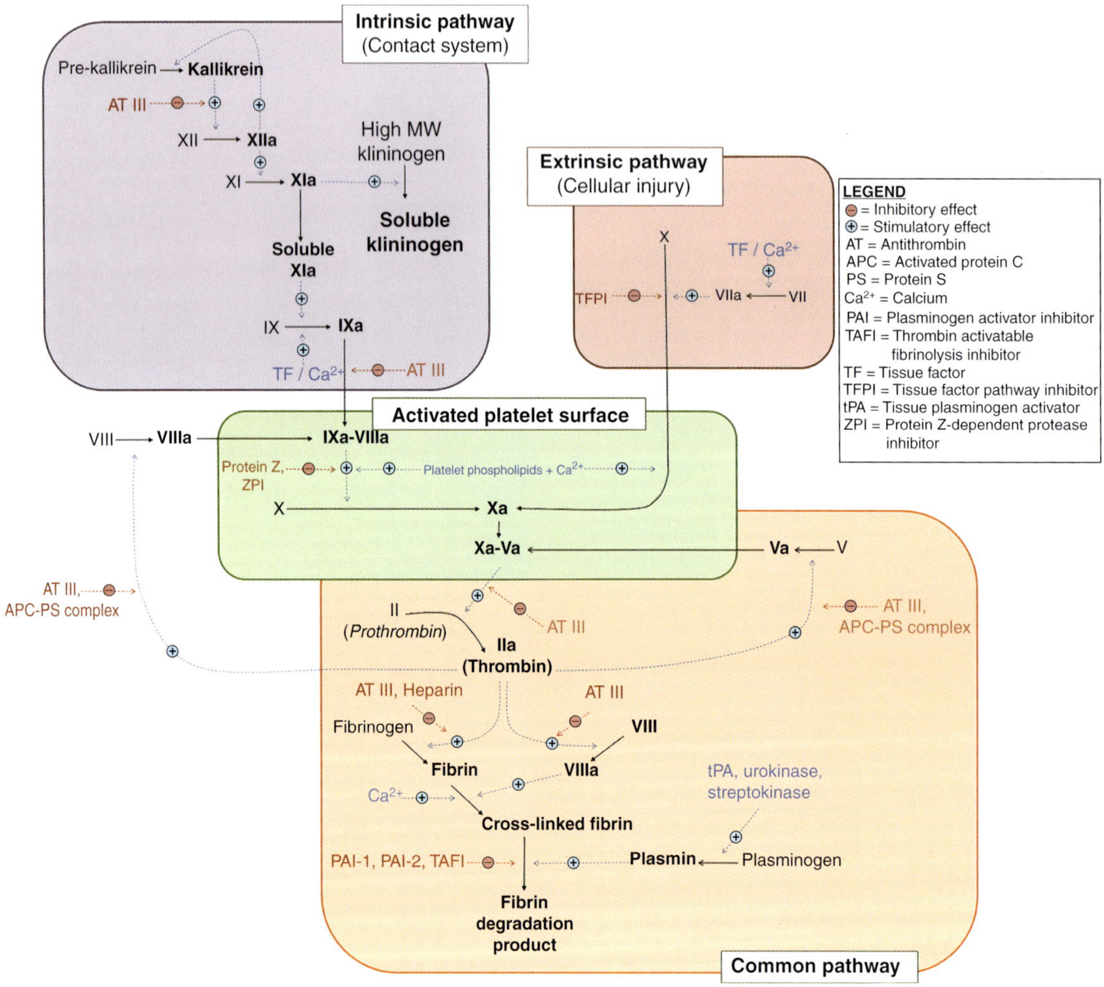

Figure 33.1 Coagulation pathway demonstrating the sites of activity for the common thrombophilias.

Acquired thrombophilia

Acquired thrombophilia or APAS is an autoimmune disorder responsible for approximately 14% of thromboembolic diseases in pregnancy. The development of antibodies to proteins associated with cell membrane phospholipids leads to endothelial dysfunction and predisposes to clot formation in APAS patients.

APAS induces a thrombophilic state via induction of procoagulant pathways, while inhibiting the actions of endogenous anticoagulant. Tissue factor, PAI-1, von Willebrand factor, and complement are essential components of the procoagulant cascade and are activated by the pathologic antibodies. In addition, antiphospholipid antibodies directly inhibit the endogenous anticoagulant effects of anionic phospholipid binding proteins, such as β2-glycoprotein-I and annexin V, and the activities of antithrombin, activated protein C, and thrombomodulin.

The diagnostic criteria for APAS were established in 2006 by a consensus panel, requiring one clinical criterion (obstetrical or nonobstetrical) and one laboratory criterion.

Clinical Criteria

1 Obstetrical outcome:
  a History of three unexplained consecutive spontaneous abortions <10 weeks' gestational age (GA), or
  b History of unexplained fetal death ≥10 weeks' GA (morphologically and karyotypically normal), or
  c History of preterm delivery < 34 weeks' GA, as a sequelae of preeclampsia or utero-placental insufficiency, including the following:
    i Nonreassuring fetal testing indicative of fetal hypoxemia (e.g., abnormal Doppler flow velocimetry waveform)
    ii Oligohydramnios with amniotic fluid index less than or equal to 5 cm
    iii Intrauterine growth restriction (IUGR) less than the 10th percentile
    iv Placental abruption
2 Non-obstetrical:
  a Thrombosis in any tissue, diagnosed by objective validated criteria, such as diagnostic imaging or histopathologic diagnosis:
  b Arterial thrombosis, including cerebrovascular accidents, transient ischemic attacks, myocardial infarction, or amaurosis fugax
  c Venous thromboembolism, including deep venous thrombosis, pulmonary emboli (PE), or small vessel thrombosis

Laboratory criteria

a Positive testing for antiphospholipid antibodies is required on two occasions, at least 12 weeks apart, and no more than 5 years prior to clinical manifestations. Any one of the following three tests fulfill the criteria:
  i Anticardiolipin antibody IgG or IgM isotype, present in medium (> 40 GPL or MPL) or high titers (> 99th percentile)
  ii Anti-β2-glycoprotein-I antibody IgG or IgM isotype (>99th percentile)
  iii Lupus anticoagulant in plasma or abnormal dilute Russell viper venom time testing

Antiphospholipid antibodies in the placenta decrease proliferation and increase apoptosis in trophoblasts, and adversely affect the formation of the utero-placental vasculature. Displacement of the protective anticoagulant annexin V protein allows deposition of fibrin on the trophoblast cell surface, increase inflammation, and elevate levels of tumor necrosis factor [1].

Clinical Pearl

The diagnosis of APAS is strongly associated with adverse pregnancy outcomes and requires both a clinical criterion and a laboratory criterion.

Adverse pregnancy outcomes

IUGR, fetal demise, recurrent pregnancy loss, placental abruption, and preeclampsia are common adverse pregnancy outcomes studied in thrombophilia. Although each of these pathologic states can be a result of other etiologies, one shared etiology for these suboptimal outcomes is placental dysfunction.

Normal placental function requires a large-capacitance, low-resistance vascular system to meet the high demands of the utero-placento-fetal unit. Preeclampsia arises from incomplete trophoblast invasion into maternal spiral arteries and suboptimal formation of this system. The retained musculoelastic vessels of the uterine spiral arteries may induce placental and fetal hypoperfusion and ischemia, as described in Chapter 32. Subsequent global maternal systemic endothelial dysfunction ensues, with secretion of antiangiogenic factors. The endothelial dysfunction and vascular hyper-reactivity comprise the stigmata of preeclampsia, with features of hypertension due to loss of normal regulation of vascular tone and proteinuria from increased glomerular vascular permeability.

Similarly, thrombophilic events involving the placental vasculature, whether on the maternal or fetal surface, may result in diminished placental function. Frequent release of microthrombi into the placental vasculature may result in a diminished functional surface area within the placenta. Several histologic findings within the vascular tree have been reported in the literature, and are theorized to provide the physiologic basis of the development of adverse pregnancy outcomes. In a large case-control study involving 205 patients with 279 late fetal losses beyond 22 weeks of gestation, vascular lesions of the placenta were found in 28% of patients without thrombophilias, whereas placental vascular lesions were found in 100% of women with both adverse pregnancy outcomes and thrombophilia [2]. Similar lesions are increased in early-onset IUGR and preeclampsia [3,4]. However, no lesion is unique or specific to thrombophilia. In fact, many placentae display similar lesions, including pregnancies affected by preeclampsia, fetal growth restriction, diabetes, sickle cell disease, or cocaine abuse, even in the absence of thrombophilia.

Clinical Pearl

Adverse pregnancy outcomes related to thrombophilia are theorized to arise from microthrombotic events occurring within the placental vascular tree.

Thrombotic locations

The arrangement of the placental vasculature provides for complete separation of the maternal and fetal circulation in humans, as described in Chapter 5. Thrombosis can thus occur in the maternal circulation, the fetal compartment, or the intervening intervillous space [5]. We will describe each location separately in the following.

Maternal vasculopathy

Histopathologic features that affect the maternal vascular compartment include decidual vasculopathy, placental infarcts, maternal floor infarction, syncytial knotting, vasculitis, and chronic villitis, as described in Chapter 14.

Decidual vasculopathy

Physiologic conversion of the intima media of the spiral arteries occur in early gestation to render the vessels refractory to vasoconstrictive mediators. Inadequate trophoblast invasion of the decidual and myometrial segments of these maternal arteries is diagnosed by the absence of fibrinoid deposition and persistence of the smooth muscle coat in the arteries. Vasculopathy of these abnormal decidual vessels is characterized by vascular smooth muscle necrosis, foamy histiocyte invasion, mural hyalinization with eosinophilic material accumulating in the vessel wall, and mononuclear infiltrate (Figure 33.2).

Placental infarcts

Proliferation of the intima and smooth muscle cells, in conjunction with vascular endothelial damage, may lead to thrombosis of arteries within the decidua basalis and infarction of the placenta (Figure 33.3). These thromboses result in necrosis and hemorrhage, which manifest clinically as retroplacental hematoma and abruptio placenta.

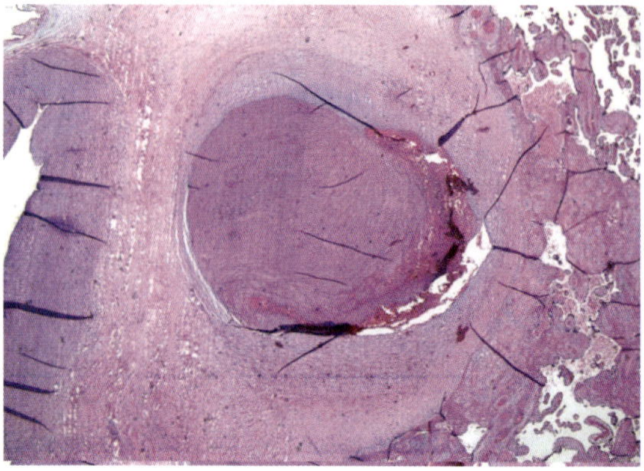

Figure 33.2 Decidual vasculopathy is characterized by vascular smooth muscle fibrinoid necrosis, foamy histiocyte invasion, mural hyalinization with eosinophilic material accumulating in the vessel walls, and mononuclear infiltrates. (From Raspollini et al., with permission.)

Gross pathologic evaluation of the placenta will reveal firm and pale areas of parenchyma. These tan-colored areas are commonly noted in normal postterm gestations and are usually only a few millimeters in diameter. In large quantities or confluent patches, these infarctions are considered to be pathologic. In addition, their presence in a placenta from the first and second trimester is also considered abnormal.

Histologic evaluation reveals villous agglutination with collapse of the intervillous space, pyknosis of trophoblasts with condensed chromatin within nuclei of apoptotic cells, karyorrhexis with fragmented and released

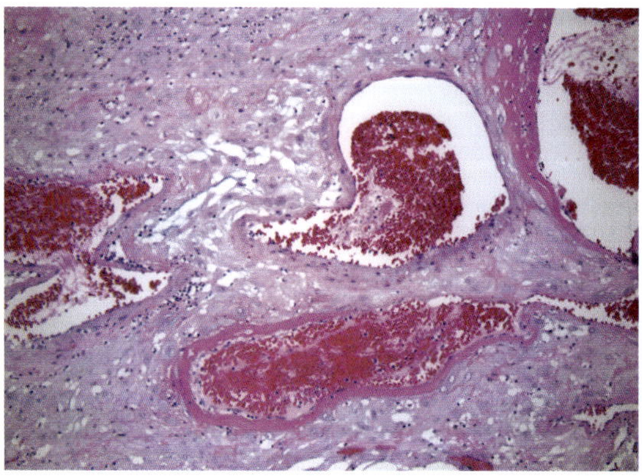

Figure 33.3 A recent thrombus is seen in this chorionic plate vessel. (From Raspollini et al., with permission.)

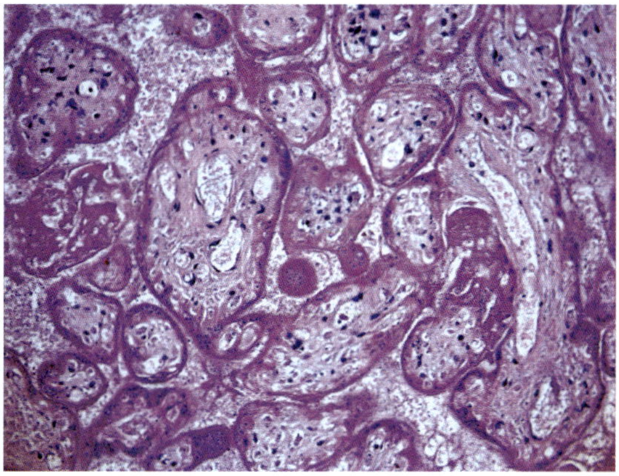

Figure 33.4 Placental infarct is characterized by clustered and necrotic trophoblastic nuclei with collapsed intervillous space. (From Raspollini et al., with permission.)

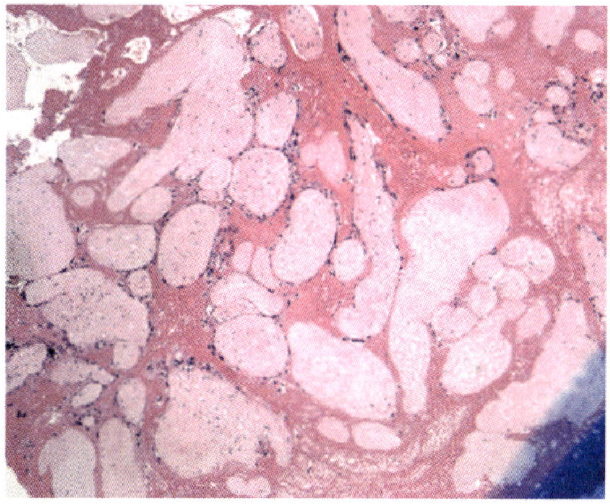

Figure 33.6 Massive perivillous fibrin deposits are seen obliterating the intervillous space. (From Raspollini et al., with permission.)

chromatin in cytoplasm, and ghost-like villi within a thin layer of fibrinoid (Figure 33.4).

Maternal floor infarction

This pathologic entity is characterized by a marked, diffuse increase in deposition of fibrinoid material along the decidua basalis and intervillous space of the basal plate. Gross pathologic examination reveals a thickened maternal floor with a network of fibrinoid material (Figures 33.5 and 33.6). This pathologic finding has been noted in thrombophilic states, particularly antiphospholipid antibody syndrome. This lesion is also seen in pregnancies with unexplained elevated maternal serum alpha-fetoprotein levels, infections, fetal growth restriction, and fetal death. Compared to gestational age-matched controls, infants born to mothers with maternal floor infarction have a higher incidence of central nervous system (CNS) injury on neonatal ultrasound examinations, have a suspicious or abnormal neurologic examination, and have lower developmental scores with neurodevelopmental impairment [6].

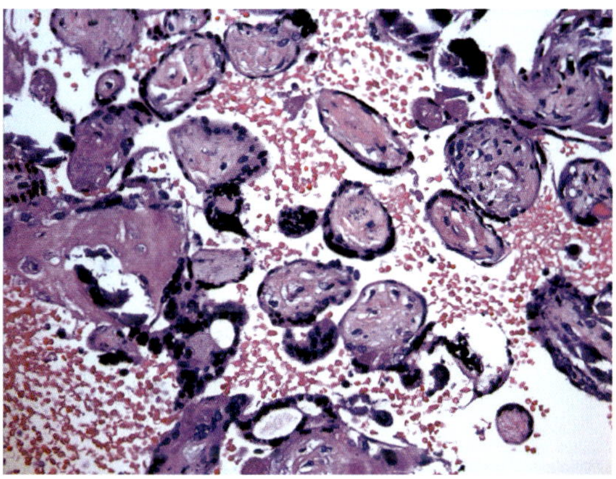

Figure 33.5 Massive perivillous fibrin deposits in a case of stillbirth at 23 weeks of gestation. (From Raspollini et al., with permission.)

Syncytial knotting

Syncytial knots are defined as aggregates of degenerating nuclei in the multinucleated syncytiotrophoblast which may protrude slightly from the villous surface. Increased numbers of syncytial knots have been reported in the placentae of pregnancies with adverse pregnancy outcomes. Similarly, hypoxic conditions, brought on by thrombotic events, may result in excess syncytial knots, capillary proliferation, and terminal villous branching (Figure 33.7).

Chronic villitis

Defined by inflammation of the villous stroma, chronic villitis often occurs with concomitant intervillositis and vasculitis. Histologic findings include infiltration of the villous stroma and adjacent intervillous spaces by polymorphous inflammatory cells (Figure 33.8). Although not a direct result of thrombophilia, chronic inflammatory

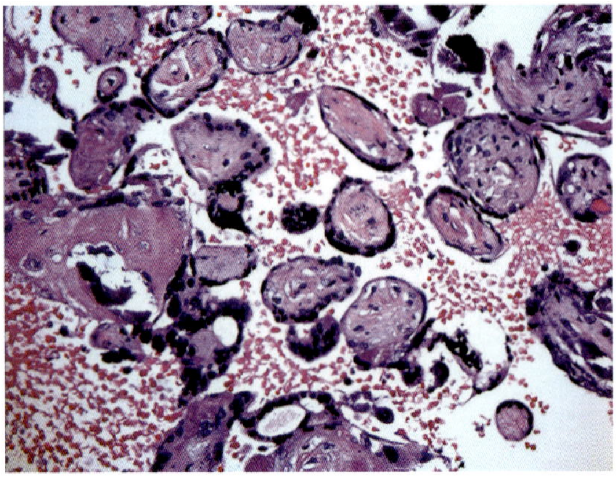

Figure 33.7 Trophoblastic knots are characterized by the clustering of nuclei. (From Raspollini et al., with permission.)

response may induce a thrombogenic environment. A thrombogenic focus that develops in the setting of chronic villitis can embolize downstream in the placental vascular tree towards the terminal villi.

Clinical Pearl

Histopathologic features of the placenta in women with thrombophilia include decidual vasculopathy, placental infarcts, maternal floor infarction, syncytial knotting, vasculitis, and chronic villitis, yet none of these lesions are unique or specific to thrombophilias.

Fetal thrombotic vasculopathy

Thrombosis of large fetal vessels may occur as a result of fetal carriage of a homozygous or compound heterozygous high- or moderate-risk thrombophilia. Fetal thrombotic vasculopathy (FTV) begins with occlusive thrombi in branches of the umbilical arteries, which lead to downstream avascular villi following the vascular distribution of a single vascular tree. FTV may occur in APAS with IgG antibodies that undergo transplacental passage into the fetal circulation. Other conditions associated with FTV include diabetes mellitus, anatomic anomalies, true knots, velamentous cord insertion, umbilical cord entanglement, perinatal liver disease, and discordant twins. FTV resulting in involvement of 40–60% of the placental mass may induce fetal demise. Another complication of FTV is embolization of the thrombotic focus to the fetus, with brain and kidney as the most likely sites. Of interest, the finding of FTV does not predict postnatal thrombotic events [7].

Histologic findings include sclerotic or avascular terminal villi, hemorrhagic endovasculitis, and inflammatory damage to vessels. Hemorrhagic endovasculitis results from disruptive extravasation of fetal erythrocytes into the vascular wall, with subsequent hemorrhage, erythrocyte fragmentation, and intravascular nucleo-cytoplasmic debris. In addition, prolonged exposure to meconium passage can lead to meconium-induced myonecrosis of the perivascular smooth muscles (Figure 33.9). The surrounding maternal spaces remain patent despite disturbance of the adjacent fetal system.

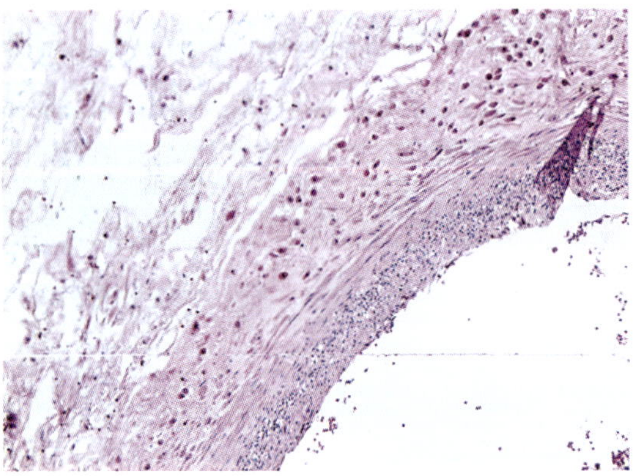

Figure 33.8 Necrosis is seen in the outer layer of the vascular smooth muscle, with pyknotic nuclei and dense, eosinophilic, smudged appearance of the cytoplasm. (From Raspollini et al., with permission.)

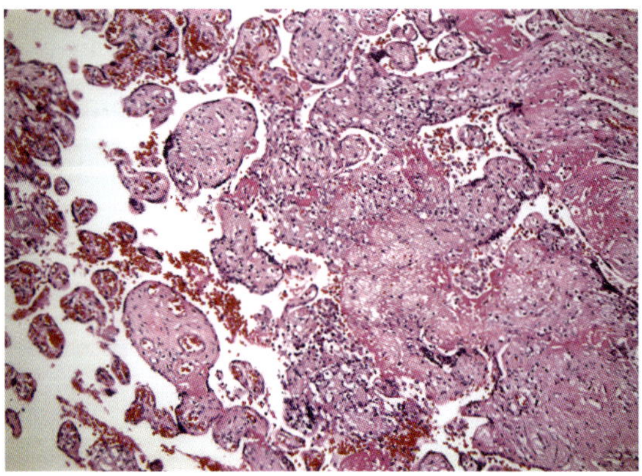

Figure 33.9 The polymorphous inflammatory composition of primarily mononuclear inflammatory cells and rare neutrophils indicates the presence of chronic villitis. (From Raspollini et al., with permission.)

Clinical Pearl

Placenta affected by FTV shows abnormalities that follow the branching vascular distribution of the umbilical artery. FTV that involves 40–60% of the placental mass results in fetal demise.

Diagnosis, management, and treatment

Evaluation for the above stated adverse pregnancy outcomes should include evaluation for APAS, namely laboratory testing for anticardiolipin antibodies, lupus anticoagulant (or dRVVT), and β2-glycoprotein-I antibodies. Conversely, the evaluation for inheritable thrombophilia should only be undertaken in women with thromboembolic events. The debatable association between inheritable thrombophilia and adverse pregnancy outcomes, and the low prevalence of some thrombophilia mutations in the general population, results in a poor yield with polymorphism testing. If screening is to be undertaken for inheritable thrombophilias secondary to a thrombotic event, the following should be tested: FVL mutation, prothrombin gene mutation, and deficiencies in antithrombin, protein C, and protein S.

Clinical Pearl

The evaluation of adverse pregnancy outcomes should include screening for APAS, but routine screening of inheritable thrombophilias is not recommended.

Given the weak association of inheritable thrombophilias with adverse pregnancy outcomes, treatment of inheritable thrombophilias is reserved for prevention of VTE. Dosing of heparin anticoagulation is based on the thrombogenic potential of the mutation and the history of prior VTE. Therapeutic-dose heparin is reserved for patients with a high-risk thrombophilic mutation and a history of prior VTE, and patients with acute thrombotic events with or without a diagnosis of inheritable thrombophilia. Prophylactic-dose heparin may be used for the following conditions:

1 Patients carrying a high-risk mutation without prior history of VTE, or in patients with moderate-risk mutations (such as compound FVL/PG heterozygosity).
2 Patients with low-risk mutations (such as FVL mutation, PG mutation, protein C deficiency, and protein S deficiency) and a history of prior venous thromboembolism.
3 Patients without mutations but with a history of prior thromboembolism in the absence of a recurring condition.

Patients with low-risk mutations without a history of thromboembolism do not require treatment in the antepartum period.

Clinical Pearl

Treatment for inheritable thrombophilia mutation in pregnancy is reserved for prevention of venous thromboembolism, and is not recommended for prevention of adverse pregnancy outcomes.

Management of APAS in pregnancy can be divided into management for maternal thrombotic outcomes or obstetrical outcomes. In patients with APAS and a history of venous thromboembolism, therapeutic-dose heparin is routinely recommended during pregnancy and the 6–8 weeks' postpartum to prevent the high risk of recurrent thrombotic events. Women with APAS without a history of VTE should receive prophylactic-dose heparin during the same period [8–11]. Additional treatment with low-dose aspirin for prevention of adverse pregnancy outcomes is debatable. Corticosteroids and intravenous immunoglobulin (IVIG) have been used to treat pregnant women with antiphospholipid syndrome, but this is not standard practice.

Long-term complications of APAS include thrombosis and stroke. In studies of women with APAS, approximately 50% women developed thromboses during 3–10 years of follow-up and 10% developed systemic lupus erythematosus. Referral for long-term follow-up should be made to a rheumatologist or hematologist after pregnancy. Patients should also be counseled against the use of estrogen-containing contraceptives or hormonal replacement.

Clinical Pearl

The mainstay of treatment of APAS in obstetrics is heparin for prevention of adverse outcomes, but low-dose aspirin may be considered for prevention of adverse pregnancy outcomes in selected patients.

Teaching Points

1. Pregnant patients with antiphospholipid antibody syndrome are at risk for adverse pregnancy and venous thromboembolism. Literature to date has not shown a causal link between inheritable thrombophilias and adverse pregnancy outcomes.
2. Placental findings in pregnancies affected by thrombophilia have significant overlap with findings in adverse pregnancy outcomes without thrombophilias.
3. The mainstay of treatment of APAS and thromboembolic events is heparin, with low-dose aspirin considered in selected patients.

References

1. Redline RW (2006) Thrombophilia and placental pathology. *Clin Obstet Gynecol* 49(4): 885–94.
2. Gris JC, Quere I, Monpeyroux F et al. (1999) Case-control study of the frequency of thrombophilic disorders in couples with late foetal loss and no thrombotic antecedent. The Nîmes Obstetricians and Haematologists Study (NOHA). *Thromb Haemost* 81: 91–9.
3. Salafia CM, Minior VK, Pezzullo JC et al. (1995) Intrauterine growth restriction in infants of less than thirty-two weeks' gestation: associated placental pathologic features. *Am J Obstet Gynecol* 173: 1049–57.
4. Ghidini A, Salafia CM, and Pezzullo JC (1997) Placental vascular lesions and likelihood of diagnosis of preeclampsia. *Obstet Gynecol* 90(4 Pt 1): 542–5.
5. Raspollini MR, Oliva E, and Drucilla JR (2007) Placental histopathologic features in patients with thrombophilic mutations. *J Matern Fetal Neonatal Med* 20(2): 113–123.
6. Adams-Chapman I, Vaucher YE, Bejar RF et al. (2002) Maternal floor infarction of the placenta: association with central nervous system injury and adverse neurodevelopmental outcome. *J Perinatol* 22(3): 236–41.
7. Leistra-Leistra MJ, Timmer A, van Spronsen FJ et al. (2004) Fetal thrombotic vasculopathy in the placenta: a thrombophilic connection between pregnancy complications and neonatal thrombosis? *Placenta 25*: S102–5.
8. Duhl AJ, Paidas MJ, Ural SH et al. (2007) Pregnancy and Thrombosis Working Group. Antithrombotic therapy and pregnancy: consensus report and recommendations for prevention and treatment of venous thromboembolism and adverse pregnancy outcomes. *Am J Obstet Gynecol* 197(5): 457. e1–21.
9. Antiphospholipid syndrome (2005) ACOG Practice Bulletin No. 68. American College of Obstetricians and Gynecologists. *Obstet Gynecol* 106: 1113–21.
10. Inherited thrombophilias in pregnancy (2010, July) ACOG Practice Bulletin No. 113. American College of Obstetricians and Gynecologists. p. 11.
11. Empson M, Lassere M, Craig JC et al. (2002) Recurrent pregnancy loss with antiphospholipid antibody: a systematic review of therapeutic trials. *Obstet Gynecol* 99: 135–44.

CHAPTER 34

Infections in the Placenta

Samuel Parry

Department of Maternal-Fetal Medicine, University of Pennsylvania, Philadelphia, PA, USA

Introduction

The transmission of infectious pathogens across the placenta from the mother to the fetus has been associated with adverse pregnancy outcomes, including congenital malformations, fetal growth restriction, miscarriage, and stillbirth. However, the impact of infections within the placenta on pregnancy outcomes has not been studied extensively, and it is biologically plausible that infections within extravillous and villous trophoblast cells impair normal placental functions and induce adverse pregnancy outcomes attributed to placental dysfunction.

In the past several years, evidence also has accumulated associating placental dysfunction with spontaneous preterm delivery. Women who deliver preterm after idiopathic preterm labor have higher rates of placental ischemia and abnormal placentation (defined as failure of physiological transformation of maternal spiral arteries resulting in reduced blood flow to the placental intervillous space) than women who deliver at term. Additionally, decreased first trimester maternal serum levels of pregnancy associated plasma protein A, which is a protease produced by trophoblast cells, are associated with an increased risk of preterm premature rupture of membranes and preterm delivery. These findings support the hypothesis that spontaneous preterm delivery, at least in part, has its origins in abnormal placental function at the beginning of pregnancy.

In this chapter, we will review the clinical significance and some current studies on infections within the placenta. We will focus on the impact of infections on placental functions.

Viral infections early in pregnancy

Cytomegalovirus (CMV)

CMV, a double-stranded DNA virus, is the most common congenital viral infection with devastating neonatal outcomes if infection occurs in the first trimester. CMV is highly contagious, and primary infection complicates up to 2% of all pregnancies. Many women of reproductive age, who have been infected previously with CMV, continue to shed viral particles during pregnancy because of its ability to reactivate after periods of latency.

> **Clinical Pearl**
>
> One of the most impressive clinical findings at delivery of an infected neonate by CMV, or other viruses, is a markedly enlarged placenta. >4 cm in thickness on ultrasound measurements and weighing a fourth or more of the neonatal weight.

CMV and the placenta

Histopathologic features of a placenta infected with CMV include clusters of viral particles and generalized inflammation (Figure 34.1). In placental villi, the syncytiotrophoblast does not become infected, but clusters of underlying cytotrophoblast cells become infected and CMV proteins can be detected in these cytotrophoblast cells following placental exposure.

The syncytiotrophoblast expresses the CMV receptor epidermal growth factor receptor but lacks integrin coreceptors, and uptake of virus occurs without replication.

The Placenta: From Development to Disease, First Edition. Edited by Helen H. Kay, D. Michael Nelson and Yuping Wang.
© 2011 Blackwell Publishing Ltd. Published 2011 by Blackwell Publishing Ltd.

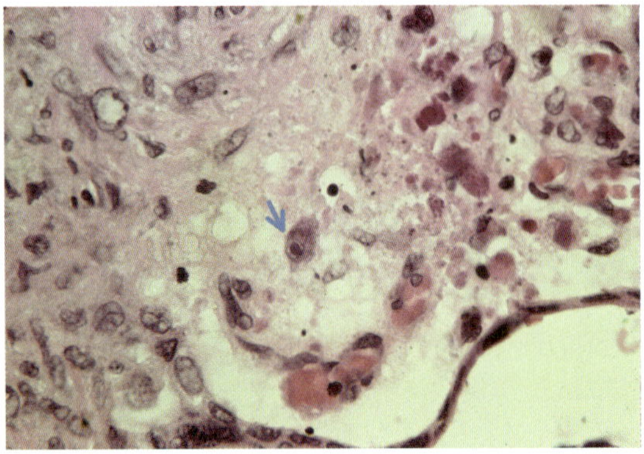

Figure 34.1 H&E stain of placental villus showing CMV inclusion (arrow) with localized recruitment of lymphocytes and histiocytes. Cytotrophoblasts are typically infected but not syncytiotrophoblasts. (Courtesy Dr. Frederick Kraus.)

Productive infection within the placenta occurs when transcytosed virions reach villous cytotrophoblast cells and extravillous (invasive) cytotrophoblast cells that express integrin co-receptors and up-regulate expression of epidermal growth factor receptor upon exposure to virus, thereby dramatically increasing susceptibility to infection.

In an experimental model, primary extravillous cytotrophoblast cells were permissive for CMV replication, and infection significantly impaired the cytotrophoblast cells' ability to differentiate and invade through an extracellular matrix [1]. Microarray analyses revealed that CMV infection strongly and reproducibly altered trophoblast gene expression, elevating expression of mitotic cell cycle genes and repressing expression of genes associated with trophoblast differentiation, particularly those associated with formation and stabilization of the extracellular matrix [2].

Adeno-associated virus (AAV)

AAV is a member of the parvovirus family, and several serotypes of AAV have been identified. Of these, types 2 and 3 infect humans, although type 3 is rare and is probably a laboratory contaminant that developed

Research Spotlight

In our laboratory, we observed that cytotrophoblast cell viability was reduced, apoptosis was increased (Figure 34.2) and secretion of the pro-inflammatory cytokines interleukin-6 and -8 was up-regulated following exposure to CMV. These results suggest that CMV infection impairs critical aspects of trophoblast function and offer testable hypotheses for explaining the deleterious effects of this virus on pregnancy outcome [1].

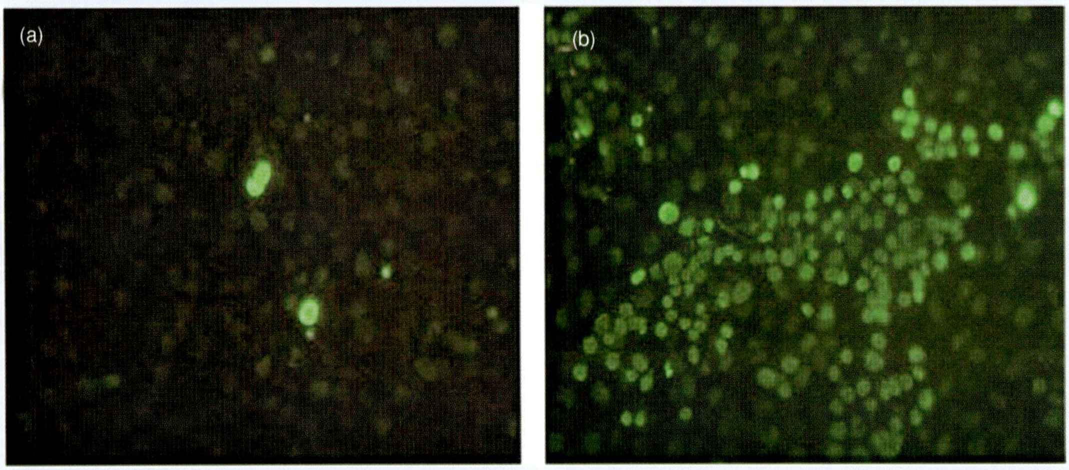

Figure 34.2 Terminal deoxynucleotidyl transferase-mediated (TdT-mediated) deoxyuridine-triphosphate-x (dUTP-X) nick end labeling assay to detect apoptosis (fluorescent signals) in trophoblast cells after infection with CMV at 1 and 5 plaque forming units (PFU)/cell 16 hours after infection. Photographs of uninfected cells (a) and cells infected by 5 PFU/cell CMV at 16 hours (b). (Adapted with permission from Chou et al. *Am J Obstet Gynecol* 2006;194: 535–41.)

Table 34.1 Rates of first trimester maternal seropositivity of IgM antibodies against AAV-2 among cases with adverse pregnancy outcomes and controls who delivered at term with no pregnancy complications.

	OD/Background (Range)[a]	P[b]	Percent Seropositive[c]	P[d]	OR (95% CI)
Controls ($N = 106$)	2.09 (0.88–15.97)	NA	17.9	NA	1.00 (reference)
SAB[e] ($N = 34$)	3.86 (0.47–7.91)	0.04	20.6	0.73	1.19 (0.45, 3.13)
SPTD[f] ($N = 24$)	9.03 (1.08–19.92)	<0.001	62.5	<0.0001	7.63 (2.91, 20.01)
Composite[g] ($N = 20$)	6.28 (0.97–32.58)	<0.001	55.0	0.0004	5.60 (2.04, 15.38)

Source: Adapted with permission from Arechavaleta-Velasco et al. (2008) Adverse reproductive outcomes in urban women with adeno-associated virus-2 infections in early pregnancy. *Hum Reprod* 23: 29–36.

OR, odds ratio; CI, confidence interval.

[a]Optical density (OD) measured by enzyme-linked immunosorbent assay to detect IgM antibodies against AAV-2 in maternal serum samples.

[b]*P*-value: Kruskal-Wallis tests, comparing each group of cases with controls.

[c]Seropositivity defined by ROC curve analysis as OD value of each sample/OD value of background signal ≥6.00.

[d]*P*-value: Chi square tests, comparing rates of seropositivity for each group of cases with controls.

[e]SAB, spontaneous miscarriage at <20 weeks' gestation.

[f]SPTD, spontaneous preterm delivery between 20 and 37 weeks' gestation.

[g]Composite group of women with pregnancies complicated by preeclampsia, fetal growth restriction, and/or intrauterine fetal demise.

during construction of recombinant AAV vectors. AAV-2 is a common human isolate (40% to 80% of adults have been exposed), and infection involves hematogenous seeding.

AAV and the placenta

The placenta may be exposed to AAV-2 during primary or reactivated maternal infection. Although productive AAV-2 infections usually require co-infection with helper viruses (including adenovirus, CMV, human papillomavirus (HPV), and herpes simplex virus), other investigators demonstrated that AAV-2 can undergo full replicative cycles in keratinocytes, and we demonstrated that trophoblast cells are susceptible to AAV-2 both in the presence and absence of helper virus co-infection. Additionally, there are several reports linking AAV-2 to adverse reproductive outcomes, including spontaneous miscarriage, gestational trophoblastic disease, and preterm labor. There are no unique histopathologic features in the placenta that are attributed to AAV infection.

Research Spotlight

We determined that transformed extravillous trophoblast (HTR-8/SVneo) cells were susceptible to AAV-2 infection both in the presence and absence of adenovirus, and that AAV-2 infection reduced invasion of HTR-8/SVneo cells through an extracellular matrix before cytopathic effects were detected.

In a case-control study, AAV-2 DNA was found more frequently in trophoblast cells from cases of severe preeclampsia than from normal term deliveries. In another study, we observed that first trimester maternal IgM seropositivity was 5.6 times more prevalent among preeclampsia/IUGR/stillbirth cases ($P = 0.0004$) and 7.6 times more prevalent among preterm deliveries ($P < 0.0001$) than among controls (Table 34.1) [3]. CMV and adenovirus IgM antibodies and chronic AAV-2 infections (IgG seropositivity) were not associated with adverse pregnancy outcomes. These results indicate that AAV-2 infection is a previously unidentified cause of placental dysfunction, and primary or reactivated AAV-2 infection (maternal IgM seropositivity) early in pregnancy is associated with adverse reproductive outcomes attributed to placental dysfunction, including preeclampsia, stillbirth, and spontaneous preterm delivery.

Human papillomavirus (HPV)

A significant proportion of women carry HPV in their genital tract. It can be transmitted transplacentally to the fetus. There are more than 100 types of HPV that are classified according to their oncogenic potential.

Similar to infection with AAV-2, we found that infection of extravillous trophoblast cells with HPV-16 induced cell death and reduced trophoblast invasion through an extracellular matrix [4]. Another group of investigators also demonstrated that HPV-16 decreased extravillous trophoblast cell viability, but they found that different strains of HPV-16 had differential effects on extravillous trophoblast cell migration and invasion [5]. There are no unique histopathologic features in the placenta that are attributed to HPV infection.

HPV in clinical disease

In a case-control study, we observed that HPV DNA was detected more frequently in placentae from spontaneous preterm deliveries than in placentae from controls [4]. Overall, HPV DNA was identified in the extravillous region of 29/108 (26.9 percent) placentae. Approximately 45% of HPV DNA corresponded with low-risk strains (HPV-6, -11) and 55% corresponded with high-risk strains (HPV-16, -18). There were no differences in detection of individual HPV types among three groups (controls, spontaneous preterm delivery, and severe preeclampsia). Identification of HPV DNA in extravillous regions of placental samples from cases of severe preeclampsia was not significantly different from that of controls (8/48 versus 6/30; $P = 0.71$). However, HPV DNA was detected more frequently in the extravillous trophoblast region of placentae from spontaneous preterm delivery cases (15/30) than from controls (6/30; $P = 0.03$), and in the subset of women who underwent spontaneous preterm delivery remote from term (<34 weeks' gestation), HPV DNA also was detected more frequently than among controls (12/22 versus 6/30; $P = 0.02$) [4].

Clinical Pearl

The relationship between cervical intra-epithelial neoplasia, cone biopsy, cervical loop electrosurgical excision procedure (LEEP), and preterm birth has been studied extensively. Our findings suggest that confounding effects between HPV infection, which causes cervical intra-epithelial neoplasia, must be considered when studying these cervical abnormalities as causes of spontaneous preterm delivery.

Potential mechanisms by which viral infections may induce failed invasion and placental dysfunction, including altered expression of cell adhesion molecules, matrix metalloproteinases, pro-inflammatory cytokines and major histocompatibility antigens, need to be explored. However, recent findings provide a solid scientific basis for the continued critical investigation of the role of common viruses in pregnancy complications related to placental dysfunction.

Common bacterial infections of the placenta

Inflammatory pathways by which bacterial infections impact placental functions likely involve toll-like receptors (TLRs), which are an evolutionarily conserved family of transmembrane proteins that play a primary role in innate immunity. TLRs recognize highly conserved pathogen-associated molecular patterns (PAMP), and ligation of TLR and PAMP triggers innate immune responses through nuclear factor-kB-dependent (NF-kb-dependent) and interferon regulatory factor-dependent signaling pathways.Examples of PAMP include lipopolysaccharide, the major component of gram-negative bacterial outer membranes, and peptidoglycan, the major component of gram-positive bacterial cell walls. TLR-4 was the first human TLR to be discovered and subsequently was identified as the specific receptor for recognition of lipopolysaccharide, while TLR-2 binds to gram-positive, gram-negative, and mycobacterial associated lipoproteins.

The possible roles of TLR in placental tissue, especially their role in protecting the conceptus from maternal infection, have been investigated, but the pathophysiological effects of bacterial infection and TLR activation on placental function have not been established.

Research Spotlight

Common bacterial pathogens, such as Group B streptococcus, and bacterial PAMP, such as lipopolysaccharide, induce trophoblast cell death, and exposure of trophoblast cells to TLR agonists affects trophoblast endocrine function, including up-regulation of human chorionic gonadotropin secretion [6].

In animal models, lipopolysaccharide interacts with TLR-4 to trigger first trimester trophoblast cells to produce high levels of cytokines, including tumor necrosis factor-α and interferon-γ. Trophoblast cells are highly sensitive to these cytokines, so while lipopolysaccharide does not directly induce trophoblast cell death, the intense inflammatory response generated by trophoblast cells following activation of TLR-4 by gram-negative bacterial pathogens may provide a mechanism for the induction of trophoblast cell death. Thus, evidence has emerged demonstrating that TLRs are expressed on trophoblast cells, and activation of these receptors by bacterial pathogens evokes both inflammatory and cell death pathways [7].

The clinical implications of bacterial infection within the placenta are demonstrated best by the association between placental infections and preterm labor, preeclampsia, and fetal growth restriction. TLRs expressed at the maternal-fetal interface may play an important role in the mechanism of pathogenesis, and intrauterine infections during pregnancy may have either a direct or an indirect effect upon trophoblast cell survival, depending upon which TLR is activated. For example, TLR-4 ligation promotes cytokine production, while ligation of TLR-2 induces apoptosis in first trimester trophoblast cells. Alternatively, soluble forms of TLR may bind to microorganisms and target them for destruction by the complement system or by phagocytosis. Therefore, soluble TLR may provide new markers of pregnancy complications as well as a potential target for therapeutic interventions. Collectively, these findings suggest that a bacterial pathogen, through TLR activation, may promote the elevated trophoblast cell death observed in a number of pregnancy complications, such as preterm labor, fetal growth restriction, and preeclampsia. How the immune system functions in the placenta during early pregnancy remains an uncertain area. The field of TLR represents an exciting area of innate immunity, and it is becoming increasingly clear that TLR signaling can generate distinct immunological outcomes. The expression and function of TLR in relation to bacterial infection at the maternal–fetal interface is a novel area of reproductive immunology with much need for future studies [7].

Chlamydia pneumoniae, Listeria monocytogenes, and Treponema pallidum

Placental infections with three other bacteria—*Chlamydia pneumoniae*, *Listeria monocytogenes*, and *Treponema pallidum*—are associated with significant pregnancy complications and warrant additional consideration here.

In the past two decades, researchers have reported an association between *Chlamydia pneumoniae* and vascular disease. *Chlamydia pneumoniae* is a common gram-negative, intracellular bacterium that is able to infect most of the cell types involved in atherogenesis, including endothelium, smooth muscle cells, and macrophages. Seropositivity for antibodies against *Chlamydia pneumoniae* (IgG class) is correlated with coronary artery disease. *Chlamydia pneumoniae* is found more frequently in atherosclerotic vascular lesions than in vascular tissue from healthy control subjects. Furthermore, patients who are seropositive for *Chlamydia pneumoniae* antibodies have a significantly greater arterial intimal medial thickness than seronegative patients. Dissemination of *Chlamydia pneumoniae* into the peripheral blood during pregnancy may expose the placenta to infection and organisms can cross the placenta to infect the fetus. *Chlamydia pneumoniae* DNA has been detected in placental tissue, and circulating maternal antibodies against *Chlamydia pneumoniae* have been found in patients with preeclampsia.

Chlamydia pneumoniae and the placenta

Recently, we studied the direct effects of the bacterium in trophoblast cells in culture and the relationship between placental infection with *Chlamydia pneumoniae* and obstetric complications resulting from placental dysfunction, such as preeclampsia. We used primary extravillous trophoblast cells isolated from first-trimester placentae to demonstrate that trophoblast cell viability and invasion through extracellular matrices were decreased after infection with *Chlamydia pneumoniae* (both $P < 0.05$) [8]. We also performed a case-control study to identify *Chlamydia pneumoniae* in trophoblast cells dissected by laser capture microscopy from placentae in women with severe preeclampsia and control subjects who delivered at term. *Chlamydia pneumoniae* DNA was detected in trophoblast cells in 15/48 cases but only 3/30 controls (odds ratio, 4.1; $P = .02$). Positive and negative controls yielded expected results. We concluded that *Chlamydia pneumoniae* infection can reduce trophoblast invasion into the uterine wall and is associated with preeclampsia.

Chlamydia pneumoniae may play a role in the pathogenesis of preeclampsia by two different mechanisms: cellular and humoral. Circulating *Chlamydia pneumoniae* during pregnancy may directly infect invasive trophoblast cells at the maternal–fetal interface and induce pathologic changes that interfere with placental invasion into the uterine wall, resulting in reduced placental perfusion, placental dysfunction, and adverse pregnancy outcomes. Meanwhile, humoral responses induced by *Chlamydia pneumoniae* could be similar to those described in the development of atherosclerosis, in which elevation of inflammatory markers and endothelial dysfunction precedes vascular injury. Enhanced intravascular inflammation is a common scenario in preeclampsia. The degree of vascular lesions in atherosclerosis correlates with levels of heat shock protein and C-reactive protein induced by *Chlamydia pneumoniae*. Elevated levels of C-reactive protein have been associated with high titers of anti-*Chlamydia pneumoniae* IgG antibodies in women with preeclampsia who delivered before term. Consequently, further investigation of the mechanisms by which *Chlamydia pneumoniae* induces trophoblast dysfunction, and the identification of therapies to prevent adverse outcomes attributed to trophoblast dysfunction, are warranted.

Listeria monocytogenes and the placenta

Listeriosis is a bacterial infection caused by a gram-positive, intracellular bacterium, *Listeria monocytogenes*. The main route of acquisition of *Listeria* is through maternal ingestion of contaminated food products (particularly raw meat, soft cheeses, unpasteurized dairy products, vegetables, and seafood), which then spread hematogenously to infect the placenta, forming microabscesses, and transplacental infection of the fetus (Figures 34.3(a, b)). Infected adults usually have only mild, flu-like symptoms; however, pregnant women are much more likely than the rest of the population to contract listeriosis, and infection during pregnancy can lead to miscarriage, still birth, preterm delivery, and infection of the neonate.

In animal models, the maternal host generates a normal adaptive immune response to *Listeria* infection, so adverse pregnancy outcomes attributed to *Listeria* infection likely involve an immunopathological response associated with placental infection. The syncytiotrophoblast, which expresses the *Listeria* host receptor E-cadherin, and extravillous cytotrophoblasts in anchoring villi are susceptible to direct invasion of extracellular *Listeria* and cell-to-cell spread. Following treatment for *Listeria*, inflammatory cytokine expression is altered and apoptosis is increased in the rodent, and these changes may contribute to preterm delivery and fetal death. More specifically, colony stimulating factor-1 (CSF-1), a macrophage growth factor, is synthesized in high concentrations by the decidua during pregnancy, where it is targeted to trophoblast bearing CSF-1 receptors. Following *Listeria* infection in mice, CSF-1 is required to recruit neutrophils to the site of infection in the decidua and placenta, and CSF-1 acts by inducing the trophoblast to synthesize neutrophil chemoattractants and macrophage inflammatory protein. Thus, during pregnancy, trophoblast cells responsive to CSF-1 act to organize the immune response to *Listeria* infection at the utero-placental interface [9]. Collectively, these observations demonstrate that the placenta functions as a pregnancy-specific component of the innate immune system, and placental infection and response to infection are critical to the development of adverse pregnancy outcomes associated with *Listeria* infections.

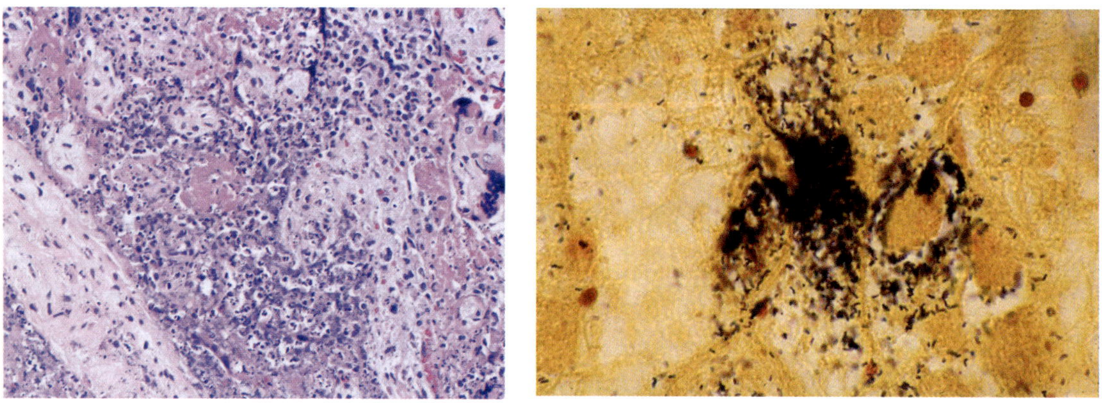

(a) (b)

Figure 34.3 (a) H&E stain of microabscess in the placenta consistent with *Listeriosis* infection. (Courtesy Dr. Aliya Husain.) (b) Silver stain of placenta showing the *Listeria* organisms within a microabscess. (Courtesy Dr. Anthony Montaq.)

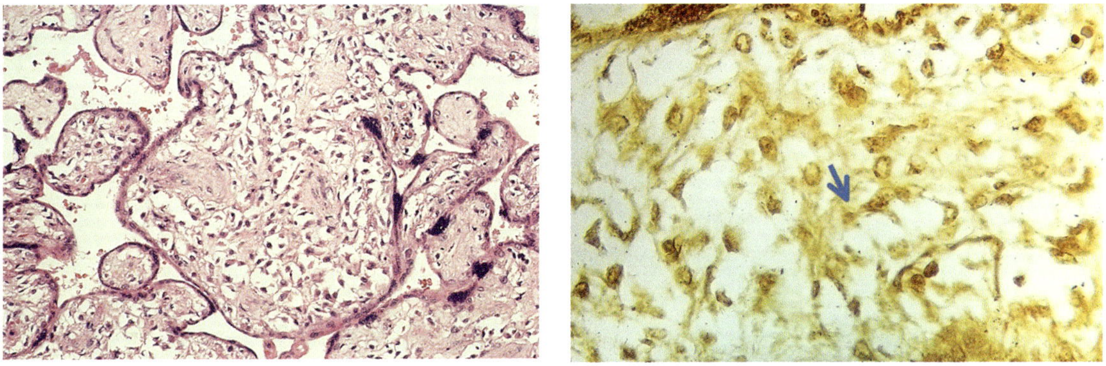

Figure 34.4 (a) H&E stain of placenta infected with *Treponema pallidum*. The villi are enlarged. (Courtesy Dr. Aliya Husain.) (b) Silver stain of enlarged placenta villi demonstrating an intravillous *Treponema pallidum* organism (arrow). (Courtesy Dr. Aliya Husain.)

Treponema pallidum and the placenta

Syphilis is caused by the spirochetal bacterium *Treponema pallidum*. The route of transmission of syphilis is almost always through sexual contact, although congenital syphilis via in utero transmission has been described extensively. Although the mechanisms by which spirochetes infect, cross, and damage the placenta are poorly understood, histopathological findings in the human placenta in cases of congenital syphilis indicate that placental infection has an integral role in the development of adverse outcomes associated with syphilis during pregnancy. In one case-control study, preterm births and stillbirths attributed to syphilis were associated with increased rates of necrotizing funisitis, placental villous enlargement, and acute villitis compared to controls [10]. (Figures 34.4(a,b)) The addition of histological evaluation of the placenta to conventional diagnostic evaluations significantly improved the detection rate for congenital syphilis in live born and stillborn infants. These results demonstrate that placental infection by *Treponema pallidum* leads to histopathologic damage within the placenta that likely contributes to the adverse outcomes associated with congenital syphilis.

Parasitic infections of the placenta

Congenital infections leading to adverse pregnancy outcomes following maternal infections with *Toxoplasma gondii* and *Plasmodium falciparum* (malaria) have been described in detail. Infection with *Toxoplasma gondii* leads to significant inflammation in the villi (Figure 34.5). Malaria during pregnancy is characterized by the sequestration of malaria-infected erythrocytes and monocyte infiltrates in the placental intervillous space and is associated with fetal growth restriction, hypertensive disorders, and pregnancy loss, although the confounding effects of maternal anemia have been difficult to distinguish (Figures 34.6(a,b)).

In experimental models, *Plasmodium falciparum* induces an innate immune response and altered gene transcription by trophoblast cells. Similarly, *Toxoplasma gondii* infections during pregnancy cause congenital malformations, neurologic damage, miscarriage, and

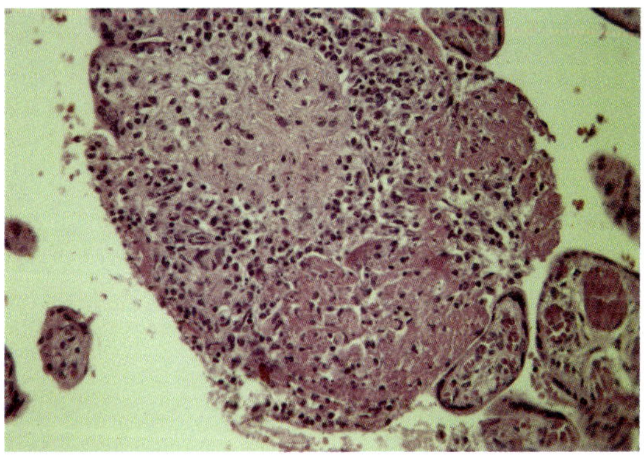

Figure 34.5 H&E stain showing chronic villitis caused by *Toxoplasmosis gondii*, with lymphohistiocytic inflammatory reaction. (Courtesy Dr. Frederick Kraus.)

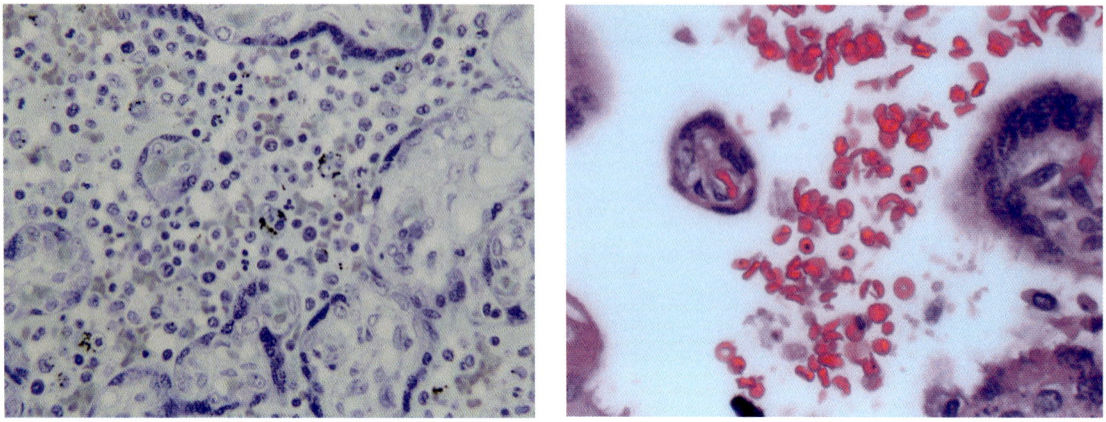

(a) (b)

Figure 34.6 (a) Giemsa stain at 20× of a case with massive chronic intervillositis, an unusual pattern associated with adverse outcomes seen in primiparous women who travel to endemic areas from cities where they have not been previously exposed. Image shows mostly monocytes, macrophages, some neutrophils, fibrin, and malaria pigment. (Courtesy Dr. Raymond Redline.) (b) H&E stain demonstrating basophilic inclusions of *Plamodium* organisms within red blood cells in the maternal intervillous space. (Courtesy Dr. Aliya Husain.)

stillbirth. Trophoblast cells can be infected by *Toxoplasma*, and noninfected, but not infected, cells undergo apoptosis, possibly secondary to cytotoxic factors such as pro-inflammatory mediators produced by infected cells. The ability of parasites to survive intra-cellularly largely depends on the blocking of different pro-apoptotic signaling cascades of the host cells. During pregnancy, however, alterations in the incidence of apoptosis are associated with abnormal placental morphology and functions. Collectively, these observations suggest that clinically relevant parasitic infections might adversely impact placental morphogenesis and functions; further investigation is warranted.

☞ Teaching Points

1. Adverse pregnancy outcomes attributed to placental dysfunction include preeclampsia, spontaneous preterm delivery, fetal growth restriction, and fetal demise.
2. Viral infection (CMV, HPV, AAV) of placental trophoblast cells can induce a pro-inflammatory response, trophoblast cell death, and failed invasion by trophoblast cells into the maternal uterine vasculature to establish normal utero-placental blood flow.
3. Rates of adverse pregnancy outcomes (i.e., preeclampsia, spontaneous preterm delivery) are increased in women with placental infections (HPV, AAV, *Chlamydia pneumoniae*).
4. Bacterial infections of the placenta early in pregnancy induce a pro-inflammatory response and are correlated with spontaneous preterm delivery.
5. Infection of the placenta by *Treponema pallidum* (syphilis) induces characteristic histopathologic damage that likely contributes to the adverse outcomes associated with congenital syphilis.

References

1. Fisher S, Genbacev O, Maidji E et al. (2000) Human cytomegalovirus infection of placental cytotrophoblasts in vitro and in utero: implications for transmission and pathogenesis. *J Virol* 74: 6808–20.
2. Schleiss MR, Aronow BJ, and Handwerger S (2007) Cytomegalovirus infection of human syncytiotrophoblast cells strongly interferes with expression of genes involved in placental differentiation and tissue integrity. *Pediatr Res* 61: 565–71.
3. Arechavaleta-Velasco F, Gomez L, Ma Y et al. (2008) Adverse reproductive outcomes in urban women with adeno-associated virus-2 infections in early pregnancy. *Hum Reprod* 23: 29–36.
4. Gomez LM, Ma Y, Ho C et al. (2008) Placental infection with human papillomavirus is associated with spontaneous preterm delivery. *Hum Reprod* 23: 709–15.

5. Boulenouar S, Weyn C, Van Noppen M et al. (2010, March) Effects of HPV-16 E5, E6 and E7 proteins on survival, adhesion, migration and invasion of trophoblastic cells. *Carcinogenesis* 31(3): 473–80. 2009 Epub.
6. Komine-Aizawa S, Majima H, Yoshida-Noro C et al. (2008) Stimuli through Toll-like receptor (TLR) 3 and 9 affect human chorionic gonadotropin (hCG) production in a choriocarcinoma cell line. *J Obstet Gynaecol Res* 34: 144–51.
7. Abrahams VM and Mor G (2005) Toll-like receptors and their role in the trophoblast. *Placenta* 26: 540–7.
8. Gomez LM and Parry S (2009) Trophoblast infection with Chlamydia pneumoniae and adverse pregnancy outcomes associated with placental dysfunction. *Am J Obstet Gynecol* 200: 526. e1–7.
9. Guleria I and Pollard JW (2000). The trophoblast is a component of the innate immune system during pregnancy. *Nat Med* 6: 589–93.
10. Sheffield JS, Sanchez PJ, Wendel GD Jr et al. (2002) Placental histopathology of congenital syphilis. *Obstet Gynecol* 100: 126–33.
11. Chou et al. (2006) *Am J Obstet Gynecol* 2006;194: 535–41.

CHAPTER 35

Aneuploidy and Polyploidy

Dan Diego-Alvarez[1,2,3] *and Wendy P. Robinson*[1,2]

[1]Department of Medical Genetics, University of British Columbia, Vancouver, BC, Canada
[2]Child and Family Research Institute, Vancouver, BC, Canada
[3]School of Biology, IE University, Segovia, Spain

Introduction

The human genome is normally packaged into 46 chromosomes in the diploid (2n) somatic cells, constituted by 22 pairs of autosomes and the sex-chromosome pair (XX in females, XY in males). During oogenesis and spermatogenesis, the diploid number of chromosomes is reduced to half by meiosis to produce haploid gametes. However, about 20% of oocytes and a few percent of spermatocytes do not have the expected number of chromosomes. Additional errors may arise during early cleavage of the embryo, resulting in chromosomal mosaicism, the situation where different cells originated from the same zygote have different chromosomal constitution. Chromosomal alterations are known to affect early embryo development from implantation to cell and tissue differentiation and function, although the underlying mechanisms are not well understood. Alterations in the deoxyribonucleic acid (DNA) content of the cell may affect its normal function and compromise cell viability, with losses of DNA generally resulting in more severe effects than gains in total DNA.

Almost half of all conceptions and 10–15% of clinically recognized pregnancies are nonviable. Chromosomal alterations are responsible for over 60% of first trimester losses and almost 10% of late spontaneous abortions. The most common error is aneuploidy, which refers to the gain (trisomy, $2n + 1$) or loss (monosomy, $2n - 1$) of one or more chromosomes in the cell. Polyploidy may also occur, which is defined by the presence of three (triploidy, 3n) or four (tetraploidy, 4n) haploid sets of chromosomes within the cell. Aneuploidy and polyploidy have different origins and causative mechanisms, clinical manifestations, incidence and recurrence risks, which will be reviewed in this chapter.

Aneuploidy

Incidence

Over 5% of all clinically recognized pregnancies are aneuploid [1]. Most of these undergo spontaneous demise in utero, making aneuploidy the leading known cause of miscarriage, and present in over 50% of first trimester miscarriages. Aneuploidy of every chromosome has been reported in early losses, although most monosomies are not observed and some trisomies (e.g., trisomy 1, 11, and 19) are quite rare, possibly because they do not survive the implantation stage. The most frequently observed monosomy is monosomy X, observed in 5–10% of miscarriage samples. The most frequently observed trisomy is trisomy 16, estimated to occur in about 1% of clinically recognized gestations; however, this aneuploidy generally ends in miscarriage between the 8th and 15th week of gestation. Trisomies involving chromosomes 13, 18, 21, X, and Y, and monosomy X can be compatible with birth even when present in the fetus. Thus, aneuploidy is also the leading known cause of congenital birth defects and mental retardation.

The Placenta: From Development to Disease, First Edition. Edited by Helen H. Kay, D. Michael Nelson and Yuping Wang.
© 2011 Blackwell Publishing Ltd. Published 2011 by Blackwell Publishing Ltd.

Origin

Most trisomies originate during oogenesis, with nondisjunction (unbalanced segregation of chromosomes leading to aneuploidy) errors at the first meiotic division (meiosis I or MI) being the most common [1]. The excess of maternal trisomy, as compared to paternally derived trisomy, could be explained by the longer duration of meiosis, lack of cell-cycle checkpoints, or more limited opportunity for gamete selection during oogenesis as compared to spermatogenesis.

Female MI is initiated during embryogenesis and completed at the time of ovulation, 20–40 years later. Meiosis II (MII) is not completed until the egg is fertilized by a sperm. In contrast, spermatogenesis occurs continuously after puberty in males, with meiosis requiring only 24 days to complete. Studies of products of conception show that some aneuploidies are more frequent than others. This suggests that risks of nondisjunction and/or their survival through implantation are chromosome-specific.

The frequencies with which errors occur at MI or MII appear to be chromosome-specific, with similar patterns for acrocentric chromosomes (13–15, 21, and 22). Virtually, all cases of trisomy 16 are linked to errors at maternal MI, while trisomy 18 is most often due to errors in maternal MII. 47,XYY cases are paternal in origin, and 47,XXY is as likely to be maternal as paternal. In 80% of 45,X cases, lack of the paternal sex chromosome has been demonstrated. This is probably a consequence of greater pairing problems between the X and Y chromosomes during male meiosis, as well as a greater tendency to somatic loss of a Y chromosome compared with an X chromosome.

Risk factors

Risk of a trisomic pregnancy is strongly affected by the age of the mother. For example, trisomy is estimated to affect less than 3% of clinically recognized pregnancies in women aged 25 years, but 35% of pregnancies in women aged 42 years. The level and distribution of chromosomal exchange during MI appears to affect the age-related susceptibility of an oocyte to undergo nondisjunction. There is also a small increase in risk for a subsequent trisomic pregnancy if a previous trisomy has occurred [2]. Risk factors for aneuploidy, other than advanced maternal age, include genetic conditions (e.g., germline mosaicism and chromosomal rearrangements) and environmental influences (e.g., occupational exposures, medical treatments, reproduction-related products, habituating agents). The latter are difficult to prove, and are relatively less important as compared to the strong maternal age effect. Balanced chromosomal translocations (i.e., interchange of chromosomal material between two or more nonhomologous chromosomes) have an incidence of 1 per 500 births. Even if they do not have an apparent phenotypic repercussion on the carrier individual, translocations have an impact on fertility and pregnancy outcome due to the increased chance to produce unbalanced gametes as a result of improper chromosomal segregation in meiosis.

Clinical Pearl

Advanced maternal age and the occurrence of a previous trisomic gestation remain the only factors incontrovertibly linked to whole chromosome aneuploidy.

Chromosomal mosaicism

Mosaic aneuploidy is the presence of two or more cell populations differing in chromosome number within one individual. Trisomy mosaicism may originate through gain of a chromosome in a normal diploid embryo (somatic origin), or loss of a chromosome from a trisomic embryo (meiotic origin; Figure 35.1). Monosomy mosaicism is rare, except for that involving the X chromosome, and this generally results from a postzygotic loss of one chromosome during mitotic cell division.

Embryos obtained after in vitro fertilization (IVF) have shown a high rate of postzygotic (mitotic) chromosomal instability in the first few cell divisions. A recent study analyzed chromosomal constitution of 23 good-quality embryos from women aged <35 years, undergoing assisted reproduction for genetic risks not related to aneuploidy, with an average of seven blastomeres per embryo. Aneuploidy was detected in 19 out of 23 embryos, with only three of them being nonmosaic [3]. In general, trisomies that arise owing to a somatic error are probably more common, but the abnormal lineage is likely eliminated by selection and, thus, of little consequence. If the abnormal cells affect the embryo or occur in a significant proportion of placental cells, there may be abnormal development.

Prenatally diagnosed confined placental mosaicism

Confined placental mosaicism (CPM) is a chromosomal abnormality, typically a trisomy that is observed in

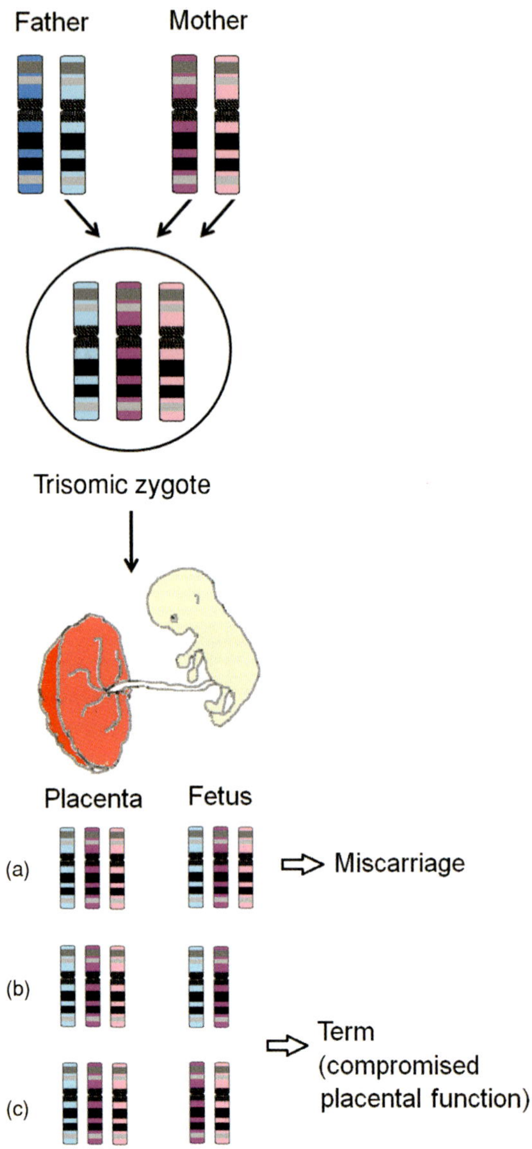

Figure 35.1 Origin and possible outcomes of meiotic trisomy. Trisomy of maternal meiotic origin is present in the zygote. This will lead to miscarriage in the majority of cases (a). If a "trisomy rescue" event occurs in the early embryo, the trisomic cell line can be confined to placental tissues (b, c), being the fetus diploid. Fetal development and growth can be compromised by an abnormal placental function in these cases. Maternal uniparental disomy in the diploid fetus (c) is the result of the loss of the paternal chromosome after a "trisomy rescue" event. Imprinting disorders may arise depending on the chromosome involved. Furthermore, if nondisjunction occurs in MII, both chromosomes inherited from the same parent will be identical, situation that can unmask recessive traits.

placental tissues, either the villous trophoblast, mesenchymal core or both, but not detected in the fetus (Figure 35.1) [4]. CPM is reported in up to 2% of pregnancies undergoing chorionic villous sampling (CVS) at 9–12 weeks of gestation. For nonviable trisomies, such as trisomy 4, 7, or 16, the presence of a normally growing embryo or fetus is suggestive that the trisomic cells are confined to the placenta, even if 100% of the placental cells analyzed by CVS show trisomy. There may be selection in such cases for chromosomally normal cells at the earliest stages of embryogenesis. Trisomy mosaicism that is observed in amniotic fluid testing is more likely to show fetal involvement; however, the pregnancy outcome in such cases can also be normal with no evidence that the resulting baby shows trisomy. In contrast, when trisomies 13 or 21 are observed in 100% of cells at CVS, the chance of the fetus being affected by the trisomy is relatively high.

Pregnancies diagnosed with CPM typically deliver at term uneventfully, but there is an increased incidence of perinatal complications, pregnancy loss, intrauterine growth restriction (IUGR), and premature labor. Placental weight after delivery in pregnancies with CPM also tends to be reduced, though fetal–placental weight ratio is normal. Clinical outcome of CPM is strongly dependent on the chromosome involved in the aneuploidy and the percentage of trisomic cells in the placenta. Pregnancies diagnosed with CPM for trisomy 2, 3, 7, and 8 are typically associated with a normal outcome. However, IUGR or fetal malformations can occur in some cases.

In the case of trisomy 16 CPM, most cases continue to term and have a good postnatal outcome, but these pregnancies display a significantly increased risk of IUGR, fetal malformation (e.g., hypospadias, cardial septal defects), maternal preeclampsia, and intrauterine or neonatal death. Long-term prognosis of trisomy 16 CPM-associated newborns is good as long as multiple malformations are not present at birth [5]. Therefore, ultrasound provides the most useful tool to predict the phenotypic outcome of the baby in these cases.

Uniparental disomy (UPD) occurs when both homologous chromosomes are inherited from the same progenitor. One-third of diploid fetuses will theoretically present with UPD in cases of CPM where there is a meiotic origin of the trisomy. UPD for certain chromosomes (e.g., 6, 7, 11, 14, 15) can cause known clinical syndromes as a consequence of an imbalance in gene expression due to genomic imprinting. Genomic imprinting is the differential expression of genes dependent on parent of origin, which occurs only at selected genes in specific chromosomes.

Confined placental mosaicism diagnosed at term

Most cases of CPM are not detected, since CVS is not routinely performed and placentas of uneventful pregnancies are not usually studied. Estimates of CPM in term placentas from uncomplicated pregnancies range from 1–5%, but higher levels of trisomy are observed in ~10% of term placentas, associated with newborns affected by IUGR. In contrast, CPM does not appear to be associated with preeclampsia in the absence of IUGR [6]. Increased maternal age and elevated maternal serum human chorionic gonadotropin (hCG) increase the chance of IUGR being associated with trisomy in the placenta.

Clinical Pearl

Defining the underlying genetic cause for IUGR can be useful in predicting the postnatal course, and in some cases testing for UPD may be warranted.

Placental development

Trisomic cells affect placental development, but little is known about the mechanisms involved. Several studies of early miscarriage samples have suggested qualitative differences in morphology and cell proliferation within both the trophoblast and mesenchymal portion of aneuploid placentas as compared to chromosomally normal placentas. However, a characteristic pathology has not been identified, and such studies are confounded by in utero demise and sampling issues.

Histomorphometric differences, identified from CVS samples from ongoing pregnancies with trisomies 13, 18, and 21, are more useful for understanding the underlying pathology [7]. Trisomy CVS samples showed measurable differences in the number of fetal vessels per villus, the amount of basophilic stippling, the percentage of double-layered villous trophoblast beyond 20 weeks, and the proportion of villous capillaries with nucleated blood cells. These parameters differed by type of trisomy, though a high rate of basophilic stippling is seen in trisomy 13, 18, and 21 and is suggested to be a marker of early placental failure [7].

Villous cytotrophoblast cultures from term trisomy 21 placentas showed delayed differentiation into syncytiotrophoblast. The cytotrophoblasts aggregated normally, but fused poorly [8]. There is an associated diminished mass of syncytiotrophoblast and decreased secretion of the syncytiotrophoblastic associated hormones, such as hCG, human placental lactogen (hPL), human placental growth hormone (hPGH), and leptin.

Clinical Pearl

Elevated maternal serum hCG, typically observed in trisomy 21 pregnancies, appears to be the result of lack of local uptake of the hCG by the placenta rather than overproduction.

Research Spotlight

The trophoblast differentiation and fusion defects of in vitro cultured trisomy 21 cells are reversible by treatment with biosynthetic hCG [8].

Molecular genetic studies

Proper embryo development and placental growth and function are processes finely regulated by a number of genetic processes. Evidence for specific gene transcriptional changes has been documented in cultured amniocytes and chorionic villous cells from pregnancies with trisomies 13, 18, and 21, showing both gene dosage effects with overexpression of some genes on the involved chromosome and a genome-wide transcriptional dysregulation with altered expression of a multitude of genes throughout the genome.

Chimerism versus mosaicism

Unlike mosaicism, where different cell populations within an individual derive from genetically identical cells from a single zygote, chimerism has traditionally been defined as the situation whereby cells from one embryo derive from more than one genetically distinct zygote. While such multiple-zygote chimerism is rare (or at any rate difficult to detect), a more common occurrence may be 'single egg chimerism', whereby mis-segregation of whole haploid chromosomal complements occurs after zygote formation (fertilization) but prior to the incorporation of paternal and maternal chromosomes into a single nucleus at the two-cell stage. This can result in chimeric embryos, whereby, for example, cells share the same maternal but different paternal haploid complement or some cells are biparental and some uniparental (androgenetic or gynogenetic) in origin.

Biparental/androgenetic chimerism (Figure 35.2) is associated with placental mesenchymal dysplasia (PMD). This is a rare placental vascular anomaly characterized by overgrowth of placental tissue, resulting in placentomegaly and grapelike vesicles ranging in size from 0.3 to 2.5 cm that resemble partial molar pregnancy by ultrasonography and by gross placental examination. These placentas differ from partial moles in the lack of trophoblastic proliferation, and, unlike molar pregnancies,

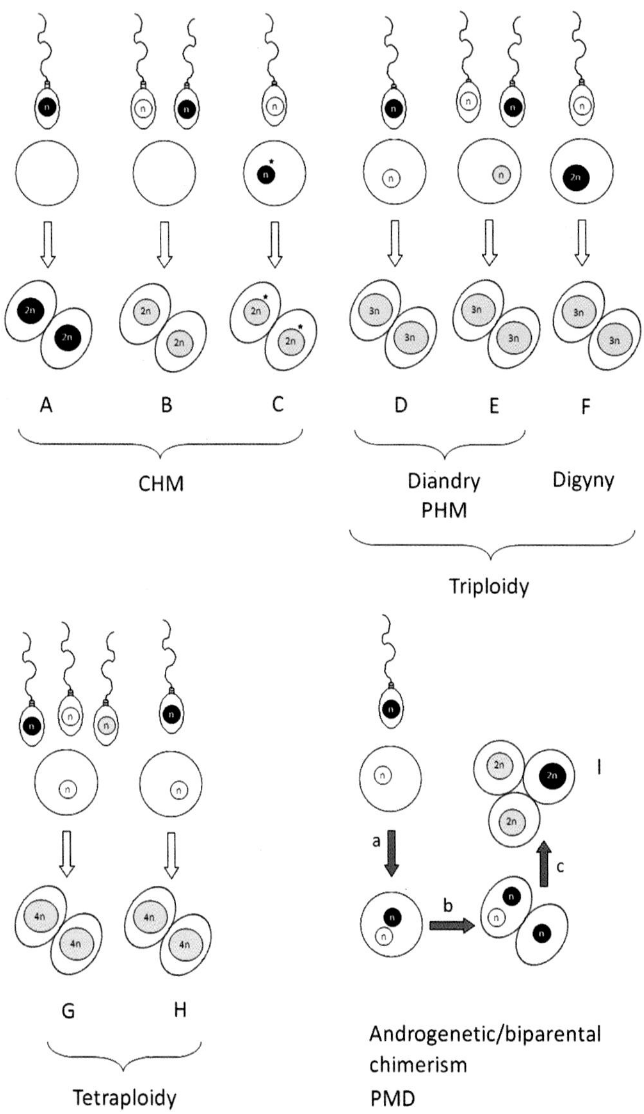

Figure 35.2 Genetic mechanisms leading to abnormal placental presentations. *Clear arrows* represent the fertilization process and the first division of the zygote (pronuclei do not become united into a single nuclear membrane until the two cell stage embryo, as represented). Ploidy constitution is noted as: n, haploid; 2n, diploid; 3n, triploid; 4n, tetraploid. Complete hydatidiform moles (CHM) may arise from: (A) the fertilization of an empty oocyte (the ovum nucleus may be either absent, inactivated, or lost) by a 23,X haploid sperm (46,YY condition is not viable), followed by duplication of the paternal chromosomes (monospermic or homozygous mole, 46,XX, 75–80% of CHM cases); (B) fertilization of an empty egg by two haploid sperms (23,X or 23,Y) (dispermic or heterozygous mole, 46,XX or 46,XY, 20–25% of CHM cases); (C) normal fertilization with mutations on *NALP7* gene on the egg (*) affecting imprinting (biparental mole, familial, and with risk of recurrence). Partial hydatidiform moles (PHM) are caused by diandric triploidy (D and E) as the parental origin of the extra chromosomes in triploidy determines the phenotype and outcome of the fetus and placenta. While digynic triploidy (F) conveys fetal asymmetric IUGR and a very small placenta, diandric triploidy shows a normally sized or mildly symmetrically growth-restricted fetus with an abnormally large placenta. Karyotype can be either 69,XXX, 69,XXY, or rarely 69,XYY. PHM may arise through fertilization of a haploid oocyte by one spermatozoon that doubles its chromosomes after fertilization (D), or by two sperms (E). Tetraploidy (G and H) is the result of fertilization of an ovum by three sperms (G) (karyotypes 72,XXXX, 72,XXXY, 72,XXYY, or 72,XYYY) or, as in the majority of cases, an early embryo cleavage error after normal fertilization (H) (72,XXXX or 72,XXYY). Placental mesenchymal dysplasia (PMD, I) can be caused by androgenetic/biparental chimerism. Failure of DNA replication and chromosome condensation in the female pronucleus after fertilization (a) may lead to the formation of diploid and haploid daughter cells after the normal segregation of the paternal genome (b) that may be endoreduplicated to become diploid, persisting in a mosaic state (c).

PMD usually features a normal fetus with the pregnancy often extending into the third trimester. However, PMD is associated with increased rates of IUGR, intrauterine fetal death, and neonatal death. A normal female karyotype (46,XX) is present in most cases of PMD, being female fetuses affected disproportionally (3.6:1, F:M). Although most cases are the result of androgenetic chimerism, mosaicism for maternal deletion, paternal duplication, or paternal UPD of the Beckwith–Wiedemann syndrome domain in chromosome 11p15.5 can cause features of PMD.

Clinical Pearl

As phenotypic changes in PMD cases may be limited to the placenta, its distinction from triploidy or CHM should be noted to prevent termination of pregnancy in cases associated with a normal fetus.

Triploidy

Incidence and origin

Triploidy is estimated to be present in 1% of all clinically recognized pregnancies, 7% of spontaneous abortions, and 0.5% of stillborn infants. Diandric triploidy indicates the extra haploid set of chromosomes is of paternal origin usually due to dispermy. Digynic triploidy indicates a maternal origin for the extra chromosomes due to failure of MI or MII divisions at meiosis (Figure 35.2). Digynic triploidy is the most common in fetuses, while diandry accounts for up to 60% of early triploid spontaneous abortions, particularly those diagnosed after 8.5 weeks with no embryo present [9].

Placental and fetal development

Two distinct phenotypes observed in triploid fetuses are associated with parental origin of the triploidy. The diandric phenotype is characterized by a normally sized or a mildly affected, symmetrically growth-retarded fetus. The placenta is abnormally large and may be cystic, with histological features of partial hydatidiform mole (PHM). Such placentas are characterized by edematous placental villi and irregular growth of the trophoblast, attributed to over-representation of the paternal genome. In contrast to PHM that is generally diandric triploid, complete hydatidiform moles (CHM) are mostly androgenetic and diploid with a 46,XX or 46,XY karyotype (Figure 35.2). The triploid digynic phenotype presents with marked, asymmetric fetal IUGR, and a very small nonmolar placenta. Although not well understood, lack of sufficient hCG production from such small digynic placentas, as documented on prenatal serum screen, may contribute, in part, to the fetal growth restriction.

Genomic imprinting is parent-of-origin and allele-specific expression of genes. The two distinct fetal and placental phenotypes in triploidy are dependent on the parental origin of the extra haploid set of chromosomes, and likely result from genomic imprinting imbalances. Interestingly, there appears to be no difference in embryonic phenotype in triploids dependent on parent of origin and, thus, many of the fetal differences may be the consequence of altered placental function. There are over 50 genes known to be imprinted in humans, most expressed in the placenta; thus, the cause of this phenotype is likely to be complex.

Risk factors

Unlike most trisomies, a maternal age effect has not been noted with triploidy, even among those cases of maternal origin. Recurrence risk is negligible; however, it has been suggested that some women may have a predisposition for meiotic errors, resulting in digyny. Some female carriers of homozygous mutations in the *NALP7* gene, typically associated with recurrent biparental CHM, also appear to be at increased risk of triploid pregnancies.

Tetraploidy

Tetraploidy is observed in approximately 2.5% of early spontaneous abortions, commonly as the result of a postfertilization cleavage error. Trispermic fertilization of an ovum has also been described. Some tetraploid conceptions show changes of PHM, and, rarely, liveborn infants with severely compromised survival have been reported. Tetraploid cells are normally present among the proliferating trophoblast cells of the first and second trimester. They may also arise in culture of CVS samples, and thus may be commonly detected in mosaic form in CVS samples from normal pregnancies. Thus, a finding of low-level (3–4%) tetraploid cells in prenatal diagnosis should be interpreted with caution.

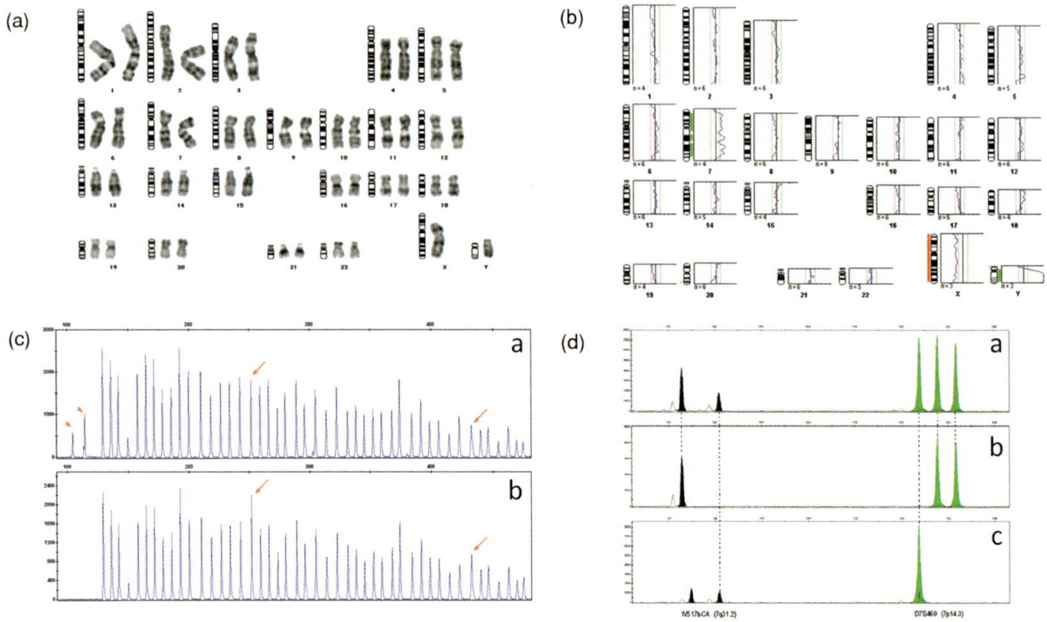

Figure 35.3 Cytogenetic and molecular techniques for the detection of chromosomal alterations. (a) Normal male karyotype (46,XY) showing the 23 pairs of metaphase chromosomes with their characteristic G-band pattern (500 bands). (b) CGH results displaying fluorescence intensity ratios of every chromosomal region between differentially labeled DNA samples (test in green, reference in red). Gains and losses of chromosomal material in the test sample are shown as green or red bars respectively. Results are compatible with trisomy 7 in a male sample using a normal female as reference. (c) MLPA results testing a region for both ends of every chromosome (P070 probe-mix). Arrowheads point to Y-chromosome-specific regions, arrows point chromosome 17 specific regions. Trisomy 17 in the test sample (b, female) can be suspected based on a 35% increase of the peak area for both regions tested of chromosome 17 when compared with those areas of a reference sample (a, male). (d) QF-PCR results for two different chromosome 7 markers in an abortion sample (a), showing the inherited alleles (peaks) from each parent (b, mother; c, father). Trisomy 7 from maternal origin in the abortion sample is noted as a trisomic diallelic pattern (peak area ratio 2:1) for marker IV517bCA and a trisomic triallelic pattern (1:1:1) for marker D7S460.

Diagnosis of placental aneuploidy and polyploidy

Karyotyping (chromosome analysis) of placentas or spontaneous miscarriages is usually performed some days after delivery or embryo demise, which can result in high rates of cell culture failure, microbial contamination, or both. Preferential growth of maternal cells can also occur. Short-term cultures of chorionic villi more likely reflect spontaneous cytotrophoblast cell divisions, while long-term cultures are mostly mesenchymal-derived fibroblasts. As detection of CPM may depend on the distribution and degree of mosaicism present on the sampled site, multiple sites should be sampled when a placenta is analyzed.

Methods that avoid cell culture are particularly useful in the analysis of miscarriages and term placenta (Figure 35.3). Ploidy changes can also be assessed by flow cytometry or fluorescence *in situ* hybridization (FISH), and molecular techniques based on the study of DNA represent a valid alternative. Comparative genomic hybridization (CGH) and multiplex ligation-dependent probe amplification (MLPA) permit the detection of aneuploidy as well as unbalanced rearrangements for every chromosome in a single assay. Chromosome-specific polymorphic marker analysis by quantitative fluorescent-polymerase chain reaction (QF-PCR) detects aneuploidy, triploidy, and UPD, and distinguishes CHM that are mono- or dispermic from PHM. Genotyping, together with p57 expression assessment by immunohistochemistry, constitute the best approach for the diagnosis and classification of hydatidiform moles, as discussed in detail in another chapter of this book [10].

Summary and future perspectives

Chromosomal alterations are frequent in the placenta. Understanding the basic mechanisms of how these alterations affect placental development and function will help prevent future risks, predict outcomes, and develop therapies for gestations at risk. Current efforts are focused on the noninvasive prenatal diagnosis (NIPD) of aneuploidies by studying the fraction of circulating cell free fetal DNA of trophoblastic origin in maternal plasma. This approach is currently limited to the detection of paternally inherited DNA sequences, fetal RhD status assessment, and fetal gender determination from the 7th week of gestation. Detection of aneuploidies by cell free fetal DNA analysis requires larger validation studies and improved, robust techniques before they can be offered to the general population. Moreover, the relatively high and still underestimated incidence of CPM and placental chimerism must be considered, since these phenomena may raise ethical concerns when NIPD becomes an affordable option.

☞ Teaching Points

1 Chromosomal errors are common in the placenta.
2 Aneuploidies that are diagnosed prenatally by chorionic villous sampling are generally confined to placental tissues.
3 Trisomy mosaicism is underdiagnosed and can contribute to placental insufficiency.
4 The majority of pregnancies that are diagnosed with placental mosaicism for trisomy 16 continue to term and have a good postnatal outcome. However, these gestations are at increased risk of IUGR, fetal malformations, and maternal preeclampsia.
5 Chromosomal studies of the placenta are important to better understand the etiology of poor gestation outcomes.

Web resources

Detailed information on chromosomal mosaicism can be found at http://mosaicism.cfri.ca/index.htm.

Acknowledgments

DDA is funded by the Interdisciplinary Women's Reproductive Health (IWRH) Research training program, a Canadian Institutes of Health Research (CIHR) funded strategic training program, and receives a postdoctoral fellowship from the Child and Family Research Institute in Vancouver, British Columbia, Canada. The authors would like to thank the rest of members of the Robinson Lab (R Jiang, C Hanna, R Yuen, D Bourque, J Blair, E Price, G Teodosio, and A Murdoch), and specially MS Peñaherrera and K Louie for the detailed review of the manuscript.

References

1. Hassold T, Hall H, and Hunt P (2007) The origin of human aneuploidy: where we have been, where we are going. *Human Molecular Genetics* 16 (Spec No. 2): R203–8.
2. Warburton D, Dallaire L, Thangavelu M et al. (2004) Trisomy recurrence: a reconsideration based on North American data. *American Journal of Human Genetics* 75(3): 376–85.
3. Vanneste E, Voet T, Le Caignec C et al. (2009) Chromosome instability is common in human cleavage-stage embryos. *Nature Medicine* 15(5): 577–83.
4. Henderson KG, Shaw TE, Barrett IJ et al. (1996) Distribution of mosaicism in human placentae. *Human Genetics* 97(5): 650–54.
5. Langlois S, Yong PJ, Yong SL et al. (2006) Postnatal follow-up of prenatally diagnosed trisomy 16 mosaicism. *Prenatal Diagnosis* 26(6): 548–58.
6. Robinson WP, Peñaherrera MS, Jiang R et al. (2010) Assessing the role of placental trisomy in pre-eclampsia and intrauterine growth restriction. *Prenatal Diagnosis* 30(1): 1–8.
7. Roberts L, Sebire NJ, Fowler D et al. (2000) Histomorphological features of chorionic villi at 10–14 weeks of gestation in trisomic and chromosomally normal pregnancies. *Placenta* 21(7): 678–83.
8. Pidoux G, Gerbaud P, Marpeau O et al. (2007) Human placental development is impaired by abnormal human chorionic gonadotropin signaling in trisomy 21 pregnancies. *Endocrinology* 148(11): 5403–13.
9. McFadden DE and Robinson WP (2006) Phenotype of triploid embryos. *Journal of Medical Genetics* 43(7): 609–12.
10. McConnell TG, Murphy KM, Hafez M et al. (2009) Diagnosis and subclassification of hydatidiform moles using p57 immunohistochemistry and molecular genotyping: validation and prospective analysis in routine and consultation practice settings with development of an algorithmic approach. *American Journal of Surgical Pathology* 33(6): 805–17.

36

CHAPTER 36

Gestational Trophoblastic Disease and Placental Tumors

Katja Gwin and Aliya N. Husain

Department of Pathology, University of Chicago, Chicago, IL, USA

Introduction

Gestational trophoblastic disease (GTD) is a heterogenous group of lesions [1] that is characterized by proliferation of the trophoblast. GTD *with* chorionic villi comprises the group of hydatidiform moles. Complete hydatidiform mole is of particular clinical importance due to the high risk of subsequent development of choriocarcinoma. GTD *without* chorionic villi covers a broad spectrum from benign, nonproliferative lesions, occasionally causing dysfunctional uterine bleeding, to highly aggressive malignant tumors.

Non-trophoblastic tumors of the placenta are uncommon and mostly incidental findings. They may evolve to clinical relevance due to complications, such as polyhydramnios or syndromic complexes. Rarely, the placenta can also be affected by metastatic tumors of either maternal or fetal origin.

Recent studies have given new insights into the pathogenesis of some types of GTD, but further research is warranted to obtain a better understanding of GTD, which may yield better treatment options in the future.

Gestational trophoblastic disease

GTD is a heterogenous group of conditions arising from abnormal trophoblast proliferation. Morphology, biologic behavior and clinical significance vary tremendously, depending on the type of lesion. GTD is traditionally classified as villous lesions with, and non-villous lesions without, chorionic villi [2]. Complete, partial and invasive hydatidiform moles constitute the villous disease category. Non-villous disease includes malignant gestational trophoblastic tumors and non-neoplastic non-molar trophoblastic lesions.

Pathophysiology

The various types of GTD originate from the different trophoblastic, morphologically and functionally distinct, cell subpopulations present during normal placental development [3,4]. Trophoblastic cells consist of three different types of cells: the cytotrophoblast, the undifferentiated stem cell of the placenta; the highly differentiated syncytiotrophoblast, which produces most of the placental hormones including human chorionic gonadotropin (hCG); and the intermediate trophoblast, a heterogeneous cell population with overlapping features of cyto- and syncytiotrophoblast. Villous intermediate trophoblast, implantation site intermediate trophoblast, and chorionic-type trophoblast are distinguished based on morphology, function, and anatomic location. Trophoblast growing in connection with chorionic villi is called villous trophoblast, and the trophoblast at other placental sites is termed extravillous trophoblast.

The Placenta: From Development to Disease, First Edition. Edited by Helen H. Kay, D. Michael Nelson and Yuping Wang.
© 2011 Blackwell Publishing Ltd. Published 2011 by Blackwell Publishing Ltd.

Table 36.1 Hydatidiform moles.

Complete hydatidiform mole
Diploid karyotype
No embryo
Elevated hCG
Large uterus
Vaginal bleeding
Product of conception has typical "bunch of grapes" appearance
Predominantly large hydropic villi with scant capillaries and edematous stroma
Circumferential proliferation of cyto- and syncytiotrophoblast with atypia
Villous stroma **negative** for $p57^{kip2}$ by immunohistochemistry
Partial hydatidiform mole
Triploid karyotype
Embryo present, usually with abnormalities
Normal hCG
Normal sized uterus
Spontaneous abortion
Product of conception looks grossly normal, occasional vesicles up to 5 mm
Variably sized chorionic villi with scalloped outlines and rare vessels
Polarized proliferation of cyto- and syncytiotrophoblast and fjord-like hyperplasia
Villous stroma **positive** for $p57^{kip2}$ by immunohistochemistry

Villous diseases

Villous lesions comprise the hydatidiform moles (Table 36.1) and originate from abnormal conceptions with characteristic chromosomal abnormalities [2,3].

Complete hydatidiform moles (CHM) are characterized by abundant placental tissue. On gross examination, the chorionic villi are easy to appreciate as round or ovoid enlarged vesicles measuring up to 2 cm. The classical appearance of a complete mole is, therefore, often described as a "bunch of grapes" (Figure 36.1(a)) and is caused by marked hydropic changes of almost all chorionic villi. On microscopic examination, typical features include vesicles with central cisterns, scant capillaries and extensive circumferential trophoblast proliferation of the cyto- and syncytiotrophoblast with atypia (Figures 36.1(b,c)) and intraepithelial lumen formation. Also, the placental implantation site containing the invasive intermediate trophoblast is usually exaggerated and shows marked cytologic atypia. Generally, no embryo or embryonal tissue is present in complete moles. Of note, the classical gross and microscopic findings of complete moles do not fully develop before 12 weeks of gestational age. Earlier, complete moles can have few diagnostic features; however, circumferential trophoblast proliferation is usually present and should raise concern.

Partial hydatidiform moles (PHM) are typically unremarkable on gross examination but occasionally can show a few vesicles measuring up to 5 mm. A gestational sac or the umbilical cord may be grossly identifiable. On microscopic examination, both normal and hydropic villi can be appreciated. The villi are frequently scalloped, leading to pseudo-inclusions in tangential sections. The trophoblast is only focally hyperplastic and often exhibits an elongated shape.

In invasive hydatidiform moles, molar villi penetrate the myometrium or are present in its vascular spaces. Invasive hydatidiform moles predominantly arise from CHM but seldom originate from PHM.

Pathophysiology

CHM develop from an anuclear ovum containing only maternal mitochondrial DNA. In most cases, fertilization with a haploid sperm (23X) and subsequent chromosome replication takes place, leading to a monospermic 46,XX karyotype of complete paternal origin. Alternatively, fertilization with two sperms (23X or 23Y) may occur, leading to a dispermic 46,XX or 46,XY karyotype. Uniparental paternal disomy with lack of maternally imprinted nuclear DNA is responsible for the failure of embryonic development and the excessive trophoblastic proliferation.

A PHM typically has a triploid karyotype and results from the fertilization of a normal oocyte with either two haploid sperms or one diploid sperm. The abundant paternal DNA is thought to be responsible for the molar changes. The triploidy in PHM is linked to fetal abnormalities and growth restriction.

Diagnosis

Most CHM are now diagnosed in the first trimester by ultrasonography and elevated concentrations of hCG. The marked hydropic villi produce a characteristic, vesicular "snow-storm" pattern by ultrasound scanning. Vaginal

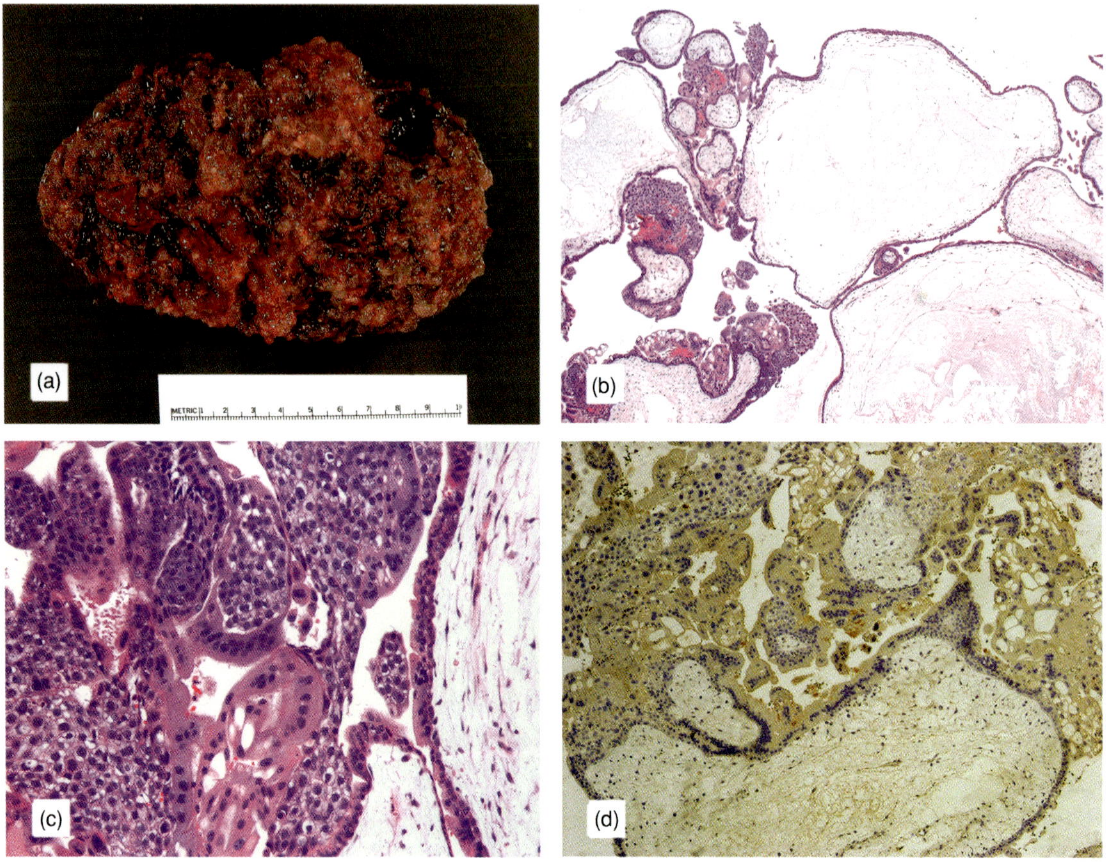

Figure 36.1 Complete hydatidiform mole. (a) Product of conception with "bunch of grapes" appearance. (b) Large hydropic villi with edematous stroma and circumferential cyto- and syncytiotrophoblast proliferation. (c) Proliferation of the cyto-and syncytiotrophoblast with atypia. (d) The villous stroma demonstrated no immunoreactivity for $p57^{kip2}$. Rare trophoblastic cells show nuclear staining.

bleeding is seen in 90% of cases; however, other "classical" findings, such as enlarged uterus for gestational age, hyperemesis and preeclampsia, are now less frequently encountered due to earlier diagnosis. Ultrasonographic findings suggestive of PHM include cystic changes of the placenta and alteration of the gestational sac shape, likely due to triploidy. Partial hydatidiform moles often result in spontaneous abortion.

Morphologic changes, seen on microscopic examination of the placental tissue, often facilitate the differential diagnosis of CHM or PHM; however, the histopathologic findings can be equivocal, especially in first trimester specimens. Immunohistochemical evaluation is useful in such cases since there is differential expression of $p57^{kip2}$ (Figure 36.1(d)), a paternally imprinted cyclin-dependent kinase inhibitor. Villous stromal cells and cytotrophoblasts in CHM do not express $p57^{kip2}$, as opposed to PHM in which > 25% of cell nuclei stain. Other methods to differentiate hydropic changes from CHM or PHM include analysis of DNA ploidy and fluorescence in situ hybridization (FISH) analysis.

Clinical management

The standard treatment for hydatidiform moles [5] is dilatation and suction curettage, with close monitoring of serum β-hCG levels for 6 months while the patient uses oral contraceptives to avoid pregnancy. Chest X-ray, liver and renal function tests, and other baseline laboratory tests should be obtained at the time of diagnosis. If an invasive mole is noted by ultrasound scanning, hysterectomy is a treatment option depending on the clinical setting. Treatment of persistent GTD includes repeated curettage, hysterectomy, and single-agent or multiple-drug chemotherapy.

Clinical Pearl

Postmolar GTD may represent a persistent mole in the uterine cavity, an invasive mole, or choriocarcinoma. Invasive hydatidiform moles can invade deeply into the myometrium and destroy the uterine wall, leading to perforation.

Risk factors

The risk of developing a hydatidiform mole is associated with age, ethnicity, and geographic location. The two peaks include women >35 or <20 years of age. Molar pregnancies are more frequent in Asia and Latin America than in North America and Europe. Women who had a prior hydatidiform mole are at risk for recurrence in a subsequent pregnancy. Risk factors for developing an invasive hydatidiform mole include diagnosis and treatment of a molar pregnancy beyond 16 weeks of gestation, large uterus, maternal age > 40 years, and a previous molar pregnancy.

Incidence

The incidence of hydatidiform moles shows significant geographic variation, ranging from 66–110 per 100,000 pregnancies in Europe and in the United States to 990 per 100,000 pregnancies in Asia. Hydatidiform moles carry a risk for persistent GTD that is up to 20% for CHM and 6% for PHM.

Research Spotlight

Analysis of a case series of familial hydatidiform mole revealed a defective recessive maternal gene mapped to chromosome 19q13.4. Two splice donor site mutations were identified as causative, and the defective protein NALP7 was part of the CATERPILLER protein family, which is an important regulator of inflammatory response [3,6].

Non-villous trophoblastic diseases

Non-villous GTD [4] ranges from benign, nonneoplastic lesions to aggressive malignant tumors. Malignant neoplasms include choriocarcinoma, placental-site trophoblastic tumor, and epithelioid trophoblastic tumor.

Gestational choriocarcinoma (CC) is a highly malignant trophoblastic epithelial tumor. The diagnosis of CC requires absence of chorionic villi. CC rarely occurs in otherwise normal term placentas (Figure 36.2(a)). On gross examination, uterine CC frequently presents as hemorrhagic or fleshy, tan masses in the endometrial cavity and myometrial wall with a variable amount of necrosis. Microscopically, CC has a characteristic biphasic pattern (Figure 36.2(b)) with clusters or sheets of mononucleate trophoblast (cyto- and intermediate trophoblast) separated by syncytiotrophoblast. Vascular invasion is frequently present. Immunohistochemical analysis of CC reveals expression of cytokeratin 18 intermediate filaments (CK18) expression in all trophoblastic elements. The syncytiotrophoblast is strongly immunoreactive for β-hCG and weakly immunoreactive for human placental lactogen (hPL), whereas the intermediate trophoblast is characterized by the opposite immunoprofile.

Clinical Pearl

Choriocarcinoma that occurs after hydatidiform mole contains only paternal DNA and is more chemosensitive than choriocarcinoma derived from molar pregnancy, which contains both paternal and maternal DNA.

Placental site trophoblastic tumor (PSTT) is a monophasic neoplasm composed of implantation site intermediate trophoblast. Grossly, PSTT is well circumscribed, shows a polypoid or exophytic growth pattern, and is generally located in the uterine corpus, although tumors occasionally involve the cervix (Figure 36.2(c)). Microscopically, these tumors are characterized by large, polyhedral, mono- or multinucleated cells with eosinophilic cytoplasm, marked atypia, and frequent mitoses. The tumor cells characteristically dissect between muscle fibers (Figures 36.2(c,d)) during myometrial invasion. Immunohistochemically, PSTT expresses CK18, inhibin, hPL, cluster of differentiation 146 (CD146), and is negative for p63 and placental alkaline phosphatase (PLAP).

Epithelioid trophoblastic tumor (ETT) is a malignant tumor originating from the chorionic type intermediate trophoblast. ETT is most commonly located in the lower uterine segment and cervix but can also occur at

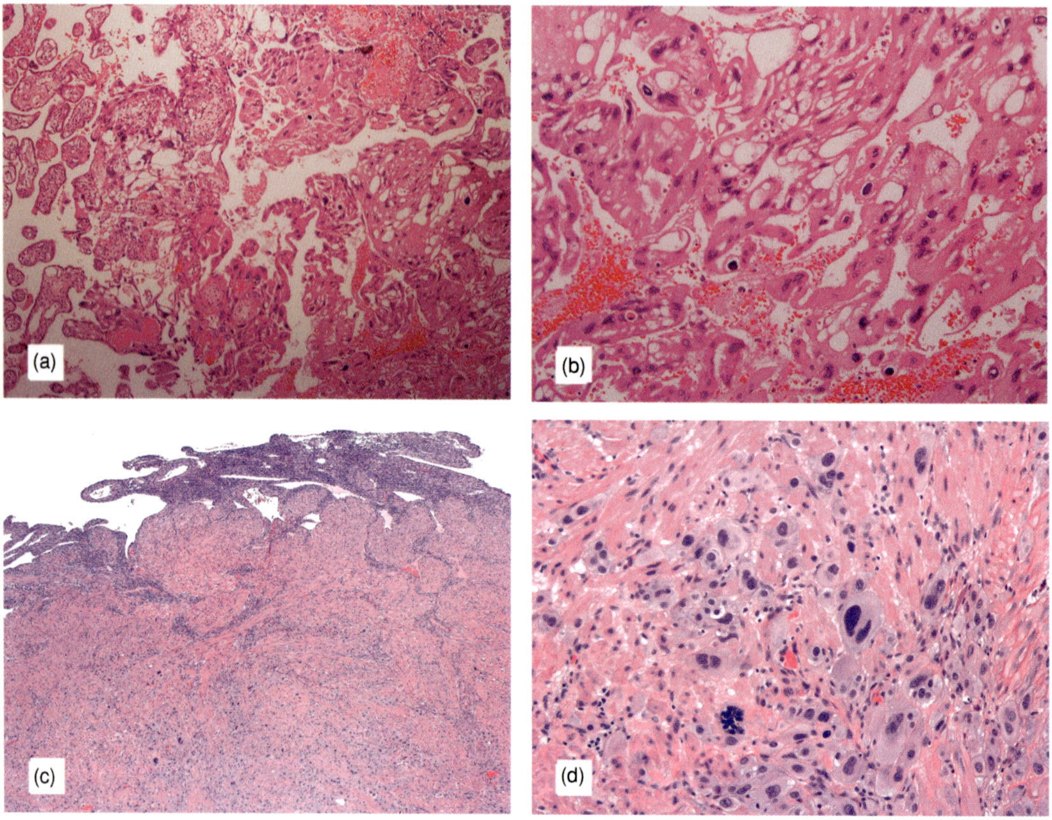

Figure 36.2 Gestational trophoblastic tumors. (a) Intraplacental choriocarcinoma: Chorionic villi (left) and choriocarcinoma in the maternal intervillous space. (b) Dimorphic pattern of choriocarcinoma: mononuclear trophoblastic cells contain moderate amounts of pale cytoplasm, large atypical nuclei with coarse chromatin, and prominent nucleoli, and are admixed with the syncytiotrophoblast exhibiting abundant eosinophilic cytoplasm and a syncytium of nuclei. (c) Placental site trophoblastic tumor extending to the cervix. (d) Placental site trophoblastic tumor: large, polyhedral, mono- and multinucleated cells with eosinophilic cytoplasm, significant atypia, and mitotic activity dissect the myometrium.

extrauterine sites. Grossly, ETT appears as hemorrhagic, tan to brown, circumscribed solitary nodules with deep myometrial invasion. ETT, morphologically, is characterized by a distinct pattern of infiltrating nests and cords of small, atypical, mononucleate cells with fine granular cytoplasm, surrounded by dense, hyalin-like material and extensive necrosis. ETT expresses immunoreactivity for p63, inhibin, hPL, CK18, and PLAP, but is usually negative for CD146.

Clinical Pearl

ETT has a predilection for the cervix and lower uterine segment and should be considered in the differential diagnosis of cervical squamous cell carcinomas.

Non-neoplastic, non-molar trophoblastic lesions include placental site nodules (PSNs) and exaggerated placental site. PSNs are small, circumscribed, yellow-tan nodules or plaques, which are usually an incidental finding in uterine specimens. Microscopically, PSN are composed of scattered, degenerative chorionic-type intermediate trophoblast cells with minimal atypia and abundant hyalinized material. Chronic inflammatory and decidual cells can be seen in the periphery of the nodules.

Exaggerated placental site (EPS) is characterized by prominent myometrial infiltration by implantation site intermediate trophoblast, which often shows multinucleation. Mitotic activity is absent, and cell proliferation is low. The presence of chorionic villi distinguishes this lesion from PSTT.

Clinical Pearl

Non-villous GTD can occur years after the antecedent pregnancy.

Risk factors

Major risk factors for CC are antecedent molar pregnancy (50%), abortion (25%), normal pregnancy (22%), and ectopic pregnancy (3%). PSTT and ETT most frequently occur after a normal pregnancy or spontaneous abortion.

Pathophysiology

Paternal alleles are found in PSTT and ETT, supporting a placental origin.

Diagnosis

Gestational trophoblastic tumors commonly present with abnormal vaginal bleeding, while women with PSTT may also present with amenorrhea. A cervical mass or uterine enlargement may be present, but uterine lesions can be restricted to the myometrium or may even be undetectable. A uterine mass may be visible on ultrasonography. β-hCG is usually elevated in CC but minimally elevated to normal in PSTT and ETT. Symptoms of metastatic disease in CC most commonly occur in the lungs and may be apparent at initial presentation. Microscopic examination of curettage or biopsy specimens and the use of selected immunohistochemical stains are normally required for a definitive diagnosis. It is important to keep in mind that PSTT and ETT can still be difficult to diagnose on a curettage specimen because involvement of the endomyometrium is not always sampled. Additional testing is based on clinical correlation.

Clinical management

Therapeutic options [5] for malignant trophoblastic tumors include hysterectomy, and chemotherapy and radiation. CC is very sensitive to chemotherapy and usually responds well to treatment, even in the setting of widespread metastatic disease. β-hCG is an important marker to monitor therapy. ETT and PSTT show variable responses to chemotherapy.

Incidence

CC occurs in North America in 1:20,000–1:40,000 pregnancies, occurring after 2–5% of complete moles in the United States and after 13% of complete moles in Japan.

PSTT and ETT are rare.

Placental tumors

Placental tumors occur infrequently and are classified as *primary*, non-trophoblastic tumors, and *secondary*, metastatic tumors of the placenta.

Primary, non-trophoblastic tumors of the placenta

The most common primary, non-trophoblastic tumor of the placenta is the placental *hemangioma*. The designation *chorangioma* describes the more frequently encountered solitary lesions, and *chorangiomatosis* describes multiple tumors or diffuse involvement of the placenta. Chorangiomas are frequently incidental, measure less than 5 mm, and can be difficult to appreciate macroscopically, especially in unfixed placental material. Large chorangiomas (> 40 mm) are rare and easier to identify. Chorangiomas, on gross examination, are firmer than the surrounding normal placental tissue, well circumscribed, and entirely intraplacental, although they can bulge from the fetal or, less frequently, from the maternal surface. Chorangiomas can also be present in the membranes or the umbilical cord. The cut surface of chorangiomas is red, congested, and flesh-colored, brown- or white-tan, depending on the degree of degenerative changes. Microscopically, chorangiomas are composed of numerous blood vessels (Figures 36.3(a,b)), surrounded by various amounts of inconspicuous mesenchymal stroma and surfaced by an attenuated trophoblast layer. Villus expansion is caused by the proliferation of blood vessels. The blood vessels are usually of capillary size, but occasionally of cavernous type if they arise from stem villi. Occasionally, chorangiomas are associated with infarction and degenerative changes, such as hyalinization, necrosis, myxoid stromal changes or calcifications.

A few chorangiomas with mitotic activity, cytologic atypia, and trophoblast proliferation have been described and designated as *chorangiocarcinoma*, but none of these reported cases have demonstrated aggressive behavior or metastasized; therefore, it is questionable whether these lesions truly represent malignant tumors.

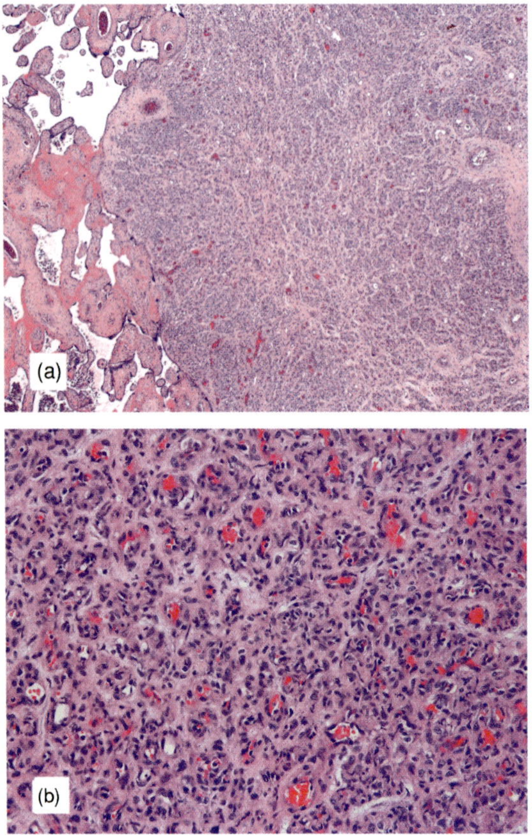

Figure 36.3 Primary tumor of the placenta. (a) Intraplacental chorangioma with villous expansion and surrounded by an attenuated trophoblast layer. (b) Chorangioma with proliferating capillary-sized blood vessels, surrounded by mesenchymal stroma.

Teratomas, germ cell tumors composed of one or more of the three germ layers, are rare tumors that can also arise as primary tumors in the placenta. They are classically located between the amnion and chorion in the chorionic plate or membranes, but can infrequently be found in the umbilical cord. These tumors likely originate from abnormal migration of mesenteric germ cells. A placental teratoma typically contains only mature elements, and can be distinguished from an acardiac fetus by the lack of organized tissue and absence of an umbilical cord. Fetal adrenal tissue (adrenal heterotopia) and hepatocellular adenomas composed of liver tissue of the fetal-type have been found in the villous parenchyma. Suggested pathogenic mechanisms include monodermal teratoma or an ectopia of embryonic hepatic and adrenal tissue.

Clinical Pearl

Chorangiomas do not occur before the second trimester. The clinical relevance depends on size, and on whether solitary or multiple/diffuse lesions are present. Most chorangiomas are incidental and < 5 mm in size. Larger chorangiomas, up to < 40 mm, are usually asymptomatic, but tumors measuring >40 mm can, like chorangiomatosis, be associated with nonimmune fetal hydrops, neonatal hemangiomatosis, oligo- and polyhydramnion, fetal cardiomegaly, growth retardation, fetal thrombocytopenia, microangiopathic hemolytic anemia as well as placental abruption and preterm delivery. Both diagnoses also associate with Beckwith–Wiedemann syndrome, hepatic hemangioendothelioma, and mesenchymal dysplasia.

Risk factors

Gestation at high altitude is correlated with the occurrence of chorangiomas, which suggests that hypoxia induces vascular growth factors.

Recurrence of chorangiomatosis in subsequent pregnancies has been described.

Pathophysiology

Chorangiomas are hamartomas arising from the primitive chorionic mesenchyme caused by abnormal angiogenesis.

Incidence

Chorangiomas occur in up to 1% of all examined placentae.

Diagnosis

Chorangiomas can be diagnosed by ultrasonography, and by gross and microscopic examination of the placenta.

Clinical management

Small chorangiomas are incidental findings and require only observation of fetal well-being. Management of larger symptomatic chorangiomas depends on fetal complications. Successful prenatal laser treatment of the vessels supplying the tumor is reported [7].

Secondary, metastatic tumors of the placenta

Metastatic tumors to the placenta are exceptionally rare but can originate from either maternal tumors or from fetal congenital neoplasms.

Although the most commonly encountered maternal malignancies in pregnancy are cervical and breast carcinoma, malignant melanoma (Figure 36.4(a)) is the most frequent tumor to metastasize to the placenta, comprising 30% of all placental metastases. Other more frequently observed metastatic maternal tumors include breast carcinomas and hematopoietic malignancies, but placental metastases may occur with ovarian, lung, gastric (Figure 36.4(b)), pancreatic, and renal carcinomas as well as Ewing's sarcomas. Pigmented malignant melanomas may be identified on gross examination, but most others are not visible during inspection of the placental parenchyma. On microscopic examination, malignant melanomas tend to infiltrate the villous stroma, which can cause transplacental metastatic extension to the fetus with a high mortality rate. Carcinomas usually form tumor cell clusters in the intervillous space.

Metastatic congenital fetal neuroblastoma (Figure 36.4(c)) is usually associated with severe hydrops or stillbirth, and the placenta is large, bulky and pale. On microscopic examination, aggregates of neuroblastoma tumor cells occlude the villous vessels.

Similarly, metastatic congenital leukemia (Figure 36.4(d)) is also frequently associated with hydrops and fetal demise. Histologic examination of the placenta reveals disseminated leukemic cells occluding villous vessels.

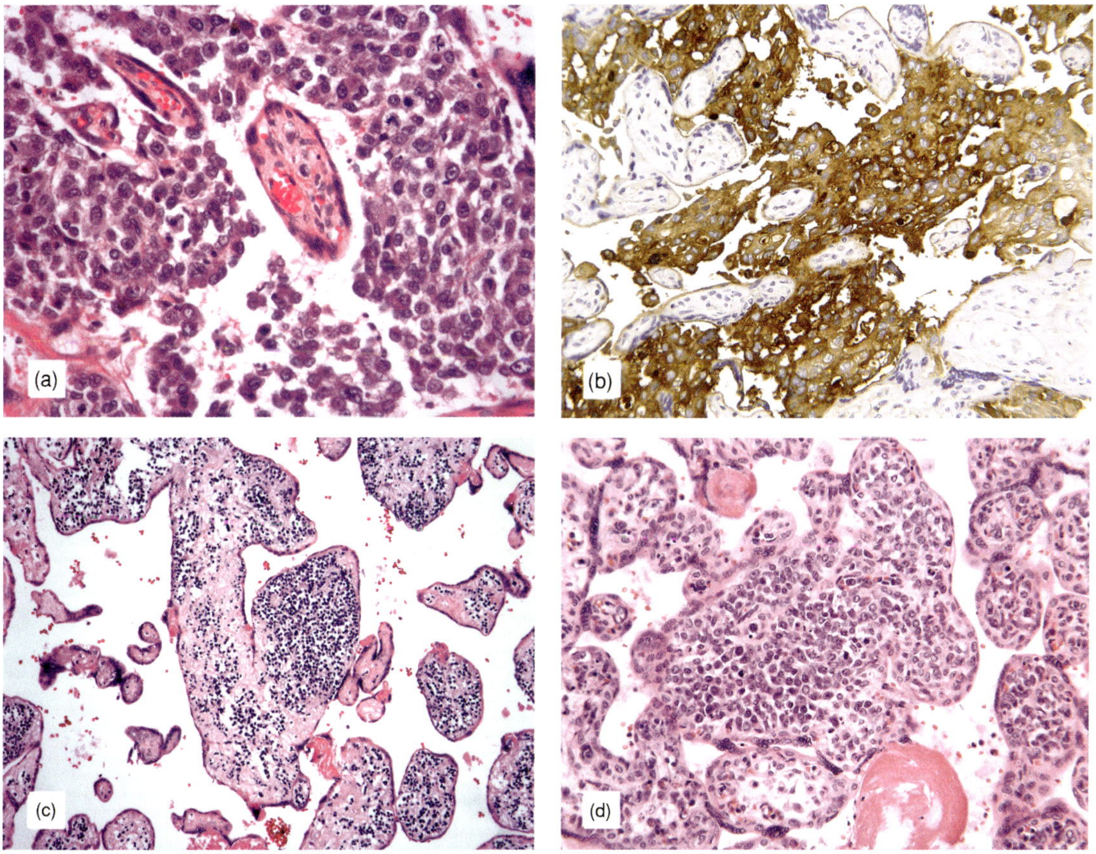

Figure 36.4 Secondary (metastatic) tumors to the placenta. (a) Metastatic malignant melanoma in intervillous space. (b) Maternal gastrointestinal adenocarcinoma, highlighted by immunohistochemical stain for carcinoembryonic antigen, in intervillous space. (c) In congenital neuroblastoma, aggregates of neuroblastoma cells are present in villous vessels. (d) Congenital leukemia, with leukemia cells occluding the villous vessels. (Parts (a) and (c): courtesy of Edwina Popek, DO, Texas Children Hospital, Houston, TX; (b) and (d): courtesy of Raymond Redline, MD, University Hospitals of Cleveland, Cleveland, OH.)

Clinical Pearl

Placentae of women with a history of malignancy should undergo pathological examination, with the pathologist being fully aware of the patient's history.

Risk factors

History of maternal malignancy or known congenital fetal neoplasm.

Incidence

Rare.

Diagnosis

Diagnosis of placental metastases is made by gross and microscopic examinations of the placenta. If indicated, selected immunohistochemical stains (Figure 36.4(b)) can be utilized to confirm the type of tumor.

Teaching Points

1 The WHO prognostic scoring index is the most commonly used classification system for GTD. Incorporated parameters are age, antecedent pregnancy type, interval from end of antecedent pregnancy to chemotherapy, hCG level, ABO blood groups of parents, largest tumor size, location and number of metastases and previously failed chemotherapy treatment.

2 Malignant gestational trophoblastic tumors need to be considered in the work-up of persistent vaginal bleeding months or even years after pregnancy.

3 Placental site nodules or plaques can be seen in endometrial biopsies or curettage years after a previous pregnancy. These lesions are benign but can be associated with dysfunctional uterine bleeding.

4 Chorangiomas of the placenta are usually incidental findings; however, large chorangiomas can cause significant fetal complications. Chorangiomas can be associated with genetic syndromes.

5 Maternal or fetal disease metastasizing to the placenta is exceedingly rare; however, some tumors such as malignant melanoma can metastasize to the fetus.

References

1. Genest DR, Berkowitz RS, Fisher RA et al. (2003) Gestational trophoblastic disease. In: Tavassoli FA and Devilee P (eds.) *World Health Organization Classification of Tumours. Pathology and Genetics of Tumours of the Breast and Female Genital Organs.* 1st edn. Lyon, France: IARC Press.
2. Lage JM (2002) Gestational trophoblastic disease. In: Robboy SJ, Anderson MC and Russel P (eds.) *Pathology of the Female Reproductive Tract.* 1st edn. London, UK: Churchill Livingstone.
3. Shih IeM (2007) Gestational trophoblastic neoplasia—pathogenesis and potential therapeutic targets. *Lancet Oncol* 8: 642–50.
4. Shie IeM (2007) Topogram, an immunohistochemistry-based algorithmic approach, in the differential diagnosis of trophoblastic tumors and tumorlike lesions. *Ann Diagn Pathol* 11: 228–34.
5. Berkowitz RS and Goldstein DP (2009) Current management of gestational trophoblastic diseases. *Gynecol Oncol* 112: 654–62.
6. Slim R and Mehio A (2007) The genetics of hydatidiform moles: new lights on an ancient disease. *Clin Genet* 71: 25–34.
7. Quarello E, Bernard JP, Leroy B et al. (2005) Prenatal laser treatment of a placental chorioangioma. *Ultrasound Obstet Gynecol* 25: 299–301.

37

CHAPTER 37

Multiple Gestation and Twin–Twin Transfusion Syndrome

Ramesha Papanna and Kenneth J. Moise Jr.
Division of Maternal-Fetal Medicine and Ultrasound-Genetics, Department of Obstetrics and Gynecology, Baylor College of Medicine, Texas Children's Fetal Center, Houston, TX, USA

Background

The influence of demographic risk factors on the incidence of twin pregnancies is mostly limited to dizygotic twins. In the United States, the incidence per 1000 live births of twin pregnancy in blacks is 15.8 compared to 11.3 in whites. The rate of twinning increases with maternal age, peaking at age 37 years. Infertility therapy has contributed significantly to the incidence of multifetal pregnancies. Multifetal pregnancies occur in 20–40% of conceptions after assisted reproductive technologies (ART), of which 70% are twins. The number of fetuses after in vitro fertilization (IVF) is directly related to the number of embryos transferred. A three-fold increase in monozygotic twinning, mostly monochorionic/diamniotic (MC/DA), after IVF has been associated with assisted hatching, intracytoplasmic sperm injection, and the late transfer of cultured blastocysts [1]. The incidence of higher order multiples with three or more fetuses has stabilized over the last 15 years (Figure 37.1), likely due to guidelines in the United States regarding the number of embryos transferred during IVF.

Embryology

A dizygotic twin pregnancy results from the release of two ova within the same menstrual cycle that are each fertilized by separate sperms. This process results in a dichorionic/diamniotic (DC/DA) twin pregnancy. Monozygotic twinning occurs when a single fertilized zygote divides into two embryos within the first 12 days after conception. If the embryo divides before the 3rd day of life, DC/DA twins result, comprising 25% of monozygotic twins. Division of the embryo between the 4th and 8th day of life results in monochorionic/diamniotic (MC/DA) twins, which comprise 75% of monozygotic twins. Division of the blastocyst into two conceptuses between the 9th and the 12th day will result in monochorionic/monoamniotic (MC/MA) twins. These represent < 1% of monozygotic twins. Division after 12th day, and up to 16th day of life will result in conjoined twins. Higher order multiples can result from fertilization of multiple ova, whether from spontaneous ovulation or ovulation induction, the transfer of multiple embryos in IVF, or the rare natural cleavage of a single fertilized conceptus.

Determining the amnionicity/chorionicity in twins

Clinical Pearl

There is no diagnosis of a twin pregnancy—twins are either monochorionic or dichorionic.

Historically, chorionicity was determined at the time of delivery through direct gross inspection of the membrane

The Placenta: From Development to Disease, First Edition. Edited by Helen H. Kay, D. Michael Nelson and Yuping Wang.
© 2011 Blackwell Publishing Ltd. Published 2011 by Blackwell Publishing Ltd.

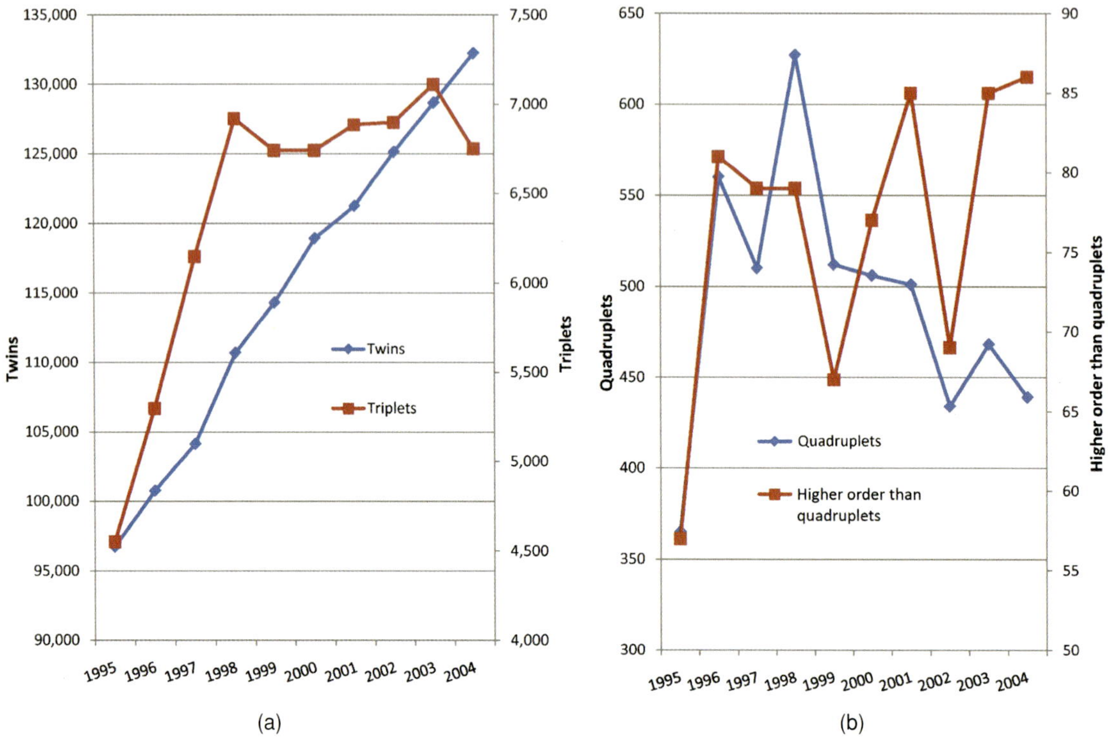

Figure 37.1 Total number of multifetal pregnancies delivered in the United States. (a) Twins and triplets. (b) Quadruplets and higher order multiples.

layers that comprised the intertwin membrane, or by obtaining a histological cross-section of the intertwin membrane (see Figure 37.2 (a,b)). Late diagnosis of twin pregnancy does not allow perinatal outcomes to be impacted. For this reason, the current approach for multifetal gestations is to determine amnionicity/chorionicity on the basis of ultrasound examination, done as early as possible in pregnancy.

Amnionicity of a twin gestation can usually be determined as early as 8 weeks of gestation by the presence of an intervening twin membrane identified by ultrasound. Although the presence of two separate yolk sacs is a good predictor of diamnionicity, a single yolk sac with two fetal poles may still result in a diamniotic pregnancy in 5–15% of cases [2].

Determining chorionicity is the most *important* step in the prenatal management of a twin gestation. DC/DA twins are associated with a perinatal mortality of 1–2%, while MC/DA twins experience a 12–20% rate of perinatal mortality. Thus, the knowledge of chorionicity assists in counseling the patient, and planning surveillance for the remainder of the pregnancy. Current guidelines from the American College of Radiology and the American Institute of Ultrasound in Medicine recommend that chorionicity be determined and documented in all multiple gestations.

A first trimester ultrasound at 10–13 weeks determines chorionicity with a sensitivity and specificity of 90% and 100%, respectively, with both negative and positive predictive values of about 98% [3]. The hallmark of dichorionicity is the presence of placental tissue between the combined chorion/amnion layers of the two opposed gestational sacs at their insertion into the placenta—so-called "lambda" or "twin peak" sign (see Figure 37.2(c,e)). In the absence of intervening placental tissue, a "T sign" indicates a single chorion surrounding two amniotic cavities (MC/DA; Figure 37.2(d,e)).

During the second trimester, determining chorionicity by ultrasound is less reliable than in the first trimester with a sensitivity, specificity, positive predictive value,

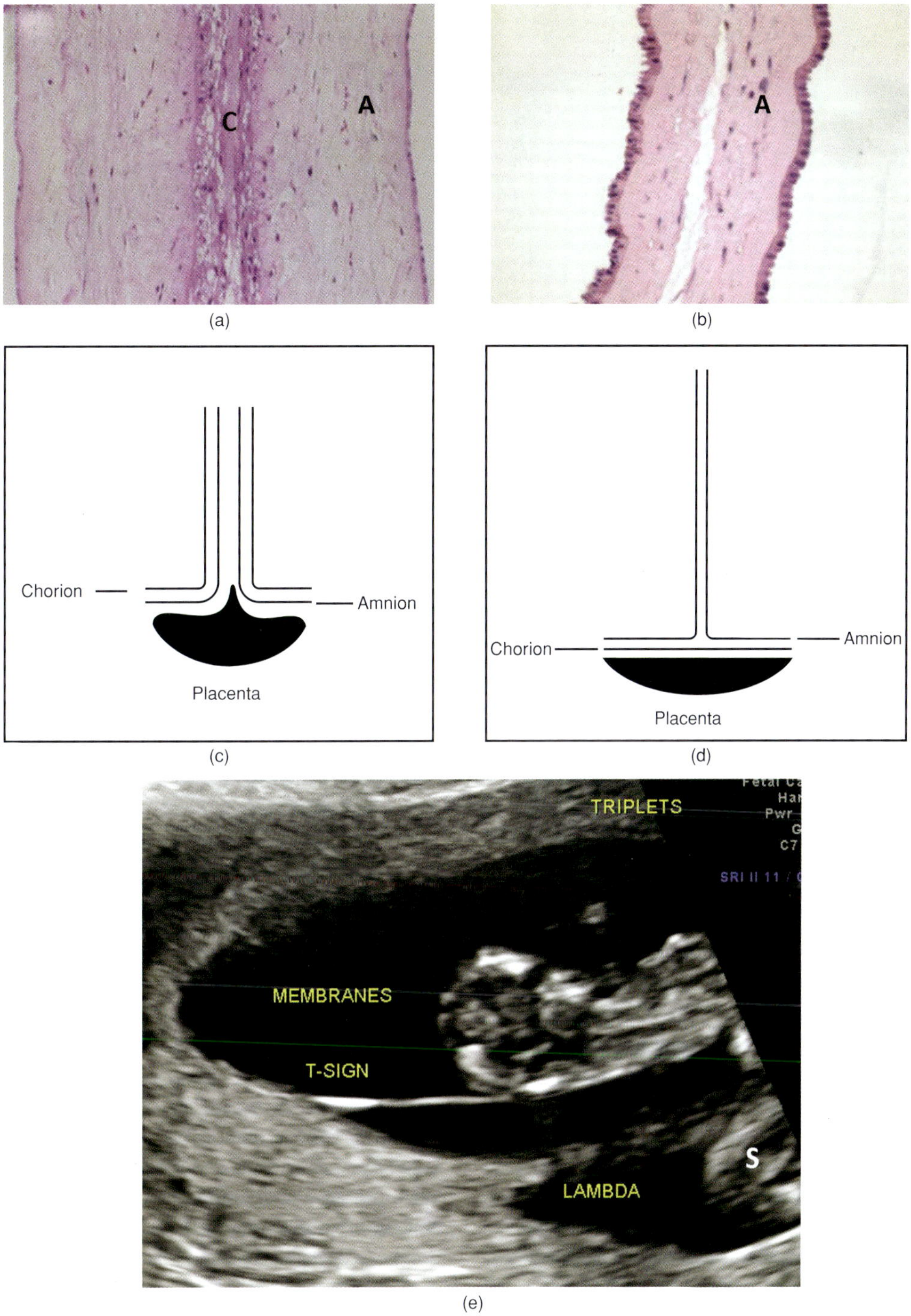

Figure 37.2 Differences in the intervening membrane in dichorionic/diamniotic and monochorionic/diamniotic twin gestations. (a) Histology of the dichorionic/diamniotic membrane. (b) Histology of a monochorionic/diamniotic membrane. (c) Diagrammatic representation of the "lambda sign" noted on ultrasound in the case of a dichorionic/diamniotic intervening twin membrane. (d) Diagrammatic representation of the " T sign" noted on ultrasound in the case of a monochorionic/diamniotic intervening twin membrane. (e) Dichorionic/triamniotic triplet gestation. Note the presence of the "T sign" between the monochorionic diamniotic twins, and the "lambda sign" between the singleton fetus in the lower right corner and the two twin sacs noted superior to this fetus. A, amnion; C, chorion; S, singleton fetus.

and negative predictive value of 88%, 95%, 88%, and 95%, respectively. Determination of fetal gender follows assessment for an intervening membrane. Dichorionicity is confirmed if a male and female are both present. The presence of two separate placental masses also confirms dichorionicity. Finally, an intervening membrane of < 2 mm thickness suggests a monochorionic gestation, while ≥ 2 mm suggests dichorionicity [4].

Dichorionic/diamniotic (DC/DA) twins

> **Clinical Pearl**
> "Two is better than one" for number of placentas in a twin gestation.

More than two-thirds of all spontaneous twins are DC/DA. These gestations can be considered "low-risk" as compared to MC/DA twins, but they are associated with slightly higher risks of congenital anomalies and selective growth restriction when compared to singleton gestations.

Clinical management

Routine comprehensive ultrasound for anatomical assessment should be undertaken at 18–20 weeks of gestation, and serial scans for fetal growth should be continued every 3–4 weeks until delivery, which is recommended by 38–39 weeks of gestation. Antenatal testing, using non-stress testing or biophysical profiles, should be initiated by 30–32 weeks of gestation if a growth discrepancy of greater than 20% is apparent in the twins.

Percentage growth discrepancy is calculated by:

$$\frac{\text{Estimated fetal weight (EFW) of large twin} - \text{EFW of small twin}}{\text{EFW of larger twin}}$$

Monochorionic/diamniotic (MC/DA) twins

Approximately one-third of spontaneous twin pregnancies are monozygotic, of which 75% are MC/DA. These pregnancies are high-risk due to complications related to placental sharing and vascular anastomoses (Table 37.1).

Table 37.1 Complications in MC/DA twin pregnancies.

Complications	Incidence
Twin–twin transfusion syndrome	10–15% of MC/DA twins
Discordant growth/selective intrauterine growth restriction	10–12% of MC/DA twins
Acardiac twin fetus	1:30,000 live births
Heterokaryotypic twin	1:40,000 live births
Molar co-twin	Rare

General clinical management

Once monochorionicity is established, preferably in the first trimester, a limited ultrasound should be undertaken at 16 weeks' gestation to assess for discordance in fetal size and amniotic fluid volumes. A routine comprehensive ultrasound for anatomical assessment should be undertaken at 18 weeks of gestation. Thereafter, limited ultrasound scans should be alternated with complete growth assessments every 2 weeks for the remainder of the pregnancy. In the case of a MC/DA twin pregnancy, delivery at 35–37 weeks of gestation should be considered.

> **Research Spotlight**
> Prospective studies are needed to determine what factors would predict which monochorionic gestation will develop complications.

Twin–twin transfusion syndrome (TTTS)

Virtually, all cases of TTTS have been reported in MC/DA twin gestations since these pregnancies share a common placental mass, and vascular anastomoses between fetuses are seen in almost 100% of cases. TTTS complicates approximately 1 in 40–65 twin pregnancies, so that approximately 2,500 cases of TTTS occur in the United States each year. About 9–15% of MC/DA twin pregnancies ultimately develop TTTS.

The following ultrasound criteria have been used for the diagnosis of TTTS:

• Polyhydramnios in the amniotic fluid compartment of the *recipient* twin: >8 cm maximum vertical pocket at < 20 weeks' gestation or >10 cm vertical pocket ≥ 20 weeks.

• Oligohydramnios in the amniotic fluid compartment of the *donor* twin: < 2 cm maximum vertical pocket.

Table 37.2 Quintero staging for TTTS.

Stage	Description
I	Oligohydramnios and polyhydramnios criteria for TTTS met, but there is a bladder still visible in the donor twin.
II	Discordant amniotic fluid volumes with the bladder not seen in the donor twin during the ultrasound evaluation.
III	Doppler blood flow studies showing absent/reverse end-diastolic velocity in the umbilical artery, reversed or absent A wave of the ductus venosus, or pulsatile flow in the umbilical vein in either fetus.
IV	One or both fetuses show signs of hydrops.
V	One or both fetuses have died.

Quintero has proposed five stages of TTTS based on additional two-dimensional (2D) and Doppler ultrasound findings [5] (see Table 37.2).

Pathophysiology

There are four types of vascular connections in the monochorionic placenta. Arterio-venous (AV) and veno-arterial (VA) anastomoses consist of feeder vessels on the surface of the chorionic plate that descend into a common cotyledon capillary network. In contrast, arterio-arterial (AA) and veno-venous (VV) anastomoses are seen exclusively on the surface of the placenta. Flow in these latter two types of connections is bidirectional, and net flow is related to opposing hydrostatic pressures of each fetus (see Figure 37.3(a)). Computer modeling has demonstrated that if the net number and diameter of connections are unbalanced, i.e., there are more AV connections between donor and recipient than there are VA connections between recipient and donor, then increasing hydrostatic and osmotic forces will result in the TTTS phenotype. In contrast, if the connections are balanced, i.e., equal numbers of bidirectional anastomoses, then TTTS does not result. Placental studies have indicated that AA anastomoses tend to be protective against the development of TTTS.

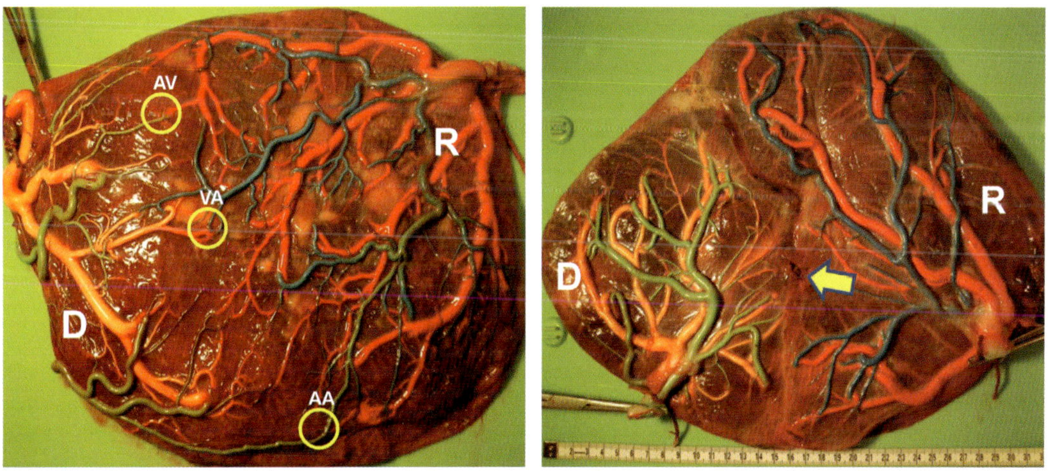

(a) (b)

Figure 37.3 Injected placenta from a monochorionic/diamniotic pregnancy with and without laser photocoagulation. (a) Placenta from untreated MC/DA twin gestation. Yellow colored vessels on the left indicate donor veins, while green colored vessels indicate donor arteries. Red colored vessels on the right side of the placenta indicate recipient veins and green colored vessels indicate recipient arteries. Anastomoses are noted as follows: AV, arterio-venous; VA, veno-arterial; AA, arterio-arterial. Multiple additional anastomoses can be noted in this placenta. (b) Placenta from MC/DA twin gestation after laser photocoagulation. Yellow colored vessels on the left indicate donor veins, while green colored vessels indicate donor arteries. Red colored vessels on the right side of the placenta indicate recipient veins and green colored vessels indicate recipient arteries. Yellow arrows indicate the "Solomnization" technique that is used by some centers after anastomotic vessels have been coagulated with the laser. D, donor cord insertion; R, recipient cord insertion. (Photos courtesy of Enrico Lopriore M.D. from the University of Leiden, Leiden, the Netherlands.)

This imbalance in vascular volume results in multiple endocrine and cardiovascular changes in both fetuses. Relative hypovolemia occurs in the *donor* twin, leading to anuria and eventual anhydramnios (Quintero stage II). Relative hypervolemia in the *recipient* fetus leads to cardiomegaly with increased production of natriuretic hormones, and subsequent polyuria leads to polyhydramnios in the *recipient's* amniotic cavity. As the disease progresses, the *donor* twin compensates by an up-regulation of its renin–angiotensin system, leading to a shunting of these vasoactive substances through placental anastomoses to the *recipient*. *Recipient* hypertension then dominates the clinical scenario leading to congestive heart failure (Quintero stage III), and eventually fetal hydrops (Quintero stage IV). Ultimately, fetal death occurs in one or both fetuses (Quintero stage V).

Although the Quintero staging represents an important tool to determine the need for therapeutic management, there are several important limitations. Atypical presentations can occur, such as an abnormal umbilical Doppler flow in the donor twin but a normal bladder seen on ultrasound (atypical Stage III). In addition, although higher Quintero stages are generally associated with a worsening perinatal prognosis, the clinical presentation of a particular case does not always follow an orderly progression of stages. As an example, a stage I case may progress rapidly over several days to stage III. In addition, regression of disease can occur in as many as 41% of stage I cases [6].

Clinical management

Historically, the overall perinatal survival rate of untreated severe TTTS was 10%. Attempts at amnioreduction and septostomy to reduce the symptoms of polyhydramnios failed to address the placental vascular anastomoses, and therefore did not improve survival. First introduced by Delia in 1990, laser photocoagulation of the problematic placental anastomoses was eventually studied in a randomized clinical trial [7]. Laser photocoagulation has improved overall perinatal survival and intact neurologic neonatal outcome, when compared to amnioreduction.

Fetoscopic laser ablation of placenta anastomoses is now accepted around the world as the standard of care for the treatment of TTTS. In the United States, patients with extreme symptoms related to extensive polyhydramnios in stage I disease, or patients with stage II–IV diseases, are considered candidates for therapy between 16 and 26 weeks of gestation. Today, a selective sequential ablation technique is used in which AV, then VA, and then AA anastomoses are coagulated. In some centers, a *Solomnization* technique follows to coagulate placental tissue between these targeted vessels to prevent the patency of small anastomoses that may be difficult to visualize (see Figure 37.3(b)). Typically, an amnioreduction is performed at the end of the procedure to normalize the amount of amniotic fluid in the *recipient's* sac.

Preterm premature rupture of the membranes complicates as many as 30% of laser cases. Preterm delivery is common, with an average gestational age at delivery of 30–32 weeks in most US studies. In experienced laser centers, survival of both fetuses occurs in approximately 60% of cases; survival of at least one fetus occurs in 90% of cases. In a two-year study from Holland, greater than 80% of survivors were without neurologic deficits [8].

Research Spotlight

New methods should be investigated to alleviate the problem of preterm premature rupture of membranes (PPROM) after fetoscopy. In addition, incorporation of echocardiographic findings into the preoperative evaluation of advanced TTTS cases may allow for medical interventions after laser therapy that will improve survival.

Selective intrauterine growth restriction (sIUGR)

Growth discordance in twins is usually defined as greater than 20% discordance in the estimated fetal weight by ultrasound parameters. When one twin is noted to be at < 10% estimated fetal weight, selective IUGR is diagnosed. This entity is as common as TTTS, complicating 10–15% of MC/DA twin gestations. The etiology is unclear, but proposed to result from an unequal division of the inner cell mass early in embryonic life. This may then result in a decreased potential for fetal growth in the affected fetus. Alternatively, an unequal split in the cytotrophoblast, that will ultimately form the placenta, can result in disproportionate placental sharing. Recently, Gratacos et al. [9] classified the sIUGR in MC/DA twins, based on the characteristics of the umbilical arterial Doppler in the smaller fetus. Type I (29%) had end diastolic flow present on Doppler waveforms, type II (22%) had absent or reversed diastolic flow, and Type III (49%) had intermittent absent or reversed end diastolic flow. Type III sIUGR was found to be associated with a greater number of large arterio-arterial placental anastomoses, when compared to the other two types of sIUGR and controls. There was also a higher incidence of fetal demise of the smaller twin fetus in conjunction with cerebral lesions on neonatal head ultrasound in the surviving co-twin.

Research Spotlight

Further studies in epigenetics and growth factors may help to elucidate the mechanisms that account for selective IUGR in monochorionic gestations.

Clinical management

The management of discordant growth depends on the gestational age at diagnosis. If detected at a previable gestational age, selective reduction should be considered for the premoribund sIUGR fetus. This can be done by occlusion of the umbilical cord through ultrasound-directed bipolar cautery or radiofrequency ablation. This will minimize the risk of death (12%) or long-term neurologic deficit (18%) in the normally grown co-fetus [10]. Laser ablation of placental anastomoses for the treatment of sIUGR is offered by some centers in an effort to protect the normal twin from the complications of death of the growth-restricted twin. However, in one study, survival of both twins was reduced to 28% in the laser group compared to 81% in the observation group [11]. If discordant growth in an MC/DA pregnancy is detected after viability has been attained, consideration for steroid administration to enhance fetal lung maturity, antenatal surveillance, and delivery should be considered.

Twin reversed arterial perfusion (TRAP) sequence

The incidence of TRAP *(acardiac twinning)* sequence is approximately 1 in 30,000 to 1 in 150,000 live births. This entity complicates approximately 1% of monochorionic twin pregnancies. There are two important ultrasound findings that are consistently noted in TRAP sequence: one of the two fetal masses has a rudimentary or absent heart; and there is reversed flow in the umbilical artery to

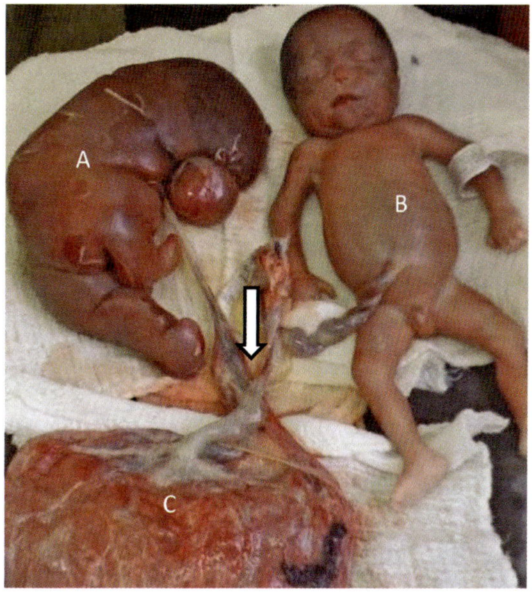

Figure 37.4 Twin reversed arterial perfusion sequence in a monochorionic twin pregnancy. White arrow points to the bifurcation of the umbilical cords. A, acardiac fetus; B, "pump twin"; C, placenta. (Photo courtesy of Saulo Molina, M.D. from the Fetal Center of Saint Joseph's Hospital—Perinatal Medicine, Bogota, Colombia.)

this fetal mass. The most common phenotype is preservation of the lower extremity structures with abnormal or absent structures in the upper half of the acardiac fetus (See Figure 37.4). This is thought to be related to deoxygenated blood perfusion from the normal, or "pump twin," to the acardiac twin via the umbilical arteries, which course first through the fetus before flowing cephalad. Proposed theories for the development of TRAP sequence include abnormal cardiogenesis in the acardiac fetus and early reversal of flow through a large placental arterio-arterial anastomosis, leading to underdevelopment of the heart in the acardiac twin.

Progressive demand on the pump twin to perfuse its own circulation as well as that of the acardiac twin results in cardiac failure and polyhydramnios. Fetal demise of the pump twin occurs in more than 50% of cases.

Clinical management

Antenatal management of TRAP sequence involves a thorough ultrasound examination of the pump twin to exclude anatomical abnormalities. An amniocentesis for karyotype in the normal twin should be considered as chromosomal abnormalities have been reported in up to 30% of cases. If serial ultrasound examinations reveal an increasing size of the acardiac fetus, ablation of flow should be considered after 16 weeks' gestation. This is usually accomplished through the use of a specialized radiofrequency ablation needle using ultrasound to target the umbilical cord insertion into the acardiac fetus. A survival rate of greater than 85% can be expected in the pump twin, although PPROM and preterm delivery are still a risk factor [12].

Research Spotlight

Targeted therapeutic ultrasound should be investigated to determine if it may play a role in the treatment of these pregnancies.

Monochorionic/monoamniotic (MC/MA) twins

Monochorionic/monoamniotic (MC/MA) twins account for 1% of all monozygotic twin pregnancies. Although the majority of monoamniotic twins occur naturally, iatrogenic or spontaneous rupture of the intervening membrane in a MC/DA pregnancy may also lead to a monoamniotic condition. MC/MA twins are at risk of developing complications similar to MC/DA twins, although the incidence of TTTS is thought to be reduced due to the usual presence of large AA anastomoses. An additional risk is entanglement of the umbilical cords (see Figure 37.5). The perinatal mortality associated with cord compromise in these pregnancies was approximately 50% in early studies; however, more recent series suggest that the perinatal mortality is ~10–20%.

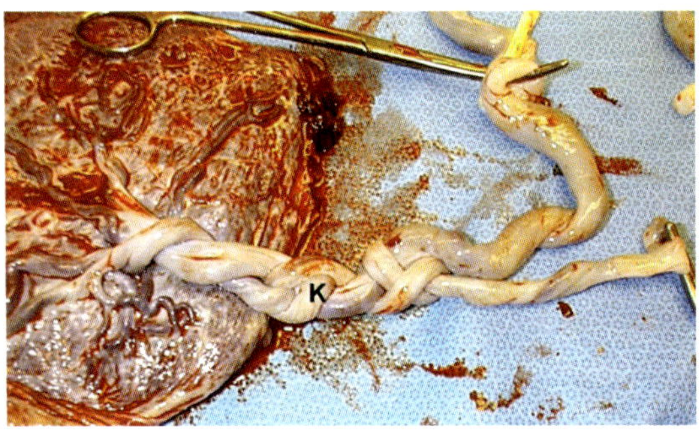

Figure 37.5 Cord entanglement in monochorionic/monoamniotic twin gestation at the time of cesarean delivery at 32 weeks' gestation. Note the proximal placental cord insertions and multiple tangled loops. K, true knot in the cords.

Clinical management

In general, most centers in the United States now offer inpatient admission for intensive fetal monitoring several times daily when the patient and her obstetrician agree that a gestational age of fetal viability has been reached. Large case series have indicated that outpatient fetal monitoring may not predict fetal compromise in a timely fashion to allow for appropriate intervention. Antenatal steroids to enhance fetal lung maturity are indicated. Delivery by cesarean section at 32–34 weeks is generally accepted as a means of preventing late perinatal loss.

Anomalous co-fetus

In multifetal gestation, discordance for a chromosomal or structural fetal abnormality can occur in both monochorionic and dichorionic twins. A chromosomal abnormality in a monozygotic gestation is called a heterokaryotypic defect. In the typical case, an X chromosome is lost soon after the early cleavage of the embryo. This results in one fetus with Turner's syndrome that typically presents with a cystic hygroma, hydrops, or both, and a co-twin that appears phenotypically normal. Assessment of the karyotype in the normal appearing twin is essential in these cases.

In utero loss of a monochorionic twin due to major abnormalities can lead to compromise of the normal co-twin. Hypotension ensues as the abnormal twin begins to die. This leads to exsanguination of the normal co-twin into the "sink" of the abnormal twin through vascular anastomoses. Death of the normal twin occurs in 12% of cases, while major neurologic deficit occurs in an additional 18% of cases when this twin survives [10].

Clinical management

In a dichorionic pregnancy, selective feticide can be performed using potassium chloride injection into the pericardial space of the anomalous twin. However, in the monochorionic twin gestation, this technique cannot be used due to the presence of placental anastomoses. In these cases, selective feticide is performed using cord occlusion techniques, such as ultrasound-guided radiofrequency ablation or bipolar cord occlusion. The success rate of such procedures is nearly 100% with 85% survival rates of the normal fetus to birth.

Teaching Points

1 Although the rate of twin pregnancies in the United States is on the rise, the incidence of higher order multiples has peaked, and more recently has decreased.

2 Monochorionic/diamniotic twins are at a 10–15-fold increased risk of perinatal mortality, secondary to unique diseases such as twin–twin transfusion syndrome, severe selective intrauterine growth restriction, discordant fetal anomalies, and twin reversed arterial perfusion sequence.

3 Twin–twin transfusion syndrome affects 1 in 10 monochorionic/diamniotic twin pregnancies, and can be successfully treated with laser photocoagulation of placental anastomoses.

4 Monoamniotic twins comprise only 1% of monozygotic twins, but they have the highest mortality rate, secondary to umbilical cord compromise after the period of viability. Therefore, intensive inpatient fetal surveillance and delivery at 32–34 weeks' gestation is recommended.

5 TRAP sequence is associated with up to 50% perinatal mortality in the normal or "pump" co-twin. Occlusion of the umbilical cord of the acardiac fetus by radiofrequency ablation is recommended if a progressive increase in the size of the acardiac twin is noted on serial ultrasound examinations.

References

1. Vitthala S, Gelbaya TA, Brison DR et al. (2009) The risk of monozygotic twins after assisted reproductive technology: a systematic review and meta-analysis. *Human Reproduction Update* 15(1): 45–55.
2. Shen O, Samueloff A, Beller U et al. (2006) Number of yolk sacs does not predict amnionicity in early first-trimester monochorionic multiple gestations. *Ultrasound in Obstetrics and Gynecology* 27(1): 53–5.
3. Shetty A and Smith AP (2005) The sonographic diagnosis of chorionicity. *Prenatal Diagnosis* 25(9): 735–39.
4. Winn HN, Gabrielli S, Reece EA et al. (1989) Ultrasonographic criteria for the prenatal diagnosis of placental chorionicity in twin gestations. *American Journal of Obstetrics and Gynecology* 161(6 Pt 1): 1540–42.
5. Quintero RA, Morales WJ, Allen MH et al. (1999) Staging of twin–twin transfusion syndrome. *Journal of Perinatology* 19(8 Pt 1): 550–55.
6. O'Donoghue K, Cartwright E, Galea P et al. (2007) Stage I twin–twin transfusion syndrome: rates of progression and regression in relation to outcome. *Ultrasound in Obstetrics and Gynecology* 30(7): 958–64.
7. De Lia JE, Cruikshank DP, and Keye WR Jr. (1990) Fetoscopic neodymium:YAG laser occlusion of placental vessels in severe twin–twin transfusion syndrome. *Obstetrics and Gynecology* 75(6): 1046–53.
8. Lopriore E, Middeldorp JM, Sueters M et al. (2007) Long-term neurodevelopmental outcome in twin-to-twin transfusion syndrome treated with fetoscopic laser surgery. *American Journal of Obstetrics and Gynecology* 196(3): 231 e1–4.
9. Gratacos E, Lewi L, Munoz B et al. (2007) A classification system for selective intrauterine growth restriction in monochorionic pregnancies according to umbilical artery Doppler flow in the smaller twin. *Ultrasound in Obstetrics and Gynecology* 30(1): 28–34.
10. Senat MV, Deprest J, Boulvain M et al. (2004) Endoscopic laser surgery versus serial amnioreduction for severe twin-to-twin transfusion syndrome. *New England Journal of Medicine* 351(2): 136–44.
11. Gratacos E, Antolin E, Lewi L et al. (2008) Monochorionic twins with selective intrauterine growth restriction and intermittent absent or reversed end-diastolic flow (Type III): feasibility and perinatal outcome of fetoscopic placental laser coagulation. *Ultrasound in Obstetrics and Gynecology* 31(6): 669–75.
12. Roman A, Papanna R, Johnson A et al. (2010) Selective reduction in complicated monochorionic pregnancies: radiofrequency ablation vs. bipolar cord coagulation. *Ultrasound in Obstetrics and Gynecology* 36(1): 37–41.

38

CHAPTER 38

Previa and Abruption

Helen H. Kay

Division of Maternal-Fetal Medicine and Ultrasound-Genetics, Department of Obstetrics and Gynecology, Washington University School of Medicine, St. Louis, MO, USA

Introduction

The placenta is a vascular organ and any developmental interference with the basal plate blood supply or architectural disruption during pregnancy can yield life-threatening bleeding, and jeopardize maternal and fetal well-being. The most critical interfaces include those between placenta and uterus, and the pipeline between placenta and fetus, the umbilical cord. Clinicians need to evaluate any bleeding during pregnancy, recognize potentially life-threatening events, and address them accordingly. Researchers should continue to shed light on etiologic contributors that predispose to abnormal placentation resulting in aberrations of placental architecture and disruption of the utero-placental interface.

Placenta previa

Placenta previa is defined as implantation of the placenta to cover the internal cervical os or be within 2 cm of the os. The presence of the previa (meaning "coming before" in Latin) predisposes to bleeding as the lower uterine segment morphoses at the choriodecidual interface with contractions in labor leading to excessive bleeding. Placenta previa was formerly described with ambiguous terms such as marginal or partial, and complete previa. The term marginal previa was used to describe a placenta whose edge was near, but not covering, the internal cervical os; partial previa pertained to the placental edge lying partially over the os; and a complete previa applied to the placenta covering the entire os. This former terminology applied to a relationship between the placenta and cervical os when the cervix was dilated, but does not apply to the relationship during most of the pregnancy when the os is closed. New technology using transvaginal ultrasound imaging allows accurate and precise assignment for the relationship between placental edge and internal cervical os, which is more useful. Terminology now used by many clinicians includes "placenta previa," "complete placenta previa," and "low lying placenta" in the third trimester. A "low lying placenta" refers to a placenta in which the edge is more than 2 cm from the internal os but still in the lower part of the uterine cavity. "Placenta previa" is defined by the presence of the inferior edge of the placenta within 2 cm of the internal os. A "complete placenta previa" is designated for those placentae that cover the internal os. All patients diagnosed with a placenta previa are delivered by cesarean section to reduce the chance of bleeding from disruption of the choriodecidual junction in the basal plate (see the chapter on placental anatomy). Such patients are most likely to have a cesarean section, but those with a distance greater than 2 cm are considered safe for a vaginal delivery (Figure 38.1). Overall, it is best to describe the distance between placental edge and cervical os in centimeters, and allow clinicians to determine how best to handle the situation at time of delivery.

Clinical Pearl

Bleeding from the site of placental attachment can be substantial at the time of cesarean section because muscle

The Placenta: From Development to Disease, First Edition. Edited by Helen H. Kay, D. Michael Nelson and Yuping Wang.
© 2011 Blackwell Publishing Ltd. Published 2011 by Blackwell Publishing Ltd.

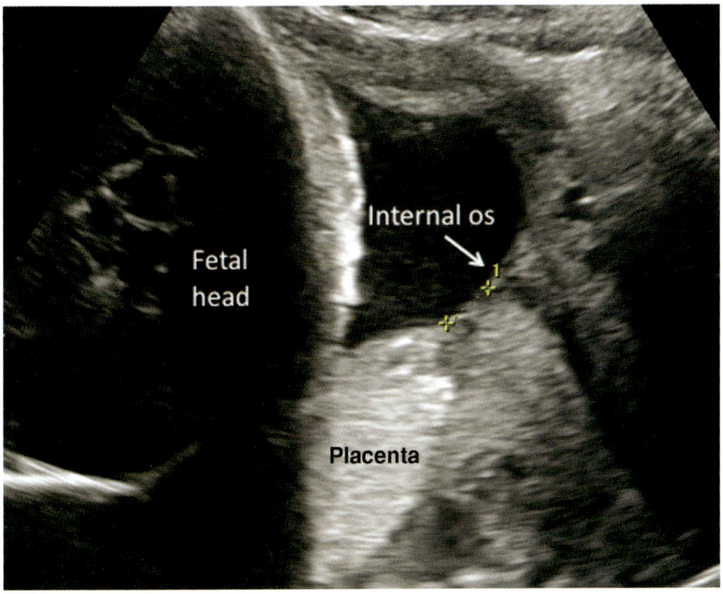

Figure 38.1 Sagittal ultrasound image of a placenta previa. The inferior edge of the posterior placenta is adjacent to the posterior cervical tissue and within 8 mm, but does not cross the internal os. Arrow points to internal os.

distribution around spiral arterioles in the placental bed may not obstruct blood flow as well as implantation in the upper uterus. Anticipate this and apply direct pressure to the denuded placental site.

Risk factors

Risk factors include those listed in Table 38.1, although some women do not have any risk factors. A significant risk is history of a cesarean section, especially with two or more previous cesarean sections. The recent rise in primary elective cesarean sections is an obvious concern in this regard.

Pathophysiology

Placenta previa is primarily a clinical diagnosis, and there are few pathologic features required to confirm the diagnosis. Because of the associated risk factors of multiparity and prior cesarean section, the predisposing pathologic abnormality is abnormal implantation in the lower uterine segment, within 2 cm of the internal cervical os. Factors regulating trophoblast invasion and deficient decidualization are involved. For example, biopsies of the implantation site in placenta previa, compared to normal implantation, show that extravillous trophoblasts migrate deeper into decidua and myometrium, there are more physiologic changes in spiral arterioles, and there is a higher incidence of inflammatory cell infiltration [1]. Repeated pregnancies in multiparous women may predispose the endometrium to abnormal healing, and hence attract implantation in the lower uterine segment. The presence of a uterine scar from previous cesarean section enhances this process.

Table 38.1 Risk factors for placenta previa.

Prior cesarean section or other uterine surgery
Advanced maternal age
High gravidity/parity
Previous abortion
Cigarette smoking and cocaine use

Incidence

The incidence of placenta previa is approximately 2–4 per 1,000 births in the United States.

Diagnosis

Diagnosis is made more frequently today because of the routine use of transabdominal and transvaginal ultrasound scanning, which is highly sensitive. Magnetic resonance imaging (MRI) can be highly sensitive as well but the complex technology involved, the high cost of imaging, and some mild safety concerns limit the usefulness of this approach.

Clinical Pearl

Placenta previa must be at the top of the diagnostic list for third trimester bleeding in women without previous ultrasound imaging.

Clinical management

Approximately 90% of the placenta previa cases diagnosed early will resolve by the third trimester, since placentae will "migrate" because of growth of the uterus and the consequent relative change in the location of the placenta to the internal cervical os. However, complete previa is unlikely to resolve. Management should include counseling on the need to report any vaginal bleeding, risks of bleeding after the sentinel bleed, high likelihood of preterm contractions leading to preterm delivery, possible use of tocolysis, potential need for blood transfusions, and possibility of hysterectomy. Bed rest is often advised in the latter part of the pregnancy, although there is no data to confirm its utility. Hospitalization may be required for larger and recurrent bleeds. Approximately one-fourth of patients do not bleed prior to 36 weeks, but complete placenta previa tends to bleed earlier. Typically, blood is maternal in origin and lighter bleeds are unlikely to cause fetal compromise. Because patients with placenta previa tend to have other complications such as preterm labor, fetal malpresentation, and postpartum hemorrhage, delivery should be achieved as soon as fetal lung is mature by amniocentesis, usually after 36 weeks' gestation. However, if there is recurrent bleeding and threat to the fetus and mother, then early administration of corticosteroids to enhance lung maturity is advised, and delivery should take place at any gestational age after viability. There are no reliable markers for bleeding, but an elevated maternal serum alpha-fetoprotein (MSAFP) level above 2.0 multiples of the median in a patient with previa and no a priori risk factor has been associated with a greater than 50% chance of hospitalization before 30 weeks' gestation and preterm delivery.

A third trimester ultrasound diagnosis of complete placenta previa confers indication for cesarean delivery. When the placental edge is greater than 2 cm from the internal os, the patient is usually considered safe to have a vaginal delivery. If the placenta is less than 2 cm from the internal os, many physicians would consider a cesarean delivery. However, discussion can take place with the patient to consider a trial of labor because the descending fetal head may tamponade the placenta and prevent excessive bleeding, particularly when the distance is between 1 and 2 cm of the os. The delivery management for this latter group of patients should be individualized [2].

Complications of placenta previa: accreta, increta, and percreta

Abnormal implantation predisposes patients with placenta previa to complications such as placenta accreta, increta, and percreta, relative to the degree of extravillous trophoblast infiltration. Placenta accreta is a condition whereby the placental interface and the myometrium at the decidua basalis are obliterated. In placenta increta, the extravillous trophoblasts invade into the myometrium. In placenta percreta, the extravillous trophoblasts invade not only into the myometrium, but also beyond the myometrium to the serosal surface of the uterus and, on occasion, into the adjacent pelvic organs such as the bladder.

Risk factors

The most significant risk factors for placenta accreta, increta, and percreta are placenta previa and previous cesarean section.

Pathophysiology

Why or how extravillous trophoblasts have enhanced invasive capacity is unknown. Immunohistochemistry and in vitro studies have suggested that cell adhesion molecules, such as carcinoembryonic antigen-related cell adhesion molecule 1 (CEACAM1), epidermal growth factor receptor (EGFR), c-erbB-2 oncoprotein, vascular endothelial growth factor (VEGF), placenta growth factor (PlGF), vascular endothelial growth factor receptors (VEGFR-1, 2, 3), among others, may play a role in abnormal placental implantation leading to this condition [3].

Research Spotlight

Research using Ki-67 as a marker of proliferation suggests that dehiscence of a uterine scar may enable the extravillous trophoblasts to gain deeper access into the myometrium through excessive proliferation, reflected by Ki-67 staining [4].

Incidence

The incidence of placenta accreta in a patient with a placenta previa and a prior low uterine segment cesarean section is reported to be on the order of 10–35%.

Diagnosis

Placenta increta or percreta are rarely diagnosed definitively prior to delivery but occurs more reliably when histology is available after a hysterectomy, often required due to an inability to deliver the placenta. Prenatal diagnosis may be successful using ultrasound imaging (sensitivity of 50–80%) or MRI (sensitivity 80–90%). Typical ultrasound findings of placenta accreta include loss of the normal hypoechoic demarcation between the placenta and myometrium at the decidual basalis, gaps in retroplacental blood flow, and thinning of the myometrium to <1 mm (Figure 38.2). In placenta percreta, there is irregularity of the linear hyperechoic delineation between the uterine serosa and the bladder wall. Some authors have also suggested that the presence of intraplacental lacunae in placenta previa is associated with a higher incidence of accreta because the lacunae represent intraplacental vascular lakes resulting from abnormal implantation. The three-dimensional (3D) color Doppler technique may enhance antepartum diagnosis in the future. MRI features include heterogeneous signal intensity in the placenta, dark intraplacental bands on T2-weighted images, thinning and interruptions of the myometrium, and invasion of placental tissue into pelvic structures such as the bladder (Figure 38.3) (see also Chapter 17 on imaging) [5].

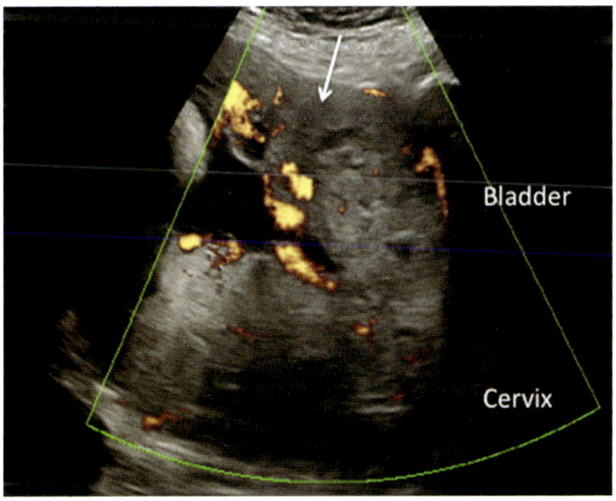

Figure 38.2 Sagittal ultrasound image and power Doppler flow of a complete placenta previa and accreta. Confirmed by pathology after hysterectomy. Heterogeneous placenta adherent to the lower uterine segment. Note the irregular intraplacental hypoechoic areas of vascular lacunae, giving the placenta a "moth-eaten" appearance. The cervical os is not clearly defined and is covered entirely by the placenta. The hypoechoic zone and echogenic decidual plate are lost in this placenta accreta. Arrow points to area of decidual basalis obliteration.

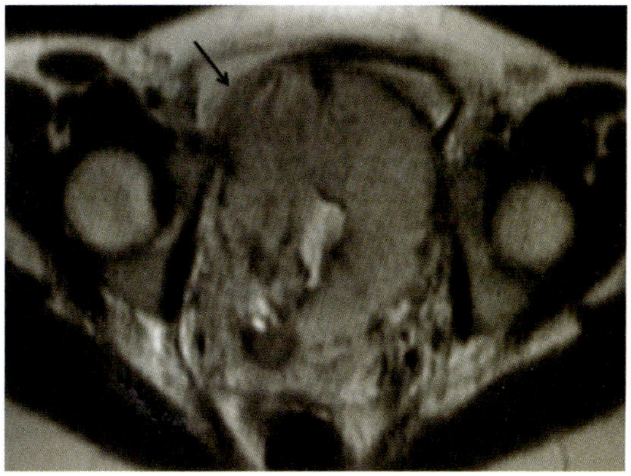

Figure 38.3 Axial MRI view of a complete placenta previa and percreta. T2-weighted single shot spin echo (SSFSE) image. Note that this image is taken low in the pelvis, and shows the circumferential placenta with a small amount of amniotic fluid centrally (bright signals). The arrow points to the area of placenta percreta demonstrating heterogeneous signal intensity and complete loss of the myometrium, plus invasion into the bladder anteriorly. These findings were confirmed by hysterectomy. (Courtesy Dr. Aytekin Oto, Department of Radiology, University of Chicago, Chicago, IL.)

Clinical management

Management of a patient with placenta accreta depends, to a large extent, on the depth of myometrial invasion. Placenta increta or percreta almost always necessitates a hysterectomy, though neoadjuvant medical therapy with methotrexate may be sufficient in some situations. A presumptive antepartum diagnosis requires a plan for appropriate anesthesia, intravenous access, and adequate blood products if hysterectomy is anticipated or required. Although controversial, interventional radiologists may place balloon catheters into the uterine arteries preoperatively to allow embolization if excessive, uncontrolled bleeding occurs from the placental site.

Research Spotlight

High levels of cell-free placental messenger RNA (mRNA) in maternal plasma may be a marker for patients with suspected placenta accreta who will require hysterectomy [6].

Vasa previa and velamentous cord insertion

Vasa previa refers to a condition whereby fetal vessels, unsupported by either the umbilical cord or placental tissue, traverse the cervical internal os. This can only occur when there is a velamentous cord insertion, where unprotected fetal vessels insert into the membranes rather than the placenta. This condition is extremely dangerous to the fetus because these vessels can rupture spontaneously in labor or during amniorrhexis, if undiagnosed antenatally, leading to rapid fetal exsanguination. The exposed fetal vessels may also be compressed by fetal movements or descent of the presenting part and heart rate decelerations may occur [7].

Risk factors

Known risk factors for vasa previa due to a velamentous cord insertion include a bilobar placenta, a succenturiate (accessory) lobe, multiple gestation, or in vitro fertilization (IVF).

Pathophysiology

The physiology of fetal vessels coalescing within the membranes to form a normal umbilical cord is unknown; thus, the etiology for abnormal membranous cord insertion is unknown. This developmental abnormality occurs in the first trimester, based on observations in some intensively monitored pregnancies from IVF. One hypothesis claims crowding within the uterine cavity predisposes to velamentous cord insertions, citing support from the increased frequency for this condition in multifetal gestations, compared to singletons. Other observations have associated vasa previa and velamentous cord insertions with low-lying placentae.

Incidence

Vasa previa is rare, occurring in approximately 1 in 1,000–5,000 deliveries.

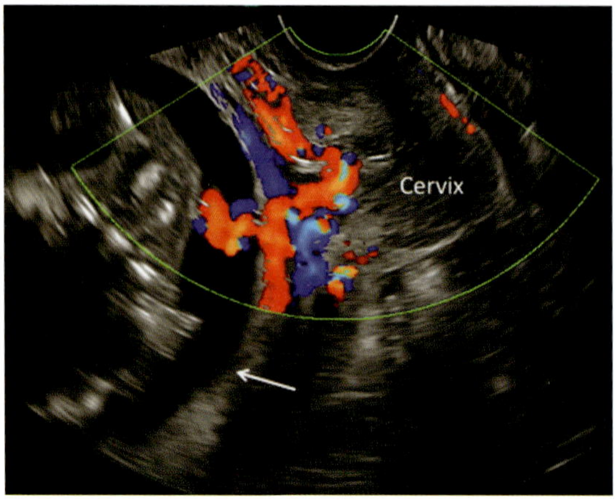

Figure 38.4 Sagittal ultrasound image of vasa previa and velamentous cord insertion. Fetal vessels seen by color Doppler coursing over the cervical internal os. The cord inserts into the membranes at a short distance from the placental edge (arrow).

Diagnosis and clinical management

Diagnosis of vasa previa is not considered part of a routine obstetrical ultrasound scan. However, if velamentous cord insertion is coincidentally suspected, transvaginal color and power Doppler assessment can evaluate the relationship between exposed vessels and cervix (Figure 38.4). The relationship should be evaluated again later in pregnancy, and the obstetrical team should be notified in order to prevent artificial rupture of the membranes and indirect rupture of fetal vessels. Delivery by cesarean section is mandated.

Clinical Pearl

When acute bleeding is seen during amniorrhexis, vasa previa should be suspected and promptly evaluated.

Placental abruption

Placental abruption is bleeding from the choriodecidual interface in the basal plate. Women with abruption most often present with complaints of bleeding, although a centrally located separation in the retroplacental space may yield a concealed abruption without vaginal bleeding. Patients may present with pain, contractions, or both if the blood seeps into the myometrium causing irritation.

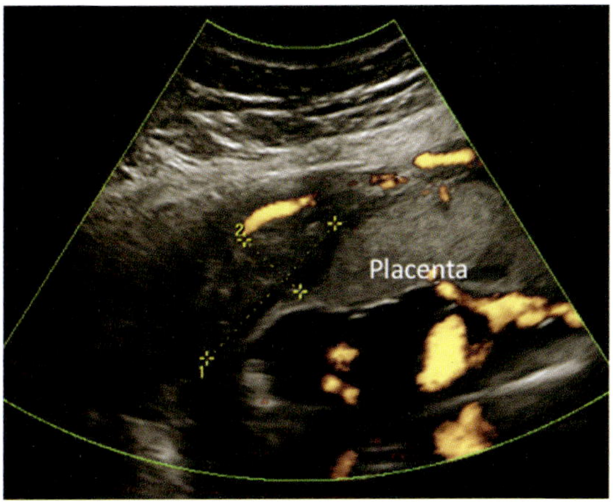

Figure 38.5 Placenta abruption. Hypoechoic region at lateral edge of the placenta (43 × 18 mm) consistent with a marginal and partially retroplacental placenta abruption. An acute abruption will appear very dark but as the clot is organized, it appears more echogenic, as in this case, but usually not as echogenic as the placenta.

Abruptions are classified as subchorionic, marginal, or retroplacental. Subchorionic abruptions originate from the choriodecidual interface. On occasion, this occurs on the maternal surface of the placenta, and the clot lies between the chorion and placenta parenchyma. Most often, it is an incidental finding by imaging and not associated with any significant clinical adverse outcomes. Marginal abruptions are also subchorionic, originating from the placental edge and tend to lead to visible blood in the vagina (Figure 38.5). Clinically, they are more concerning because blood can serve as a focus for inflammation, if not infection. These sites predispose to premature rupture of the membranes or preterm labor, possibly via thrombin-enhanced interleukin production and recruitment of neutrophil infiltration into the decidua. Most concerning is a marginal abruption that leads to blood dissection into the retroplacental space. These abruptions can lead to significant separation of the placenta from the uterine wall, compromising blood flow to the fetus and leading to fetal demise, especially common if more than 50% of the placental attachment to the basalis is disrupted. In rare and extreme cases, blood dissects extensively into the myometrium giving a bluish tinge to the uterus, known as Couvelaire's uterus, and is associated with uterine atony.

Table 38.2 Risk factors associated with placental abruption.

Obstetric
Prior pregnancy complicated by abruption
High parity
Infertility treatment
Uterine myomas or anatomic defects
Prior cesarean section
Medical disorders
Chorioamnionitis
Hypertension
Antiphospholipid syndrome
Diabetes
Thrombophilias
Iatrogenic
Blunt trauma
Car accidents
Cigarette smoking
Cocaine and alcohol abuse
Invasive procedures such as amniocentesis
External cephalic version for breech

Risk factors

There are many risk factors associated with abruption (Table 38.2), but the most common are a history of an abruption in a previous pregnancy, chorioamnionitis, trauma, prior cesarean section, cigarette smoking, cocaine abuse, and thrombophilia.

Pathophysiology

These risk factors converge in a common pathophysiology pathway involving ischemia and hypoxia, which are responsible for cell apoptosis in the decidua basalis. This necrosis leads to vascular disruption and bleeding. Infection and chorioamnionitis contribute to the pathophysiology through release of free oxygen radicals that are cytotoxic [8]. Trauma leads to direct tissue necrosis and hemorrhage. Cigarette smoking and cocaine abuse cause vasoconstriction and hemorrhage. Finally, thrombophilia may lead to abruption via thrombosis, infarction, necrosis, and hemorrhage in the basal plate. Both acquired and inherited thrombophilias have been implicated, including anticardiolipin antibodies, hyperhomocysteinemia, deficiencies in protein C, protein S and antithrombin III, and mutations in the factor V Leiden and prothrombin *20210 A* gene.

> **Research Spotlight**
>
> Recent research on molecular mechanisms strongly suggests that localized blood clotting, inflammation, and subsequent cell death at the decidua basalis or the choriodecidual interface is a leading cause of abruption.

Incidence

Placenta abruption is reported in 1/50–1/200 unselected pregnancies and deliveries at term.

Diagnosis

Diagnosis of an abruption is often based on clinical criteria of pain and vaginal bleeding. Blood is not always easily visualized on ultrasound. MRI is not practical in the setting of acute bleeding. When suspected clinically, careful inspection of the utero–placental junction with ultrasound and Doppler assessment may yield the diagnosis. Earlier in pregnancy, the presence of an elevated maternal serum alpha-fetoprotein (MSAFP) level may be a marker for abruption in women without an elevated a priori risk for a neural tube defect, reflecting placental maldevelopment at the decidua basalis.

Clinical management

Management should focus on hemodynamic stability of the mother, fetal well-being, gestational age at diagnosis, and presence or absence of preterm labor. When a small abruption is encountered in a premature fetus, corticosteroids should be administered to enhance fetal lung maturity. Tocolysis may be considered until corticosteroid course is complete. Delivery can and should be delayed if there is no imminent danger to mother or fetus. If the abruption is advanced, delivery of the fetus should ensue, especially if the abruption is large enough to induce a consumptive coagulopathy with disseminated intravascular coagulation. Unfortunately, there are no reliable means to prevent or reverse the process. Anticoagulation and folic acid may be beneficial when there is a known underlying thrombophilia. Patients should always be counseled regarding the ill effects of smoking and cocaine abuse.

> **Teaching Points**
>
> 1 Patients with placenta previa should be delivered by cesarean section, but those in the intermediate range with the edge between 1 and 2 cm of the os may be considered for vaginal delivery.
> 2 Placenta accreta, increta, and percreta are best diagnosed by ultrasound or MRI, but neither is significantly superior to the other.
> 3 When there is velamentous insertion of the umbilical vessels into the placental membranes, there is a higher risk for vasa previa.
> 4 Placental abruptions can be caused by a multitude of factors and all point to apoptosis, necrosis, and vascular disruption at the decidua basalis.
> 5 The incidence of placenta previa, placenta accreta, and placental abruption is on the rise due to the increasing cesarean section rate.

References

1. Biswas R, Sawhney H, Dass R et al. (1999) Histopathological study of placental bed biopsy in placenta previa. *Acta Obstet Gynecol Scand* 78: 173–79.
2. Vergani P, Ornaghi S, Pozzi I et al. (2009) Placenta previa: distance to internal os and mode of delivery. *Am J Obstet Gynecol* 201: 266–68.
3. Tseng JJ, Chou MM, Hsieh YT et al. (2004) Differential expression of vascular endothelial growth factor, placenta growth factor and their receptors in placentae from pregnancies complicated by placenta accreta. *Placenta* 27: 70–78.
4. Tantbirojn P, Crum CP, and Parast MM (2008) Pathophysiology of placenta creta: the role of decidua and extravillous trophoblast. *Placenta* 29: 639–45.
5. Baughman WC, Corteville JE, and Shah RR (2008) Placenta accreta: spectrum of US and MR imaging findings. *Radiographics* 28: 1905–16.
6. Miura K, Miura S, Yamasaki K et al. (2008) Increased level of cell-free placental mRNA in a subgroup of placenta previa that needs hysterectomy. *Prenat Diagn* 28: 805–9.
7. Lee W, Lee VL, Kirk JS et al. (2000) Vasa previa: prenatal diagnosis, natural evolution, and clinical outcome. *Obstet Gynecol* 95: 572–76.
8. Nath CA, Ananth CV, Smulian JC et al. (2007) Histologic evidence of inflammation and risk of placental abruption. *Am J Obstet Gynecol* 197: 319–24.

39

CHAPTER 39

The Placenta as a Functional Barrier to Fetal Drug Exposure

Tatiana N. Nanovskaya[1], *Gary D.V. Hankins*[1], *and Mahmoud S. Ahmed*[1,2,3]

[1]Department of Obstetrics and Gynecology, University of Texas Medical Branch, Galveston, TX, USA
[2]Department of Biochemistry and Molecular Biology, University of Texas Medical Branch, Galveston, TX, USA
[3]Department of Pharmacology and Toxicology, University of Texas Medical Branch, Galveston, TX, USA

Introduction

Treatment of the pregnant patient for a medical or substance abuse disorder, such as opiate or nicotine dependence, is complicated by the following: (1) the pregnancy-induced physiological changes that could affect the pharmacokinetics of administered medication; (2) growth and development of the fetus and placenta that constitute an additional compartment for drug distribution; and (3) the continuous changes in the functions of the placenta throughout gestation. Accordingly, dose adjustment of a medication given during pregnancy is often required to achieve therapeutic levels of the medication in the maternal system. In cases of substance abuse disorders, this requires careful consideration of the dose needed to maintain the mother from withdrawal without adverse effects to fetal development or neonatal outcome. This chapter will provide an overview of the role of the human placenta in the biodisposition of the medications utilized for opiate and nicotine dependence during pregnancy.

Opiate dependence and addiction

Opiates are classified into five groups of compounds according to their chemical structure: phenanthrenes (e.g., morphine and hydrocodone), phenylethylamines (methadone), morphinans (levorphanol), phenylpiperidines (meperidine), and benzomorphans (pentazocine). Morphine is a mu-opiate agonist and is currently the most widely used analgesic. Chronic abuse of morphine, or any other opiate agonist, results in development of tolerance, dependence, and addiction. However transient administration of an opiate to relieve pain from a pathological condition, as opposed to recreational use/abuse, is less likely to cause addiction but will result in development of tolerance. Moreover, there is cross-tolerance and dependence among the different opiates.

The molecular basis underlying addiction to opiates is not clearly understood. Therefore, women who are addicted to opiates and who become pregnant have limited opportunities to "kick the habit" due to a lack of proven and effective psychosocial programs. Abrupt and complete cessation of opiate intake during pregnancy is generally not recommended because of withdrawal complications for the woman and her fetus. On the other hand, the use of methadone, and more recently buprenorphine, in maintenance programs for the pregnant opiate addict significantly improves maternal and neonatal outcomes.

> **Clinical Pearl**
>
> Opiate addiction during pregnancy places both mother and fetus at risk for medical, social, and psychological harm. During the last 60 years, methadone has become the gold standard for maintenance of the pregnant opiate addict. However, the significant improvement in maternal and neonatal outcomes of these patients is often associated with neonatal abstinence syndrome (NAS).

The Placenta: From Development to Disease, First Edition. Edited by Helen H. Kay, D. Michael Nelson and Yuping Wang.
© 2011 Blackwell Publishing Ltd. Published 2011 by Blackwell Publishing Ltd.

Neonatal abstinence syndrome (NAS)

NAS can lead to serious complications that include fever, irritability, hyperactive reflexes, dehydration, poor weight gain, and, in severe cases, seizures and death. Moreover, intensive care treatment is required for 10%–30% of the neonates. The reports on whether the incidence and severity of NAS correlate with the dose of methadone administered to the mother are conflicting. This lack of correlation suggests that the concentration of the opiate in the fetal circulation is not proportional to that in the mother. A major determinant of methadone concentration in the fetal circulation is its disposition by the placenta during pregnancy. Therefore, a better understanding of the biodisposition of opiates by placental tissue might clarify the relationship between maternal dosing and the incidence and severity of NAS.

Research Spotlight

Since the late 1990 s, the authors hypothesized that the human placenta acts as a functional barrier that decreases fetal exposure to metabolic waste products, environmental toxins, and xenobiotics (compounds foreign to the body), including medications.

Human placenta as a functional barrier between the maternal and fetal circulations

For decades, the human placenta was assumed to act as an impermeable barrier to drugs. However, the thalidomide-induced birth defects found in the 1960s dispelled this concept. Currently, the placenta is viewed as a "permeability barrier" which allows small molecular weight compounds <900kDa, such as most of our current medications, to cross from the maternal to the fetal circulation by simple or facilitated diffusion. Additionally, placental uptake and efflux transporters, present on the basal and apical membranes, can transfer medications by energy-dependent mechanisms. Therefore, the human placenta acts as a functional barrier between the maternal and fetal circulations by virtue of the activity of its metabolic enzymes and efflux transporters. The function of the barrier is dependent on the following:

1 The activity of trophoblast enzymes responsible for the biotransformation of xenobiotics including most medications. These metabolic enzymes are often identical in their functions to those in the liver, but with lower activity.

2 Activity of uptake and efflux transporters that are localized at the apical and basal membranes. These transporters are usually unidirectional and each spans the phospholipid bilayer of the cell. These transporters facilitate the transfer of their substrates from the maternal to fetal circulation (e. g., certain nutrients). The efflux transporters extrude their substrates from the feto-placental compartment to the maternal circulation (e.g. waste products). Uptake and efflux transporters are also involved in the transfer of intermediates from several metabolic pathways catalyzed by maternal, fetal, and placental enzymes.

In addition, the activity of placental metabolic enzymes and transporters are subject to modifications by:

1 Induction or inhibition due to their exposure to chemicals (environmental toxins or medications). For example, maternal exposure to smoking during pregnancy results in induction of placental CYP 1A1 isozymes and an increase in their activity [1,2].

2 Single nucleotide polymorphisms (SNPs) can occur in the genes encoding the metabolic enzymes and efflux transporters, thus affecting their activity.

3 Changes associated with gestational age. For example, the expression and activity of CYP 19/aromatase, the enzyme responsible for placental biotransformation of methadone, increases with the progress of gestation [3]. On the other hand, the expression of placental efflux transporter P-gp decreases with gestational age [4].

Research Spotlight

Human placental metabolic enzymes and efflux transporters are major determinants of the concentration of a medication in the fetal circulation.

Placental disposition of medications

Placental disposition of a medication refers to its transplacental transfer, distribution into trophoblast tissue, biotransformation by metabolic enzymes, and elimination/extrusion back to the maternal circulation by transporters. The disposition of a compound depends on its physicochemical properties, ionization, polarity, and partition coefficient, as well as its susceptibility to derivatization by metabolic enzymes. Placental disposition of medications can be studied and measured using in vitro methods, and the data obtained provides valuable information on the extent of fetal exposure to a medication during pregnancy.

Research Spotlight

Data on placental disposition of medications should be obtained from human or primate placental derived preparations. Data from other animal models, especially nonprimates, should not be extrapolated to human because of the differences in the anatomy and physiology of their placentas.

In vitro placental transfer of medications and their quantification

The technique of dual perfusion of the placental lobule is the closest in vitro model to simulate in vivo placental transfer of medications, as described in another chapter of this book. Detection of medication in placental tissue and both circulations provides information on the rate and extent of drug transfer from the maternal to the fetal circulation. The minimum concentration detected for a compound during its dual perfusion depends on the analytical method used. The following analytical methods are typically used and each is at least two orders of magnitude more sensitive than the following: radioactive isotopes (femto to pico grams) > mass spectrometry (LC/MS; pico to nanograms) > fluorescence spectroscopy (nano to micro grams) > visible or UV spectrometry (micrograms).

Biotransformation/metabolism of medications administered during pregnancy by human placental enzymes

During pregnancy, the placenta becomes an additional site for extra-hepatic metabolism of medications. Notably, the activity of placental enzymes in the biotransformation of a medication is only 10% of maternal hepatic enzyme activity. This is in agreement with the role of the placenta as a second line of defense to protect the fetus. The volume of fetal circulation is less than 10% of the volume of the mother's circulation, and fetal weight is significantly less than 10% of the maternal weight. Therefore, the activity of placental enzymes are most likely adequate for protecting the fetus from xenobiotics present in the maternal circulation.

Information on placental metabolism of medications can be obtained by utilizing the technique of dual perfusion or by preparations of subcellular fractions. The limitations of utilizing this technique for metabolism investigations include: (1) restricted access of the medication to the metabolizing sites due to the small size of the perfused cotyledon; (2) the relatively short duration of the perfusion period (typically 4 hours); (3) a medication concentration used during perfusion is usually similar to that achieved in vivo, which is, in most cases, below its affinity to the enzyme (i.e., lower than its Km); (4) the amounts of metabolite(s) formed may be lower than the detection limits of the analytical method used.

Therefore, subcellular fractions of trophoblast tissue obtained from term and preterm placentas are the preferred in vitro method for investigating the biotransformation of medications. Several enzymes responsible for the biotransformation of xenobiotcs, including medications, have been identified in placental tissue through gestation. These enzymes are either localized in the cytoplasm, mitochondria, or microsomes of preterm and term placentas. The identification of these enzymes is performed at the level of its mRNA or its expressed protein. However, these two methods do not provide information on the activity of the enzymes involved in the biotransformation of a specific medication/compound.

Most biotransformation enzymes convert the medication to a metabolite that is more water soluble than the parent compound. This is achieved by the introduction of a polar group (hydroxyl group) as is the case for numerous Cytochrome P 450 (CYP) isozymes or an ionizable group. In a few cases, CYP isozymes reduce the lipophilicity of a medication by its dealkylation (removal of a hydrocarbon chain). Alternatively, the enzyme could conjugate the medication with a compound that possesses hydroxyl or ionizable groups, e. g., glucuronic acid. Other metabolic enzymes identified in placental tissue include glutathione S-transferase, N-acetyltransferase, and uridine diphospho-glucuronosyltransferase.

The subcellular localization of an enzyme is identified by determining its activity in preparations of mitochondrial, microsomal, and cytosolic fractions. The affinity of the substrate to the enzyme and its activity are characterized by determining the kinetic parameters of the reaction (Km and Vmax, respectively), as well as the metabolites formed. Therefore, it is essential to identify the major placental enzyme (s) responsible for the biotransformation of each medication given to a pregnant woman because of possible drug interactions.

Examples of the differences between placental and hepatic metabolism of particular medications:

1 In a few cases, placental and hepatic enzymes form identical metabolites of the drug as reported for methadone and buprenorphine [5–7].

2 In other cases, placental microsomes form a metabolite previously unidentified for hepatic enzymes as was reported by glyburide [8].

3 Alternatively, different hepatic and placental enzymes form the same metabolite of a drug. For example, the major placental enzyme responsible for the biotransformation of methadone and buprenorphine was identified as CYP 19/aromatase, while the hepatic enyme was CYP 3A4 and 2B6.

4 The activity of placental mitochondrial enzymes involved in the biotransformation of 17-hydroxyprogesterone caproate was significantly higher than the microsomal enzymes. On the other hand, the activity of hepatic mitochondrial enzymes was a small fraction of the microsomal.

5 Both hepatic and placental enzymes metabolize bupropion to hydroxy-, threo-, and erythrohydrobupropion. Notably, the major metabolite of bupropion formed by hepatic enzymes was hydroxybupropion, whereas the major metabolites formed by the placenta were threo- and erythrohydrobupropion.

6 Placental metabolic enzymes can be sites for drug interactions. This was evident from the metabolism of methadone and bupropion by CYP 19/aromatase which is a key enzyme in the biosynthesis of estrogens. The recent identification of this interaction site [5–7] provided an explanation for the lower-than-control estrogen levels in pregnant women treated with methadone reported earlier [9].

Research Spotlight

The activity of placental enzymes in the biotransformation of a medication is <10% of that in the liver. The cellular localization of the enzyme, the responsible isoform catalyzing the reaction, as well as the metabolites formed by placental tissue, could be either identifical or different from the liver. However, the metabolites formed in the placenta have greater access to the fetal circulation, which is also <10% of the maternal circulation volume.

Efflux transporters

Placental efflux transporters are localized in the apical membranes of the syncytiotrophoblast. Their function is to extrude their substrates from the fetoplacental unit to the maternal circulation, thus decreasing fetal exposure to the medication. Three highly characterized efflux transporters are expressed in the placental apical membranes namely, P-glycoprotein (P-gp), Breast Cancer Resistance Protein (BCRP), and Multi Drug Resistance-associated Proteins (MRP). These three transporters are members of the ATP Binding Cassette family (ABC) and utilize ATP hydrolysis to provide the metabolic energy necessary for extrusion of the medication. The functions of placental efflux transporters could be determined by using several techniques/preparations, including dual perfusion of placental lobules and inside-out vesicles (IOV) prepared from apical membranes.

Role of glycoprotein (P-gp) in the efflux of methadone and buprenorphine (BUP)

Methadone transfer across term placenta, as determined by the technique of dual perfusion of placenta lobule, was greater than BUP which was retained extensively by trophoblast tissue. In addition, the transfer of methadone across preterm placenta was 70% of that transferred across term placentas. To identify the role of the efflux transporters in the transfer of methadone and BUP, two in vitro techniques were utilized. The first is dual perfusion of placental lobule, and the second is inside-out vesicle preparations from placental apical membranes. The addition of an inhibitor selective for P-gp in the maternal circulation during the perfusion of methadone resulted in an increase in the amount of the opiate transferred to the fetal circulation. However, perfusing BUP in presence of the inhibitor did not affect the amount of the opiate transferred to the fetal circulation. This data suggested that methadone, but not BUP, is a transport substrate of P-gp. However, neither the rate of transfer (V, Vmax) nor the affinity (Kt) of the substrate to the transporter can be determined using this method. In order to determine these kinetic parameters, an inside-out vesicle preparation from placental apical membranes was developed. The activity of P-gp in the IOV preparation was characterized by the uptake of its prototypic substrate paclitaxel (taxol) using its radiolabelled isotope to maximize its detection limits and quantification. The data obtained revealed typical saturation kinetics, thus validating the method. The uptake of the radioactive isotopes of methadone and BUP were used, and the data obtained demonstrated that methadone is transported by P-gp, while BUP only binds to the transporter but is not transferred.

Notably, the extent of P-gp protein expression in placental apical membranes did not correlate with its activity, as higher amounts of the protein did not correlate with a higher Vmax that would reflect enhanced activity [3]. Moreover, single nucleotide polymorphisms (SNPs) in the MDR 1 gene encoding P-gp, namely, C1236T, C3435T, and G2677T/A, are associated with a decrease in the expression of P-gp protein. Therefore, the expression of P-gp in a particular placenta regulates the extent of methadone transfer from the maternal to the fetal circulation and most likely correlates with the incidence and severity of neonatal withdrawal (NAS).

Research Spotlight

The role of efflux transporters in placental apical membranes is to decrease fetal exposure to xenobiotics, including medications.

Nicotine addiction

Nicotine is the addictive compound in cigarette smoke and is the primary factor in continued and compulsive use. Nicotine binds to the nicotinic acetylcholine receptors located in the mesolimbic dopaminergic system of the brain (the reward center). Stimulation of these receptors increases dopamine release and consequently stimulation of the brain-reward system. The latter interaction is the impetus for the most "pleasure" producing and addiction behavior of a drug. The rapid peak in the level of nicotine in blood after smoking is quickly followed by a steady decline to the withdrawal stage, which triggers the need for the next cigarette. This repetitive cycle of stimulation and withdrawal relief is the basis for nicotine addiction in both the nonpregnant and pregnant patient.

Nicotine replacement therapy (NRTs)

The goal of NRT in the pregnant individual is to provide a level of nicotine just above that associated with withdrawal symptoms by delivering nicotine at a constant rate. The available forms of NRT include the nicotine transdermal patch, nasal spray, gum, inhaler, sublingual tablet, and lozenge. Transdermal patches produce lower, longer-lasting, steadier concentrations of nicotine instead of higher concentrations of a drug for shorter periods of time. As a result, the transdermal patches have less potential for addiction, making them the preferred NRT both in the pregnant and nonpregnant patients.

Efficacy of NRT during pregnancy

In an investigation of 250 pregnant women who smoked 10+ cigarettes a day and used the 15 mg 16-hour NRT transdermal patch, the benefit observed in pregnant women was less than nonpregnant patients with the standard clinical dose of 21 mg [10]. The reasons why nicotine replacement therapy was not effective was explained later by Dempsey et al. These authors demonstrated that lower plasma levels of nicotine in pregnant women were associated with its faster metabolism due to the induction of the enzyme CYP2A6 activity and the increase in hepatic blood flow during pregnancy [11]. Thus, 15-mg nicotine patches were not adequate for pregnant women who metabolize nicotine faster than nonpregnant women.

Maternal and fetal side effects

NRT can cause dose-related increases in maternal blood pressure and heart rate. Nicotine freely crosses the placenta and may have similar effects on the fetus, but to a lesser degree [12]. However, these changes are less significant than the effect of continued smoking on the fetus.

Clinical Pearl

(1) The risk of cigarette smoking during pregnancy is far greater than the risk of exposure to nicotine from nicotine therapy; (2) Physiological changes accompanying the onset and progression of pregnancy affect pharmacokinetics of nicotine, thus requiring dose adjustment of NRT for pregnant smokers.

Bupropion

Bupropion (amfebutamone) was initially developed for the treatment of depression. It has since been developed as a nonnicotine aid for smoking cessation. It is considered an alternative for individuals who cannot tolerate NRT or who prefer nonnicotine treatment. The clinical effects of bupropion are mediated by the weak inhibition of the neuronal uptake of norepinephrine and dopamine.

Placental transfer and metabolism of bupropion

Bupropion crosses the human placenta as determined by an ex vivo model system [13]. It is extensively metabolized by human hepatic CYP 2B6 to hydroxybupropion (OH-bupropion, the major metabolite) as well as threohydrobupropion and erythrohydrobupropion. Bupropion is also metabolized by the human placental 11β-hydroxysteroid dehydrogenases to predominantly threobupropion [13].

Research Spotlight

The major metabolic pathway for the biotransformation/metabolism of bupropion is by reduction in the placenta and by oxidation in the liver.

Teaching points

1 The pharmacokinetics of a medication is altered by pregnancy. Human placental disposition of a medication is one of the factors affecting these changes.

2 The molecular mechanisms underlying addiction to a drug are not clearly understood. Therefore, maintenance of the pregnant patient on a medication is necessary and usually improves maternal and neonatal outcomes.

3 Dose of the medication (e.g., methadone) used for maintenance of the pregnant opiate addict varies widely between patients. The dose used in a nonpregnant patient cannot be extrapolated to the pregnant woman and should be carefully considered.

4 The concentration of a medication in the fetal circulation throughout pregnancy should not be assumed as equal to that in the maternal circulation even if it is the same at delivery/birth.

5 Human placental enzymes could biotransform a medication to metabolites that are different in their structure from those formed by hepatic enzymes (e.g., glyburide [15] and 17-hydroxyprogestronecaproate [16]) Therefore, identification of each metabolite formed by the placenta should be determined and not assumed.

6 The metabolites formed by the placenta have greater access to the fetal circulation than those formed by hepatic enzymes and are present in the maternal circulation. Therefore, their pharmacologic effects, as compared to the parent compound, should be identified.

7 The promiscuous nature of the majority of metabolic enzymes to their substrates (e.g., cytochrome P 450, CYP) requires the identification of each placental enzyme responsible for the biotransformation of a medication administered during pregnancy. For example, hepatic CYP 3A4 is responsible for metabolizing approximately 50% of the current medications. This enzyme is not present in human placenta but CYP 19 biotransforms many of its known hepatic substrates.

8 The activity of placental efflux transporters should be determined for each medication administered to a pregnant patient, i.e., in preterm and term placentas. Determination of their expression can not be assumed to correlate with activity.

Reference

1. Sesardic D, Pasanen M, Pelkonen O et al. (1990) Differential expression and regulation of members of the cytochrome P450IA gene subfamily in human tissues. *Carcinogenesis* 11(7): 1183–8.
2. Manchester DK and Jacoby EH (1981) Sensitivity of human placental monooxygenase activity to maternal smoking. *Clin Pharmacol Ther* 30(5): 687–92.
3. Hieronymus TL, Nanovskaya TN, Deshmukh SV et al. (2006) Methadone metabolism by early gestational age placentas. *Am J Perinatol* 23(5): 287–94.
4. Hemauer SJ, Patrikeeva SL, Nanovskaya TN et al. (2009) Opiates inhibit paclitaxel uptake by P-glycoprotein in preparations of human placental inside-out vesicles. *Biochem Pharmacol* 78(9): 1272–8.
5. Deshmukh SV, Nanovskaya TN, Ahmed MS (2003) Aromatase is the major enzyme metabolizing buprenorphine in human placenta. *J Pharmacol Exp Ther* 306(3): 1099–105.
6. Nanovskaya TN, Deshmukh SV, Brooks M et al. (2002) Transplacental transfer and metabolism of Buprenorphine. *Pharmacology* 300(1): 26–33.
7. Nanovskaya TN, Deshmukh SV, Nekhaeva IA et al. (2004) Methadone metabolism by human placenta. *Biochem Pharmacol* 68: 583–91.
8. Zharikova OL, Ravindran S, Nanovskaya TN et al. (2007) Kinetics of glyburide metabolism by hepatic and placental microsomes of humans and baboon. *Biochem Pharmacol* 73: 2012–19.
9. Facchinetti F, Comitini G, Petraglia F et al. (1986) Reduced estriol and dehydroepianrosterone sulphate plasma levels in methadone-addicted pregnant women. *Eur J Obstet Gynecol Reprod Biol* 23: 67–73.
10. Wisborg K, Henriksen TB, Jespersen LB et al. (2000) Nicotine patches for pregnant smokers:a randomized controlled study. *Obstet Gynecol* 96: 967–71.
11. Dempsey DA and Benowitz NL (2001) Risks and benefits of nicotine to aid smoking cessation in pregnancy. *Drug Saf* 24(4): 277–322. Review
12. Rore C, Brace V, Danielian P et al. (2008) Smoking cessation in pregnancy. *Expert Opin Drug Saf* 7(6): 727–37.

13. Earhart AD, Patrikeeva S, Wang X et al. (2010) Transplacental transfer and metabolism of bupropion. *J Matern Fetal Neonatal Med* 23(5): 409–16.
14. Wang X, Abdelrahman DR, Zharikova OL et al. (2010) Bupropion metabolism by human placenta. *Biochem Pharmacol* 79(11): 1684–90.
15. Zharikova OL, Fokina VM, Nanovskaya TN et al. (2009) Identification of the major human hepatic and placental enzymes responsible for the biotransformation of glyburide. *Biochem Pharmacol* 78(12): 1483–90.
16. Yan R, Nanovskaya TN, Zharikova OL et al. (2008) Metabolism of 17alpha-hydroxyprogesterone caproate by hepatic and placental microsomes of human and baboons. *Biochem Pharmacol* 75(9): 1848– 57.

40

CHAPTER 40
Placental Drug Transport

Clifford W. Mason and Carl P. Weiner
Department of Obstetrics and Gynecology, School of Medicine, University of Kansas Medical Center, Kansas City, KS, USA

Introduction

The placenta is a portal for drug transmission between mother and fetus. Depending on the effect and designated use, a drug may be harmful, beneficial, or nonthreatening to the fetus. The FDA has an imperfect classification of risk for use during pregnancy (Table 40.1) and this is slated for replacement. The physiochemical characteristics of most chemical substances, including therapeutic agents, enable their permeation across the placenta. Other factors such as drug transport proteins, determine the rate and extent of placental drug transfer.

Structural features in the placenta relevant to drug transport

The placenta is the first fetal organ a drug encounters. The multinucleated, polarized syncytiotrophoblast serves as a rate-limiting barrier for permeation due to the presence of transport proteins and metabolic enzymes. Drugs that permeate the syncytiotrophoblast layer must then cross the underlying basement membrane of the fetal capillary endothelial cells before gaining access to the fetal circulation.

Modes of placental drug transfer

Passive diffusion

The chemical composition of most drugs enables transplacental transfer via passive diffusion. In general, drug properties such as molecular weight, ionization (pKa), lipid solubility, and protein binding determine placental transfer by passive diffusion. Substances that transfer by a mechanism other than passive diffusion, such as facilitated diffusion or active transport, may not necessarily possess these characteristics. Few drugs are transported across the placenta by facilitated diffusion. The quantity of drug that crosses is dependent on the concentration of the drug in the maternal and fetal circulation, physiochemical properties of the molecule, and characteristics of the placenta (i.e., surface area and thickness of the placental membrane). Drug distribution from the maternal circulation is primarily a function of both uterine blood flow and placental membrane permeability. Decreased blood flow limits the transfer of drugs from mother to fetus, but will also reduce the clearance of drugs from the fetal compartment, a double edge sword in terms of fetal toxicity [1].

Clinical Pearl

Some placental transfer is inevitable with any drug, and the potential for fetal toxicity must be considered before prescribing any medication.

Active transport

Active transport requires the use of energy provided by either adenosine triphosphate (ATP) hydrolysis or transmembrane electrochemical gradients of Na^+, Cl^-, or H^+ to fuel the saturable transporter proteins to move molecules against a concentration gradient [1]. Both the apical microvillous membrane (maternal-facing brush

The Placenta: From Development to Disease, First Edition. Edited by Helen H. Kay, D. Michael Nelson and Yuping Wang.
© 2011 Blackwell Publishing Ltd. Published 2011 by Blackwell Publishing Ltd.

Table 40.1 Pregnancy drug categories set by US food and drug administration.

Category	Pregnancy Category Definition	Example
A[a]	Adequate, well-controlled studies in pregnant women have not shown an increased risk to the fetus in any trimester of pregnancy, and there is no evidence of later risk either *Very few medications have been tested to this level*	Folic acid, magnesium sulfate
B[b]	Animal studies have revealed no evidence of harm to the fetus, however, there are no adequate and well-controlled studies in pregnant women **OR** Animal studies have shown no adverse effect, but adequate and well-controlled studies in pregnant women have failed to demonstrate a risk to the fetus in any trimester.	Metformin PI, NVRT
C[b]	Animal studies have shown an adverse effect and there are no adequate and well-controlled studies in pregnant women. **OR** No animal studies have been conducted and there are no adequate and well-controlled studies in pregnant women.	SSRI[d], Glyburide, labetalol, nifedipine
D[c]	Adequate well-controlled or observational studies in pregnant women have demonstrated a risk to the fetus, but the benefits may outweigh the risk for pregnant women who have a serious condition that cannot be treated effectively with a safer drug.	ACE inhibitors, paroxetine
X[c]	Adequate well-controlled or observational studies in animals and pregnant women have demonstrated positive evidence of fetal abnormalities or risks and the risks outweigh any potential benefits for women who are (or may become) pregnant.	Isotretinoin, thalidomide

[a]Drugs grouped as probably safe.
[b]Drugs grouped as potentially harmful.
[c]Drugs grouped as clearly harmful.
[d]Except paroxetin.

border) and basal membrane (fetal-facing) of the syncytiotrophoblast and fetal capillary endothelial cells express active transporters. Some transporters facilitate the transfer of drugs to the fetal compartment, while others prevent their entry into the fetoplacental unit. The small distribution volume in the fetus and low abundance of placental cytochrome P450 (CYP) metabolizing enzymes suggest that drug transporters play an important role in the overall pharmacokinetics of placental drug transfer.

Placental drug transporters

The human placenta is enriched with a variety of influx and efflux transporters (Figure 40.1) (Table 40.2). Once a drug is absorbed into the syncytiotrophoblasts, based on its physical properties, the efflux transporters return some of the drug to the maternal circulation and the influx transporters guide some drug to the fetal circulation. Among them, the ATP-binding-cassette (ABC) and solute carrier (SLC) superfamilies are the major transporters. The types of transporters, and their activity and expression across gestation can have a profound effect [2]. ABC transporters extensively limit the transfer of drugs to the fetus, while SLC transporters generally use electrochemical solute gradients to regulate the cellular uptake and efflux of drugs. Together, these transporter families have an integral role controlling the chemical environment of the fetus.

Clinical Pearl

The interaction of drugs with placental transporters determines the clinical utility, side effects, and toxicity of drugs.

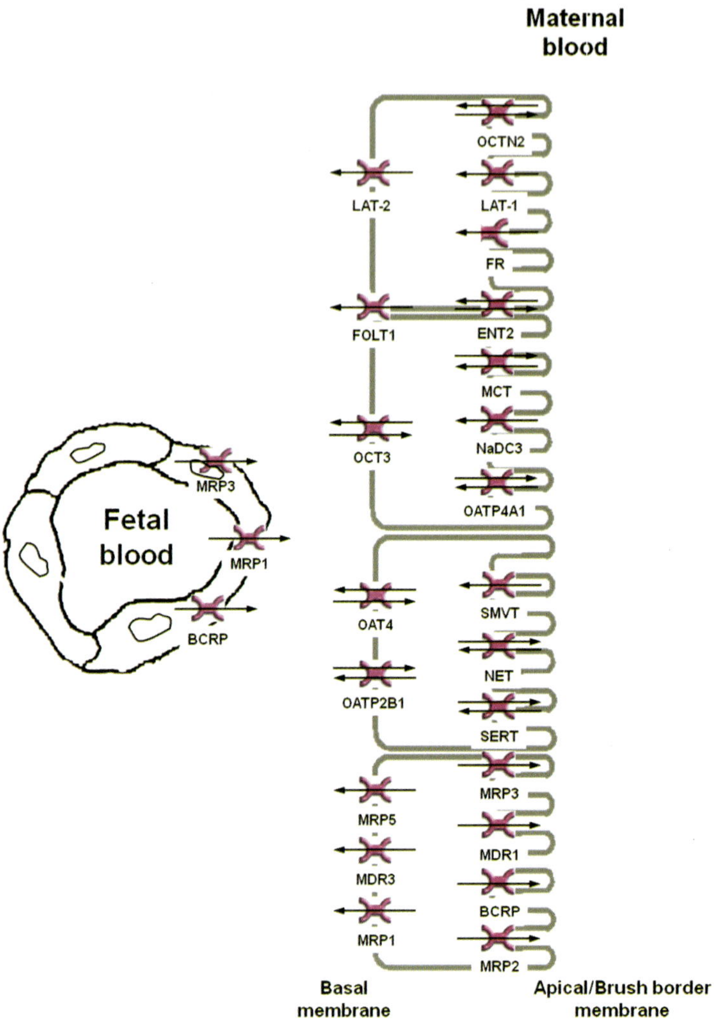

Figure 40.1 Schematic representation of the putative localization and function of the major placental drug transport proteins. The placenta expresses various drug transport proteins in the apical (brush border) and basal membrane that function through influx and efflux mechanisms to regulate the passage of various drugs and xenobiotics across the placenta. Drug transporter proteins (mostly efflux transporters) are also expressed in the fetal capillary endothelial cells. Several transporters such as OCTN1 and ENT1 are expressed but localization is unknown.

Efflux (ABC) transporters involved in placental drug transfer

ABC transporter expression is tissue dependent; placental transporters include ABCB1 (P-glycoprotein, P-gp, multidrug resistant protein [MDR1]), ABCB4 (MDR3), ABCC1–3 (multidrug-resistant associated protein [MRP1–3]), and ABCG2 (breast cancer resistance protein [BCRP]). P-gp and BCRP at the apical brush-border microvillous membrane serve as regulators of drug efflux, limiting drug transfer to the fetus. P-gp in the placenta is perhaps best characterized. A large number of drugs or drug metabolites are recognized as P-gp substrates. These include anticancer, immunosuppressive, antiretroviral, cardiac, and cholesterol-lowering drugs [3].

One ABC transporter, BCRP, is highly expressed on the apical side of the syncytiotrophoblast and on fetal vascular endothelial cells where the transporter may aid removal of fetal byproducts. BCRP transports a broad spectrum of substrates such as anticancer drugs, antibiotics, antihypertensives, and hypoglycemic agents. BCRP also transports organic anions such as estrone-3-sulfate, 17β-estradiol, and dehydroepiandrosterone, suggesting that the transporter may be an important regulator of estrogen synthesis [4].

Table 40.2 Drug transporters and their putative function.

Drug Transporter	Transporter Name	Placental Localization	Putative Function
P-gp	P-glycoprotein	Apical syncytiotrophoblast	Efflux
BCRP	Breast cancer resistance protein	Apical syncytiotrophoblast, fetal capillaries	Efflux
MRP1	Multidrug resistance associated protein 1	Basal membrane, fetal capillaries	Efflux
MRP2	Multidrug resistance associated protein 2	Apical syncytiotrophoblast	Efflux
MRP3	Multidrug resistance associated protein 3	Apical syncytiotrophoblast, fetal capillaries	Efflux
MRP5	Multidrug resistance associated protein 5	Basal membrane	Efflux
OATP2B1	Organic anion transporter polypeptide 2B1	Basal membrane	Influx/Efflux
OATP4A1	Organic anion transporter polypeptide 4A1	Apical syncytiotrophoblast	Influx/Efflux
OATP3A1	Organic anion transporter polypeptide 3A1	Unknown	Influx/Efflux
OAT4	Organic anion transporter 4	Basal membrane	Influx/Efflux
SERT	5-HT transporter	Apical syncytiotrophoblast	Influx/Efflux
NET	Noraderenaline transporter	Apical syncytiotrophoblast	Influx/Efflux
LAT1	L-type amino acid transporter 1	Apical syncytiotrophoblast	Influx
LAT2	L-type amino acid transporter 2	Basal membrane	Influx
OCT3	Organic cation transporter 3 / extraneuronal monoamine transporter	Basal membrane	Influx/Efflux
OCTN1	Organic cation transporter 1/Carnitine transporter	Unknown	Influx/Efflux
OCTN2	Organic cation transporter 3/Carnitine transporter	Apical syncytiotrophoblast	Influx/Efflux
MCT	Monocarboxylate transporter	Apical syncytiotrophoblast	Influx/Efflux
NaDC3	Dicarboxylate transporter	Apical syncytiotrophoblast	Influx
ENT1	Equilabrative nucleoside transporter 1	Apical syncytiotrophoblast	Influx/Efflux
ENT2	Equilabrative nucleoside transporter 2	Unkown	Influx/Efflux
SMVT	Sodium multivitamin transporter	Apical syncytiotrophoblast	Influx
FOLT1	Folate transporter	Apical syncytiotrophoblast	Influx
FR	Folate receptor	Basal membrane	Influx

Clinical Pearl

If the target is maternal disease, drugs that are P-gp or BCRP substrates are preferable rather than drugs that are not P-gp or BCRP substrates, since the latter more easily cross the placenta to the fetus.

Another ABC efflux transporter, MDR3, encodes a membrane glycoprotein with relatively unknown function but with a structure similar in sequence to P-gp and a localization to the basal membrane of term and preterm human placenta. Among the multidrug resistance (MDR) proteins, MRP1 and MRP3 by immunolocalization are expressed in endothelium of fetal blood vessels and along the basal membrane of syncytiotrophoblasts. MRP2 differs in immunolocalization along the apical membrane of the syncytiotrophoblast. The protective function of these MRP proteins involves the transportation away from the fetus of organic anions such as sulfate, glucuronide, and glutathione conjugates. These transporters act interchangeably with each other.

Placental transfer of antidiabetic drugs

Many pregnant women develop gestational diabetes, and a large percentage will benefit from treatment with hypoglycemic agents. There are several medication options. The high molecular weight (6000 Da) of insulin precludes passive transport across the placenta, although insulin bound to anti-insulin antibodies can cross the placental barrier [5].

Glyburide (glibenclamide) is a second generation sulfonylurea effective for the treatment of most women with gestational diabetes, and some Type II diabetic women. The drug has minimal to modest maternal-fetal transfer due to a high-protein binding of nearly 99.8% to yield less free drug to cross the placenta [5]. Glyburide is neither immunogenic nor significantly metabolized by the placenta, despite specificity for placental CYP19/aromatase. Glyburide has a short elimination half-life, low volume of distribution, and rapid clearance [5] suggesting a limited opportunity for the drug to reach the placental membrane and the ABC efflux transporters. Glyburide is preferentially effluxed out of the placenta by BCRP and MRP3, and may also interact with P-gp and MRP2 [6].

Metformin is another antidiabetic agent commonly prescribed to pregnant women that does not stimulate insulin secretion. However, metformin is not selectively effluxed by any known transporter, and the drug may cross the placenta to concentrate in the fetal compartment. Metformin is not teratogenic and is extensively used in women with metabolic syndrome seeking to conceive and as an adjunct to either glyburide or insulin in resistant women.

Clinical Pearl

Glyburide is an attractive therapy for hyperglycemia during pregnancy from gestational or type II diabetes and is a good example of a drug that preferentially targets maternal distribution without significant transport to the fetal compartment.

Placental transfer of antiretroviral drugs

Maternal drug transport is increasingly used as a portal for fetal therapy. One example is the use of antiretroviral agents in HIV-infected women to prevent perinatal infection. Multiple antiretroviral drugs are used during pregnancy to treat maternal HIV infection and prevent transmission to the fetus. The most frequently prescribed regimen combines a protease inhibitor(s) (PI) and nucleoside reverse transcriptase inhibitors (NRVT). PI drugs (i.e., nelfinavir, ritonavir, saquinavir, lopinavir) do not cross the placenta to an appreciable extent and are unlikely to provide any direct protection to the fetus. The limited placental transfer of PI drugs results from their high degree of plasma protein binding and their substrate specificity for efflux transporters, specifically P-gp. This class of agents seeks a reduction in the maternal viral load and should be used in multiple-doses in a regimen for prophylaxis. In contrast, the placental transfer of NVRTs is unimpeded and sufficient to ensure suppressive fetal blood levels. These drugs are less bound by protein and there is no apparent interaction with drug efflux transporters. Use of this combination has dramatically reduced (<2%) perinatal transmission and failures are due mostly to omission. However, there is an increased risk of short-term toxicity for the fetus and newborn and an unknown long-term impact on the mother and the child [7].

Newer medicines with greater potency and improved safety profiles open the possibility for enhancing long-term use of first-line antiretroviral therapy. However, a number of clinical questions remain to be answered, particularly those regarding placental transfer and safety.

Clinical Pearl

Best practice indicates that maternal viral load levels be monitored. The doses of antiretroviral drugs may require modification to achieve optimal maternal and fetal antiretroviral activity due to changes in maternal pharmacokinetics.

Influx/efflux transporters involved in placental drug transfer

Apart from the major ABC efflux transporters, the placenta expresses a number of other drug transporters responsible for the transfer of a wide variety of therapeutic agents. These include organic anion and cation, monoamine, equilibrative nucleoside, mono- and dicarboxylate, vitamin, amino acid, and carnitine transporters, in addition to the receptor and transporter for folate.

Research Spotlight

The maternal-to-fetal transport of vitamins, like folate, is mediated by the apical folate receptor and the basal folate transporter (FOLT1). Drugs could be chemically conjugated to folate (vitamin B9) to facilitate placental transfer and delivery to the fetus.

Placental transfer of antidepressant drugs

Approximately 7–10% of women have depression during pregnancy and many patients benefit from pharmacologic therapy if diagnosed. Pregnancy poses a unique challenge for the ongoing treatment of depression. Selective serotonin reuptake inhibitors (SSRI) are often prescribed antidepressants; they do cross the placenta but to date have little evidence for concern. SSRIs including citalopram, fluoxetine, paroxetine, and sertraline block monoamine transporters, serotonin transporter (SERT), and noradrenaline transporter (NET), which improves the clinical symptoms of depression. However, NET and SERT are also expressed on placental brush border membrane where they regulate stable blood flow to the placenta and fetus by controlling placental transfer of vasoactive compounds such as norepinephrine and serotonin [1]. Blockade of placental NET and SERT by SSRI could predispose to conditions such as preeclampsia and IUGR.

Organic cation transporter 3 (OCT3) is the only OCT isoform found in the placenta. In contrast to NET and SERT, OCT3 is expressed on the basal membrane of human trophoblast cells. OCT3 also transports serotonin, dopamine, norepinephrine, and histamine, as well as cationic compounds that include antidepressant agents such as amphetamines, imipramine, and desipramine. This suggests OCT3 may also be important in maintaining optimal blood flow to the fetus.

Placental transfer of antihypertensive drugs

Hypertension is one the most common complications of pregnancy affecting more than 10% of all pregnancies. Several classifications have been suggested and each may require different antihypertensive treatments. A wide variety of drugs have been advocated (i.e., β-adrenergic blockers, α-adrenergic agents, calcium channel blockers, and vasodilators) to treat chronic hypertension, gestational hypertension, and preeclampsia and all appear to cross the placental barrier to some extent. Methyldopa and β-adrenoceptor antagonists have been used most extensively.

Methyldopa is a substrate for the L-type amino acid transporters (LAT-1 and LAT-2) that are expressed on both the brush border and basal membrane of the placenta where they may facilitate transfer of methyldopa across the placenta [8]. Methyldopa is historically considered safe, but is a weak antihypertensive that must be given three or four times a day, creating adherence issues. Treatment with methyldopa may require the use of an additional medication. Labetalol (third-generation β-adrenoceptor antagonist) and nifedipine (calcium channel blocker) are the most frequently employed agents for the rapid reduction of acute severe hypertension. Both drugs are substrates for the P-gp efflux transporter. Nifedipine is also a substrate for the CYP3A4 drug metabolizing enzyme and affinity of this drug for CYP3A4 may predispose it to drug interactions. For example, P-gp mediated efflux into maternal circulation could prolong nifedipine exposure and increase its metabolism by CYP3A4, resulting in reduced placental absorption. Labetalol is well absorbed and has a relatively high permeability suggesting it may overcome the P-gp mediated efflux. Magnesium sulfate remains the drug of choice for the prevention and treatment of eclampsia. All these compounds are relatively safe despite their ability to transverse the placenta. All angiotensin converting enzyme inhibitors or angiotensin receptor antagonists should be avoided during pregnancy for fetal indications.

Clinical Pearl

From a placental transport perspective, there is no basis for recommending any particular antihypertensive drug over any other in pregnancy since most have some affinity for one or another transporter. The choice should be based on the clinician's experience with the drug.

Significance of drug-drug interactions

The administration of multiple drugs to the mother potentiates the risk of significant drug interactions in the placenta [1], which are enhanced by the high number of active transporters. Multidrug therapy yields competition with endogenous and exogenous substrates for the above transporters, and fetal drug concentrations depend on whether the transporter induces or inhibits these interactions. Concentrations could differ from those originally predicted, ultimately affecting treatment outcomes [1]. At present, these mechanisms are not fully understood.

Clinical Pearl

The potential for drug-transporter and drug-drug interactions to occur in the placenta should be researched and monitored accordingly to ensure no harm is done to either the mother or the fetus; identification of drug interactions will greatly facilitate dosage adjustments during pregnancy.

Clinical relevance of placental transporter regulation

There are clinical conditions that regulate placental transporters. The patterns of expression of drug transporters appear to vary with gestational age and medical condition during pregnancy. Changes in transporter activity during pregnancy may contribute to different maternal and fetal drug concentrations. For example, P-gp and BCRP expression levels decline, whereas MRP2 and MDR3 levels increase with gestational age. The discovery of mechanisms mediating gestational change in placental drug transporters continues to be a major area of research. Hereditary variation in these transporter genes could partially explain interindividual differences in transporter expression and pharmacokinetics that influence drug efficacy and fetal toxicity. Additionally, infection, inflammation, or both have a negative effect on placental P-gp expression and function, and possibly other transporters. Finally, hypoxia, which affects various efflux transport proteins, has been studied in tumor biology, but few studies have focused on this interaction in placentas of women with preeclampsia or fetal growth restriction even though hypoxia is believed to be an important variable in these syndromes.

Clinical Pearl

Factors that modulate placental transporter activity, such as interindividual variability, gestation, and medical condition, should be factored into the risk-benefit analysis when prescribing drugs during pregnancy.

Models to study placental drug transport

In vitro models

A variety of in vitro systems have been established to study placental drug transfer. While in vitro models resolve some of the ethical and methodological problems encountered with in vivo studies, they cannot fully account for the physiological and biochemical variations in the mother, placenta, and fetus and the gestational regulation of these variables. In fact, most in vitro systems are often derived from term placentas and may not represent early pregnancy when drug exposure is critical for the developing fetus.

Tissue culture

Human trophoblast culture systems, both primary cultures and immortalized cell lines, have frequently been used to study uptake and transport mechanisms of drugs at the cellular and molecular levels. Human placental choriocarcinoma cells, such as BeWo, JAr, and JEG, share many properties with villous trophoblasts in terms of morphology, biochemical markers, hormone secretion, and invasiveness. BeWo cells undergo syncytialization, leading to changes that model primary syncytiotrophoblasts derived from placenta, and these cells are commonly used for studies of the placental barrier to dissect transport mechanisms and evaluate transporter activity [9].

Perfused placental cotyledon

The placental perfusion method is the only experimental method used to study human placental transfer and pharmacokinetics of drugs in organized placental tissue and thus is the optimal in vitro system. Experiments can either be conducted using a closed (recirculating) method where both maternal and fetal perfusates are recirculated, or in an open model (single pass, nonrecirculating) where a period of equilibration is required to achieve steady state and maternal-to-fetal clearance can be calculated [1].

In vivo models

Pregnant women are usually excluded from clinical trials unless a direct benefit is expected. The fetal-to-maternal blood drug concentration ratio is the simplest index of placental transfer in vivo. This is calculated from blood samples taken from a peripheral vein (maternal blood) and from the umbilical cord (fetal blood) at delivery after a single maternal dose. This provides the most pragmatic current approach to in vivo measurements of maternal-to-fetal drug transfer.

Animal models are often used as surrogates for drug transfer studies in humans, as human fetal studies are typically opportunistic. Animal models also have limitations related to the anatomical and functional differences among placentas of the animal kingdom and this requires all to have a cautious approach when extrapolating drug transfer data from animals to humans. When testing only the transfer of a compound, guinea pigs and primates, such as rhesus macaques and baboons, are the best models since they have placentas that are hemochorial with endocrine functions similar to the human. However, differences in gestational length and maternal physiological changes during pregnancy likely do not perfectly replicate pharmacokinetic measurements that would be observed in humans.

Research Spotlight

Mice offer unique advantages in the study of placental drug transfer, toxicology, and fetal drug disposition because genetic manipulation of the animals allows development of knockout models that are null for a given transporter.

Teaching Points

1 The choice of therapy during pregnancy should depend on a drug's efficacy in treating the maternal condition, transplacental passage, the risk of teratogenicity, and factors influencing compliance.

2 The nature and regulation of placental influx and efflux transporters will help predict the transfer of drugs and guide the selection and dose for maternal and fetal drug treatment.

3 The potential for drug interactions, which are mediated by inhibition and induction of transporter proteins, can have a profound effect on placental drug transfer and fetal exposure; a thorough evaluation of the medical history and current medication will help determine the potential risk-benefit of a specific drug administration during pregnancy.

References

1. Syme MR, Paxton JW, and Keelan JA (2004) Drug transfer and metabolism by the human placenta. *Clin Pharmacokinet* 43(8): 487–514.
2. Unadkat JD, Dahlin A, and Vijay S (2004) Placental drug transporters. *Curr Drug Metab* 5(1): 125–31.
3. Ceckova-Novotna M, Pavek P, and Staud F (2006) P-glycoprotein in the placenta: expression, localization, regulation and function. *Reprod Toxicol* 22(3): 400–10.
4. Mao Q (2008) BCRP/ABCG2 in the placenta: expression, function and regulation. *Pharm Res* 25(6): 1244–55.
5. Gedeon C and Koren G (2006) Designing pregnancy centered medications: drugs which do not cross the human placenta. *Placenta* 27(8): 861–8.
6. Gedeon C, Behravan J, Koren G et al. (2006) Transport of glyburide by placental ABC transporters: implications in fetal drug exposure. *Placenta* 27(11–12): 1096–102.
7. Gulati A and Gerk PM (2009) Role of placental ATP-binding cassette (ABC) transporters in antiretroviral therapy during pregnancy. *J Pharm Sci* 98(7): 2317–35.
8. Ganapathy V, Prasad PD, Ganapathy ME et al. (2000) Placental transporters relevant to drug distribution across the maternal-fetal interface. *J Pharmacol Exp Ther* 294(2): 413–20.
9. Evseenko DA, Paxton JW, and Keelan JA (2006) ABC drug transporter expression and functional activity in trophoblast-like cell lines and differentiating primary trophoblast. *Am J Physiol Regul Integr Comp Physiol* 290(5): R1357–65.

VI

PART VI

Future Clinical Applications

41

CHAPTER 41
Umbilical Cord Blood Banking

Gilad A. Gross[1], *Thinh Nguyen*[1], *and Laura Meints*[2]

[1]Division of Maternal-Fetal Medicine and Ultrasound-Genetics, Department of Obstetrics, Gynecology and Women's Health, St. Louis University School of Medicine, St. Mary's Health Center, St. Louis, MO, USA
[2]Department of Obstetrics and Gynecology, Barnes-Jewish Hospital, Washington University School of Medicine, St. Louis, MO, USA

Introduction

Human umbilical cord blood, once viewed as biologic waste, is now considered a highly valued commodity. Umbilical cord blood is a rich source of hematopoietic stem cells, and, since the inaugural use of these cells 1988 [1], there have been an estimated 8,000 transplants [2]. As of November 2009, a total of 52 facilities adhere to the standards of the American Association of Blood Banks and are accredited cord blood facilities. Twenty-seven of these facilities are within the United States and 25 are located internationally [3]. The growing number of individuals with ailments amenable to stem cell transplantation has captured the attention of legislators across America. In 2004, Illinois became the first state to pass legislation addressing cord blood donation, enacting Section 6.21 of the Hospital Licensing Act that mandates women delivering babies have the option to donate umbilical cord blood for stem cells a public repository at no cost to the patient [4]. In 2007, Arizona became the first state to require health care professionals to inform women in their midtrimester about the availability of both private and public cord blood storage facilities. Twenty states have enacted legislation in response to guidelines of the Institute of Medicine [5] that were established by request of the Health Resources and Services Administration [5]. Providers of obstetrical care must be familiar with the current state of umbilical cord blood donation. The goal of this chapter is to provide basic and contemporary information that educates clinicians and researchers about the potential uses of umbilical cord blood donation.

Why umbilical cord blood?

Stem cells are categorized as embryonic or adult, and each stem cell population possesses the ability to differentiate into diverse cell types. Traditionally, stem cells have been harvested from bone marrow or peripheral blood. Importantly, the list of diseases successfully treated with stem cell transplantation grows monthly (Table 41.1). Both *allogeneic* (related or unrelated) and *autologous* (self) bone marrow, and peripheral blood have been used as sources of hematopoietic progenitor cells to achieve cures or remission. Allogeneic stem cells are most successful for use in indicated treatments. The closest HLA-matched donor (usually a sibling) is chosen to improve the graft success and to lessen graft versus host disease.

Umbilical cord blood contains ample hematopoietic stem cells for transplantation, and cord blood stem cells proliferate more than cells from marrow or peripheral blood [6]. By early 2010 there were over 5500 unrelated

The Placenta: From Development to Disease, First Edition. Edited by Helen H. Kay, D. Michael Nelson and Yuping Wang.
© 2011 Blackwell Publishing Ltd. Published 2011 by Blackwell Publishing Ltd.

Table 41.1

Leukemias, Lymphomas, other Blood Cancers	Other Cancers	Bone Marrow Disorders	Hemoglobinopathies
Acute leukemias	Brain tumors	Amegakaryocytosis	Beta Thalassemia Major
Chronic leukemias	Ewing sarcoma	Aplastic anemia	Sickle cell
Hodgkin's lymphoma	Neuroblastoma	Backfan-diamond Anemia	Histocytic disorders
Multiple myeloma	Ovarian cancer	Congenital cytopenia	Familial Erythrophagocytic Lymphohistiocytosis
Non-Hodgkin's lymphoma	Renal cell carcinoma	Congenital dyserythropoietic Anemia	Hemophagocytosis
Waldenstrom's macroglobulinemia	Rhabdomyosarcoma	Dyskeratosis Congenita	Langerhans' Cell Histiocytosis (Histiocytosis X)
	Small-cell lung cancer	Fanconi anemia	
	Testicular cancer		
	Thymic carcinoma		
Myelodysplastic/ Myeloproliferative Disorders	**Inherited Metabolic Disorders**	**Other Inherited Disorders**	**Other**
Acute myelofibrosis	Adrenoleukodystrophy	Wolman disease	Chronic active Epstein Barr
Agnogenic myeloid metaplasia (Myelofibrosis)	Fucosidosis	Cartilage-hair Hypoplasia	Evans syndrome
Amyloidosis	Gaucher disease	Conital Erythropoietic Porphyria	Rheumatoid arthritis
Chronic myelomonocytic leukemia	Hunter syndrome	DiGeoge syndrome	Systemic lupus Erythematosus
Essential thrombocytopenia	Hurler syndrome	Osteoporosis	Thymic dysplasia
Polycythemia vera	Krabbe disease		
Refractory anemias	Lesch-Nyhan syndrome		
Paroxysmal nocturnal Hemoglobinuria	Mannosidosis		
Pure red cell aplasia	Maroteaux-Lamy syndrome		
Inherited immune system disorder	Mucolipidosis		
Chronic granulomatous disease	Neuronal ceroid lipofuscinosis		
Congenital neutropenia	Niemann-Pick disease		
Leukocyte adhesion deficiency	Sandhoff disease		
Severe combined immunodeficiencies	Sanfilippo syndrome		
Wiskott-Aldrich syndrome	Scheie syndrome		
X-linked lymphoproliferative disorder	Sly syndrome		
	Tay sachs		

Source: Adapted from cord blood registry website (6-17-10); http://www.cordblood.com/cord_blood_banking_with_cbr/banking/diseases_treated.asp?fbid=dworpp9KtPC

donor cord blood stem cell transplants, with success rates as high as 90% after sibling HLA-matched cord stem cell transplants and as high as 80% after unrelated cord blood stem cell transplantation [7]. Umbilical cord blood, therefore, emerged as a limitless source for procurement of stem cells, as there is no pain involved, unlike bone marrow retrieval, and cost is minimal. Importantly, stem cells from umbilical cord can be transplanted within two days of retrieval [8]. There are reduced risks of blood borne infections from umbilical cord blood [9], less HLA matching is required for recipient acceptance, and a lower risk of lethal graft versus host disease [10]. Proposed mechanisms for this acceptance include reduced concentration of CD8+ lymphocytes in cord blood and a reduced ability of these lymphocytes to produce cytokines secondary to their immature status [11].

Clinical Pearl

Transplant with cord blood stem cells produce less graft versus host disease. However, even with a sibling donor, there is only a 25% of a perfect match.

Currently, many ethnic and racial minorities, as well as multiple-race patients, are at significant disadvantage in finding matches [12]. Sixty percent of individuals who require bone marrow transplantation cannot find a donor. Caucasians have an 80% chance of finding an unrelated donor, compared to African-Americans whose chances are no greater than 30%. By increasing the number of donors from racial and ethnic minorities, patients of these persuasions will have better chances of finding appropriate donors.

Disadvantages of using cord blood?

A major concern about use of cord stem cells is that the number of cells available per sample donated is limited. The volume collected from cord blood is finite, which limits patient eligibility, in contrast to the limitless cells available from a bone marrow source. The cell dose for transplantation is based on the weight of the recipient, and only small children were initially considered candidates for cord stem cell transplantation. However, recent successes in older children and adults indicate cell volume may not be a limiting factor. The use of multiple, cryopreserved units from separate donors can be used to treat adults. A recent trial demonstrated that 82% of child and adolescent leukemia patients achieved donor-type engraftment using umbilical cord blood stem cell transplantation from two different donors [13]. In 2008 investigators in Germany reported that adults now receive more transplants than children, highlighting the widening pool of recipients for this valuable resource.

Cord blood banks

Public banks collect, type, screen for infection, and cryogenically store cord blood for use in unrelated recipients. This is akin to adults donating blood to the Red Cross at no cost to the donor and any abnormality found will be conveyed to the donor. Programs are funded by the National Institutes of Health, the National Marrow Donor Program, the American Red Cross, and other academic programs that are not for profit. Facilities within some public banks now provide the means for patients to donate directly. One program run by the NIH was created exclusively for sibling donors of first degree relatives who are diagnosed with diseases amenable to allogeneic stem cell transplantation [14].

In contrast to public banks, private umbilical cord blood banks are for-profit companies seeking patients to bank their newborn's blood for autologous use or for allogeneic directed donation for a family member should a future need arise. Some consider this to be a form of "biologic insurance." Patients pay an initial processing fee, and then incur annual storage fees. The range for process and annual storage fees is $1,000–$2,000 and $100–$200, respectively, provided by multiple companies.

Clinical Pearl

The likelihood of a patient's child ever needing their stored cord blood stem cell sample is uncertain but reported to range from 1 in 1000 to 1 in 200,000 [7]. Therefore, private storage for self or family members for future use has been discouraged because the condition to be treated, i.e., leukemia, may already be genetically present within those stored stem cells. However, cord blood banking directed to a sibling with a known disorder that can be treated with stem cell transplantation should be encouraged because the more likely HLA matching will make this worthwhile.

Obtaining the cord blood sample

Umbilical cord blood are procured from deliveries that meet screening criteria for donation. Generally, pregnancies beyond 34 weeks yield an adequate cell count. Multiple gestations pose a concern for cross contamination, labeling error, and reduced cell numbers. Infection from chorioamnionitis and active herpes disqualify a donor, given the risks of transmission of infectious pathogens, and screening for HIV is now done. Fetuses with chromosomal abnormalities or structural malformations cannot be used as donors. Mothers are also screened for medical and familial conditions that preclude donating umbilical cord blood from her placenta.

Patients contributing to either public or private banks best give consent prior to labor as the consent process is detailed, and the consent must be verified at delivery. Counseling should be noncoercive, unrelated to fiduciary relationships, and links between cord blood to donors must avoid disclosure of abnormal screening test obtained during the process [9].

Cord blood can be collected following vaginal delivery or cesarean section, but safe obstetric practice must be ensured during the collection process so as not to endanger the patient. Because the collection process adds up to three minutes operative time to cesarean section, physicians must use judgment in deciding whether or not to perform the collection. Some advocate collecting during the third stage of labor with the placenta in situ, while others prefer to deliver the placenta and then obtain the sample. Antiseptic cleanser is used at the puncture site and a 17 gauge needle is inserted into the umbilical vein, which is connected to a bag under vacuum and containing citrate phosphate dextrose anticoagulant. A term placenta yields approximately 110 milliliters [15]. Studies have shown that in situ collection results in a cord blood sample of larger volume, higher CFU, and CD34 cell counts [16]. In the processing facility, red cell and plasma components are removed in preparation for cryopreservation. A cell cryoprotectant containing dimethyl sulfoxide (DMSO) is added, cooling is done in a controlled manner, and the specimen is transferred to a liquid nitrogen tank at -196°C or -320°F for long-term storage. Reports of marrow transplants done following many years of storage have shown that cord blood that has been cryopreserved for 15 years maintains biologic properties similar to freshly harvested samples [17]. The shelf life and expiration dates for cord blood is yet to be determined.

Appropriate uses

Stem cell transplantation is used to reconstitute a patient's hematopoietic cell lines. In 1989 Gluckman reported the first successful umbilical cord blood transplantation donated from an HLA-identical sibling to a child with severe Fanconi's anemia [1]. Since then, hematopoietic stem cells from allogeneic cord blood have been successfully used to treat more than 70 diseases (see Table 41.1). Indications for cord blood stem cell transplantation include the following conditions: (1) malignancies of the hematopoietic and lymphatic systems; (2) metabolic disorders; (3) immunodeficiencies; (4) oncologic disorders; (5) and hematologic disorders (including hemoglobinopathies and sickle-cell disorders). For many common conditions, such as thalassemia major and sickle-cell disease, hematopoietic stem cell transplantation is currently the only treatment known to be curative [18]. The National Cord Blood Program (NCBP) lists the conditions that have been treated with donated NCBP units, as well as the national and international transplant centers that performed them [19].

Research Spotlight

In treating children with leukemia, some concerns have been raised regarding the suitability of their autologous cord stem cells. In some cases DNA mutations have been identified, and in others, advisability of gene therapy has been questioned. Further research should be performed to better understand behavior of these stem cells. Reports of mutations in cord blood stem cells may preclude their use for autologous transplant in children who subsequently develop leukemia.

Currently, hematopoietic stem cells are the only stem cells used to treat disease. While this treatment is still in its early stages, much attention, research, and promise have been given to the use of umbilical cord blood stem cells in regenerative medicine. Umbilical cord blood that has not been previously frozen is also a potential source of nonhematopoietic stem cells. These cells are scarce in marrow and peripheral blood and cannot be harvested following cryopreservation and thawing. Other components of cord blood include unrestricted somatic stem cells that can be amplified and differentiated into tissue specific cell lines. Pluripotent somatic stem cells have essentially the same capacity to differentiate as embryonic stem cells. Stem cells for regeneration have shown promise in the treatment of several diseases, especially cardiac and neurologic diseases. Stem cells from fresh cord blood have the ability to differentiate into neurons, microglial cells, and astrocytes, and these cells have been used experimentally in models for the treatment of stroke, amyotrophic lateral sclerosis, Parkinson's disease, Alzheimer's disease, spinal cord injuries, and other cerebral disease processes. These same pluripotent cells can be stimulated to become myocytes that promote recovery from myocardial infarction and regenerate specialized epithelium associated with cardiac valves.

Research Spotlight

Although umbilical cord blood stem cells may have a role in regenerative medicine, many treatments are still in the research stages. Donors should be counseled that there is no current scientific assurance that their donated samples can be used for future regenerative medical treatments for their child.

Unresolved issues

There remain several unanswered questions about the use of umbilical cord blood stem cells that challenge obstetric providers worldwide. Most of these revolve around the issue of consent. The American College of Obstetricians and Gynecologists (ACOG) recommends counseling patients if they request information on umbilical cord banking [2]. However, focus group studies have shown that patients are frequently unaware of the possibility of umbilical cord blood donation and may experience regret if they are not informed by their health care team about the opportunity for donation [20]. Because pregnant women are considered by some to be emotionally vulnerable, the consent process must be done with awareness and sensitivity.

Patients must be given accurate information about potential benefits and limitations of public and privately donated cord blood. Providers should familiarize themselves with the standard list of conditions currently treated with allogeneic stem cells. Women also need to be told that there is currently no proven benefit in using stem cells for regenerative medicine and that models of their use are experimental. Most experts do not recommend that patients store their cord blood in private facilities unless there is an appropriate family history. A cross-sectional survey of pediatric hematopoietic cell transplantation physicians in the United States and Canada revealed that few specialists endorse private banking in the absence of an identified recipient, even for mixed-ethnicity children for whom finding a suitably matched unrelated donor may be difficult [21].

Patients should understand that the chance of a privately donated unit of blood being used by a offspring or by a relative is very low. Researchers from the University of California-San Francisco (UCSF) concluded that there was an additional $1,374,246 per life-year gained and that the procedure was only cost-effective for families with a child with a very high likelihood of needing a stem cell transplant. A survey of private banks conducted by the American Society of Blood and Marrow Transplantation found that in approximately 460,000 cord blood units banked, only 99 were distributed for clinical use [22].

Future of cord blood banking

Future research for this technology will focus on methods to expand stem cell counts and alternate sources for stem cell procurement. Studies are underway to evaluate how to expand cell numbers ex vivo [23]. Other investigators are experimenting with stem cell mobilizing agents, such as AMD3100, in order to improve stem cell number at the time of collection from the cord/placenta [24]. One final promising area of research that does not involve cord blood stem cells is the procurement of pluripotent stem cells from amniotic fluid and numerous studies have demonstrated their ability to differentiate into cells of all three embryonic germ layers [25,26].

Teaching Points

1 Human umbilical cord blood is a rich, easy-to-obtain, source of hematopoietic stem cells.
2 Stem cells have been used to successfully treat and cure a number of cancers and inherited diseases.
3 There are benefits and drawbacks to using stem cells obtained from umbilical cord blood, one being the lower number of stem cells and its limited one time source.
4 Both public and private cord blood collection systems exist. No charges are incurred by the donor in public banks but no specified and directed future use can be dictated. However, such need for a directed sample for self or a relative is very unlikely.
5 The clinician should be knowledgeable about the uses and collection of umbilical cord blood in order to help their patient make an informed decision about donating to a public bank versus personal banking at a private bank.

References

1. Gluckman E, Broxmeyer HA, Auerbach AD et al. (1989) Hematopoietic reconstitution in a patient with fanconi's anemia by means of umbilical-cord blood from an HLA-identical sibling. *N Engl J Med* 321(17): 1174–8.
2. Committee on Obstetric Practice, Committee on Genetics (2008) ACOG committee opinion number 399, February

2008: umbilical cord blood banking. *Obstet Gynecol* 111 (2 Pt 1): 475–7.

3. Accredited Cord Blood Facilities. Website: www.aabb.org/sa/facilities/celltherapy/pages/CordBloodAccrfac.aspx
4. Illinois General Assembly. Website: www.ilgagov/legislation/96/sb/09600sb3448.htm
5. Cord Blood Awareness. Website: www.cordbloodawareness.org/iom_study.htm
6. Hao QL, Shah AJ, Thiemann FT et al. (1995) A functional comparison of CD34 +CD38- cells in cord blood and bone marrow. *Blood* 86(10): 3745–53.
7. Lubin BH and Shearer WT (2007) Cord blood banking for potential future transplantation. *Pediatrics* 119(1): 165–70.
8. Reimann V, Creutzig U, and Kogler G (2009) Stem cells derived from cord blood in transplantation and regenerative medicine. *Dtsch Arztebl Int* 106(50): 831–6.
9. Armson BA (2005) Umbilical cord blood banking: implications for perinatal care providers. *J Obstet Gynaecol Can* 27(3): 263–90.
10. Varadi G et al. (1995) Umbilical cord blood for use in transplantation. *Obstet Gynecol Surv* 50(8): 611–7.
11. Moise KJ Jr (2005) Umbilical cord stem cells. *Obstet Gynecol* 106(6): 1393–407.
12. Brunstein CG and Wagner JE (2009) Chapter 105 – Umbilical cord blood transplantation. *Hematology: Basic Principles and Practice.*. 5th edn. Philadelphia: Churchill Livingston Elsevier.
13. Hyoung J (2010) Double umbilical cord blood transplantation for children and adolescents. *Ann Hematol* 89(10): 1035–44
14. Reed W, Smith R, Dekovic F et al. (2003) Comprehensive banking of sibling donor cord blood for children with malignant and nonmalignant disease. *Blood* 101(1): 351–7.
15. Kurtzberg J, Lyerly AD, and Sugarman J (2005) Untying the gordian knot: policies, practices, and ethical issues related to banking of umbilical cord blood. *J Clin Invest* 115(10): 2592–7.
16. Solves P, Perales A, Moraga R et al. (2005) Maternal, neonatal and collection factors influencing the haematopoietic content of cord blood units. *Acta Haematol* 113(4): 241–6.
17. Broxmeyer HE, Srour EF, Hangoc G et al. (2003) High-efficiency recovery of functional hematopoietic progenitor and stem cells from human cord blood cryopreserved for 15 years. *Proc Natl Acad Sci U S A* 100(2): 645–50.
18. Smiers FJ, Krishnamurti L, and Lucarelli G (2010) Hematopoietic stem cell transplantation for hemoglobinopathies: current practice and emerging trends. *Pediatr Clin North Am* 57(1): 181–205.
19. NCBP List of Centers. Website: www.nationalcordbloodprogram.org
20. Rucinski D (2010) Exploring opinions and beliefs about cord blood donation among hispanic and non-hispanic black women. *Transfusion* 50(May): 1057–1063.
21. Thornley I, Eapen M, Sung L et al. (2009) Private cord blood banking: experiences and views of pediatric hematopoietic cell transplantation physicians. *Pediatrics* 123(3): 1011–7.
22. Kaimal AJ, Smith CC, Laros RK Jr. et al. (2009) Cost-effectiveness of private umbilical cord blood banking. *Obstet Gynecol* 114(4): 848–55.
23. Lu JAR, Pompili VJ, and Das H (2010) A novel technology for hematopoietic stem cell expansion using combination of nanofiber and growth fibers. *Recent Pat Nanotechnol* 4(2): 125–35.
24. Cashen AF, Nervi B, and DiPersio J (2007) AMD3100: CXCR4 antagonist and rapid stem cell-mobilizing agent. *Future Oncol* 3(1): 19–27.
25. Perin L, Sedrakyan S, Da Sacco S et al. (2008) Characterization of human amniotic fluid stem cells and their pluripotential capability. *Methods Cell Biol* 86: 85–99.
26. Siegel N, Rosner M, Hanneder M et al. (2008) Human amniotic fluid stem cells: a new perspective. *Amino Acids* 35(2): 291–3.

42

CHAPTER 42
Stem Cells from the Placenta

Thaddeus G. Golos

Departments of Comparative Biosciences, Obstetrics, and Gynecology, The Wisconsin National Primate Research Center, University of Wisconsin-Madison, Madison, WI, USA

Introduction

The placenta has the primary function of providing the fetus with nutrients to sustain its growth and survival throughout gestation. Derangements in placental function can be deleterious to fetal survival and, appropriately, a major focus of placental research has been on its endocrine, metabolic, and transport functions as they impact on fetal growth. These areas are comprehensively covered in other chapters in this volume. In recent years, a critical focus of placental research has been in the area of stem cell biology. This reflects growing interest and technical ability to identify, isolate, and expand rare populations of stem cells applied to organs beyond the bone marrow. Since there have been many recent reviews of this topic [1–3], we will only briefly describe current knowledge and areas of need for further research.

Within the placenta, three major populations of stem cells have received significant experimental attention. In most placentas, but particularly in hemochorial placentas, the trophoblast population is highly diverse, with morphological and functional specialization. Since the trophectoderm of the blastocyst is the preimplantation progenitor, studies have revealed that trophoblast stem cells (TSC) have the capacity to give rise to all trophoblasts of the definitive placenta. Two other lines of investigation have revealed that the placenta is a source not only of its own self-renewal through the TSC, but as a source of cell renewal with therapeutic potential. In the past decade it has been well established that the placenta harbors additional multipotent cells not related to the trophoblast lineage. Both hematopoietic stem cells (HSC) and mesenchymal stem cells (MSC) have been well characterized from mouse and human placentas. What is unknown is whether these cells serve as progenitors for the constituents of the placental villous stroma in normal development, or perhaps serve as a reservoir of multipotent regenerative cells in the event of developmental, chemical, or metabolic insult to the fetus. Cells resembling MSC have also been isolated from the fetal membranes. We will review the characteristics of these populations, their placental niches recently described, and discuss current speculation on their therapeutic potential as autologous therapeutic cells for transplantation and regenerative medicine. Figure 42.1 summarizes major points established by the studies that will be discussed in this review.

Trophoblast stem cells in placental development

Methodologies for the study of TSC were dramatically advanced in 1997 when Tanaka et al. [4] reported that a trophoblast population could be isolated from the mouse implantation site or preimplantation blastocyst and maintained with fibroblast growth factor (FGF4) and heparin on a fibroblast feeder layer. The cells were capable of extended proliferation under these conditions, yet upon withdrawal of FGF4, the cells differentiated preferentially to trophoblast giant cells and syncytiotrophoblasts (a population distinct from human syncytiotrophoblasts). The stem cell identify of these cells was revealed by

The Placenta: From Development to Disease, First Edition. Edited by Helen H. Kay, D. Michael Nelson and Yuping Wang.
© 2011 Blackwell Publishing Ltd. Published 2011 by Blackwell Publishing Ltd.

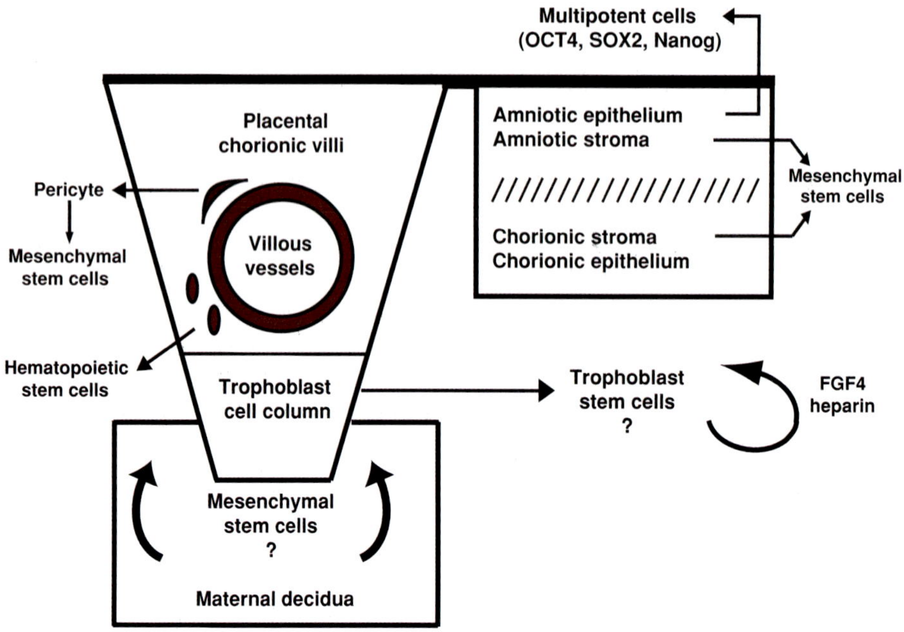

Figure 42.1 Schematic depiction of domains of the human placenta and current research on stem cell populations based on cell culture and histological experiments discussed in this review. The maternal decidua may contribute MSC to the placenta, as demonstrated by studies isolating XX MSC from male placentas [26,27]. The chorionic villi and fetal membranes are both sources of stem cells. MSC-like populations can be isolated from amniotic and chorionic stroma, and cells expressing pluripotency markers can be isolated from amniotic epithelium and demonstrate differentiation plasticity [28]. Cells with MSC and HSC phenotypes can be isolated from the stroma of the chorionic villi; histological analysis indicates that these stem cell niches are in close association with the vessels of the villi [16,17,25]. The cytotrophoblasts of the proximal cell column may have trophoblast stem cell-like characteristics and their differentiation may be modulated by FGF4 and heparin, similar to mouse TSC [4,13]. Question marks indicate concepts less firmly established at this time.

experiments in which they were mixed with mouse preimplantation embryos in tetraploid aggregation. Trophoblasts were found to be solely derived from the TSC, while the fetus proper was derived from the embryonic inner cell mass. In this experiment, all trophoblast populations of the mouse placenta, but not the allantois, yolk sac, or amnion, were derived from the TSC. These and other studies have confirmed that the TSC population gives rise to all trophoblast populations of the mouse placenta. The TSC are thus committed to this lineage. Subsequent studies have shown that mouse TSC can also be derived directly from embryonic stem cells, under appropriate experimental conditions [5].

Research Spotlight

Mouse TSCs have proven to be a valuable platform to understand mouse trophoblast differentiation, both in vitro and in vivo. For example, the ability to selectively modify gene expression in the placenta without altering the fetal genome allows the direct study of the roles that specific genes may play in placental function, without the additional confounder of changing gene expression in the fetus [6].

The human placenta likely also contains a multipotent TSC that can give rise to the villous and extravillous populations, but TSC derived directly from human preimplantation embryos have not been reported. Apparently, human-specific TSC culture conditions have been difficult to define [7]. The conditions for human embryonic TSC derivation are not similar to those that successfully sustain mouse TSC. Therefore, an alternative to the direct use of embryos is the use of human embryonic stem cells (hESC) as a pluripotent embryonic surrogate. Indeed, several approaches for the differentiation of trophoblasts directly from hESC have been established. In the first approach, Xu et al. [8] demonstrated that hESC treated with bone morphogenetic protein 4 (BMP4), or related ligands that bind the BMP receptor BMPR-IB, differentiate to a homogeneous population of cells with a gene expression profile indicating a trophoblastic phenotype. These cells demonstrate characteristics of endocrine differentiation in that they secrete hormone chorionic gonadotropin (hCG), progesterone, and estradiol-17β, generally considered major secretory products of the human placental syncytiotrophoblasts. On the other hand, they clearly are not identical to villous cytotrophoblasts, which undergo widespread spontaneous morphological differentiation to multinuclear syncytiotrophoblasts in culture, a phenotype not seen in the BMP4-treated cells although some multinuclear structures have been noted in other studies [9]. Thus, the phenotype of these cells remains somewhat unclear, and not all human ESC lines respond in this way to BMP ligands [10]. For example, formation of embryoid bodies, formed as spherical aggregates of ESC in suspension culture, has also been reported to give rise to trophoblasts that migrated outwardly from the embryoid bodies in adherent cultures [11,12]. Some investigators have suggested that these cells represent a population with human trophoblast stem cell characteristics. Indeed, under some culture conditions, the expression of HLA-G can be detected as a marker of extravillous trophoblasts at the human implantation site, and the cells have some migratory characteristics [12]. One of the difficulties in confirming this "human TSC" phenotype is that the phenotype of trophoblasts present at the implantation site during the first weeks of the human gestation is not readily established because such specimens are not available for experimental interrogation. The trophoblasts derived from hESC have a complex phenotype. An important area for further study is to define the culture conditions, such as extracellular matrix, endometrial/placental cell coculture, soluble factors, among others, that determine the differentiation decisions that define the phenotype of their final differentiation.

A recent study [13] has supported the possibility that FGF4 may support human stem cytotrophoblast renewal, suppressing differentiation towards either the extravillous or villous lineage. Using an explant system in which villous stroma and cell column cytotrophoblasts are maintained in organ culture, investigators have suggested that FGF4 and heparin decreased the repopulation of villous cytotrophoblasts and ensuing regeneration of the syncytial layer, as well as the differentiation of extravillous trophoblasts expressing HLA-G and integrins alpha 1 and beta 1 upon enzymatic removal of villous trophoblasts. This suggested that TS-like FGFR2-expressing trophoblasts reside in the human placental cell column. Further studies are warranted to extend this concept.

Hematopoietic stem cells in the placenta

The placenta has long been suspected of being a source of HSC. The use of cord blood cells as a source of HSC for hematologic therapy is covered in a separate chapter in this volume and will not be covered here except to note that the presence of these fetal HSC in the cord blood supports a placental origin. However, this was not carefully investigated until fairly recently. Initial studies were performed in the mouse, where fetal development is much more readily accessed. The yolk sac is the initial organ of hematopoiesis in early development, with later appearance of HSC in the aorta-gonadal-mesonephros (AGM) region, and eventually with major hematopoiesis in the fetal liver. The ontogeny of HSC in fetal development first intrigued placental biologists in 2003, as HSC progenitors increased in the placenta more dramatically than in the fetal AGM, and the placental HSC's preceded the increase in the liver [14]. Experiments with green fluorescent protein transgene-bearing mice showed that the substantial majority of HSC from the placenta were of fetal origin, and not from contaminating maternal blood. Gerkas et al. [15] confirmed and extended these studies, providing further support for the hypothesis that the placenta may be a source of HSC, which then seeds the HSC in the liver. Indeed, this latter study indicated that the placental HSC were more rapidly expanding than those in the AGM, unlike the adult HSC niche, which in the bone marrow restricts proliferation. The placental niche promotes expansion would be logical in fetal development. The labyrinthine placenta was then identified as the likely placental niche in the mouse.

Research Spotlight

In the absence of fetal blood circulation in genetically modified mice with a cardiac defect, active HSC proliferation was still demonstrated in the placenta, indicating that the placenta itself, and not other organs were the source of these HSC [16]. Moreover, genetically marked HSC were associated with large blood vessels in the placenta, suggesting the location of the physical niche that gave rise to or sustained these cells.

More recently, the hematopoietic niche in the human placenta has been investigated as well. The placenta is an attractive source of HSCs for therapeutic purposes, because this organ makes an easily obtained population of autologous cells available without the complications of bone marrow access. In 2009 several groups reported the isolation of cells with HSC characteristics from human placentas between 5 and 39 weeks of gestation [17–19]. One group demonstrated that placental HSC have clonogenic multilineage potential at term, supporting their therapeutic potential. In addition, these cells demonstrated engraftment in immunodeficient mice, an important biological characteristic similar to that of bone marrow HSC. As with the studies discussed above in mice, histological studies indicated the presence of HSC in the chorionic villi, closely associated with vessels. Placental stromal cells supported the proliferation of these HSC [17], suggesting (as with the mouse placenta) that villous stromal vessels represent the niche for human placental HSC, a feature emerging as a characteristic of adult tissue stem cells.

Mesenchymal stem cells in the placenta

MSCs are cells of multipotent differentiation potential that initially were characterized as having a commitment to the formation of mesodermal differentiated derivatives, including chondrogenic, osteogenic, and adipogenic lineages. Recent studies have noted that these cells can have much broader multipotency and may give rise to cardiomyocytes, endothelial cells, hepatocytes, neural stem/progenitor cells, and neurons. MSC early on were identified in cord blood (e.g., [20]), and the placenta was shown to be a source of MSC, trafficking to maternal blood and tissues and persisting long after pregnancy [21]. Maternal-fetal microchimerism is covered in a separate chapter in this volume. In direct comparison with bone marrow-derived MSC, placental MSC have almost identical adhesion molecule and chemokine receptor profiles, but they may exhibit enhanced VLA-4-mediated engraftment properties [22] and enhanced proliferative potential, compared to bone marrow MSC.

Clinical Pearl

MSC, including those isolated from the placenta, have immunosuppressive and immunoregulatory activity, making them potential immunologically privileged transplantation candidates. Thus, along with the multipotential differentiation properties, placental MSC have generated substantial interest as agents of regenerative medicine and cell therapy.

Recent studies have sought to identify the tissue niche where the MSC reside. Intriguingly, a vessel-associated cell with contractile properties, the pericyte, is a strong candidate as the in vivo MSC [23,24]. Another recent study identified the pericyte of the placental villous vessels as the likely MSC source [25]. Thus, the placental vessels appear to be the niche where both placental MSC as well as HSC reside, indicating that the placental vasculature may be an important source of progenitors not only supporting placental and fetal growth and development, but also as a source for postnatal regenerative medicine with further therapeutic development.

There are also areas that need greater attention regarding the characteristics of placental MSC. Barlow et al. [26] noted placental MSC chromosomal changes, including generation of trisomies, with passage in culture. Thus, careful optimization of culture conditions that will support maintenance of karyotype stability are essential.

Research Spotlight

Recent studies [26,27] evaluated the karyotype of placental MSC, and unexpectedly noted that they were actually of maternal rather than fetal origin. This may indicate that residual decidual tissue was the actual origin of the maternal cells, or perhaps maternal MSC are trafficking to the placenta during pregnancy. These intriguing observations require further study.

Stem cells from the fetal membranes

The fetal membranes have also been the focus in the search for stem cells. This area has recently been extensively reviewed by Ilancheran et al. [28] and the reader is referred to that review for detailed discussion of stem cell populations isolated from the amniotic stroma and epithelium, and more limited studies from the chorionic stroma. Briefly, amnion stromal cells and chorion stromal cells can be shown in vitro to have MSC-like characteristics, including the expression of bone marrow MSC-like cell surface marker characteristics. With in vitro assays, both amniotic and chorionic stromal cells can differentiate into the characteristic mesodermal lineages (chondrogenic, osteogenic, adipogenic). In addition, a range of other differentiated outcomes have been reported, including the formation of endothelial cells, hepatocytes, cardiomyocytes, and ectodermal neural derivatives [28]. Amniotic epithelial cells have also been investigated as sources of stem cells. Interestingly, a small number of these cells express stem cell pluripotency markers, including Oct4, Sox2, and nanog. However, it is difficult to correlate the expression of these genes with the differentiation state of the cells, and in transplantation experiments, it may be that amniotic epithelial cells act not as a source of differentiated cells for tissue regeneration, but to promote tissue repair and/or regeneration within the local microenvironment.

Epilogue

The use of stem cells isolated from the placenta or fetal membranes has attracted substantial attention because of their potential for autologous transplantation. While specific cellular or therapeutic advantages have not been clearly demonstrated, the relative ease of preparing substantial numbers of MSC or HSC from placental tissues, universally available at delivery, contrasts with the more invasive collection of bone marrow from patients. In addition, the number of stem cells decreases as patients age, also underscoring the opportunity available from placental stem cells. Finally, an advantage of MSC or HSC over embryonic stem cells for cell therapy and regenerative medicine is that they have not been shown to form teratomas with transplantation to immunodeficient mouse hosts, whereas that remains a potential risk for even the well-differentiated derivatives of embryonic stem cells.

Complexities remain to be addressed with future studies. Cord blood from first trimester but not term placentas contains MSC [29]. Thus, placental tissue may be the tissue of choice for MSC, since cord blood from term placentas may not provide all needed cell types. There are also fundamental areas where further research is needed. First, most in vivo studies undertaken so far are limited in scope. That is, transplantation of human placental stem cells into mouse hosts can provide limited insight into their true therapeutic opportunity. Advancement with nonhuman primate models should be an important goal. The role(s) of stem cells through 9 months of human pregnancy is unclear. The multipotent differentiation potential would not seem necessary within the chorionic villi, so do they serve as a physiologically meaningful "in-house" regenerative cell population for the fetus? If so, how are they mobilized from the placenta? How do they home and engraft to sites of need, if indeed this is their role, and what are their limitations?

Research Spotlight

Placental and other MSCs may not serve to directly provide regenerative building blocks for tissue, despite intense efforts into defining their differentiation potential in this regard [28,30]. Rather, regenerative cell therapy may act by exerting beneficial trophic effects on host cells: activating local stem cell populations, improving angiogenesis, and opposing deleterious inflammation.

In conclusion, the placenta, harvested at birth, has not been exposed to the pathogens, toxins, or other genetic digressions that impact on autologous bone marrow or other tissue stem cells over the lifespan of the host. Clinicians and scientists have been fascinated with the role of the placenta in sustaining and nurturing fetal development, and more recently, its pivotal role in intrauterine programming with consequences to adult life. The significance of the placenta to human health and well-being may now be extended to the provision of therapeutic tools that are capable of regenerating and rejuvenating us through the challenges of the physiology and pathophysiology of adult life.

Teaching Points

1 Trophoblast and nontrophoblast compartments of the placenta contain stem cell populations.
2 TSC differentiate only into trophoblast lineage derivatives, whereas MSC and HSC of the placenta have the ability to differentiate into diverse cell populations.

3 The placental role of the trophoblast stem cell is clearly defined as the source of the terminally differentiated trophoblasts in the definitive placenta. The HSC of the placenta may be a source of fetal hematopoiesis in early development before hematopoiesis is initiated in the liver. The endogenous role of MSC in the placenta is unknown.

4 Consistent with emerging concepts in the stem cell field, histological studies indicate the presence of hematopoietic and MSC in the chorionic villi, closely associated with vessels.

Acknowledgements

TGG thanks Maria Giakoumopoulos for assistance with figure preparation, and Mark Garthwaite for assistance with preparation of this manuscript. This research was supported by NIH grants HD046919 and HD038843 to TGG, by the WNPRC P51 base grant RR000167, and was conducted in part at a facility constructed with support from Research Facilities Improvement Program grants RR15459–01 and RR020141–01. This publication's contents are solely the responsibility of the author and do not necessarily represent the official views of NCRR or NIH.

References

1. Douglas GC, VandeVoort CA, Kumar P et al. (2009) Trophoblast stem cells: models for investigating trophectoderm differentiation and placental development. *Endocrine Reviews* 30: 228–40.
2. Himeno E, Tanaka S, and Kunath T (2008) Isolation and manipulation of mouse trophoblast stem cells. *Curr Protoc Stem Cell Biol.* Chapter 1:Unit 1E.4.
3. Rielland M, Hue I, Renard JP et al. (2008) Trophoblast stem cell derivation, cross-species comparison and use of nuclear transfer: new tools to study trophoblast growth and differentiation. *Dev Biol* 322: 1–10.
4. Tanaka S, Kunath T, Hadjantonakis AK et al. (1998) Promotion of trophoblast stem cell proliferation by FGF4. *Science* 282: 2072–2075.
5. Niwa H. Miyazaki J, and Smith AG (2000) Quantitative expression of Oct-3/4 defines differentiation, dedifferentiation or self-renewal of ES cells. *Nat Genet* 24: 372–376.
6. Natale DR, Starovic M, and Cross JC (2006) Phenotypic analysis of the mouse placenta. *Methods Mol Med* 121: 275–93.
7. Rossant J (2007). Stem cells from the mammalian blastocyst. *Stem Cells* 19: 477–482.
8. Xu RH, Chen X, Li DS et al. (2002) BMP4 initiates human embryonic stem cell differentiation to trophoblast. *Nat Biotechnol* 20: 1261–1264.
9. Schulz LC, Ezashi T, Das P et al. (2008) Human embryonic stem cells as models for trophoblast differentiation. *Placenta* 22: S10–S16.
10. Pera MF, Andrade J, Houssami S et al. (2004) Regulation of human embryonic stem cell differentiation by BMP-2 and its antagonist noggin. *J. Cell Sci* 117: 1269–1280.
11. Gerami-Naini B, Dovzhenko OV, Durning M et al. (2004) Trophoblast differentiation in embryoid bodies derived from human embryonic stem cells as a model for trophoblast differentiation. *Endocrinology* 145: 1517–1524.
12. Harun R, Ruban L, Matin M et al. (2006) Cytotrophoblast stem cell lines derived from human embryonic stem cells and their capacity to mimic invasive implantation events. *Hum Reprod* 21: 1349–1358.
13. Baczyk D, Dunk C, Huppertz B et al. (2006) Bi-potential behaviour of cytotrophoblasts in first trimester chorionic villi. *Placenta* 27: 367–74.
14. Alvarez-Silva M, Belo-Diabangouaya P, Salaün J et al. (2003) Mouse placenta is a major hematopoietic organ. *Development* 130: 5437–44.
15. Gekas C, Dieterlen-Lièvre F, Orkin SH et al. (2005) The placenta is a niche for hematopoietic stem cells. *Dev Cell* 8: 365–75.
16. Rhodes KE, Gekas C, Wang Y et al. (2008) The emergence of hematopoietic stem cells is initiated in the placental vasculature in the absence of circulation. *Cell Stem Cell* 2: 252–63.
17. Bárcena A, Kapidzic M, Muench MO et al. (2009) The human placenta is a hematopoietic organ during the embryonic and fetal periods of development. *Dev Biol* 327: 24–33.
18. Serikov V, Hounshell C, Larkin S et al. (2009) Human term placenta as a source of hematopoietic cells. *Exp Biol Med* 234: 813–23.
19. Robin C, Bollerot K, Mendes S et al. (2009) Human placenta is a potent hematopoietic niche containing hematopoietic stem and progenitor cells throughout development. *Cell Stem Cell* 5: 385–95.
20. Kögler G, Sensken S, Airey JA et al. (2004) A new human somatic stem cell from placental cord blood with intrinsic pluripotent differentiation potential. *J Exp Med* 200: 123–35.
21. O'Donoghue K, Chan J, de la Fuente J et al. (2004) Microchimerism in female bone marrow and bone decades after fetal mesenchymal stem-cell trafficking in pregnancy. *Lancet* 364: 179–82.
22. Brooke G, Tong H, Levesque JP et al. (2008) Molecular trafficking mechanisms of multipotent mesenchymal stem cells derived from human bone marrow and placenta. *Stem Cells Dev* 17: 929–40.

23. Crisan M, Yap S, Casteilla L et al. (2008) A perivascular origin for mesenchymal stem cells in multiple human organs. *Cell Stem Cell* 3: 301–13.
24. Chen CW, Montelatici E, Crisan M et al. (2009) Perivascular multi-lineage progenitor cells in human organs: regenerative units, cytokine sources or both? *Cytokine Growth Factor Rev* 20: 429–34.
25. Castrechini NM, Murthi P, Gude NM et al. (2010) Mesenchymal stem cells in human placental chorionic villi reside in a vascular Niche. *Placenta* 31: 203–12.
26. Barlow S, Brooke G, Chatterjee K et al. (2008) Comparison of human placenta- and bone marrow-derived multipotent mesenchymal stem cells. *Stem Cells Dev* 17: 1095–107.
27. Semenov OV, Koestenbauer S, Riegel M et al. (2010) Multipotent mesenchymal stem cells from human placenta: critical parameters for isolation and maintenance of stemness after isolation. *Am J Obstet Gynecol* 202: 193. e1–193.e13.
28. Ilancheran S, Moodley Y, and Manuelpillai U (2009) Human fetal membranes: a source of stem cells for tissue regeneration and repair? *Placenta* 30: 2–10.
29. Portmann-Lanz CB, Schoeberlein A, Portmann R et al. (2010) Turning placenta into brain: placental mesenchymal stem cells differentiate into neurons and oligodendrocytes. *Am J Obstet Gynecol* 202: 294. e1–294.e11.
30. Parolini O, Alviano F, Bergwerf I et al. (2010) Toward cell therapy using placenta-derived cells: disease mechanisms, cell biology, preclinical studies, and regulatory aspects at the round table. *Stem Cells Dev* 19: 143–54.

43

CHAPTER 43
Fetal DNA, RNA, and Prenatal Diagnosis

Olav Lapaire[1] *and Wolfgang Holzgreve*[1,2]

[1]Department of Obstetrics/Department of Biomedicine, University of Basel, Basel, Switzerland
[2]Institute for Advanced Study, Wallotstrasse, Berlin, Germany

Introduction

The fast-growing field of global postgenomic research offers many promising perspectives for noninvasive prenatal diagnosis, especially with the use of gender-independent sequences, and may very likely become a reality in a few years.

Developments in the field of noninvasive prenatal diagnosis

Fetal material, covering a spectrum from intact cells to cellular debris and cell-free fetal DNA (cffDNA), crosses the placental barrier into the maternal circulation, and has been a focus of intense research over the last 20 years. The goal was to develop noninvasive prenatal diagnostic markers for the detection of fetal aneuploidies, and this objective was made possible when molecular technologies became available. Today, the presence of fetal material in the maternal circulation of pregnant women is not only of interest for prenatal diagnosis, but also may have an immediate impact on maternal health in cases of preeclampsia.

Cells and subcellular particles trafficking between the fetus and mother provide indirect clues to the underlying pathophysiology affecting a particular pregnancy. This material also provides specimens for noninvasive prenatal diagnosis. Georg Schmorl, a German pathologist, first documented the presence of fetal cells in the maternal body in 1893, and emphasized the importance of the placenta in eclampsia. He also recognized that fetomaternal trafficking occurred in normal gestations but was increased in pregnancies affected by eclampsia. Using sophisticated molecular techniques, we can now precisely confirm what Schmorl so elegantly described [1].

Similar findings were reported in the 1950s by Gordon Douglas and his colleagues in New York. They hypothesized that "low-grade" cell traffic from the fetus to the mother might be a physiologic phenomenon that is elevated in preeclampsia and eclampsia. However, they were unable to prove their theory based on cytological methods available at that time. Technical advances in sophisticated molecular techniques allow detection of fetal cells and their debris to revisit the problem quantitatively. We now know that an average of one out of a million cells in the maternal circulation is of fetal origin.

In 1997, the group of Dennis Lo showed that cffDNA extracted from maternal circulation can be analyzed, and that this phenomenon can be used clinically for the noninvasive diagnosis of some genetic conditions in the fetus. The methodology to detect very small amounts of "foreign" DNA sequences in maternal plasma and serum has been further improved since then. New generations of noninvasive diagnostic procedures in sequencing, and digital polymerase chain reaction (PCR), may move noninvasive prenatal diagnosis from bench to bedside.

In the first phase of the research for noninvasive prenatal diagnostic markers, many years and enormous efforts

The Placenta: From Development to Disease, First Edition. Edited by Helen H. Kay, D. Michael Nelson and Yuping Wang.
© 2011 Blackwell Publishing Ltd. Published 2011 by Blackwell Publishing Ltd.

were spent on cell enrichment and depletion techniques as well as on searching for the "ideal" fetal target cell. During this phase, syncytiotrophoblast cells were found to be technically disadvantaged since they were often multinucleated with no specific antibody for their enrichment. Diana Bianchi and her colleagues highlighted the advantages of using fetal nucleated erythrocytes because of the enrichment achieved by the specific antitransferrin antibody, CD71. Fetal nucleated erythrocytes have a short half-life, and this excludes interference from contaminating cells from previous pregnancies. Considerable worldwide efforts were subsequently undertaken to develop efficient enrichment and depletion techniques, but each step aimed to increase the specificity of cell selection yielded loss of some of the rare fetal cells. The rarity of fetal cells in the maternal circulation mandated rigorous testing before a widespread clinical application could be considered. The National Institute of Health (NIH) initiated a large-scale multicenter study to evaluate cell-based techniques for noninvasive prenatal diagnosis of fetal aneuploidies, and to further develop the existing methods [2]. This study prevented dissemination of the approach inappropriately in nonstudy locations. The results of this so-called NIFTY trial (National Institute for Child Health and Development Fetal Cell Isolation Study) revealed that the detection rate of fetal cells was 74.4%, with a false-positive rate estimated to be between 0.6% and 4.1%, using cell-based methods. This was inadequate for clinical implementation as a tool for fetal aneuploidy detection because of the difficulty in reliably detecting a third copy of a chromosome in a background of abundant disomic maternal cells.

In contrast to the disappointing experience using intact fetal cells, the discovery of cell-free fetal DNA in the maternal circulation opened a new avenue for the noninvasive assessment of fetal genetic traits. Importantly, this is successful in identification of simple loci in clinical practice.

Technical advances from individual laboratories, and the development of international groups such as the European Union's Special Advances in Fetal Evaluation (SAFE) network, have allowed multicenter studies to proceed. These examine diagnostic aspects related to quality assurance and explore issues related to accuracy, efficiency, and costs. Noninvasive prenatal diagnosis of fetal Rhesus D is currently transitioning in a controlled manner from the research arena to standard clinical care in Europe.

Maternal DNA complicates the analytic conditions for fetal DNA, and diagnosis has more recently focused on alleles that do not occur in the maternal genome, for example, paternal dominant alleles. The best example of this is prenatal detection of the fetal Rhesus status. Approximately 15% of Caucasian women are at risk of Rhesus incompatibility. Analogous to the amplification of specific sequences of the Y chromosome, the Rhesus constellation of the fetal Rhesus status can be determined through the use of cell-free fetal DNA probes. A meta-analysis pooled data from 37 publications that reported noninvasive Rhesus genotyping using fetal DNA from maternal plasma or serum. This meta-analysis confirmed a high accuracy of 94.8%, and included 16 studies that reported 100% diagnostic accuracy in their fetal Rhesus D genotyping [3]. Providers in some European countries may offer this new noninvasive test to all Rhesus-negative women antepartum as a cost-effective approach in order to save the prepartum anti-Rhesus D prophylaxis in those cases where the child has been found to be Rhesus-negative. In some centers such as Bristol and Amsterdam, the noninvasive Rhesus test has transitioned from the research to the service laboratories, primarily within blood banks.

Clinical Pearl

To date, two applications of cell-free fetal DNA, namely, gender determination for X-linked genetic disorders and the noninvasive prenatal diagnosis of the fetal Rhesus D status, have already been translated from bench to bedside.

After separation of fetal DNA, monogenic diseases such as myotonic dystrophy, achondroplasia, cystic fibrosis, and congenital adrenal gland hyperplasia can be diagnosed. Recently, cell-free fetal DNA (cffDNA) was separated from the mother's DNA according to fragment sizes as fetal fragments are generally smaller than those of maternal origin. The majority of fetal DNA in maternal blood consists of less than 300 base pairs (bp), whereas the maternal DNA consists of more than 500–1,000 bp. The size difference is probably the result of the origin of the cell-free (cf) DNA. These findings may be due to differences in the apoptotic mechanisms involved in the release of cffDNA by the syncytiotrophoblast. The latter villous component contains a multitude of highly apoptotic nuclei, whilst maternal cf DNA is most likely due to release by cells of the hemopoietic system.

Separation of maternal DNA from fetal DNA according to size simplifies the examination of paternally inherited point mutations. Addition of mass spectrometry permits the determination of specific alleles, including point mutations and differences of single-nucleotide polymorphisms.

> **Clinical Pearl**
>
> The field of prenatal diagnosis using maternal blood has not met the original goal of a noninvasive diagnostic tool to reliably detect fetal chromosomal anomalies. At the same time, an ever-increasing list of high-risk single gene diseases can now be detected by using cffDNA as the source.

Cell-free fetal DNA as a marker for preeclampsia

Cell-free fetal DNA is a promising marker for preeclampsia. Preeclampsia is discussed in more detail in Chapter 32. Currently, there is no single reliable parameter for the prediction of preeclampsia, and much attention has turned to noninvasive testing methods, including ultrasound examination and the quantification of various blood-borne and urinary biomarkers. Circulating cf nucleic acids in plasma and serum are novel biomarkers with promising clinical applications in different medical fields, including prenatal diagnosis. Quantitative changes of cffDNA in maternal plasma, as an indicator for impending preeclampsia, have been measured by real-time quantitative PCR for the *SRY* gene and the *DYS 14* gene on the Y chromosome. The levels were increased fivefold in women with preeclampsia, compared to the normotensive controls. Levels may be elevated as early as the first trimester in pregnancies that develop early onset preeclampsia.

The largest study to date of cffDNA, as a predictor of preeclampsia, was conducted by Levine et al., using stored samples of 120 pregnant women who developed preeclampsia and 120 controls, who were enrolled as part of the *Two-stage elevation of cell-free fetal DNA inmaternalsera before onset of preeclampsia* [4]. This study showed a two- to fivefold increase of cffDNA levels, starting from week 17 of gestation, in women who subsequently developed the disorder, compared to gestational age matched controls. In addition, the authors demonstrated that the elevation of cffDNA was biphasic. An initial elevation was seen between 17 and 28 weeks of gestation, and the second elevation was observed beginning 3 weeks before the onset of the clinical symptoms. The increased levels of cffDNA before the onset of symptoms may be due to hypoxia with reoxygenation within the intervillous space, leading to tissue oxidative stress and increased placental apoptosis and necrosis. In addition to the evidence for increased shedding of cffDNA into the maternal circulation, there is also evidence for reduced renal clearance of cffDNA in preeclampsia. As the amount of fetal DNA is currently determined by quantifying Y-chromosome-specific sequences, alternative approaches are needed. Promising alternatives include the measurement of total cf DNA or the use of gender-independent fetal epigenetic markers, such as DNA methylation. Through the use of gender-independent sequences, the universal incorporation of fetal nucleic acids into routine obstetric care and into screening or diagnostic settings using combined markers may soon become a reality.

> **Research Spotlight**
>
> The data suggest that cffDNA measured between 20–25 weeks of gestation and cffRNA extracted from the maternal blood could be used as potential biomarkers to predict the development of preeclampsia before the onset of symptoms in high-risk patients.

Noninvasive prenatal diagnosis and screening with cell-free fetal RNA from maternal plasma

The detection of fetal-derived DNA and RNA molecules in maternal plasma is a promising approach for the development of noninvasive prenatal diagnostic strategies. Circulating fetal RNA analysis has the additional advantage of being applicable to pregnancies involving fetuses of both genders, unlike the conventionally used Y-chromosomal fetal DNA markers, such as *DYS 14* or *SRY*. Tsui et al. showed that endogenous RNA is quite stable in comparison to extracted and purified RNA from cells [5]. Furthermore, endogenous plasma RNA molecules are associated with subcellular particles that protect them from degradation. Not only fetal DNA, but also fetal RNA, such as messenger RNA (mRNA) from corticotrophin releasing hormone (CRH), are present in elevated levels in pregnant women with preeclampsia. Increased values of mRNA of the b-subunit of Human chorionic gonadotropin (HCG) are elevated in pregnant women with aneuploid fetuses. The ability to measure fetal RNA affords the opportunity to explore the expression of certain genes, analogous to RNA markers used in oncology. Placentally derived mRNA is rapidly and simply determined by use of the microarray technique.

Technical aspects

Since the first detection of fetal nucleic acid in maternal plasma, many laboratories search for new diagnostic applications and evolve sophisticated methods for determination of cffDNA and RNA. Variations in centrifugation steps, different primers, and hydrolysis probes with either tetramethyl-6-carboxyrhodamin (TAMRA) or "minor groove binder (MGB) probes" with a nonfluorescent quencher make the comparison between laboratories difficult. Fetal DNA extraction from maternal probes was evaluated in different laboratories with a unified, standardized method [6]. Although all involved centers were able to extract fetal male DNA, there was a great variance in the sensitivity (31–97%) and specificity (93–100%). New methods, such as the addition of formaldehyde, promise to increase the yield of fetal DNA, but these must be critically evaluated before they are in daily use.

Future prospects

The discovery of cff nucleic acids, circulating in the maternal circulation, has opened a new avenue for the noninvasive assessment of fetal genetic traits, and has successfully been implemented for simple loci such as Rhesus D and the Y chromosome. The fast-growing knowledge from biologic behavior and the potential clinical uses for fetal nucleic acids in maternal plasma have brought us closer to the goal of finding noninvasive diagnostic markers in fetal screening, and diagnostic tests for such use in the clinic.

Teaching Points

1. Circulating cf nucleic acids in plasma and serum are novel biomarkers with promising clinical applications in different medical fields, including prenatal diagnosis.
2. Elevated levels of cffDNA and fetal RNA in maternal plasma have been reported to be an indicator for impending preeclampsia.

References

1. Lapaire O, Holzgreve W, Oosterwijk JC et al. (2007) Georg Schmorl on trophoblasts in the maternal circulation. *Placenta* 28(1): 1–5.
2. Bianchi DW, Simpson JL, Jackson LG et al. (2002) Fetal gender and aneuploidy detection using fetal cells in maternal blood: analysis of NIFTY I data. National Institute of Child Health and Development Fetal Cell Isolation Study. *Prenat Diagn* 22: 609–15.
3. Geifman-Holtzman O, Grotegut CA, and Gaughan JP (2006) Diagnostic accuracy of noninvasive fetal Rh genotyping from maternal blood – a meta-analysis. *Am J Obstet Gynecol* 195(4): 1163–73.
4. Levine RJ, Qian C, Leshane ES et al. (2004) Two-stage elevation of cell-free fetal DNA in maternal sera before onset of preeclampsia. *Am J Obstet Gynecol* 190(3): 707–13.
5. Tsui NB, Ng EK, and Lo YM (2002) Stability of endogenous and added RNA in blood specimens, serum, and plasma. *Clin Chem* 48: 1647–53.
6. Johnson KL, Dukes KA, Vidaver J et al. (2004) Interlaboratory comparison of fetal male DNA detection from common maternal plasma samples by real-time PCR. *Clin Chem* 50: 516–21.

Index

Note: Page numbers followed by f and t indicates figures and tables respectively.

The Placenta: From Development to Disease, First Edition. Edited by Helen H. Kay, D. Michael Nelson and Yuping Wang.
© 2011 Blackwell Publishing Ltd. Published 2011 by Blackwell Publishing Ltd.